The Sinus Bone Graft

Second edition

The Sinus Bone Graft

Second edition

Edited by

Ole T. Jensen, DDS, MS
Private Practice
Oral and Maxillofacial Surgery
Denver, Colorado

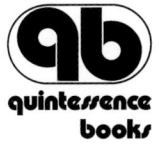

Quintessence Publishing Co, Inc

Chicago, Berlin, Tokyo, London, Paris, Milan, Barcelona, Istanbul,
São Paulo, New Delhi, Moscow, Prague, and Warsaw

The sinus bone graft / edited by Ole T. Jensen. -- 2nd ed.
    p. ; cm.
   Includes bibliographical references and index.
   ISBN 0-86715-455-1 (hardcover)
   1. Maxillary sinus. 2. Maxillary sinus--Surgery. 3. Bone-grafting.
I. Jensen, Ole T.
   [DNLM: 1. Maxillary Sinus--surgery. 2. Bone Transplantation
--methods. 3. Reconstructive Surgical Procedures.   WV 345
S618 2006]
RF421.S55 2006
617.5'2--dc22

                                                   2005032653

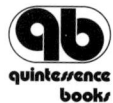

© 2006 Quintessence Publishing Co, Inc

All rights reserved. This book or any part thereof may not be reproduced, stored in a retrieval system, or transmitted in any form or by any means, electronic, mechanical, photocopying, or otherwise, without prior written permission of the publisher.

Quintessence Publishing Co, Inc
4350 Chandler Drive
Hanover Park, Illinois 60133
www.quintpub.com

Editor: Lisa C. Bywaters
Production: Sue Robinson
Cover and internal design: Dawn Hartman

Printed in China

Dedicated to Dr Philip J. Boyne

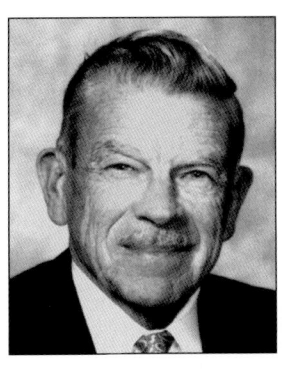

In 1956, Dr Philip Boyne published what would be the first of some 125 papers (and counting) on the subject of surgery, grafting, and healing of bone. It is now 2006, and he is still going strong. One day this 40-year period will surely be referred to as the Golden Age of Discovery in osseous surgery.

Dr Boyne has long ranked as one of the great orthopedic thinkers and teachers of the age. His contemporaries include Marshall Urist, who first characterized the elusive bone morphogenetic protein; Harold Frost, whose analytic mechanico-adaptive bone-healing hypotheses had a profound impact on the field of orthopedic science; and Per-Ingvar Brånemark, whose provocative findings on hard tissue osseointegration to titanium permanently altered the course of dentistry. Emerson's dictum—"do not require a description of the country toward which you sail"—serves as Phil Boyne's guiding principal. Taking a conceptual and biological rather than a technical or "cookbook" approach, Dr Boyne has modified and improved nearly every osseous surgical protocol ever developed within the scope of oral and maxillofacial surgery. It is not only for his contributions as the inventor of the sinus bone graft, but for his creative and imaginative approach to reconstructive surgery that we honor Dr Boyne by dedicating this book to him.

Dr Boyne has described a startling number of firsts. He studied the use of xenograft, freeze-dried bone, and autograft for bone defect treatment as early as 1957! He advocated the use of autogenous bone marrow aspirate in dental reconstruction (1970) and reported the first proven technique for secondary bone grafting of alveolar clefts (1972) as well as the first described use of sinus elevation to augment alveolar bone mass for implants (1980). He reported the use of socket preservation grafts in 1987. He was first to use recombinant human BMP-2 for mandibular discontinuity treatment (1996), for sinus grafting (1997), for alveolar cleft repair (1998), and most recently as part of dental implant surfaces (2005).

As Dr Boyne continues his journey in this age of discovery, we know that what was once a far-away country—the complete understanding of bone biology—is closer now than we ever imagined it would be, and that this is due in great measure to Dr Philip J. Boyne.

Preface

Inveni quod deficiens. . . .

Despite its relatively brief history, the sinus bone graft today constitutes one of the most popular and successful bone-grafting procedures undertaken in the maxillofacial region. Moreover, the maxillary sinus serves as the subject of more research, both in animal and clinical trials, than any other single bone-grafting site, culminating in a variety of modifications to the procedure and hence its role as the graft site most often used to establish efficacy for emerging dental implant technologies.

The sinus floor, and to a smaller extent the elevated sinus membrane, offers an ideal environment for bone formation. Though it would seem intuitively counterproductive to bone graft healing, especially if the sinus membrane becomes perforated during the course of graft placement, this area is instead remarkably forgiving of complication, infection, resorption, or rejection.

As we enter a new era and contemplate the likely reality of avoiding bone grafts altogether with CAT scan–derived treatment plans based on available bone, or the use of zygomaticus implants, or a return to cantilever prosthetics, one cannot help but wonder how the story of the history of sinus grafting will end.

This second edition subscribes to the concept *inveni quod deficiens*, "recover what is lost." The restorative dentist's charge is to reconstruct lost bone and restore lost function.

The as-yet unknowable potential of exogenous recombinants, cell-based therapies, gene-transfer technology, and, ultimately, tooth-germ transplantation will likely be pursued beneath elevated sinus membrane. The sinus floor in "end times" will host bioengineered dental lamina; in place of polished titanium, gleaming enamel will re-emerge through gingiva.

To this end, I would like to acknowledge Dr Hilt Tatum for teaching me how to do a sinus graft, and Dr Per-Ingvar Brånemark for showing me how to do an implant.

A book of this complexity and magnitude would not have been possible without the excellent work and diligent care of Lisa Bywaters, who helped edit and organize the manuscript into a coherent book.

I also express appreciation to Karen Shoop, my implant coordinator, the heart and soul of this 2-year experience.

I must also acknowledge my surgical assistants, Cindy Formaneck, Anna Dykes, and Kristin Stifflear, who during the course of this work assisted with both surgery and photographic documentation.

Research assistants who contributed to the book include Steve Tanberg, David Baer, and Brent Kimball.

Though section editors were avoided, I give special thanks to Drs Phil Boyne and Bo Rangert, who informally advised me at critical stages of the book.

And of course I must thank my family as well: my wife Marty, my sons Sverre and Trygve, and my daughter Autumn—even my grandchildren, Abigail, Sierra, and Ole Tait, for whom it is I work.

Table of Contents

Dedication v
Preface vii
Contributors xi

Section I Biologic, Biomechanical, and Prosthetic Considerations

1 History of Maxillary Sinus Grafting *3*
   Philip J. Boyne

2 Biologic Basis of Sinus Grafting *13*
   Georg Watzek, Gabor Fürst, and Reinhard Gruber

3 Vital Biomechanics of Bone and Bone Grafts *27*
   Harold M. Frost and Ole T. Jensen

4 Indications for and Classification of Sinus Bone Grafts *41*
   Carl E. Misch, Matteo Chiapasco, and Ole T. Jensen

5 Sinus Floor Augmentation: Simultaneous Versus Delayed Implant Placement *53*
   Ronald M. Achong and Michael S. Block

6 Sinus Floor Augmentation at the Time of Tooth Removal *67*
   Paul A. Fugazzotto and Ole T. Jensen

7 Prosthetic Management of the Sinus Graft Patient *75*
   Ira D. Zinner, Stanley A. Small, and Lloyd S. Landa

8 Contraindications for Sinus Graft Procedures *87*
   Matteo Chiapasco, Joel L. Rosenlicht, Salvatore L. Ruggiero, and Ronald F. Schneider

9 Complications of Maxillary Sinus Augmentation *103*
   Michael A. Pikos

10 Sinus Reactions to Invasive Surgery *115*
    Chantal Malevez

Section II Graft Sources and Materials

11 Maxillofacial Donor Sites for Sinus Floor and Alveolar Reconstruction *129*
Craig M. Misch

12 Tibia Bone Grafting for Sinus Augmentation *147*
Robert E. Marx

13 Sinus Augmentation with Bone Harvested from the Ilium *157*
R. Gilbert Triplett and Sterling R. Schow

14 Sinus Augmentation with Bone Harvested from the Calvarium *171*
Jean F. Tulasne

15 Safety and Efficacy of Bone Allograft for Sinus Grafting *183*
Laureen Langer, Burton Langer, and James T. Mellonig

16 Use of Alloplasts for Sinus Floor Grafting *201*
Ole T. Jensen, Giuliano Garlini, Dieter Bilk, and Fabian Peters

17 Use of Xenografts for Sinus Augmentation *211*
Stuart J. Froum, Stephen S. Wallace, Sang-Choon Cho, and Dennis P. Tarnow

Section III Technical Variations and Auxiliary Procedures

18 Effect of Surface Morphology on Implant Survival in the Grafted Maxillary Sinus *223*
Dennis P. Tarnow, Sang-Choon Cho, Stephen S. Wallace, and Stuart J. Froum

19 Use of Barrier Membranes in Sinus Augmentation *229*
Stephen S. Wallace, Stuart J. Froum, and Dennis P. Tarnow

20 Le Fort I Downgraft with Sinus Elevation *241*
Ole T. Jensen and Richard Branca

21 Trans-Alveolar Sinus Elevation Combined with Ridge Expansion *251*
Daniel R. Cullum and Ole T. Jensen

22 Osteotome Technique for Site Development and Sinus Floor Augmentation *263*
Robert B. Summers

23 Piezoelectric Bone Surgery for Sinus Bone Grafting *273*
Tomaso Vercellotti, Myron Nevins, and Ole T. Jensen

24 Le Fort I and Alveolar Distraction Osteogenesis with Sinus Bone Grafting *281*
Ole T. Jensen and Zvi Laster

25 PRP and BMP: A Comparison of Their Use and Efficacy in Sinus Grafting *289*
Robert E. Marx

26 Zygomatic Implants: A Viable Alternative to the Sinus Bone Graft *305*
Steven M. Sullivan, Chantal Malevez, and Daniel Henrichson

27 Graftless Rehabilitation of the Atrophied Maxilla Using Tilted and Short Implants and Immediate Function *315*
Bo Rangert, Carlos Aparicio, Chantal Malevez, Edmond Bedrossian, Franck Renouard, Paul Maló, and Roberto Calendriello

Section IV Looking to the Future

28 Stromal Stem Cell Preparation from Iliac Bone Marrow Aspirate for Sinus Bone Grafting *327*
Ole T. Jensen

29 Tissue Engineering for Maxillary Sinus Augmentation *333*
Ronald Schimming and Rainer Schmelzeisen

30 Use of Tissue-Engineered Bone Cells for Sinus Augmentation with Simultaneous Implant Placement *341*
Minoru Ueda, Yoichi Yamada, Morimich Ohya, and Hideharu Hibi

31 Gene Therapy of Growth Factors for Tissue Engineering and Regenerative Medicine *349*
William V. Giannobile, Brent Y. Kimball, and Li-Xing Man

Index *355*

Contributors

Ronald M. Achong, DMD, MD
Former Chief Resident
Department of Oral and Maxillofacial Surgery
School of Dentistry
Louisiana State University Health Sciences Center
New Orleans, Louisiana

Carlos Aparicio, MD, DDS, DLT, MS
Private Practice
Periodontics
Barcelona, Spain

Edmond Bedrossian, DDS
Director, Surgical Implant Training
Oral and Maxillofacial Surgery Residency Program
Alameda County Medical Center
Oakland, California

Director, Post-Doctoral Implant Training Program
School of Dentistry
University of the Pacific
San Francisco, California

Dieter Bilk, DDS
Private Practice
Muenzenberg, Germany

Michael S. Block, DMD
Professor
Department of Oral and Maxillofacial Surgery
School of Dentistry
Louisiana State University Health Sciences Center
New Orleans, Louisiana

Philip J. Boyne, DMD, MS
Professor Emeritus
Department of Oral and Maxillofacial Surgery
School of Dentistry
Loma Linda University
Loma Linda, California

Richard Branca, DDS, MS
Private Practice
Oral and Maxillofacial Surgery
Loveland, Colorado

Arnold S. Breitbart, MD
Associate Clinical Professor
Division of Plastic Surgery
Department of Surgery
Columbia University Medical Center
New York, New York

Roberto Calandriello, DDS
Private Practice
Oral and Maxillofacial Surgery
Bologna, Italy

Matteo Chiapasco, MD
Chairman, Oral and Maxillofacial Surgery Unit
Department of Medicine, Surgery and Dentistry
San Paulo Institute of Biomedical Sciences
University of Milan
Milan, Italy

Sang-Choon Cho, DDS, BDS, MS
Clinical Assistant Professor and Associate Research
    Scientist
Ashman Department of Implant Dentistry
College of Dentistry
New York University
New York, New York

Daniel R. Cullum, DDS
Private Practice
Oral and Maxillofacial Surgery
Coeur d'Alene, Idaho

Harold M. Frost, MD, DSc
Department of Orthopedic Surgery
Southern Colorado Clinic
Pueblo, Colorado

Stuart J. Froum, DDS
Clinical Professor and Director of Clinical Research
Ashman Department of Implant Dentistry
College of Dentistry
New York University
New York, New York

Paul A. Fugazzotto, DDS
Private Practice
Periodontics
Milton, Massachusetts

Gabor Fürst, MD, DDS
Senior Resident
Department of Oral Surgery
School of Dentistry
University of Vienna
Vienna, Austria

Giuliano Garlini, DDS
Tutor
Department of Oral Implants
Dental Clinic Instituti Clinici Perfectionarento
University of Milan
Milan, Italy

William V. Giannobile, DDS, DMedSc, MS
Professor and Director of Center for Craniofacial Regeneration
Department of Periodontics, Prevention, and Geriatrics
School of Dentistry
University of Michigan
Ann Arbor, Michigan

Associate Professor
Department of Biomedical Engineering
College of Engineering
University of Michigan
Ann Arbor, Michigan

Reinhard Gruber, PhD
Professor
Department of Oral Surgery
School of Dentistry
University of Vienna
Vienna, Austria

Daniel Henrichson, DMD
Private Practice
Oral and Maxillofacial Surgery
Lancaster, Pennsylvania

Hideharu Hibi, DDS, PhD
Center for Genetic and Regenerative Medicine
Graduate School of Medicine
Nagoya University
Nagoya, Japan

Ole T. Jensen, DDS, MS
Private Practice
Oral and Maxillofacial Surgery
Denver, Colorado

Brent Y. Kimball, BS
Department of Medicine
Columbia University
New York, New York

Lloyd S. Landa, DDS, MSD
Clinical Professor
Blatterfein Department of Prosthodontics
College of Dentistry
New York University
New York, New York

Burton Langer, DMD, MSD
Private Practice
Periodontics
New York, New York

Laureen Langer, DDS
Associate Clinical Professor
Division of Periodontics
School of Dental and Oral Surgery
Columbia University Medical Center
New York, New York

Zvi Laster, DMD
Chairman
Department of Oral and Maxillofacial Surgery
Poriya Hospital
Tiberias, Israel

Chantal Malevez, MD, DDS
Professor
Free University of Brussels, ULB
Erasme Hospital
Brussels, Belgium

Paulo Maló, DDS
Private Practice
Oral and Maxillofacial Surgery
Lisbon, Portugal

Li-Xing Man, MD, MSc
General Surgery Resident
Department of Surgery
Hospital of the University of Pennsylvania
Philadelphia, Pennsylvania

Robert E. Marx, DDS
Professor and Chief
Division of Oral and Maxillofacial Surgery
Department of Surgery
Miller School of Medicine
University of Miami
Miami, Florida

James T. Mellonig, DDS, MS
Professor
Department of Periodontics
School of Dentistry
University of Texas Health Science Center at San Antonio
San Antonio, Texas

Carl E. Misch, DDS, MDS
Clinical Professor and Co-Director of Oral Implantology
Department of Periodontology
School of Dentistry
Temple University
Philadelphia, Pennsylvania

Craig M. Misch, DDS, MDS, PA
Private Practice
Oral and Maxillofacial Surgery and Prosthodontics
Sarasota, Florida

Myron Nevins, DDS
Clinical Associate Professor
Department of Periodontology
Harvard School of Dental Medicine
Harvard University
Boston, Massachusetts

Morimich Ohya, DDS, PhD
Department of Oral and Maxillofacial Surgery
Graduate School of Medicine
Nagoya University
Nagoya, Japan

Fabian Peters, PhD, MS
Head of Technical Development
Curasan
Frankfurt am Main, Germany

Michael A. Pikos, DDS
Private Practice
Oral and Maxillofacial Surgery
Palm Harbor, Florida

Bo Rangert, PhD, MechEng
Chief Scientist
Nobel Biocare
Gothenburg, Sweden

Associate Professor
Department of Biomedical Engineering
Rensselaer Polytechnic Institute
Troy, New York

Franck Renouard, DDS
Private Practice
Oral and Maxillofacial Surgery
Paris, France

Joel L. Rosenlicht, DMD
Associate Clinical Professor
Ashman Department of Implant Dentistry
College of Dentistry
New York University
New York, New York

Salvatore L. Ruggiero, DMD, MD
Chief of Oral and Maxillofacial Surgery
Department of Dental Medicine
Long Island Jewish Medical Center
New Hyde Park, New York

Ronald Schimming, MD, DMD, PhD
Private Practice
Oral and Maxillofacial Surgery
St Gallen, Switzerland

Rainer Schmelzeisen, MD, DMD, PhD
Professor and Chairman
Division of Oral and Maxillofacial Surgery
University Dental Hospital
University of Freiburg
Freiburg, Germany

Ronald E. Schneider, DDS
Residency Program Director
Oral and Maxillofacial Surgery
Department of Dental Medicine
Long Island Jewish Medical Center
New Hyde Park, New York

Sterling R. Schow, DMD
Professor and Director of Graduate Education
Department of Oral and Maxillofacial Surgery and
    Pharmacology
Baylor College of Dentistry
Texas A&M University System Health Science Center
Dallas, Texas

Stanley A. Small, DDS
Associate Clinical Professor
Department of Oral and Maxillofacial Surgery
College of Dentistry
New York University
New York, New York

Steven M. Sullivan, DDS
Professor and Chair
Department of Oral and Maxillofacial Surgery
College of Dentistry
University of Oklahoma
Oklahoma City, Oklahoma

Robert B. Summers, DMD
Private Practice
Periodontics
Narberth, Pennsylvania

Dennis P. Tarnow, DDS
Professor and Chairman
Ashman Department of Implant Dentistry
College of Dentistry
New York University
New York, New York

R. Gilbert Triplett, DDS, PhD
Regents Professor and Chairman
Department of Oral and Maxillofacial Surgery and
    Pharmacology
Baylor College of Dentistry
Texas A&M University System Health Science Center
Dallas, Texas

Jean F. Tulasne, MD
Private Practice
Oral and Maxillofacial Surgery
Paris, France

Minoru Ueda, DDS, PhD
Professor and Chairman
Department of Oral and Maxillofacial Surgery
Graduate School of Medicine
Nagoya University
Nagoya, Japan

Tomaso Vercellotti, MD, DDS
Private Practice
Periodontics
Genova, Italy

Stephen S. Wallace, DDS
Associate Clinical Professor
Ashman Department of Implant Dentistry
College of Dentistry
New York University
New York, New York

Georg Watzek, MD, DMD, PhD
Head
Department of Oral Surgery
School of Dentistry
University of Vienna
Vienna, Austria

Yoichi Yamada, DDS, PhD
Center for Genetic and Regenerative Medicine
Graduate School of Medicine
Nagoya University
Nagoya, Japan

Ira D. Zinner, DDS, MSD
Clinical Professor
Division of Restorative and Prosthodontic Sciences
College of Dentistry
New York University
New York, New York

Section 1

Biologic, Biomechanical, and Prosthetic Considerations

chapter 1
History of Maxillary Sinus Grafting

Philip J. Boyne, DMD, MS, DSc

Traditionally, the maxillary sinus has been an area that has been avoided by most dentists. General practitioners and oral and maxillofacial surgeons generally entered the maxillary sinus from the oral cavity only when absolutely necessary. Even otolaryngologists usually would consider undertaking an antrostomy only as part of a more involved nasal sinus procedure. That such an anatomic structure should now be entered almost routinely for sinus floor grafting in preparation for implant placement is quite extraordinary.

Bone grafting of the maxillary sinus in cases of trauma, however, has been well established. Comminuted fractures involving the maxilla, orbital floor, lateral nasal wall, and maxillary alveolus are treated by open reduction. Through primary or secondary bone grafting, these damaged bones have been completely restructured and restored to their original anatomic conformation. The application of grafting procedures for osseous restoration after oncologic partial resection of the maxilla or after traumatic avulsion also is common. Bone grafting of the maxillary sinus for prosthodontic rehabilitation, however, has been very rare.

Early Bone-Grafting Procedures for Conventional Prostheses

The use of bone grafting of the maxillary sinus to increase osseous tissue for prosthodontic purposes was first proposed in the 1960s by Boyne (US Navy Dental School lectures to postgraduates, 1965–1968). Grafting of the maxillary sinus was used at that time to increase the bulk of bone for subsequent maxillary posterior ridge reduction for optimal prosthodontic interarch distance. Some patients presenting for conventional complete maxillary and mandibular prostheses had bulbous or enlarged tuberosities that impinged on the interarch space, making it impossible to construct complete mandibular and maxillary prostheses. Because removal of bone from the mandible was not feasible, removal of bone from the maxillary tuberosity was the obvious option. However, some of these patients presented with large, pneumatized sinuses that would not permit bone removal to produce the necessary interarch accommodation. Therefore, construction of a functional prosthesis was difficult or impossible.

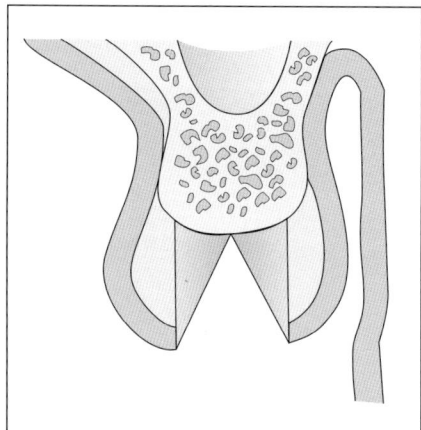

Fig 1-1a Excision of soft tissue preparatory to reduction of bone of a large maxillary tuberosity.

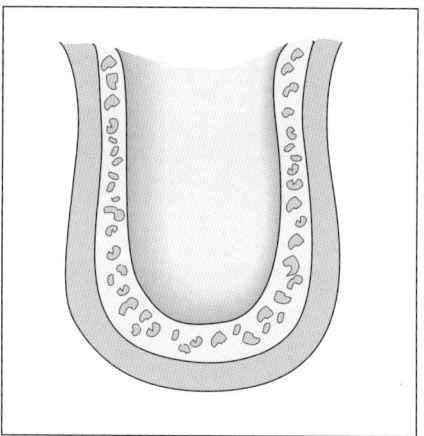

Fig 1-1b Enlarged posterior maxilla, which has a pneumatized antrum and insufficient bone to sustain osseous reduction of the tuberosity.

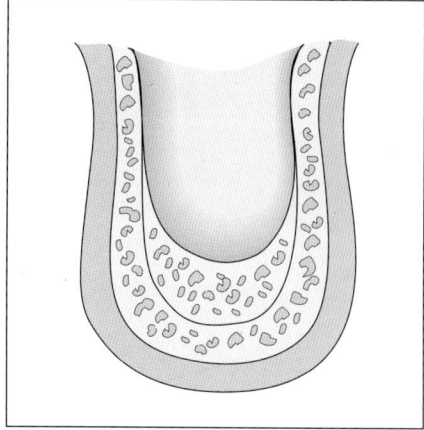

Fig 1-1c Sinus bone graft placed to increase the thickness of the sinus floor. The entire tuberosity can be reduced approximately 3 months later to obtain sufficient interarch space.

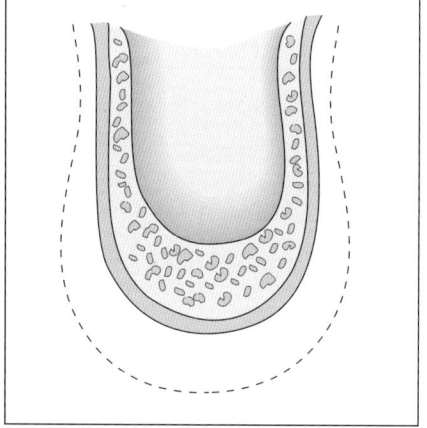

Fig 1-1d Adequate interarch space (*dashed line*) obtained through surgical reduction of the posterior maxilla and tuberosity.

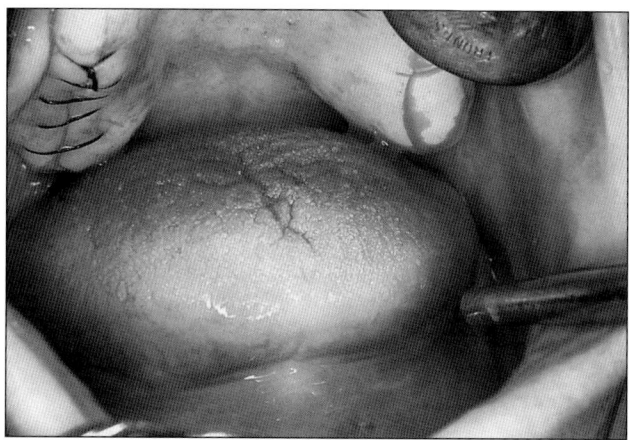

Fig 1-1e Reduction of the maxillary tuberosities after grafting to obtain sufficient protective height of the sinus floor. (The same type of high Caldwell-Luc approach for sinus grafting was used in the 1970s by Boyne and James[1] for placement of blade implants.)

To address this situation, a Caldwell-Luc opening was made in the maxillary antrum, the sinus membrane was elevated, and then an autogenous particulate marrow cancellous bone graft was placed in the sinus floor. Approximately 3 months later, the bone of the tuberosity (along with excess soft tissue) could be reduced without the risk of opening into the antrum, which is now protected by the additional osseous structure. This unique surgical treatment enabled many patients, who otherwise would have been denied adequate reconstruction, to have conventional prostheses. Thus, the first sinus elevation bone graft procedure was undertaken for placing a conventional denture (Fig 1-1).

Bone Grafting of the Maxillary Sinus for Metallic Implants

Blade implants

During the late 1970s, grafting of the maxillary sinus as described for conventional prostheses was undertaken for patients who had large, pneumatized antra in preparation for blade implant placement to enable construction of fixed, semifixed, or removable prostheses for the posterior maxilla. Autogenous particulate iliac bone was usually used as the grafting material. After a postoperative period of approximately 3 months, the blade implants were placed and subsequently used as abutments for removable or fixed prostheses. In 1980, Boyne and James[1] published the first report detailing the surgical technique and the results of three such cases. The same report also described successful results for 11 additional cases of antral grafting for the construction of conventional prostheses.

Root form implants

With the advent of titanium root-form implants, it became apparent that many potential posterior maxillary sites were too deficient in vertical bone height and width for placement of implants. Augmentation of the alveolar ridge was one option for correcting this deficit, but in many situations the antrum also required bone grafting. Several practitioners undertook various surgical techniques designed to enter the antrum, elevate the sinus membrane, and place a bone graft of one type or another. Three major differences in technical approach to the surgical procedure were reported[2]:

1. The type of graft material used varied markedly from one practitioner or surgeon to another[2–4]
2. The technique used for the anatomic site of the antrostomy varied with each surgeon[3,5]
3. The amount of sinus membrane elevation varied markedly with each surgeon[5]

In general, entrance to the antrum was made from three anatomic sites:

1. The classic superior position of the Caldwell-Luc opening, located just anterior to the zygomatic buttress[3]
2. A mid-maxillary position, between the level of the crest of the alveolar ridge and the level of the zygomatic buttress area[3,5]
3. A low position along the anterior surface of the maxilla, very near the level of the existing alveolar ridge[5,6]

The third entrance site became quite popular because it provided quick access to the sinus floor and enabled the practitioner to make an antral window, infracture the buccal osseous plate into the antrum, expeditiously place the bone graft material, and close the incision. However, it also posed a problem: Should there be any infection, large hematoma, or pre-existing sinus disease, the resulting drainage would collect in the area of the osteotomy and tend to produce an oroantral fistula. Thus the midposition antrostomy and the high classic Caldwell-Luc opening were the ones recommended by most oral and maxillofacial surgeons.[1,3]

Additionally, the handling of the lateral cortical plate, which represented the window of the antrostomy, varied with the surgical technique. Many surgeons eliminated it, using a bur to thin the cortical plate down to a paper-thin cortex and removing the thin bone carefully with a mosquito hemostat prior to elevation of the sinus membrane. Others used the infractured cortical plate as a superior limit to the window, leaving it attached to the mucosa. Still others removed the infractured cortical plate and then replaced it on the lateral surface as a graft at the end of the procedure. The rationale was that the antrostomy window would not completely heal without the replacement of the cortical plate. Many have since demonstrated, however, that the antrostomy window will heal with the apposition of bone without the use of the cortical bone window graft.[7,8]

Regarding the elevation of the sinus membrane, some practitioners used minimal elevation, others elevated all of the sinus membrane, while still others elevated the membrane only from the lower half of the antral cavity. The advantage of membrane elevation is that it allows the membrane to collapse over any laceration made in the sinus soft tissue lining, thus facilitating healing. If the membrane is not elevated, the laceration or opening will tend to persist because of the tightness of the membrane in the area.

The results of these various approaches to bone grafting and types of bone graft materials were reported at the 1996 Sinus Consensus Conference.[2]

Indications for the Use of Graft Materials in the Antrum

How to diagnose the need for grafting when implants are placed is a difficult question to answer. It is generally acknowledged that the alveolar ridge should be at least 4 to 5 mm in height to effectively immobilize the implant during the period when the sinus bone graft is maturing.[2] There is a great difference of opinion, however, regarding the need for grafting if implants protrude into the antrum.[7]

Some believe that any protrusion of an implant into the antrum necessitates bone grafting and hence entrance into the antrum for surgical osseous reconstruction. Others

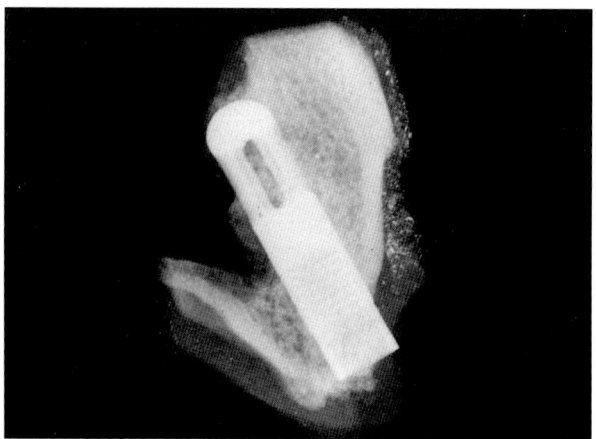

Fig 1-2 Spontaneous bone repair covering about 50% of the surface of an implant that was placed without a bone graft. The round cylindrical surface of the implant is titanium plasma sprayed.

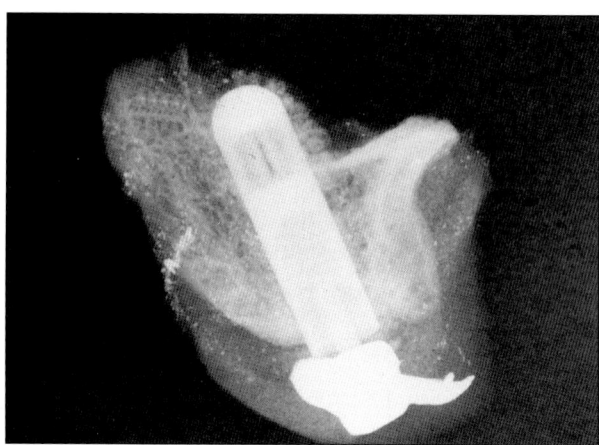

Fig 1-3 New bone covering the entire surface of an implant that was placed without a bone graft. (Specimen taken after 14 months of occlusal function.)

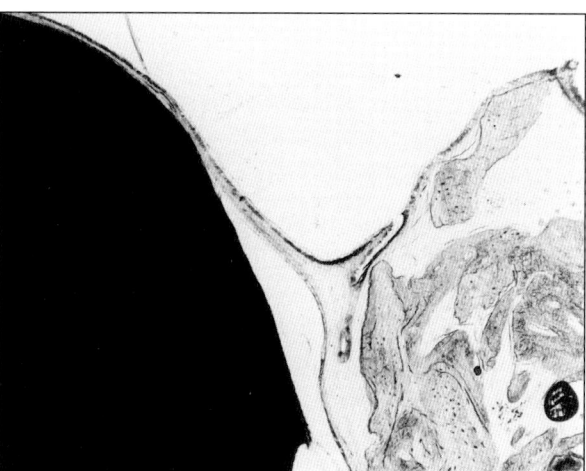

Fig 1-4 Microscopic view of an implant that was placed without a bone graft and was protruding 5 mm into the antrum. Spontaneous growth of bone has migrated up the implant from the sinus floor, covering more than half of the implant surface. Penetration of the antrum by an implant does not, therefore, necessitate a bone graft. (Specimen taken after 14 months of function.)

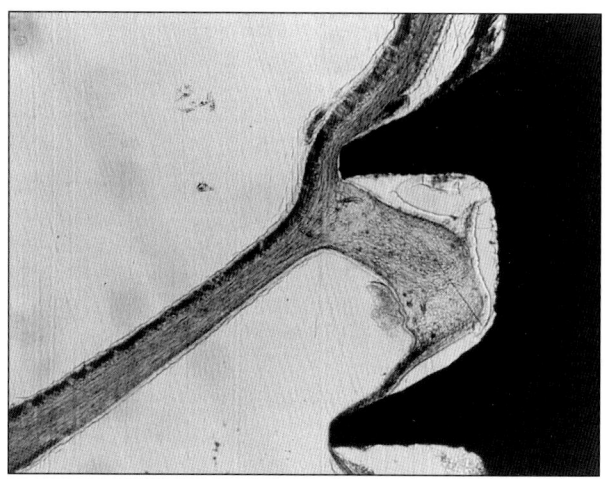

Fig 1-5 Implant with sharp surface angles enters the sinus floor and protrudes 5 mm. New bone does not tend to spontaneously regenerate over such penetrating implants. Only the sinus membrane is visible over the implant surface. (Specimen taken after 14 months of function.)

believe that a certain amount of protrusion into the antrum by the root form implant may not require grafting, provided that the prosthodontic load on the implant is within acceptable limits and will be shared by other teeth or other implants.[7]

Studies involving Rhesus monkeys (*Macaca fascicularis*) have shown that implants protruding up to 5 mm in the antrum without a graft may be subjected to occlusal forces for more than 14 months and yet function and perform as well as implants placed into grafted sinuses.[7] The governing factor appears to be *distribution of the occlusal load* among other implants or natural teeth, not the mere protrusion of the implant into the antrum. Implants protruding 5 mm into the antrum without grafting of the sinus floor exhibited spontaneous bone regeneration over more than half of their surface[3] (Figs 1-2 and 1-3). Thus, the

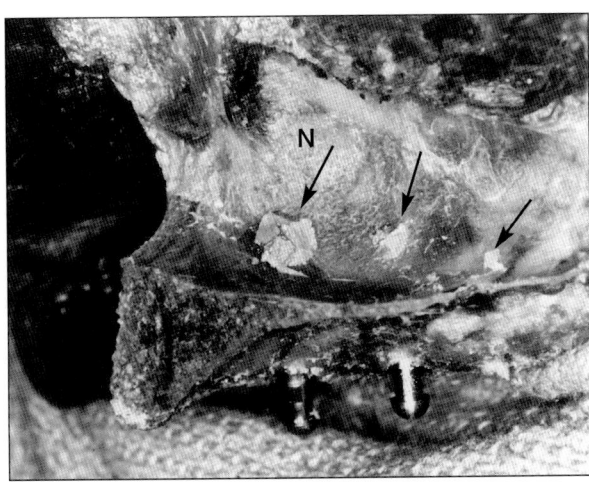

Fig 1-6a Implants *(arrows)* placed in an edentulous atrophic posterior maxilla of a cadaver skull penetrate into the nasal fossa (N) rather than the maxillary sinus.

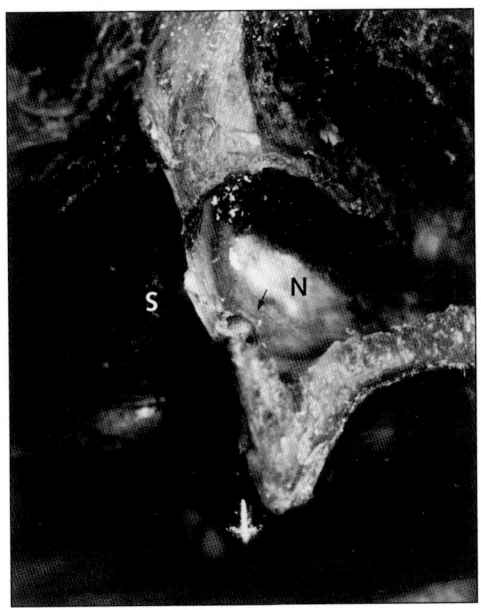

Fig 1-6b Implants placed on the crest of the alveolar ridge penetrate *(arrow)* into the nose (N) despite having been placed lateral to the ridge crest for antral penetration. It appears that with advancing atrophy, the maxilla resorbs from buccal to palatal, and consequently the residual crest of the ridge "moves" palatally. Implants placed on the atrophic crest will, as a result, usually penetrate the nasal floor rather than the sinus floor (S).

mere protrusion of an implant into the sinus floor does not appear to be an indication of a need for bone grafting (see chapter 27).

It appears that the configuration of the implant is the most significant factor governing the effects of penetration of the sinus floor. Some implants with open-ended apices or deep-threaded configurations have exhibited very little spontaneous bone regeneration in Rhesus monkeys. Under the same conditions, round cylindrical implants tend to invite spontaneous growth of bone from the sinus floor over their surface in the absence of any bone-grafting procedure.[7] Titanium plasma-sprayed round cylindrical implants protruding 2 to 3 mm into the antrum were found to have complete spontaneous regeneration of bone over their surfaces. When the same type of implant protrudes up to 5 mm, it is found to have a partial growth of bone toward the apex, but not complete coverage by osseous repair.[7] When open-ended or deep-threaded implants protrude up to 5 mm, little bone regeneration is produced (Figs 1-4 and 1-5).

Edentulous Posterior Maxilla

As the popularity of sinus grafting in preparation for implant placement increased, some investigators began to raise questions about the anatomic characteristics of resorption of the alveolar ridge following the loss of teeth. It has been shown that edentulous areas of the posterior maxilla lose bone buccally, leading to the palatal displacement of the central portion of the residual resorbed ridge.[8] When implants are then placed in the midportion of the ridge, the apex of the implant is positioned in the nasal wall of the antrum or *in the nasal floor itself,*[8] as has been demonstrated in studies of cadaver material (Fig 1-6). This knowledge reinforces the importance of adhering to presurgical and pregrafting diagnostic criteria to identify the correct area to be grafted for maximum support of the implant system being used.

Surgical Innovations in Sinus Floor Grafting

Over the past 15 years, various changes in surgical techniques have been applied to bone grafting of the floor of the maxillary sinus, mostly related to the use of different types of bone graft materials and different intraoperative techniques.

Osteotome technique

In the osteotome technique, a small osteotomy is made at the inferior portion of the sinus, either through the crest of an edentulous alveolar ridge or at the apex of a fresh extraction socket, and the mucoperiosteum of the antral floor is elevated using specially designed osteotomes. Reported outcomes have been mixed. Some surgeons have used it extensively with great success,[9] while others have reported failures related to tearing of the sinus membrane caused by the apices of the implants. If the membrane is torn during a lateral approach when making a window osteotomy, elevating it at the periphery allows it to collapse upon itself for adequate healing, as described earlier. In the intrusion osteotomy technique, however, this is not possible because the intrusion of the antral floor is done blindly. If the antral membrane is not tented up, it is likely to be torn. Since the antral membrane will be in a very taut state, the tear will remain open and may in fact widen to expose the ends of the implant.

The intrusion osteotomy procedure has been used to tent up the antral floor so as to allow room for bone graft materials, which are placed blindly into the surgical bony socket at the alveolar crest and forced into the submembrane area of the sinus. In many cases, graft particles, especially autografts, have undergone bone formation at their periphery. Again, the drawback of this technique is not knowing whether the antral membrane has been punctured.

When this application of the osteotome technique was performed under direct nasal endoscopic evaluation, it was found to produce two types of elevation of the sinus membrane[10]:

1. Limited elevation to the area immediately surrounding the implant apices
2. Extensive elevation with detachment from the sinus floor over a broader area

It was concluded that tearing of the sinus membrane is not uncommon in the first type of elevation. Of the two types of elevation, the potential for perforation, according to proponents, is higher following localized vertical augmentation (as in no. 1 above). This observation confirms the work of other investigators, who have noted the same descriptive characteristics.

Most prudent investigators believe that when using the "blind" osteotome technique, only a certain amount of elevation of the sinus membrane is possible without significant tearing of the soft tissue lining. Beyond that amount, there tends to be an increase in clinical problems associated with this procedure. Additionally, as noted by Berengo et al,[10] direct vertical elevation of the sinus membrane without lateral release from the adjacent bony floor tends to produce perforations.

The use of various bone graft materials in the intrusion osteotomy technique appears to produce two effects:

1. Effective stimulation of host stem cells in the periosteal antral membrane to form osteoblasts, leading to new bone formation
2. "Tenting up" of the antral membrane with the bone graft material to maintain space until bone forms as a result of the surgical stimulation of antral membrane stem cells. (Some investigators have used materials such as calcium sulfate or demineralized freeze-dried bone allograft to produce this type of effect. The problem with calcium sulfate is that it is resorbed in a relatively short period [ie, 5 to 8 weeks]. This is probably insufficient time for replacement osseous repair if the surgical space extends very far from the sinus floor [Boyne PJ, Herford AS, unpublished data, 2003].)

The osteotome technique is effective in certain cases and apparently has been very successful (see chapter 22). However, it can produce an acute or chronic infection in the floor of the antrum, where tears of the antral membrane lead to subsequent dehiscence of bone graft material. The use of nonresorbable ceramics, spilled onto the floor of the sinus, poses a potentially hazardous complication. The main problem with the technique is that it is *blind*, and the surgeon cannot be expected to investigate membrane status or take local countermeasures to prevent infection when perforation is confirmed.

A second matter to consider is that the technique produces an opening into the sinus in a highly dependent position. Inflammatory exudate from any inflammation of the antrum spills dependently onto the area of the disrupted graft and the exposed, protruding implants. Therefore the osteotomy site is unfavorably situated to invite complication. The fact that these potential complications have not been prominently reported in the literature indicates that the procedure may be more successful clinically than one would expect based on the anatomy involved or that most intrusions measure only a few millimeters, well within the self-repair capacity of the sinus.

Pathophysiology of the Maxillary Sinus Floor

Effect on bone repair of implants placed just below the sinus floor

Despite claims about the significance of various types of implants and about healing responses attributed to particular bone-grafting systems, the most significant factor in the overall success of implants placed in grafted sinuses is physiologic bony sinus floor repair phenomena.

In response to the multitude of anecdotal reports of disparate bone response to implants placed at, near, and through the sinus floor, a study[11] was undertaken in mature M fascicularis monkeys to observe the host osseous response to the placement of root form implants, the apices of which were located just beneath the sinus floor.

The implants were placed 1 to 2 mm below the actual bony floor of the sinus (n = 8). Evaluation of the biomechanical reaction of host bone at the apex of these implants under load was believed to be important in assessment of the true role played by bone grafting, choice of implant, or technical modification of surgical treatment protocol. In addition, the purposes of the study were: (1) to evaluate the capacity of an implant to stimulate bone formation in the antral floor, (2) to evaluate osseous repair capacity and sustained capacity of the osseous floor under load, and (3) to obtain information on the possibility of adverse reactions, such as migration of implants superiorly or increased pneumatization of the sinus floor.[11]

Materials and methods

In this study, implants were placed 1 to 2 mm (by radiographic measurement) below the sinus floor in four mature M fascicularis monkeys. Beginning 4 months after placement, the implants were brought into prosthetic function for 5 months (Fig 1-7). Intravital labeling with intramuscular tetracycline (20 mg/kg of body weight) 5 weeks after implant placement and again 9 months after implant placement (1 week before sacrifice) measured the amount of late bone remodeling under function. The implants were in function with the animals masticating a normal diet for 5 months. At sacrifice, the status of the osseous floor of the sinus and the characteristics of bone repair and remodeling between the apex of the implant and the antral floor were measured and evaluated histologically.

Results

All implants placed within 2 mm of the sinus floor resulted in enhanced vertical bone formation of the sinus floor. There was increased distance (average .5 mm) between the sinus floor and the apex of the implants (Figs 1-7 to 1-10). As indicated by tetracycline-induced fluorescence from intravital labeling, proliferative osseous repair apparently augmented bone volume in a long-term remodeling process. Cancellous bone formation in the marrow vascular spaces of the bone above the implant apices condensed into a more lamellar structure after 4 months of function as compared to adjacent marrow vascular spaces not subject to direct implant function (see Fig 1-10). This observed increase in bone density was seen routinely and indicates the favorable effect of the implant.

Significant osteoblastic activity was observed at the periosteal surface of the sinus membrane and was still prominent 9 months after placement of the implants (Fig 1-11).

Discussion

Based on the findings of this study, it is reasonable to expect that implants placed clinically in close proximity to the sinus floor will provide increased osseous support at the sinus floor in a vertical direction from the apex of a subsinus-placed implant.

The animal study observations indicate that the amount of bone formation following placement of sinus bone graft material onto the maxillary sinus floor may be due in part to the intrinsic capacity of the surgical procedure and subsequent implant loading and not to the load-bearing capacity of sinus-grafted bone.

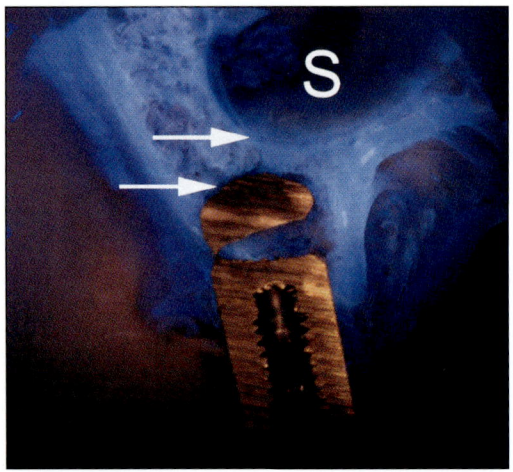

Fig 1-7 Implant placed 2 mm below the sinus floor (S). *Arrows* indicate the amount of bone that was maintained and remodeled during 5 months of function. The increased bone density at the apex of the implant indicates the response of the bone to function and good osteogenetic capability of the antral membrane. These findings demonstrate the maxillary sinus's capacity to form bone and to serve as an excellent environment for long-term osseous remodeling without a bone graft (magnification ×10).

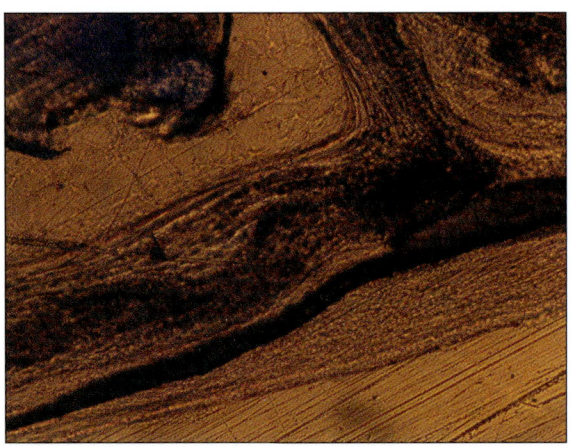

Fig 1-8a Histologic specimen under incandescent light showing the sinus membrane *(top)*, as well as formation of new bone, increased density of cancellous bone, and formation of lamellar bone after 5 months of masticatory function (magnification ×100).

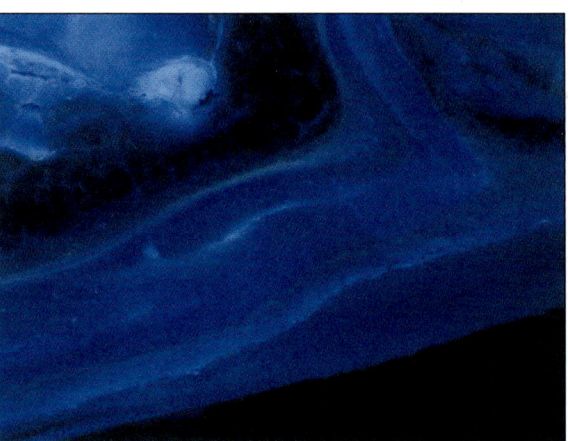

Fig 1-8b Specimen shown in Fig 1-8a under ultraviolet light showing tetracycline-induced fluorescence with new bone formation and increased sinus floor density. The distance between the two labels indicates the amount of bone formed over a 1-month period.

This type of functional mechanical stimuli, perhaps on the order of 2,000 to 3,000 microstrain, to the osseous sinus floor induces available stem cells beneath the sinus membrane and also within the marrow vascular space to differentiate, proliferate, and augment host bone (see chapter 3).

Thus, the atrophic maxillary sinus floor, once believed to be inactive and without significant reparative potential, has been demonstrated to be capable of forming significant reparative bone when adequately functionally stimulated.[12] The physiology of the host bone clearly must be factored into any analysis of results from the use of various bone graft modalities because the underlying load-bearing repair may be primarily physiologic, deriving minimal contribution from the sinus bone graft. The stimulation of stem cells by biomechanical strain as well as the initial surgery may be the true explanation for the sinus floor augmentation phenomenon.

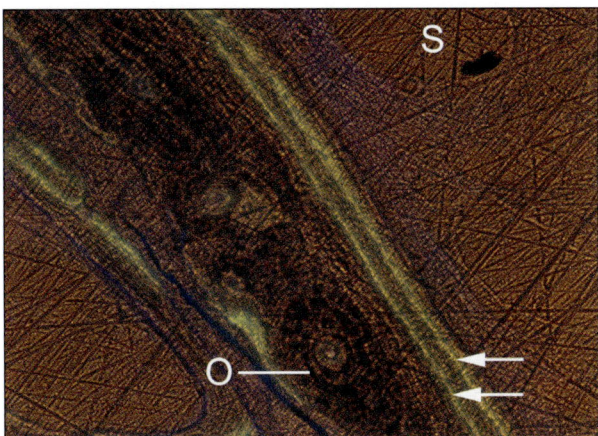 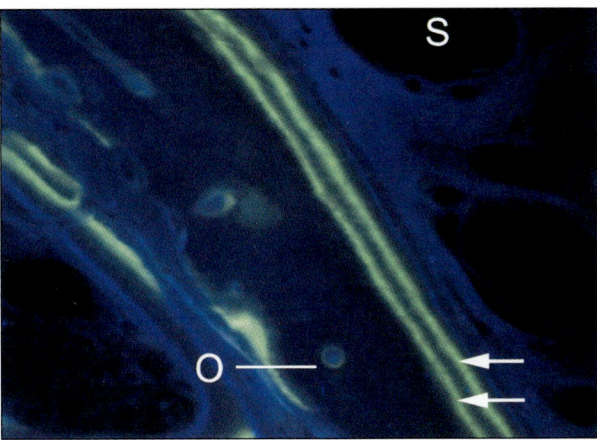

Fig 1-9a Similar view after 5 months of function in the same *M fascicularis* monkey with the implants placed 2 mm from the sinus floor. New bone has formed in the sinus (S) floor *(arrows)* and in remodeling marrow vascular spaces, forming new osteons (O) adjacent to the sinus floor. These are indications of continuing appropriate anabolic remodeling under occlusal function (incandescent light).

Fig 1-9b Same specimen viewed under ultraviolet light showing increased density and lamellar bone formation after 5 months of function. *Arrows* indicate two labels of tetracycline-induced fluorescence showing the amount of lamellar bone formed between 5 weeks and 1 week prior to sacrifice after 5 months of function. Note also the new osteons (O) forming a new cortical bone surface beneath the sinus floor (S).

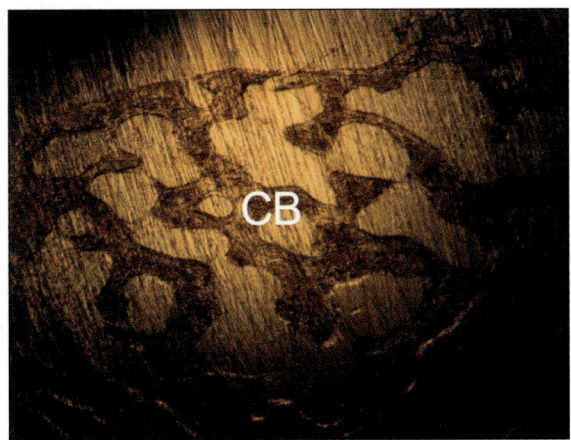 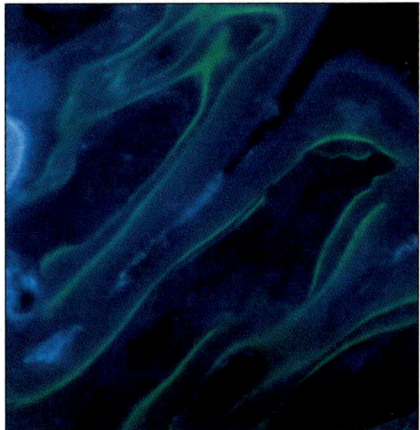

Fig 1-10a Marrow vascular spaces adjacent to the functioning implant shown in Fig 1-9 after 9 months. There is very little increase in the density of the cancellous bone (CB) in this non–implant-supporting area.

Fig 1-10b Similar area in the same animal showing the bone above the apex of an adjacent implant. There is increased cancellous bone density with new lamellar bone formed from remodeling of the cancellous trabeculae.

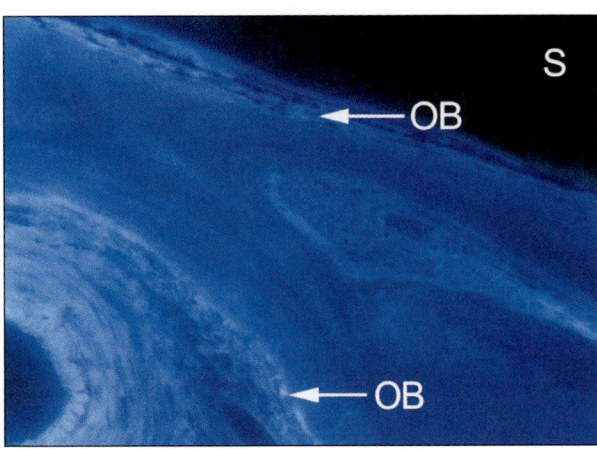

Fig 1-11 Histologic sections observed 9 months after implant placement and after 5 months of occlusal function. A row of osteoblasts (OB) from the periosteal layer of the sinus membrane area indicates significant osteogenic activity in the sinus floor (S) over a sustained period of time (eg, 5 months of function). Active osteoblasts are also observed in the underlying marrow vascular spaces (magnification ×120).

Present and Future Aspects of Sinus Grafting

Researchers are now investigating the possibility of incorporating bone graft inductor materials into suitable carriers placed in the antrum to regenerate bone without the need for conventional bone graft materials (autogenous, allogeneic, or alloplastic). It has been shown that when placed in an appropriate collagen carrier, bone morphogenetic protein will cause a complete regeneration of bone in large discontinuity defects of the mandible,[13] in surgically created "cleft" defects in the maxilla,[14] and on the sinus floor.[15] A multicenter investigation has been successful in using a bone morphogenetic protein (rhBMP-2) in sinus grafting for the placement of implants in clinical patients.[15] Herford and Boyne have reported the successful use of rhBMP-2 in osseous clefts of children, some of whom received root form implants in the restored areas (Joint Meeting of the American College of OMS and the Canadian Association of OMS; June 22–25, 2005; Nova Scotia, Canada). Thus, a significant research thrust of the future will be in the appropriate application of morphogenetic cytokines to induce adult mesenchymal stem cells existing in the sinus floor.[16]

Advances in sinus bone grafting have been interesting and exciting for prosthodontic reasons. Future areas of research offer the opportunity for development of better methods of treating prosthodontic patients with significant maxillary deficiencies in need of osseous reconstruction as part of their overall root form implant-supported prosthodontic rehabilitation.

Where technologic innovation of the sinus bone graft will lead in the future, as clinicians enter the age of tissue engineering, remains to be seen. One can only stipulate, as Aristotle did, that all future inquiry must be based on critical observation and experimental validation, always putting first our responsibility to take utmost care of the patients we serve.

References

1. Boyne PJ, James R. Grafting of the maxillary sinus floor with autogenous marrow and bone. J Oral Surg 1980;38:613–618.
2. Jensen OT, Shulman LB, Block MS, Iacono VJ. Report of the Sinus Consensus Conference of 1996. Int J Oral Maxillofac Implants 1998;13(suppl):11–45.
3. Lazzara RJ. The sinus elevation procedure in endosseous implant therapy. Curr Opin Periodontol 1996;3:178–183.
4. Triplett RG, Schow SR. Autologous bone grafts and endosseous implants: Complementary techniques. J Oral Maxillofac Surg 1996;54:486–494.
5. Zitzmann NU, Schärer P. Sinus elevation procedures in the resorbed posterior maxilla: Comparison of the crestal and lateral approaches. Oral Surg Oral Med Oral Pathol 1998;85:8–17.
6. Summers RB. The osteotome technique: Part 3—Less invasive methods of elevating the sinus floor. Compendium 1994;15:698, 700, 702–704.
7. Boyne PJ. Analysis of performance of root-form endosseous implants placed in the maxillary sinus. J Long Term Eff Med Implants 1993;3:143–159.
8. Boyne PJ. The use of bone graft systems in maxillary implant surgery. Proceedings of the 50th Annual Meeting of the American Institute of Oral Biology, Palm Springs, CA, Oct 29–Nov 2. Madison, WI: Omni, 1993:107–114.
9. Kaufman E. Maxillary sinus elevation surgery: An overview. J Esthet Restorative Dent 2003;15:272–283.
10. Berengo M, Sivolella Z, Majzoub G, Cordioli G. Endoscopic evaluation of the bone-added osteotome sinus floor elevation procedure. Int J Oral Maxillofac Surg 2004;33:189–194.
11. Andreana S, Cornelini R, Edsberg LE, Natiella JR. Maxillary sinus elevation for implant placement using calcium sulfate with and without DFDBA: Six cases. Implant Dent 2004;3:270–277.
12. Iida S, Tanaka N, Kogo M, Matsuya T. Migration of a dental implant into the maxillary sinus. A case report. Int J Oral Maxillofac Surg 2000;29:358–359.
13. Boyne PJ. Animal studies of the application of rhBMP-2 in maxillofacial reconstruction. Bone 1996;19(suppl):83S–92S.
14. Boyne PJ, Nath R, Nakamura A. Human recombinant BMP-2 in osseous reconstruction of simulated cleft palate defects. Br J Oral Maxillofac Surg 1998;36:84–90.
15. Boyne PJ, Marx RF, Nevins M, et al. A feasibility study evaluating rhBMP-2/absorbable collagen sponge for maxillary sinus floor augmentation. Int J Periodontics Restorative Dent 1997;17:11–25.
16. Boyne PJ, Lilly LC, Marx RE, Moy PK, Nevins M, Spagnoli DB, Triplett RG. De novo bone induction by recombinant human bone morphogenetic protein-2 (rhBMP-2) in maxillary sinus floor augmentation. J Oral Maxillofac Surg 2005;63:1693–1707.

chapter 2
Biologic Basis of Sinus Grafting

Georg Watzek, MD, DMD, PhD
Gabor Fürst, MD, DDS
Reinhard Gruber, PhD

Implant Survival at Sinus Augmentation Sites

The volume of the maxillary sinus, which increases with age and tooth loss, ranges from 4.5 to 35.2 cm^3. Maxillary bone loss accompanies enlargement of the sinus and is mainly observed in the horizontal rather than the vertical dimension. Based on the Cawood and Howell classification of bone loss, the residual alveolus may be classified in gradations of I (dentate) to VI (paper-thin).[1] In classes IV to VI, vertical bone volume is the primary factor limiting implant placement.[2]

Grafting of the maxillary sinus floor increases the vertical height of the posterior maxillary bone prior to implant placement. The 1996 Sinus Consensus Conference deemed this therapeutic modality highly predictable and effective.[3] In the augmented sinus, reports of implant survival under functional loading varied from 36%[4] to 61.7%,[5] even reaching 100% in recent meta-analyses. The overall success rate is 91.6% for implants with a rough surface and 92.3% for particulate bone grafts.[5] Both of these parameters, along with the application of guided bone regeneration techniques, were found to positively affect the long-term stability of loaded implants.[5] Whether or not other parameters—eg, aging, systemic diseases, lifestyle factors, one- or two-stage procedures, vertical height of residual bone—influence implant survival in the augmented sinus was not stated.[4,5] Moreover, aborted or failed sinus grafting procedures, instances where primary stability was not obtained or implants were lost in the early stages of osseointegration, were not covered by these meta-analyses.

Failures before loading were reported to occur in 3.6% of patients when implants are placed in nongrafted bone.[6] These cases may lower considerably the overall success rate of the sinus-grafting procedure.

Osseointegration, which is a prerequisite for long-term stability of dental implants under functional loading, depends on the dynamic process of bone regeneration as originally defined by Brånemark et al[7] and revised by Schenk and Buser.[8] Bone regeneration is initiated by the formation of a peri-implant blood clot, which is replaced first by granulation tissue, then by woven bone, and finally by lamellar bone.[9,10] Dental implants must consequently be placed in vital bone that provides a blood supply, osteogenic cells, growth and differentiation factors, and a provisional extracellular matrix.[11,12] Moreover, primary stability must be achieved for intramembranous bone formation around dental implants.[7,13] However, primary stability cannot easily be achieved.

Early failure rates of 32% are reported for implants placed with inadequate primary stability.[14,15] Type 4 bone, which is characterized by a thin cortex and loose trabeculae, does not possess the mechanical properties that allow implants to achieve primary stability with a high rate of success.[16] The molar region of the maxilla has a trabecular bone volume of 17% in women and 23% in men, with wide variations in each group.[17] Type 4 bone predominates

> **BOX 2-1 Regulation of osteogenic differentiation and blood vessel formation**
>
> Upon sinus elevation, blood vessel disruption leads to the immediate development of a blood clot that entraps the graft within a provisional extracellular fibrin-rich matrix. Accumulating platelets and, later, neutrophils and macrophages serve as a source for growth factors, including PDGF, VEGF, and bFGF, as well as a broad spectrum of other bioactive molecules.[30] PDGF is a potent mitogen and chemoattractant for osteogenic cells and can temporarily suppress their differentiation.[31–33] PDGF induces blood vessel formation and acts in concert with VEGF and bFGF in this process.[34,35] The phospholipid sphingosine-1-phosphate, which is released from activated platelets, has a potent angiogenic activity.[36] *Angiogenesis*, the formation of new capillaries from existing blood vessels, is a multistep process initiated by degradation of the basal membrane by proteases such as matrix metalloproteinases. Once endothelial cells are released, they migrate into the interstitial stroma, where they proliferate and form capillary-like structures before they produce a basal membrane and attract pericytes.[37,38] In parallel, endothelial progenitor cells that originate from the bone marrow are transported via the bloodstream to the site of blood vessel formation, where they contribute to capillary sprouting by a process termed *vasculogenesis*.[39] Once the blood clot is replaced by the blood vessel–rich granulation tissue, the differentiation of mesenchymal progenitor cells into functional osteoblasts is initiated as observed in tooth extraction sites[40] and during osseointegration of dental implants.[9] Although the mechanisms that regulate osteogenic differentiation in this particular time frame are not known in detail, they are likely to involve the response to differentiation factors such as members of the BMP family,[41] Hedgehog proteins, and factors affecting wingless-type (Wnt) signaling.[42,43] Activation of these signaling pathways can modulate the expression of transcription factors, such as RUNX-2 and Osterix, that drive the differentiation process.[44] Chondrogenic differentiation of mesenchymal progenitor cells in the grafted area will likely be initiated by mechanically unstable conditions that prohibit blood vessel formation.[45] Moreover, osteoblasts provide a niche for hematopoietic stem cells, suggesting that they are involved in the formation of bone marrow in the augmented area (Fig 2-1).[46]

in the molar region of the edentulous maxilla (68% in women and 62% in men).[17] Primary stability can be moderately increased by means of bone condensation and modification of implant design and surface.[18] Unfortunately, these methods have limited potential to compensate for the severely resorbed posterior maxilla of poor structural integrity (see chapter 27).

The Dynamic Process of Graft Consolidation

Sinus grafting aims to restore the resorbed posterior maxilla to allow placement of stable dental implants through the dynamic process of osseointegration. Consolidation of the graft material with host bone is prerequisite to osseointegration. *Graft consolidation* describes graft material that is surrounded and invested by newly modeled bone and incorporated into the vital host vascular bed followed by functional remodeling. Consolidation involves the formation of a graft–woven bone complex that remodels into lamellar bone and further adapts based on functional load. Graft consolidation requires an ample supply of blood and osteogenic cells, which deposit new bone onto a solid surface.[19] Continuous delivery of osteogenic cells is necessary because mature osteoblasts either end up as osteocytes and lining cells or undergo apoptosis.[20] Blood vessel formation, osteoblast function, and graft consolidation, therefore, share a functional linkage.

The dense vascular network of the maxilla diminishes after tooth loss and advancing age. Because 70% to 100% of the blood vessels in the maxilla originate from the periosteum,[21] much care must be taken to ensure atraumatic elevation of the mucosa. Disruption of the sinus mucosa also impairs local blood flow, which can compromise graft consolidation and implant survival.[22] Depending on the processing of graft material, blood vessels sprout into the haversian channels of block grafts or in the spaces between particulated materials of bone during the early stages of bone graft incorporation. Blood vessels are

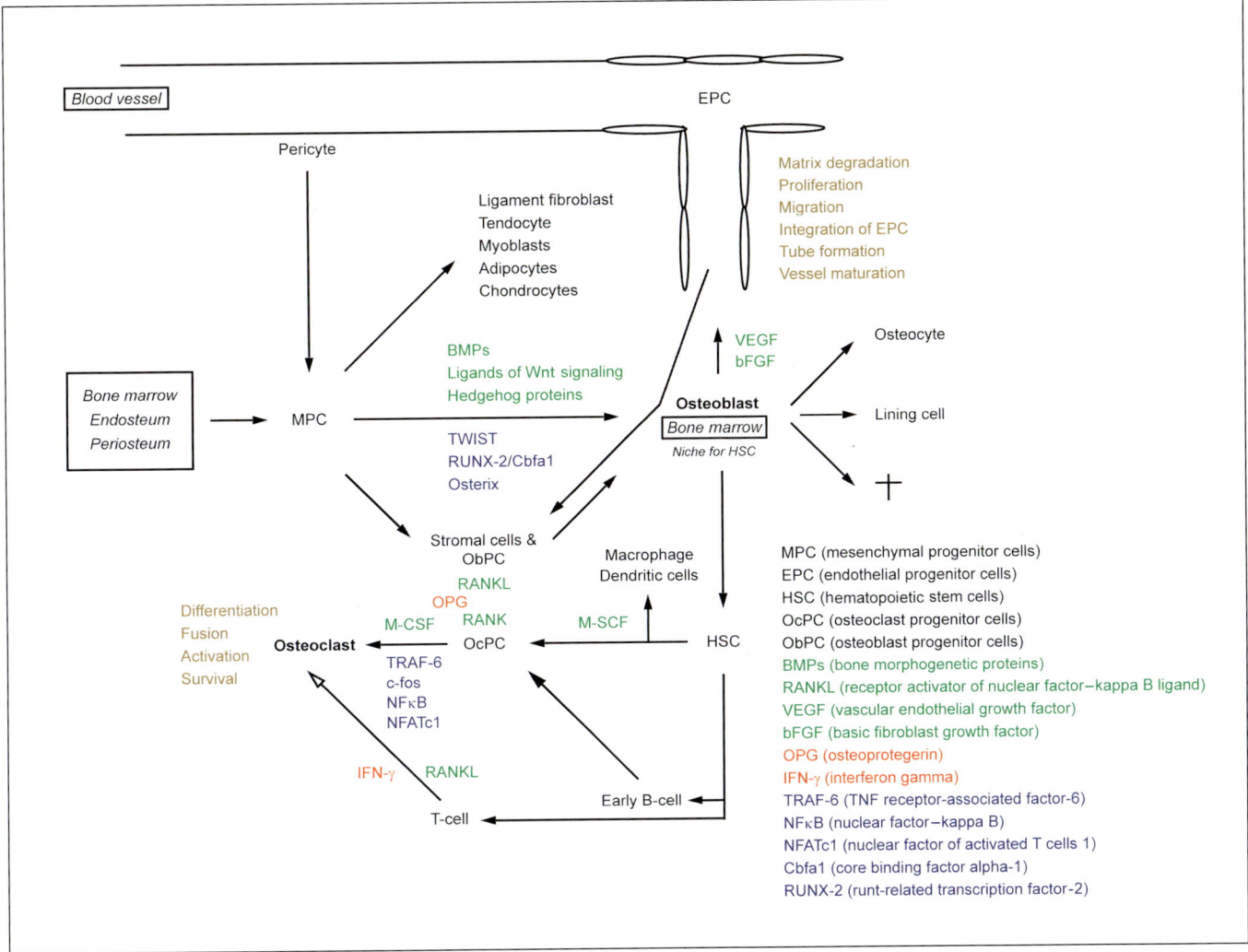

Fig 2-1 Sequence and functional relationship of blood vessel formation, osteogenic differentiation, and osteoclastogenesis, as described in Boxes 2-1 and 2-2. Blood vessels provide a source of circulating hematopoietic progenitor cells and vascular pericytes, progenitors of osteoclasts and osteoblasts, respectively. Recent findings suggest that osteogenic cells are transported via the bloodstream.[47] Independent of their origin, mesenchymal progenitor cells require autocrine and paracrine signals that regulate migration, proliferation, and differentiation into bone-forming osteoblasts. A less differentiated phenotype of the osteogenic lineage supports the process of osteoclastogenesis by providing M-CSF and the key factor RANKL. Under physiologic conditions, osteoclastogenesis is regulated by the balance between the concentration of the decoy receptor OPG and RANKL. At sites of chronic inflammation, T-cell–derived IFN-γ directly counteracts the osteoclastogenic effects of RANKL and TNFα, and early stages of B-cells can serve as osteoclast progenitor cells. Whether this osteoimmunologic scenario takes place during graft consolidation remains to be determined. Osteoblasts can establish a favorable microenvironment for hematopoietic stem cells, osteogenic cells can interact with endothelial cells and vice versa, and osteoclasts can stimulate bone formation. It becomes obvious that all of these processes are highly interrelated and are important in the orchestration of graft consolidation.

organized by angiogenic signal molecules released at the defect site from activated platelets,[23] migrating macrophages,[24] and osteogenic cells.[25] Hypoxic conditions in the early graft site provide a further stimulus for the expression of angiogenic molecules by macrophages[26] and osteogenic cells.[27] The blood clot serves as a reservoir of angiogenic factors, such as vascular endothelial growth factor and basic fibroblast growth factor.[28] Capillary sprouting into a defect site is abundant, usually exceeding the formation of newly formed bone. In vitro studies suggest that endothelial cells provide a stimulus to attract osteogenic cells into granulation tissue at the defect site (Box 2-1).[29]

> **BOX 2-2** Regulation of osteoclastic differentiation
>
> Osteoclasts are highly specialized bone-resorbing cells.[59] These cells originate from the hematopoietic lineage and form large multinucleated cells, a process that is strictly controlled by the triad of receptor activator of NF-kappa B ligand (RANKL), receptor activator of NF-kappa B (RANK), and osteoprotegerin (OPG).[60] Cells of the mesenchymal lineage, T-cells, B-cells, and monocytes produce RANKL, which binds to its corresponding receptor RANK on hematopoietic cells.[61] This binding activates a signaling cascade that induces *(1)* the differentiation of progenitor cells into the osteoclastogenic lineage, *(2)* the fusion of the osteoclast progenitors, *(3)* stimulation of the resorptive activity, and *(4)* increased survival.[62,63] OPG acts as a soluble decoy receptor for RANKL and is released by a large number of cell types, including osteoblasts. The stochiometric ratio between RANKL and OPG is consequently a parameter for the formation, activation, and survival of osteoclasts. Other locally produced factors such as IL-1, tumor necrosis factor-alpha (TNF-α), and transforming growth factor-beta (TGF-β), which are highly expressed at sites of chronic inflammation, can enhance the RANKL-RANK–mediated effects and further increase bone resorption.[64]
>
> Osteoclastogenesis and activity is required for bone remodeling of the entire skeleton but also at sites of graft placement. Remodeling of bone grafts requires the biologic activity of RANKL and VEGF, suggesting that both osteoclasts and blood vessels are essential in this process (see Fig 2-7).[65] Fracture healing studies indicate that the expression of RANKL was nearly undetectable in unfractured bone but strongly induced throughout the healing period.[66] Osteoclasts are further required during early stages of osseointegration where dead bone is to be replaced by vital bone and during adaption of peri-implant bone tissue under functional loading.[11] Osteoclasts are necessary when microcracks in the peri-implant bone, which result from loading, are repaired.[67] Cells staining positive for the tartrate-resistant acid phosphatase, a characteristic marker for osteoclasts, were reported in augmented sinuses.[68,69] Tartrate-resistant acid phosphatase–positive cells were detected near the elevated sinus membrane and close to the local host bone.[68] Osteoclasts can originate from hematopoietic progenitors within the graft and blood vessels sprouting into the augmented area from the mucosa and local host bone. More information is required to know whether treatment regimens that affect systemic bone resorption have an impact on graft consolidation and the early and later stages of osseointegration. It is also unclear why autograft is sometimes completely resorbed and not remodeled into bone.

Osteogenic cells within the autograft contribute to its early consolidation provided that nutrients and growth factors diffuse through the blood clot.[48,49] For this reason, the processing of autograft must be considered. Neither grinding nor morselizing of autograft disturbs the viability of osteogenic cells,[50,51] which will survive in a hypoxic environment for at least 3 days (unpublished observations). However, blood vessels are apparently needed to provide a continuous source of osteogenic cells. The origin of osteogenic cells at sites of bone regeneration is not entirely clear, although vascular pericytes and blood-derived cells are potent candidates.[47,49] Migration, proliferation, and differentiation of osteogenic cells are orchestrated by autocrine-paracrine factors released from activated platelets,[31,52] neutrophils,[53] macrophages,[30] osteogenic cells,[25] and endothelial cells,[29] as well as from components in the extracellular matrix.[54] Bone morphogenetic proteins can adsorb to extracellular matrix proteins, such as collagens I and IV and heparin, thereby increasing local threshold levels to initiate osteogenic differentiation.[55] The main source of osteogenic cells during graft consolidation is the periosteum, which has mesenchymal progenitor cells in the cambium layer and provides a rich source of blood vessels. The sinus mucosa also contains osteogenic cells, but what they contribute to graft consolidation is unclear (see Box 2-1).[56]

Osteoclastogenesis is required for remodeling of the graft–woven bone complex. Progenitor cells of hematopoietic lineage are transported via the bloodstream, indicating that a continuous supply of osteoclasts at the graft site also requires blood vessel formation. Osteoclastogenesis requires a microenvironment provided by mesenchymal cells triggered into the osteogenic lineage.[57] Recent findings suggest that osteoclasts also are involved in the coordination of bone formation.[58] Although the signals that control osteoclast formation, activation, and survival are known in great detail (Box 2-2), the main signal coordinating bone resorption during graft consolidation remains unknown.

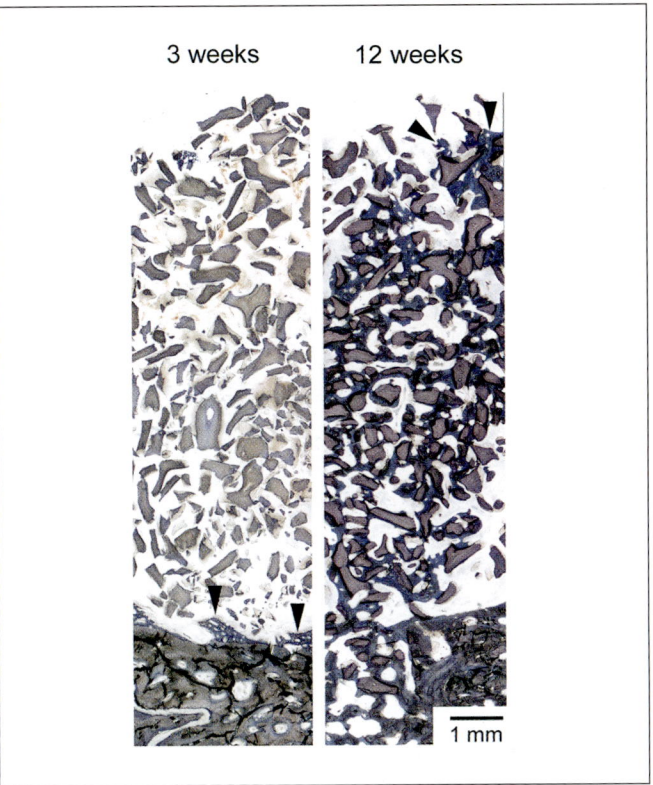

Fig 2-2 Histologic specimens of minipig sinus augmented with bovine bone mineral. New bone originating from the sinus bony wall continuously grows into the augmented area toward the sinus membrane. Consolidation is reached after approximately 3 to 4 months. This figure confirms that xenograft is osteoconductive, allowing newly formed bone to "jump" from one particle to the next. At all time points, large osteocyte lacunae characteristic of woven bone are visible in the mineralization front, which grows at approximately 1 mm per week into the augmented area. (*Arrowheads* designate the upper limit of newly formed bone.)

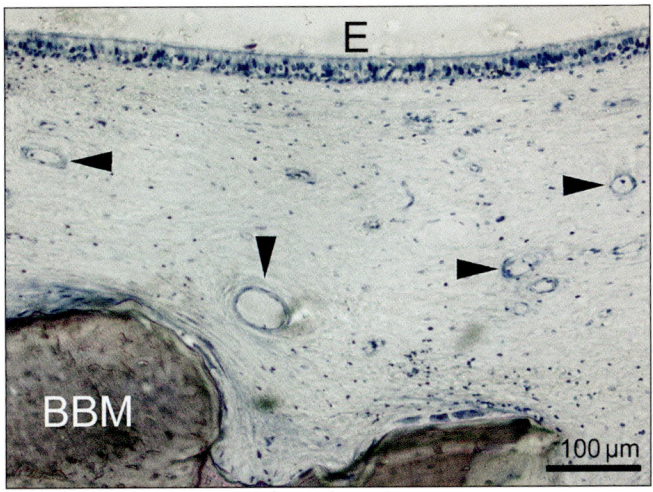

Fig 2-3 Sinus membrane covering a sinus graft of bovine bone mineral. The space between the epithelium and the xenograft contains blood vessels (*arrowheads*) embedded in loose connective tissue of the lamina propria. No bone formation is visible on the surface of the xenograft particle. This figure demonstrates that the microenvironment of a vital bone surface is necessary to initiate bone formation. (BBM, bovine bone mineral; E, epithelium; toluidine blue stain.)

Grafting Materials, Membranes, and the Consolidation Process

Consolidation depends on the properties of the graft material and the osteogenic potential of the recipient bed. The graft material should allow ingrowth of blood vessels and formation of bone on its surface for integration into the recipient bed. Autografts provide a source of both osteogenic cells and growth and differentiation factors to support bone regeneration. Iliac crest bone is still considered the osteogenic gold standard for sinus grafting; however, harvesting can cause morbidity and does not always provide an adequate amount of bone. Ceramic bone substitutes lack osteogenic capacity and are therefore limited to regenerating bone through osteoconduction.[70,71] Unlike osteogenesis, osteoconduction involves the accumulation of plasma components such as fibronectin and vitronectin on the surface of the bone substitutes, which allows osteogenic cell attachment via integrin and heparan sulfate receptors (Figs 2-2 and 2-3).[72–75] The use of bone substitutes that have been coated with arginine-glycine-aspartic acid (RGD)-containing peptides is one approach to encourage this process.[76] Bone substitutes as well as autograft have also been supplemented with growth factors, extracellular matrix, and osteogenic cells,[77–80] but whether

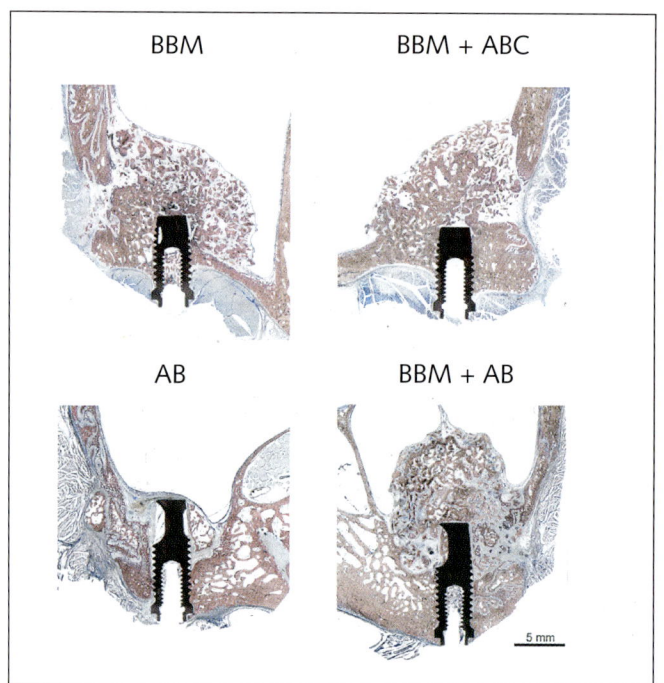 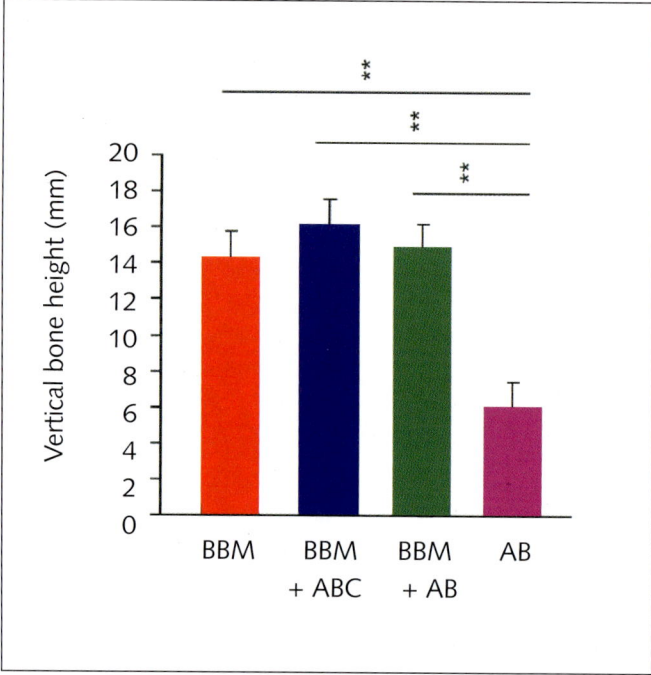

Fig 2-4a Histologic specimens of grafted minipig sinuses after 12 weeks of healing. Implants were placed at the time of sinus augmentation in a one-stage procedure. In this model, the sinuses grafted with autogenous bone were severely resorbed. Note that fibrous tissue originating from the bone window invades the augmented side. (BBM, bovine bone mineral; ABC, autogenous bone cells; AB, autogenous bone; Levai-Laczko stain.)

Fig 2-4b Histogram illustrating the corresponding vertical height of the grafted area. Data are given as least square means and corresponding standard deviations. (BBM, bovine bone mineral; ABC, autogenous bone cells; AB, autogenous bone; **$P < .01$.)

these therapies are substantially more efficacious is currently unclear (see chapter 30).

Barrier membrane coverage of the lateral window is reported to improve long-term implant survival.[5] The membrane stabilizes the blood clot at the grafted site and serves as a barrier against the immigration of nonosteogenic cells from the soft tissue into the defect site (Fig 2-4).[81] Further research is needed to determine which membrane type is preferred and whether their use should be recommended (see chapter 19).

Disease Background and Graft Consolidation

The number of patients with age-related bone diseases, among which osteoporosis is highlighted here, has steadily increased within recent decades.[82,83] The estimated lifetime risk of hip fracture is 17% for white women and 6% for white men.[82,84] A transient but disproportional bone loss of 20% to 30% in trabecular bone and 5% to 10% in cortical bone occurs in women during the first postmenopausal decade. The following slow phase accounts for 20% to 30% of trabecular and cortical bone loss in aged individuals of both sexes.[85] In sinus grafting, the reduced amount of mineral matrix per volume of bone is an important factor to consider. In a retrospective study, implant loss after one-stage sinus augmentation was higher in patients with low bone mineral density when compared to age- and sex-matched controls.[86] These results suggest that osteoporosis is a possible risk factor for implant survival in the augmented sinus. However, more research is needed to establish a relationship between the disproportional remodeling cycle in osteoporosis, graft consolidation, and implant survival. Ovariectomized sheep, goats, and dogs may serve as a suitable model for this purpose.[87–89] Moreover, evaluation of the effects of therapeutic regimens for osteoporosis—such as hormone replacement therapy, selective estrogen receptor modulators, parathyroid hormone, and bisphosphonates—on graft consolidation and implant survival in the augmented sinus should be performed.[90] For example, bisphosphonates can increase bone mineralization,[91] which may add to implant stability; however, a reduced remodeling rate may have a negative effect on graft consolidation (see chapter 8).

Age-related bone loss is associated with a declining number of osteogenic progenitor cells in the bone marrow,[92] decreased chondrogenic potential of the periosteum,[93] and limited proliferation and differentiation capacity of osteogenic cells.[94,95] In an ectopic model, bone formation resulting from the bone marrow of a young animal was approximately fivefold greater than that resulting from bone marrow of old rats.[96] Age of the recipient had only minor influence, suggesting that the number and responsiveness of osteogenic cells within the bone marrow was the key factor in bone formation.[96] Other animal models indicate that angiogenesis and vasculogenesis are impaired with increasing age.[97,98] Prolonged healing periods and modulation of the bioactive properties of the grafting material may compensate for the age-related decline in graft consolidation, as described in Box 2-3.

Diabetes also is associated with impaired angiogenic potential, which may be the cause of suboptimal osseointegration of dental implants in long bones.[117,118] However, diabetic patients with controlled glucose levels had success

---

BOX 2-3 Possible strategies to support graft consolidation

Natural and recombinant growth factors have been tested for their potential to support bone formation in augmented sinuses. Platelet-rich plasma (PRP) is an autologous source of platelet-released molecules. Supernatants from activated platelets are highly mitogenic and chemotactic for mesenchymal progenitor cells; their osteogenic differentiation is temporarily suppressed[31] in the presence of BMPs.[99] Platelets can induce the formation of osteoclast-like cells in vitro and may contribute to early bone remodeling.[100] Animal experiments and clinical studies showed no or only a weak stimulation of bone regeneration and osseointegration in augmented sinuses.[101–103] It is possible that the accumulation of physiologic quantities of platelets during blood clot formation are sufficient to induce the healing cascade in young and healthy patients. In compromised patients who have undergone tumor resection, PRP can increase the process of bone remodeling, as observed by the greater amount of lamellar bone in the grafted area. Among the recombinant growth factors, PDGF has been approved for treatment of chronic ulcers in diabetic patients[104] and is a potential treatment option for periodontal disease.[105] Studies on bone regeneration in sinus elevation surgery have not been performed so far. Osteoinductive BMP-2 and BMP-7 were tested in sinus-grafting applications; however, the carrier has a limited space-providing potential.[106,107] When applied together with bovine bone mineral, BMP-7 induced homogenous bone formation throughout the augmented area in minipigs.[108] Also, the surfaces of the dental implants, which where placed simultaneously, showed bone-implant contact of up to 81%.[108] This is a promising approach because implants can survive functional loading in bone tissue induced by BMP-2.[109]

Another strategy to enhance graft consolidation is through supplementation of osteogenic cells of autologous origin.[110,111] Osteogenic cells can be isolated from periosteum, iliac crest, or bone marrow, expanded ex vivo, and seeded onto the grafting material.[112] The expanded cells can also be mixed with the grafting material immediately before sinus augmentation.[113] The construct of grafting material, osteogenic cells, and a mineralized extracellular matrix is not vital bone, however, and requires remodeling similar to that required in transplanted autografts.

Gene therapy approaches are based on the concept that the cells to be transplanted serve as bioreactors to produce growth factors over a prolonged period, acting via an autocrine-paracrine mode of action.[78,114] This method has led to promising results in regeneration of mandibular defects[115] and discontinuity defects in long bones[116] of animal models. No studies have been reported for gene therapy–stimulated graft consolidation in the maxillary sinus. Numerous questions remain open to discussion—in particular: which group of patients will benefit from enhanced biotechnology? What treatment has the best cost-efficacy ratio? What approach results in consistent graft consolidation for long-term performance?

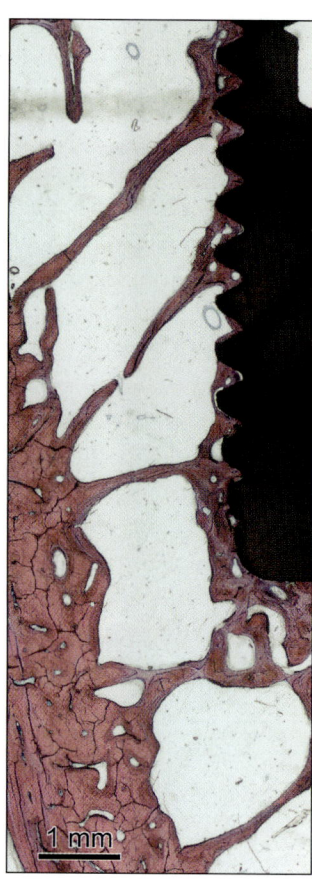

Fig 2-5 Implant placed in mandibular bone of nonhuman primate after 18 months of functional loading. Bone trabeculae have modeled so that functional stress is transferred to the surrounding bone. The trabecular structure leaves space for the bone marrow, which holds all components necessary for bone remodeling to repair microcracks that form under loading. This is an example of adaptation of peri-implant bone to mastication force.

originates from the implant bed.[11] This can explain their higher degree of bone-implant contact during early osseointegration. Intimate peri-implant bone is a prerequisite to strain adaptation, which occurs in trabecular bone as well as in cortical bone in the form of remodeling and modeling. This mechanism is based on signal sensing from mechanical strain, leading to cellular mechanotransduction. Conversion of mechanical forces into cellular response involves activation of intercellular signals induced by stretched cytoskeletal molecules and piezoelectric potentials. Surface roughness provides the intimate connection to peri-implant bone that initiates functional loads and consequent adaptive remodeling and modeling (Fig 2-5).

Type 4 bone in the posterior maxilla has insufficient volume and density to withstand occlusal force. Normal bite force should not exceed the peri-implant bone microdamage threshold of approximately 3,000 microstrains (a bone subjected to 3,000 microstrains is shortened by 0.3% of its original length). Optimal peri-implant bone modeling occurs at about 1,000 microstrains.[124,125] Loading of implants positively influences the peri-implant bone reaction,[126] with one exception. In type 4 bone quality with insufficient load-bearing capacity, even osseointegrated implants with a rough surface can fail. The aim of sinus grafting, therefore, is to increase bone volume and bone mineral density enough to allow interconnection between the bone and implant. This intimate interconnection distributes functional forces within physiologic parameters. Again, functional strain limits transferred by dental implants to bone are based on adequate osseointegration, which depends on bone remodeling, which in turn requires the presence of vital bone tissue established by graft consolidation.

Loss of autograft bone mass occurs when resorption exceeds formation during the consolidation phase. Such a situation increases the risk of implant loss because the compromised bone graft fatigues to failure. To overcome excessive, at times even complete, resorption of autograft and to reduce the volume of bone that must be harvested, bone substitutes that are chosen for their capacity to resorb slowly are added to the graft. Animal models show that the use of a bone substitute such as bovine bone mineral, either alone or in combination with autograft, preserves the vertical height of the augmented sinus over time. In this indication, slowly resorbing bone substitutes serve a space-maintaining function during consolidation. Host bone, which invests the bone substitutes, retains its capacity to respond to mechanical forces via adaptive re-

rates similar to those of healthy patients.[119,120] Studies are needed to determine whether diabetes is a risk factor for implant survival in augmented areas. Smoking is a risk factor for implant survival, generally including those placed in the augmented sinus.[121–123] More clinical studies are required to identify patients who are at potential risk of impaired graft consolidation in the augmented sinus.

Graft Consolidation and Implant Loading

Implants with rough surfaces perform better than implants with smooth surfaces under functional loading over the long term.[5] Rough-surfaced implants support the attachment of the developing blood clot after placement. The provisional extracellular matrix of the blood clot allows osteogenic cells to migrate to the implant surface, where they can lay down new bone to supplement the bone that

TABLE 2-1 Graft consolidation factors (GCFs) and their theoretical effects on healing times

Systemic diseases and treatment	Osteoporosis (×1.3)	Diabetes (×1.2)	Chemotherapy (×1.3)
Age	< 20 y (×0.8)	21–60 y (×1.0)	> 61 y (×1.2)
Residual bone height	< 6 mm (×1.2)	6–8 mm (×1.0)	> 8 mm (×0.8)
Augmentation material	Autograft (×1.0)	Bone substitute (×1.4)	Autograft + bone substitute (×1.2)
Rupture of sinus mucosa	Yes (×1.1)	No (×1.0)	
Material properties	Block (×1.2)	Particulated (×1.0)	
Supplements	BMP (×0.7)	PRP (×0.9)	
Lifestyle factors	Smoking (×1.2)	Alcohol abuse (×1.1)	

modeling and modeling. A greater interconnection between bone and implant is observed in these settings, and consequently the distribution of functional forces within physiologic limits remains achievable despite the addition of a partially nonvital admixture. Meta-analysis of sinus grafting procedures indicates that autografts and bone substitutes make it possible to achieve a similar long-term survival rate for implants under functional loading.[5]

Theoretical Concept for Management of Risk Factors

It is often difficult to consider all patient-related and therapeutic variables before making a decision about the duration of healing for graft consolidation. One theoretical concept is to begin with a standard 4-month graft consolidation period that is then modified by a graft consolidation factor (GCF), which takes into account such variables as health status, aging, disparate properties of graft materials, implant surface properties, and surgical technicalities (Table 2-1). The GCF, which is based on the experience of each surgeon, is then multiplied with the "standard" healing time of 4 months. When this formula is used, graft consolidation in osteoporotic patients would be expected to take 4 months × 1.3 (GCF for osteoporosis) for a total of 5.2 months. If autograft is used in combination with a bone substitute, the graft consolidation phase is prolonged by a factor of 1.2 (GCF for bone substitute), resulting in a 6.2-month healing time. Alternatively, the addition of BMP-2 or BMP-7 to bone substitutes in osteoporotic patients would decrease healing time to 4.4 months. Of course, these calculations are based on a theoretical concept and must be confirmed by evidence-based data. Moreover, augmentation height, not to mention other potential risk factors such as genetic background and mental disease, are not included in the calculation. Possible synergistic and antagonistic effects are also not considered in this simplified model. However, with the use of more sophisticated data, calculation of the approximate time required for graft consolidation is possible, just as calculation of shorter healing times associated with the use of various implant surfaces have been confirmed by clinical and animal studies.

Summary

Clinician surgical experience and a controlled surgical field are undoubtedly important to the success of the sinus augmentation procedure. Because the multistep process of graft consolidation provides the foundation for osseointegration, understanding the biology of bone graft consolidation is of increasing importance, especially if we wish to maximize treatment understanding of osseointegration in the sinus floor graft. Graft consolidation is also a prerequisite for attaining peri-implant bone that has the capacity

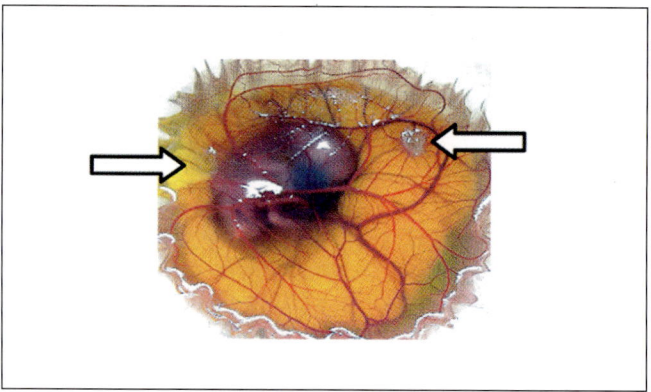

Fig 2-6 Chorioallantoic membrane (CAM) assay. Gelatin sponges were immersed in concentrated supernatants of marrow-derived stromal cells and placed on top of the CAM *(right arrow)*; sponges containing low-serum medium served as controls *(left arrow)*. The figure shows CAM at day 12 after fertilization. Allantoic vessels grew radially toward the sponges soaked with concentrated bone marrow stromal cell supernatant, but not toward the sponges soaked with low-serum medium. These findings suggest that transplanted cells, either within autograft or as a supplement via tissue engineering, can support the growth of blood vessels into augmented areas.

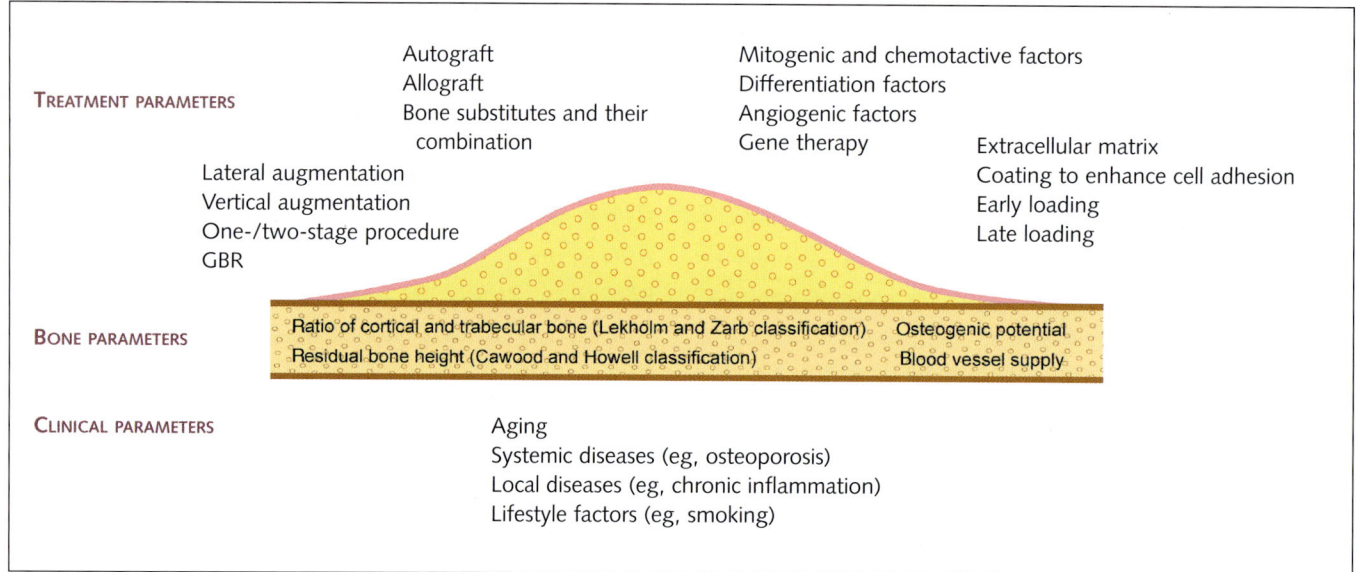

Fig 2-7 Graft consolidation can be divided into three levels. The first level, termed *clinical parameters*, represents patient characteristics such as health or disease status and lifestyle factors, which may impact on level two, the *bone parameters*. Bone parameters include the osteogenic and angiogenic potential as well as the local morphology of host bone. At the third level are *treatment parameters*. Surgeons must make decisions about the type of grafting material to use, whether a one- or two-stage grafting procedure is to be performed, which surgical approach to take, and the possible application of growth and differentiation factors. All three levels of parameters affect graft consolidation and consequently osseointegration in both short-term and long-term function.

for functional adaptation to load, which improves bone mineral density in the latter stages of osseointegration.

Understanding graft consolidation is a challenge because of the complex interplay between host- and graft-derived osteogenic cells. Graft materials, implant properties, local and systemic signaling molecules, and mechanical forces all play a critical role in this process. Moreover, medical status and lifestyle factors influence this interplay and therefore modulate the healing time for graft consolidation. Anamnesis criteria may help us establish a patient's potential risk or compromise to graft consolidation. This area of study may shed light on disparate healing results and provide evidence for an enhanced approach using tissue engineering (Fig 2-6). In this way, the requirements of bone graft consolidation may be *individualized* to overcome a compromised biologic state (Fig 2-7). Future efforts should also focus on developing a sinus-grafting procedure that is minimally invasive and yet still allows for predictable, long-term survival of dental implants in the augmented sinus floor.

Acknowledgment

The authors want to thank Dr Jeffrey O. Hollinger (Bone Tissue Engineering Center, Carnegie Mellon University, Pittsburgh, PA) for his critical reading of the manuscript.

References

1. Cawood JI, Howell RA. A classification of the edentulous jaws. Int J Oral Maxillofac Surg 1988;17:232–236.
2. Cawood JI, Howell RA. Reconstructive preprosthetic surgery. I. Anatomical considerations. Int J Oral Maxillofac Surg 1991;20:75–82.
3. Jensen OT, Shulman LB, Block MS, Iacono VJ. Report of the Sinus Consensus Conference of 1996. Int J Oral Maxillofac Implants 1998;13(suppl):11–45.
4. Graziani F, Donos N, Needleman I, Gabriele M, Tonetti M. Comparison of implant survival following sinus floor augmentation procedures with implants placed in pristine posterior maxillary bone: A systematic review. Clin Oral Implants Res 2004;15:677–682.
5. Wallace SS, Froum SJ. Effect of maxillary sinus augmentation on the survival of endosseous dental implants. A systematic review. Ann Periodontol 2003;8:328–343.
6. Esposito M, Hirsch JM, Lekholm U, Thomsen P. Biological factors contributing to failures of osseointegrated oral implants. (I). Success criteria and epidemiology. Eur J Oral Sci 1998;106:527–551.
7. Brånemark P-I, Hansson BO, Adell R, et al. Osseointegrated implants in the treatment of the edentulous jaw. Experience from a 10-year period. Scand J Plast Reconstr Surg Suppl 1977;16:1–132.
8. Schenk RK, Buser D. Osseointegration: A reality. Periodontol 2000 1998;17:22–35.
9. Berglundh T, Abrahamsson I, Lang NP, Lindhe J. De novo alveolar bone formation adjacent to endosseous implants. Clin Oral Implants Res 2003;14:251–262.
10. Botticelli D, Berglundh T, Buser D, Lindhe J. The jumping distance revisited: An experimental study in the dog. Clin Oral Implants Res 2003;14:35–42.
11. Davies JE. Understanding peri-implant endosseous healing. J Dent Educ 2003;67:932–949.
12. Albrektsson T, Johansson C. Osteoinduction, osteoconduction and osseointegration. Eur Spine J 2001;10(suppl 2):S96–S101.
13. Albrektsson T, Brånemark P-I, Hansson HA, Lindstrom J. Osseointegrated titanium implants. Requirements for ensuring a long-lasting, direct bone-to-implant anchorage in man. Acta Orthop Scand 1981;52:155–170.
14. Friberg B, Jemt T, Lekholm U. Early failures in 4,641 consecutively placed Brånemark dental implants: A study from stage 1 surgery to the connection of completed prostheses. Int J Oral Maxillofac Implants 1991;6:142–146.
15. Lazzara R, Siddiqui AA, Binon P, et al. Retrospective multicenter analysis of 3i endosseous dental implants placed over a five-year period. Clin Oral Implants Res 1996;7:73–83.
16. Lekholm U, Zarb GA. Patient selection and preparation. In: Brånemark P-I, Zarb GA, Albrektsson T (eds). Tissue-Integrated Prostheses: Osseointegration in Clinical Dentistry 1985:199–209.
17. Ulm CW, Solar P, Gsellmann B, Matejka M, Watzek G. The edentulous maxillary alveolar process in the region of the maxillary sinus—A study of physical dimension. Int J Oral Maxillofac Surg 1995;24(4):279–282.
18. Martinez H, Davarpanah M, Missika P, Celletti R, Lazzara R. Optimal implant stabilization in low density bone. Clin Oral Implants Res 2001;12:423–432.
19. Schenk RK, Hunziker EB. Histologic and ultrastructural features of fracture healing. In: Brighton CT, Friedlaender G, Lane JM (eds). Bone Regeneration and Repair. Rosemont, IL: American Academy of Orthopedic Surgeons, 1994:117–146.
20. Manolagas SC. Birth and death of bone cells: Basic regulatory mechanisms and implications for the pathogenesis and treatment of osteoporosis. Endocr Rev 2000;21:115–137.
21. Chanavaz M. Anatomy and histophysiology of the periosteum: Quantification of the periosteal blood supply to the adjacent bone with 85Sr and gamma spectrometry. J Oral Implantol 1995;21:214–219.
22. Proussaefs P, Lozada J, Kim J, Rohrer MD. Repair of the perforated sinus membrane with a resorbable collagen membrane: A human study. Int J Oral Maxillofac Implants 2004;19:413–420.
23. Kandler B, Fischer MB, Watzek G, Gruber R. Platelet-released supernatant increases matrix metalloproteinase-2 production, migration, proliferation, and tube formation of human umbilical vascular endothelial cells. J Periodontol 2004;75:1255–1261.
24. Sunderkotter C, Steinbrink K, Goebeler M, Bhardwaj R, Sorg C. Macrophages and angiogenesis. J Leukoc Biol 1994;55:410–422.
25. Gruber R, Kandler B, Watzek G. Hypoxia does not impair BMSC survival—No effect on angiogenic potential—in vitro. Dent J 2005:(in press).
26. Knighton DR, Hunt TK, Scheuenstuhl H, Halliday BJ, Werb Z, Banda MJ. Oxygen tension regulates the expression of angiogenesis factor by macrophages. Science 1983;221(4617):1283–1285.
27. Steinbrech DS, Mehrara BJ, Saadeh PB, et al. VEGF expression in an osteoblast-like cell line is regulated by a hypoxia response mechanism. Am J Physiol Cell Physiol 2000;278:C853–C860.
28. Sahni A, Francis CW. Vascular endothelial growth factor binds to fibrinogen and fibrin and stimulates endothelial cell proliferation. Blood 2000;96:3772–3778.
29. Kandler B, Watzek G, Gruber R. Endothelial cell–Conditioned medium stimulates migration of osteogenic cells. Dent J 2005:(in press).
30. Singer AJ, Clark RA. Cutaneous wound healing. N Engl J Med 1999;341:738–746.
31. Gruber R, Karreth F, Kandler B, et al. Platelet-released supernatants increase migration and proliferation, and decrease osteogenic differentiation of bone marrow–derived mesenchymal progenitor cells under in vitro conditions. Platelets 2004;15:29–35.

32. Fiedler J, Roderer G, Gunther KP, Brenner RE. BMP-2, BMP-4, and PDGF-bb stimulate chemotactic migration of primary human mesenchymal progenitor cells. J Cell Biochem 2002;87:305–312.
33. Hsieh SC, Graves DT. Pulse application of platelet-derived growth factor enhances formation of a mineralizing matrix while continuous application is inhibitory. J Cell Biochem 1998;69:169–180.
34. Cao R, Brakenhielm E, Pawliuk R, et al. Angiogenic synergism, vascular stability and improvement of hind-limb ischemia by a combination of PDGF-BB and FGF-2. Nat Med 2003;9:604–613.
35. Richardson TP, Peters MC, Ennett AB, Mooney DJ. Polymeric system for dual growth factor delivery. Nat Biotechnol 2001;19:1029–1034.
36. English D, Welch Z, Kovala AT, et al. Sphingosine 1-phosphate released from platelets during clotting accounts for the potent endothelial cell chemotactic activity of blood serum and provides a novel link between hemostasis and angiogenesis. FASEB J 2000;14:2255–2265.
37. Carmeliet P. Mechanisms of angiogenesis and arteriogenesis. Nat Med 2000;6:389–395.
38. Risau W. Mechanisms of angiogenesis. Nature 1997;386(6626):671–674.
39. Asahara T, Kawamoto A. Endothelial progenitor cells for postnatal vasculogenesis. Am J Physiol Cell Physiol 2004;287:C572–C579.
40. Cardaropoli G, Araujo M, Lindhe J. Dynamics of bone tissue formation in tooth extraction sites. An experimental study in dogs. J Clin Periodontol 2003;30:809–818.
41. Barnes GL, Kostenuik PJ, Gerstenfeld LC, Einhorn TA. Growth factor regulation of fracture repair. J Bone Miner Res 1999;14:1805–1815.
42. Hu H, Hilton MJ, Tu X, Yu K, Ornitz DM, Long F. Sequential roles of Hedgehog and Wnt signaling in osteoblast development. Development 2005;132:49–60.
43. Westendorf JJ, Kahler RA, Schroeder TM. Wnt signaling in osteoblasts and bone diseases. Gene 2004;341:19–39.
44. Harada S, Rodan GA. Control of osteoblast function and regulation of bone mass. Nature 2003;423(6937):349–355.
45. Haas R, Donath K, Fodinger M, Watzek G. Bovine hydroxyapatite for maxillary sinus grafting: Comparative histomorphometric findings in sheep. Clin Oral Implants Res 1998;9:107–116.
46. Taichman RS. Blood and bone: Two tissues whose fates are intertwined to create the hematopoietic stem-cell niche. Blood 2005;105:2631–2639.
47. Eghbali-Fatourechi GZ, Lamsam J, Fraser D, Nagel D, Riggs BL, Khosla S. Circulating osteoblast-lineage cells in humans. N Engl J Med 2005;12:352:1959–1966.
48. Pittenger MF, Mackay AM, Beck SC, et al. Multilineage potential of adult human mesenchymal stem cells. Science 1999;284(5411):143–147.
49. Doherty MJ, Ashton BA, Walsh S, Beresford JN, Grant ME, Canfield AE. Vascular pericytes express osteogenic potential in vitro and in vivo. J Bone Miner Res 1998;13:828–838.
50. Gruber R, Baron M, Busenlechner D, Kandler B, Fuerst G, Watzek G. Proliferation and osteogenic differentiation of cells from cortical bone cylinders, bone particles from mill, and drilling dust. J Oral Maxillofac Surg 2005;63:238–243.
51. Springer IN, Terheyden H, Geiss S, Harle F, Hedderich J, Acil Y. Particulated bone grafts—Effectiveness of bone cell supply. Clin Oral Implants Res 2004;15:205–212.
52. Oprea WE, Karp JM, Hosseini MM, Davies JE. Effect of platelet releasate on bone cell migration and recruitment in vitro. J Craniofac Surg 2003;14:292–300.
53. Hubner G, Brauchle M, Smola H, Madlener M, Fassler R, Werner S. Differential regulation of pro-inflammatory cytokines during wound healing in normal and glucocorticoid-treated mice. Cytokine 1996;8:548–556.
54. Browder T, Folkman J, Pirie-Shepherd S. The hemostatic system as a regulator of angiogenesis. J Biol Chem 2000;275:1521–1524.
55. Paralkar VM, Nandedkar AK, Pointer RH, Kleinman HK, Reddi AH. Interaction of osteogenin, a heparin–binding bone morphogenetic protein, with type IV collagen. J Biol Chem 1990;265:17281–17284.
56. Gruber R, Kandler B, Fuerst G, Fischer MB, Watzek G. Porcine sinus mucosa holds cells that respond to bone morphogenetic protein (BMP)-6 and BMP-7 with increased osteogenic differentiation in vitro. Clin Oral Implants Res 2004;15:575–580.
57. Abe E, Yamamoto M, Taguchi Y, et al. Essential requirement of BMPs-2/4 for both osteoblast and osteoclast formation in murine bone marrow cultures from adult mice: Antagonism by noggin. J Bone Miner Res 2000;15:663–673.
58. Martin TJ, Sims NA. Osteoclast-derived activity in the coupling of bone formation to resorption. Trends Mol Med 2005;11:76–81.
59. Teitelbaum SL. Bone resorption by osteoclasts. Science 2000;289(5484):1504–1508.
60. Suda T, Takahashi N, Udagawa N, Jimi E, Gillespie MT, Martin TJ. Modulation of osteoclast differentiation and function by the new members of the tumor necrosis factor receptor and ligand families. Endocr Rev 1999;20:345–357.
61. Eghbali-Fatourechi G, Khosla S, Sanyal A, Boyle WJ, Lacey DL, Riggs BL. Role of RANK ligand in mediating increased bone resorption in early postmenopausal women. J Clin Invest 2003;111:1221–1230.
62. Teitelbaum SL, Ross FP. Genetic regulation of osteoclast development and function. Nat Rev Genet 2003;4:638–649.
63. Rho J, Takami M, Choi Y. Osteoimmunology: Interactions of the immune and skeletal systems. Mol Cells 2004;17:1–9.
64. Udagawa N, Kotake S, Kamatani N, Takahashi N, Suda T. The molecular mechanism of osteoclastogenesis in rheumatoid arthritis. Arthritis Res 2002;4:281–289.
65. Ito H, Koefoed M, Tiyapatanaputi P, et al. Remodeling of cortical bone allografts mediated by adherent rAAV-RANKL and VEGF gene therapy. Nat Med 2005;11:291–297.
66. Kon T, Cho TJ, Aizawa T, et al. Expression of osteoprotegerin, receptor activator of NF-kappaB ligand (osteoprotegerin ligand) and related proinflammatory cytokines during fracture healing. J Bone Miner Res 2001;16:1004–1014.

67. Trisi P, Rebaudi A. Progressive bone adaptation of titanium implants during and after orthodontic load in humans. Int J Periodontics Restorative Dent 2002;22:31–43.
68. Xu H, Shimizu Y, Asai S, Ooya K. Grafting of deproteinized bone particles inhibits bone resorption after maxillary sinus floor elevation. Clin Oral Implants Res 2004;15:126–133.
69. Tadjoedin ES, de Lange GL, Bronckers AL, Lyaruu DM, Burger EH. Deproteinized cancellous bovine bone (Bio-Oss) as bone substitute for sinus floor elevation. A retrospective, histomorphometrical study of five cases. J Clin Periodontol 2003;30:261–270.
70. Bucholz RW. Nonallograft osteoconductive bone graft substitutes. Clin Orthop 2002;395:44–52.
71. Bauer TW, Muschler GF. Bone graft materials. An overview of the basic science. Clin Orthop 2000;371:10–27.
72. McFarland CD, Mayer S, Scotchford C, Dalton BA, Steele JG, Downes S. Attachment of cultured human bone cells to novel polymers. J Biomed Mater Res 1999;44:1–11.
73. Kilpadi KL, Chang PL, Bellis SL. Hydroxylapatite binds more serum proteins, purified integrins, and osteoblast precursor cells than titanium or steel. J Biomed Mater Res 2001;57:258–267.
74. Kilpadi KL, Sawyer AA, Prince CW, Chang PL, Bellis SL. Primary human marrow stromal cells and Saos-2 osteosarcoma cells use different mechanisms to adhere to hydroxylapatite. J Biomed Mater Res A 2004;68:273–285.
75. Clark RA, Lin F, Greiling D, An J, Couchman JR. Fibroblast invasive migration into fibronectin/fibrin gels requires a previously uncharacterized dermatan sulfate-CD44 proteoglycan. J Invest Dermatol 2004;122:266–277.
76. Degidi M, Piattelli M, Scarano A, Iezzi G, Piattelli A. Maxillary sinus augmentation with a synthetic cell-binding peptide: Histological and histomorphometrical results in humans. J Oral Implantol 2004;30:376–383.
77. Meyer U, Joos U, Wiesmann HP. Biological and biophysical principles in extracorporal bone tissue engineering. Part I. Int J Oral Maxillofac Surg 2004;33:325–332.
78. Wiesmann HP, Joos U, Meyer U. Biological and biophysical principles in extracorporal bone tissue engineering. Part II. Int J Oral Maxillofac Surg 2004;33:523–530.
79. Meyer U, Joos U, Wiesmann HP. Biological and biophysical principles in extracorporal bone tissue engineering. Part III. Int J Oral Maxillofac Surg 2004;33:635–641.
80. Jadlowiec JA, Celil AB, Hollinger JO. Bone tissue engineering: Recent advances and promising therapeutic agents. Expert Opin Biol Ther 2003;3:409–423.
81. Hammerle CH, Jung RE. Bone augmentation by means of barrier membranes. Periodontol 2000 2003;33:36–53.
82. Cummings SR, Melton LJ. Epidemiology and outcomes of osteoporotic fractures. Lancet 2002;359(9319):1761–1767.
83. Clark S. Osteoporosis—The disease of the 21st century? Lancet 2002;359(9319):1714.
84. Melton LJ III. Who has osteoporosis? A conflict between clinical and public health perspectives. J Bone Miner Res 2000;15:2309–2314.
85. Riggs BL, Melton LJ III. Involutional osteoporosis. N Engl J Med 1986;314:1676–1686.
86. Blomqvist JE, Alberius P, Isaksson S, Linde A, Obrant K. Importance of bone graft quality for implant integration after maxillary sinus reconstruction. Oral Surg Oral Med Oral Pathol Oral Radiol Endod 1998;86:268–274.
87. Newton BI, Cooper RC, Gilbert JA, Johnson RB, Zardiackas LD. The ovariectomized sheep as a model for human bone loss. J Comp Pathol 2004;130:323–326.
88. Leung KS, Siu WS, Cheung NM, et al. Goats as an osteopenic animal model. J Bone Miner Res 2001;16:2348–2355.
89. Frenkel SR, Jaffe WL, Valle CD, et al. The effect of alendronate (Fosamax) and implant surface on bone integration and remodeling in a canine model. J Biomed Mater Res 2001;58:645–650.
90. Delmas PD. Treatment of postmenopausal osteoporosis. Lancet 2002;359(9322):2018–2026.
91. Roschger P, Rinnerthaler S, Yates J, Rodan GA, Fratzl P, Klaushofer K. Alendronate increases degree and uniformity of mineralization in cancellous bone and decreases the porosity in cortical bone of osteoporotic women. Bone 2001;29:185–191.
92. D'Ippolito G, Schiller PC, Ricordi C, Roos BA, Howard GA. Age-related osteogenic potential of mesenchymal stromal stem cells from human vertebral bone marrow. J Bone Miner Res 1999;14:1115–1122.
93. O'Driscoll SW, Saris DB, Ito Y, Fitzimmons JS. The chondrogenic potential of periosteum decreases with age. J Orthop Res 2001;19:95–103.
94. Bellows CG, Pei W, Jia Y, Heersche JN. Proliferation, differentiation and self-renewal of osteoprogenitors in vertebral cell populations from aged and young female rats. Mech Ageing Dev 2003;124:747–757.
95. Pfeilschifter J, Diel I, Pilz U, Brunotte K, Naumann A, Ziegler R. Mitogenic responsiveness of human bone cells in vitro to hormones and growth factors decreases with age. J Bone Miner Res 1993;8:707–717.
96. Inoue K, Ohgushi H, Yoshikawa T, et al. The effect of aging on bone formation in porous hydroxyapatite: Biochemical and histological analysis. J Bone Miner Res 1997;12:989–994.
97. Shimada T, Takeshita Y, Murohara T, et al. Angiogenesis and vasculogenesis are impaired in the precocious-aging klotho mouse. Circulation 2004;110:1148–1155.
98. Rivard A, Fabre JE, Silver M, Chen D, et al. Age-dependent impairment of angiogenesis. Circulation 1999;99:111–120.
99. Gruber R, Kandler B, Fischer MB, Watzek G. Bone morphogenetic protein–induced osteogenic differentiation in vitro can be suppressed by platelet-released supernatants. Clin Oral Implants Res (in revision) 2005.
100. Gruber R, Karreth F, Fischer MB, Watzek G. Platelet-released supernatants stimulate formation of osteoclast-like cells through a prostaglandin/RANKL-dependent mechanism. Bone 2002;30:726–732.
101. Jakse N, Tangl S, Gilli R, et al. Influence of PRP on autogenous sinus grafts. An experimental study on sheep. Clin Oral Implants Res 2003;14:578–583.
102. Fuerst G, Gruber R, Tangl S, et al. Sinus grafting with autogenous platelet-rich plasma and bovine hydroxyapatite. A histomorphometric study in minipigs. Clin Oral Implants Res 2003;14:500–508.

103. Wiltfang J, Schlegel KA, Schultze-Mosgau S, Nkenke E, Zimmermann R, Kessler P. Sinus floor augmentation with beta-tricalciumphosphate (beta-TCP): Does platelet-rich plasma promote its osseous integration and degradation? Clin Oral Implants Res 2003;14:213–218.
104. Perry BH, Sampson AR, Schwab BH, Karim MR, Smiell JM. A meta-analytic approach to an integrated summary of efficacy: A case study of becaplermin gel. Control Clin Trials 2002;23:389–408.
105. Nevins M, Camelo M, Nevins ML, Schenk RK, Lynch SE. Periodontal regeneration in humans using recombinant human platelet-derived growth factor-BB (rhPDGF-BB) and allogeneic bone. J Periodontol 2003;74:1282–1292.
106. Boyne PJ, Marx RE, Nevins M, et al. A feasibility study evaluating rhBMP-2/absorbable collagen sponge for maxillary sinus floor augmentation. Int J Periodontics Restorative Dent 1997;17:11–25.
107. van den Bergh JP, ten Bruggenkate CM, Groeneveld HH, Burger EH, Tuinzing DB. Recombinant human bone morphogenetic protein-7 in maxillary sinus floor elevation surgery in 3 patients compared to autogenous bone grafts. A clinical pilot study. J Clin Periodontol 2000;27:627–636.
108. Terheyden H, Jepsen S, Moller B, Tucker MM, Rueger DC. Sinus floor augmentation with simultaneous placement of dental implants using a combination of deproteinized bone xenografts and recombinant human osteogenic protein-1. A histometric study in miniature pigs. Clin Oral Implants Res 1999;10:510–521.
109. Jovanovic SA, Hunt DR, Bernard GW, et al. Long-term functional loading of dental implants in rhBMP-2 induced bone. A histologic study in the canine ridge augmentation model. Clin Oral Implants Res 2003;14:793–803.
110. Cancedda R, Dozin B, Giannoni P, Quarto R. Tissue engineering and cell therapy of cartilage and bone. Matrix Biol 2003;22:81–91.
111. Caplan AI, Bruder SP. Mesenchymal stem cells: Building blocks for molecular medicine in the 21st century. Trends Mol Med 2001;7:259–264.
112. Schmelzeisen R, Schimming R, Sittinger M. Making bone: Implant insertion into tissue-engineered bone for maxillary sinus floor augmentation—A preliminary report. J Craniomaxillofac Surg 2003;31:34–39.
113. Fuerst G, Tangl S, Gruber R, Gahleitner A, Sanroman F, Watzek G. Bone formation following sinus grafting with autogenous bone–derived cells and bovine bone mineral in minipigs: Preliminary findings. Clin Oral Implants Res 2004;15:733–740.
114. Dai J, Rabie AB, Hagg U, Xu R. Alternative gene therapy strategies for the repair of craniofacial bone defects. Curr Gene Ther 2004;4:469–485.
115. Park J, Ries J, Gelse K, Kloss F, von der Mark K, Wiltfang J, et al. Bone regeneration in critical size defects by cell-mediated BMP-2 gene transfer: A comparison of adenoviral vectors and liposomes. Gene Ther 2003;10:1089–1098.
116. Lieberman JR, Daluiski A, Stevenson S, et al. The effect of regional gene therapy with bone morphogenetic protein-2–producing bone-marrow cells on the repair of segmental femoral defects in rats. J Bone Joint Surg Am 1999;81:905–917.
117. Nevins ML, Karimbux NY, Weber HP, Giannobile WV, Fiorellini JP. Wound healing around endosseous implants in experimental diabetes. Int J Oral Maxillofac Implants 1998;13:620–629.
118. Siqueira JT, Cavalher-Machado SC, Arana-Chavez VE, Sannomiya P. Bone formation around titanium implants in the rat tibia: Role of insulin. Implant Dent 2003;12:242–251.
119. Farzad P, Andersson L, Nyberg J. Dental implant treatment in diabetic patients. Implant Dent 2002;11:262–267.
120. Abdulwassie H, Dhanrajani PJ. Diabetes mellitus and dental implants: A clinical study. Implant Dent 2002;11:83–86.
121. Woo VV, Chuang SK, Daher S, Muftu A, Dodson TB. Dentoalveolar reconstructive procedures as a risk factor for implant failure. J Oral Maxillofac Surg 2004;62:773–780.
122. Kan JY, Rungcharassaeng K, Lozada JL, Goodacre CJ. Effects of smoking on implant success in grafted maxillary sinuses. J Prosthet Dent 1999;82:307–311.
123. Widmark G, Andersson B, Carlsson GE, Lindvall AM, Ivanoff CJ. Rehabilitation of patients with severely resorbed maxillae by means of implants with or without bone grafts: A 3- to 5-year follow-up clinical report. Int J Oral Maxillofac Implants 2001;16:73–79.
124. Frost HM. Wolff's Law and bone's structural adaptations to mechanical usage: An overview for clinicians. Angle Orthod 1994;64(3):175–188.
125. Frost HM. A 2003 update of bone physiology and Wolff's Law for clinicians. Angle Orthod 2004;74:3–15.
126. Gotfredsen K, Berglundh T, Lindhe J. Bone reactions adjacent to titanium implants with different surface characteristics subjected to static load. A study in the dog (II). Clin Oral Implants Res 2001;12:196–201.

chapter 3
Vital Biomechanics of Bone and Bone Grafts

Harold M. Frost, MD, DSc
Ole T. Jensen, DDS, MS

A bone graft can become a mechanically functioning part of host bone if the surrounding hard and soft tissue host bed is viable and has a good blood supply. Grafts to nonvital host bone do not succeed. In the weeks after grafting, new vessels, interstitial cells, and osteoblasts produce woven bone in which to embed the graft, creating a graft–woven bone complex.[1,2] Cement lines "weld" woven bone to the graft and host bone to achieve biologic as well as mechanical continuity. Autogenous cancellous bone remains the best material available to achieve integration of the graft–woven bone complex and the host bed.

Bone Graft Healing

Incorporation

The process of graft incorporation, which varies in duration depending on the graft material used, consists of cellular proliferation, migration, differentiation, gene expression, adhesion, and apoptosis. For autograft, this phase generally lasts 4 months, for allograft 7 or 8 months, and for alloplast 1 year or longer. The end goal of this nonmechanical process is to make functionally adaptable bone.[3,4]

Replacement

Even before incorporation is finished, *basic multicellular unit* (BMU) *remodeling* begins to replace the graft–woven bone complex with lamellar bone. Remodeling slowly removes incorporated graft that does not experience mechanical strain; however, the graft–woven bone complex that is subjected to a suitable degree of mechanical strain is replaced with load-bearing bone. When bone graft is not strained, as in the case of sinus floor autografts that never receive dental implants, it is resorbed.

Modeling

Bone strain activates modeling to reshape the graft–woven bone complex internally and externally. It aligns the grain of any new lamellar bone to satisfy the local mechanical needs; and it aligns, shapes, and strengthens the complex's trabeculae and cortex to satisfy those needs.[5] Cement lines weld new lamellae to graft material and host bone. Completion of this process takes 1 year or longer, depending on host variables.

Regional acceleratory phenomenon

Osseous surgical trauma accelerates all regional tissue processes within the host bed.[6-8] This *regional accelerator phenomenon* (RAP) begins on the day of surgery and lasts for more than 2 years. The RAP accelerates all phases of bone graft healing. Failed RAPs occur in chronic diseases such as Type I diabetes or hepatic cirrhosis. They reduce healing and resistance to infection, often resulting in a biologic failure of bone healing known as *atrophic nonunion*.[6,9-11] Nonsteroidal anti-inflammatory drugs (NSAIDs) can depress an RAP and retard the graft's replacement and modeling phases.[12,13]

When successful, these four phases of graft healing create a host bone–graft bone complex that functions mechanically for life.

Emergence of Vital Biomechanics

In early views, the success of bone grafts was thought to depend not on mechanical factors but on osteoblasts and the factors that affect them, including:

- Estrogen
- Growth hormone
- Somatomedins
- Parathyroid hormone
- Vitamin D
- Other vitamins
- Growth factors
- Mitogens
- Membrane receptors
- Other cytokines
- Autocrine effects
- Amino acids
- Gene expression
- Androgens
- Calcitonin
- Insulin
- Thyroxine
- D metabolites
- Dietary calcium
- Morphogens
- Membrane pumps
- Apoptosis
- Paracrine effects
- Cell-cell interactions
- Lipids
- Drugs/other artificial agents

What we now know is that osteoblasts and osteoclasts, though necessary for bone growth and repair, *do not control* these processes. Nonmechanical factors are clearly essential,[14] but equally essential are vital biomechanics. In fact, the nonmechanical and vital biomechanical facets of skeletal physiology are interdependent[8,15,16]; their relationship reveals the indissoluble mutual dependence of cell and molecular biology on tissue- and organ-level physiology.[17–20]

Physical Determinants of Bone Strength

The strength of bone grafts and of the host bone–graft bone complex depends on numerous factors.

Mass and architecture

Stiffness, ultimate strength, and yield point determine the strength of bone.[8] Lamellar bone surpasses woven bone in these respects. These material properties are primarily genetically determined and vary little by age, sex, species, or (for the most part) disease state. Another important factor is bone mass. The more bone, and the more lamellar bone in proportion to woven bone, the stronger the graft. The shape and size of a mature graft as well as the distribution of its cortical and trabecular components affect its strength. Making a bone graft stronger usually requires improved architecture and a greater quantity of bone instead of better material properties.

Microdamage

Microscopic fatigue damage, or *microdamage*, weakens bone without affecting its architecture or mass.[21–23] Visible as cracks and delamination under the light microscope, ultramicroscopic microdamage can cause stress and spontaneous fractures of trabeculae and loosening of load-bearing implants. Under parallel-grain loads that cause about 2,000 microstrain, normal lamellar bone endures about 10 million loading cycles before it breaks; under loads that cause 4,000 microstrain, however, normal lamellar bone can break in fewer than 20,000 loading cycles. As loads and strains double, microdamage increases more than 400 times.[24]

Remodeling repair by BMUs normally keeps up with microdamage caused by strains below about 2,000 microstrain. Larger strains cause damage too great to repair, so microdamage accumulates to cause fatigue fractures.[22] Hence, the range of 2,000 to 4,000 microstrain defines an operational *microdamage threshold* range (MESp), which centers near 3,000 microstrain. For purposes of comparison, normal bone can be expected to fracture at about 25,000 microstrain.

In the early phase of a sinus graft restoration with implants, the host bone–graft bone complex exhibits reduced stiffness. Thereafter, biting forces cause strains in the bone-supporting implants to reach the microdamage threshold. The reduced stiffness of the complex stems from the excessive remodeling space and the high rate of bone turnover from the postoperative RAP; these, in turn, are the results of the incomplete replacement of the graft complex by stiffer lamellar bone, the incomplete modeling of the graft, and the reduced quantity of host bone caused by the demineralization RAP.

Implants provide adequate surface touching bone so that *total loads* transferred from implant to bone maintain *unit loads* on the bone below its microdamage threshold.[6,25] Where too little host bone exists to satisfy this criterion, increased bone stock is needed from grafts.

Fig 3-1 Bone modeling by drifts. (A) Infant's long bone with its original size and shape in solid lines. To keep this shape as it grows in length and diameter, its surfaces must move in tissue space as the dashed lines suggest. *Formation drifts* make and control new osteoblasts to build some surfaces up (as shown in Fig 3-4). Separate and independent *resorption drifts* make and control new osteoclasts to remove material from other surfaces. (B) A different drift pattern can correct the fracture malunion *(solid line)* in a child. The cross-sectional view to the right shows the cortical-endosteal and the periosteal drifts that do that. (C) The drifts in (B) move the whole segment to the right (R = resorption; F = formation). Large forces from voluntary activities, such as in weight lifting, make modeling strengthen bone far better than do smaller voluntary forces, no matter how frequent, as in marathon running. Drifts can also thicken and strengthen trabeculae. They are created anew when and where they are needed, and they include capillaries, precursor and "supporting" cells, and some wandering cells. They are multicellular entities in the same sense as renal nephrons and hepatic lobules. The old idea that osteoblasts alone can add to and strengthen bone is no longer tenable; modeling drifts do it instead. (From Frost HM. Strain and other mechanical influences on bone strength and maintenance. Curr Opin Orthop 1997;8:60–70. Reprinted with permission.)

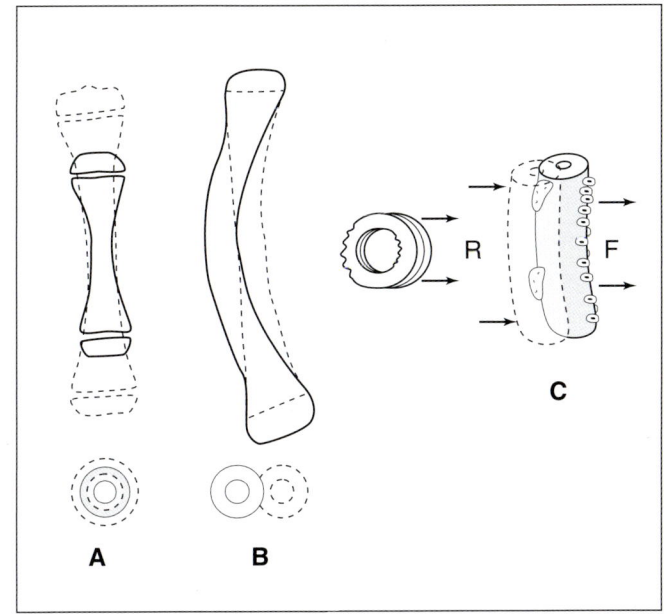

Bone cannot predict future load, so its biologic mechanism is to adjust strength to fit previous and ongoing loads (strain-rate history).

Vital Biomechanical Determinants of Bone Strength

Bone modeling by drifts

Macromodeling

Macromodeling is the chief mechanism by which bone strength and mass are increased (Fig 3-1).[6,15,26] Bone formation and resorption drifts use osteoblasts and osteoclasts, respectively, to move bone surfaces within tissue space to define bone shape, cross-sectional area, and strength. Whole bone macromodeling (henceforth called *modeling*) is operative during growth but also pertains to adult bone. It is a slow process[27] that is averaged over the whole bone.

When bone strains near 1,000 microstrain, the *modeling threshold* range (MESm) is exceeded and modeling is turned on in order to strengthen bone and reduce later strains.[28–30] When bone strains remain below the modeling threshold, mechanically controlled modeling turns off. An MESm below the microdamage threshold maintains bone strains comfortably below the microdamage threshold. Macromodeling thus determines where, when, and how much bone is added to meet mechanical needs. Strains near and above the microdamage threshold stimulate woven bone formation drifts.[30–32]

Macromodeling strengthens implant-loaded bone grafts to keep bone strain from exceeding MESm and hence from exceeding MESp.

Micromodeling

Micromodeling is cellular-level activity that determines what *kind* of bone—that is, woven or lamellar—is formed in a given place.[33] Micromodeling would be analogous to the person who determines whether a home should be made of bricks or of stone; macromodeling is the use of that material to construct arches, posts, and walls. Normally, micromodeling also orients the "grain" of lamellar bone in parallel alignment with the strain of the bone on which it is formed; this allows the grain to be oriented so as to withstand the load to which it was subjected while bone was forming.[34] Woven bone can form even in places where no bone previously existed, whereas lamellar bone can form only on pre-existing bone (either woven or lamellar). Strain of dead bone has no known effect on modeling except as it affects live bone that is attached to dead bone. The sinus bone graft complex begins as an admixture of living and dead bone.

Remodeling by basic multicellular units

Whole bone graft remodeling by BMUs (rather than by osteoclasts alone) is the chief mechanism by which bone strength and mass are reduced. It rarely increases them. BMUs also repair microdamage (Fig 3-2). In the activation → resorption → formation sequence, a BMU replaces a small "packet" of old bone (either woven or lamellar) with new lamellar bone over a period of 3 months or longer. This slow process continues over the course of a lifetime, continually creating new BMUs to replace those that have been completed, so these creations control bone turnover by remodeling. BMUs revitalize bone and turn admixture bone grafts into vital bone.

Remodeling works by one of two modes. A *remodeling threshold* strain range (MESr), about 50 to 100 microstrain, controls the switch between them. Where strains stay below this threshold, remodeling BMUs make less bone than they resorb. This *disuse mode* removes bone, reduces bone strength and mass, and increases the remodeling space. Edentulous jaw bone, for example, becomes atrophic via the disuse mode of remodeling. Where strains exceed the remodeling threshold strain range, resorption and formation by BMUs tend to be equal. This *conservation mode* maintains bone strength and mass and prevents osteopenia and progressive bone loss.[29]

BMUs repair microdamage in living bone,[21,35] but in dead bone microdamage accumulates undetected and unrepaired. Because remodeling BMUs replace the original graft with lamellar bone,[9,10] agents that depress BMU creations (such as bisphosphonates) could impair this process (see chapter 8). These agents could potentially interrupt repair of microdamage associated with load-bearing implants or lead to fatigue failure of a bone graft.[7,36,37] Strains of dead bone have no known effect on remodeling.

Disuse bone remodeling

When teeth are lost, the disuse mode of remodeling[6,15,30] turns on, causing increased bone loss, osteopenia, and a reduction in the stiffness of the bone. If, after osteopenia develops, the bone still carries some load, the conservation mode of remodeling takes over to minimize further bone loss. Even without teeth, the remaining jaw bone continues to bear a certain amount of functional load. Because rather small strains turn conservation mode on, small bite forces strain the bone-graft complex to minimize bone loss during the replacement phase of graft remodeling. For more than two centuries, physicians knew that too much strain (motion between the fracture fragments) impairs bone healing. Only recently did it become apparent that small strains not only improve healing but may indeed be essential to it.[38–41]

Small strains refer to those in the 50 to 1,000 microstrain range. However, even loads that are less than 1% of the size of normal peak biting forces cause strain favorable to healing. In the months immediately following simultaneous implant placement and bone grafting, regularly applied *small* bite forces probably improve both graft replacement and modeling phases. Excess force, however, is harmful. Although we do not yet know how to apply optimal forces to grafted bone, the concept is sound.

In bone grafts, remodeling replaces woven bone with lamellar bone and conserves bone where strains exceed the remodeling threshold; otherwise, mechanically unneeded bone will be removed. The undefinable concept of progressive loading of dental implants placed in grafted bone is derived from these principles (see chapter 7).

Mechanical "overload"

Because they lack a periodontal ligament, dental implants overload bone whereas teeth do not. Implants upshift strains beyond the remodeling threshold to turn modeling on, thus thickening trabeculae and producing compact bone. In a steady-state conservation mode, remodeling preserves this added bone, as demonstrated by observations of increased bone density around implants. Bone strength improves as much as needed to fit the increased loads. Anabolic modeling then turns off, and bone strength and bone mass plateau at higher levels for conservation-mode remodeling.[42,43] Modeling's responses to mechanical usage by dental implants strengthens bone grafts to accomodate the loads placed on them; without this, the graft fails.

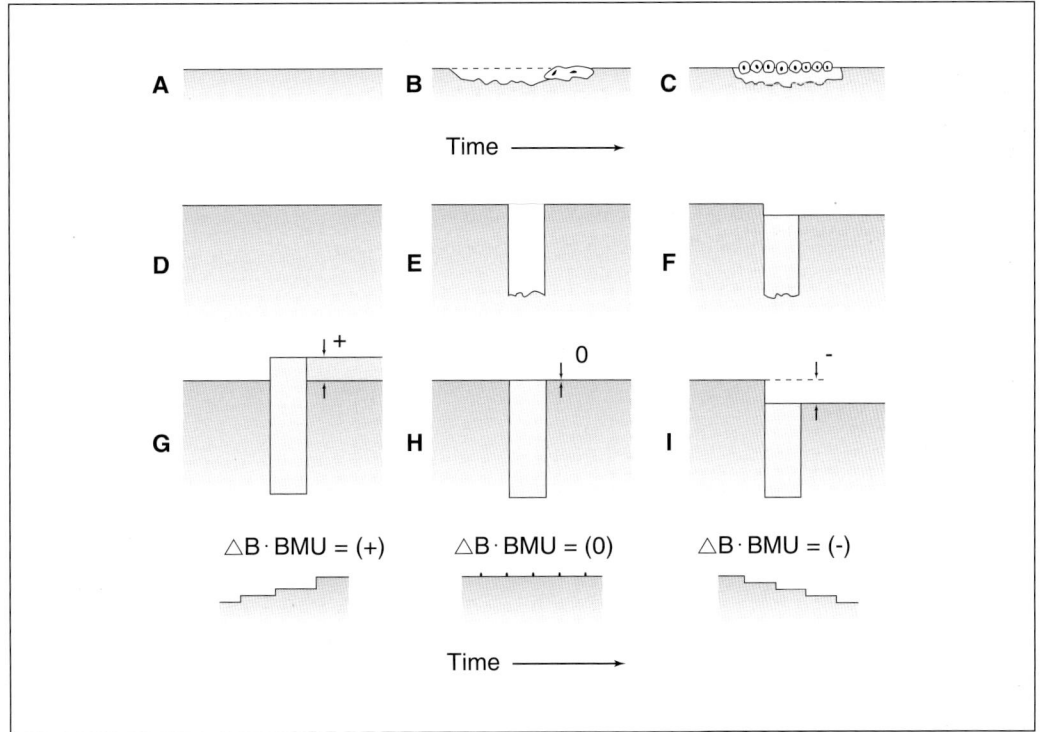

Fig 3-2 Bone-remodeling BMUs. *(Top row)* An activation event on a bone surface (A) causes a packet of bone resorption (B), and then replacement of the resorbed bone by osteoblasts (C). The BMU makes and controls the new osteoclasts and osteoblasts that do this. *(Second row)* Idealization of those activation events (D) maximizes the amounts of bone resorbed (E) and formed (F) by completed BMUs. *(Third row)* BMU graphs (after Frost). (G) Small excess of formation over resorption as, perhaps, on periosteal surfaces. (H) "Conservation mode," or equalized resorption and formation, as on haversian surfaces. (I) "Disuse mode," or deficit of formation, as on cortical-endosteal and trabecular surfaces. *(Bottom row)* These stair graphs (after P. J. Meunier) show the effects on the local bone balance and mass of a series of BMUs of the kind shown immediately above. BMUs are created anew when and where they are needed, and they include capillary, precursor, and "supporting" cells and some wandering cells. They are true multicellular entities in the same sense as renal nephrons and intestinal villi. The old idea that osteoclasts alone cause net bone losses is no longer tenable; BMUs do it instead. (From Frost HM. Strain and other mechanical influences on bone strength and maintenance. Curr Opin Orthop 1997; 8:60–70. Reprinted with permission.)

Adaptational lag time

As bone loads in growing children steadily increase, the strengthening of bone is characterized by a sluggish, "error-driven" bone modeling[44] lag time. This lag time allows strains to exceed modeling threshold to maintain modeling during growth. Bone loads plateau in young adults and bone adaptation catches up to turn modeling off. The largest strains in long bones from voluntary activity range from 2,000 to 4,000 microstrain in most growing subjects compared to 800 to 1,300 microstrain in most adults.[23,29,32,45–47] Bone strain associated with loading of dental implants exceeds 3,000 microstrain, but is gradually reduced as bone density around the implants increases to reduce overall bone strain.

Bone adapts to nearly any mechanical challenge *if given adequate time*. With dental implants placed in bone graft, the key is to manage the process of adaptation so that strain never exceeds the bone's relatively narrow physiologic window. Otherwise, hyperphysiologic load will lead to implant loss and graft resorption.

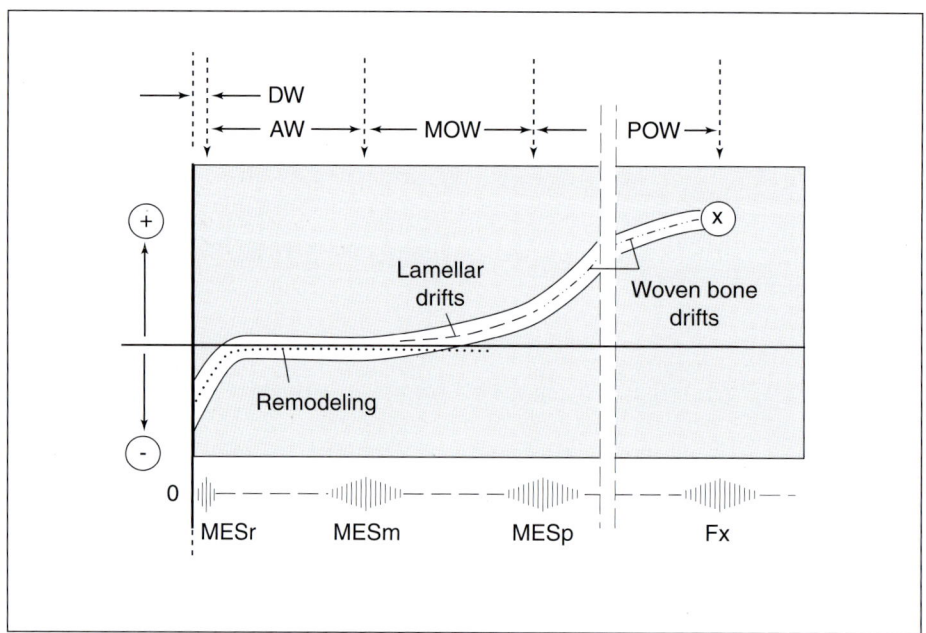

Fig 3-3 Combined modeling and remodeling effects on bone strength and mass. The horizontal line at the bottom suggests typical peak bone strains, from 0 on the left to the fracture strain (near 25,000 microstrain) on the right (Fx), plus the locations of the remodeling (MESr), modeling (MESm), and microdamage (MESp) thresholds. The horizontal axis represents no net gains or losses of bone strength or mass. The dotted line curve suggests how remodeling responses to bone strains remove and weaken bone where strains stay below the MESr range, but otherwise tend to keep bone and its strength. The middle dashed line curve suggests how modeling responses to bone strains begin to increase bone strength where strains enter or exceed the MESm range. The solid outlines suggest the combined effects of modeling and remodeling on bone strength. At and beyond the MESp range, woven bone formation drifts usually replace lamellar bone formation drifts. In the nearly flat comfort zone or adapted window (AW), as in normally adapted adults, bone strength and mass change little as typical strains change. (DW, disuse window; MOW, mild overload window as in growing mammals; POW, pathologic overload window.) The increasing body weight and muscle loads on children's bones can upshift some bone strains above the MESm range, to turn modeling on. Because these seem to be fundamental properties of living extremity bones, it can be inferred that this would be analogous to the healing of maxillary bone grafts. (From Frost HM. Strain and other mechanical influences on bone strength and maintenance. Curr Opin Orthop 1997;8:60–70. Reprinted with permission.)

Combined modeling and remodeling effects

Accumulated evidence suggests that bone adapted to mechanical usage strains everywhere (E) stays in the zone between the remodeling and modeling thresholds (the so-called comfort zone), well below the microdamage threshold (MESp), and far below fracture strain (Fx) (Figs 3-3 and 3-4). That relationship defines a successful graft based on the vital biomechanical criterion, which describes the adapted state as follows:

$$MESr \ldots < \ldots E \ldots < \ldots MESm \ll MESp \lll Fx$$
$$/\text{adapted state}/$$

Strain "Windows"

Both normal and healing bone function in three broad strain windows, a concept that can be illustrated through provisional strain values (see Fig 3-3).[6,48] Where strains (E) remain too small, bone is removed (the disuse window: E < about 50 to 100 microstrain). In a somewhat larger, narrow window or comfort zone, bone strength is maintained or even increased (the adapted and mild overload windows: E > about 50 to 100 to about < 2,000 microstrain). At larger strains bone healing can break down, but the window is quite broad: E = 3,000 to 25,000 microstrain.

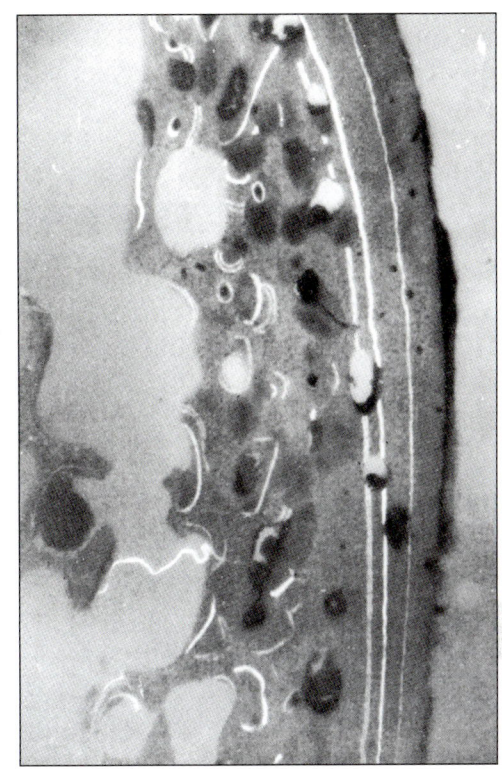

Fig 3-4 Tetracycline bone labeling. Ultraviolet fluorescence microscopy of an undecalcified cross section of the middle third of the left seventh rib. The patient was an adolescent girl who took tetracycline antibiotics for respiratory infections on three occasions before a thoracotomy for cardiac surgery provided this sample. This is the cutaneous cortex of the rib as viewed from the front of the patient, so its cutaneous-side periosteal surface lies on the right and the marrow cavity to the left. Tetracyclines deposit where new bone mineralizes. They are fluorescent under ultraviolet or blue light, so they provide a bone tissue time marker suitable for use in humans and animals. The three long, curved vertical bright lines to the right reveal tetracycline deposited on three occasions in a periosteal formation drift of lamellar bone. Its additions of new layers of bone gradually moved this periosteal surface to the reader's right in tissue space (this is normal in this part of this rib during growth). Knowing the time intervals between those "labels," one can measure the rate of bone formation by this modeling drift and its osteoblasts. In life, a companion resorption drift acted on the left (marrow cavity side) of this cortex, so this whole cortex drifted to the reader's right. The situation corresponds exactly to the cortical drifts shown in the right-hand cortex in Fig 3-1(C). The shorter curved lines inside the cortex are labels deposited in secondary osteons that were being formed when the labels in the formation drifts were deposited. BMUs made these osteons. They are elongated cylinders, parallel to the bone's length, seen in cross section here. The labeled osteons formed some time before the surgery at which this bone was resected, and newer ones partly replaced most of them. That explains the broken arcs. Because of the above drift pattern, the left half of this cortex is older than the right half. This helps to explain why the left half contains more secondary osteons; it had more time to accumulate them. The white curlicue in the marrow space in the lower part of the figure is a stray cotton fiber caught in the mounting medium. (Original magnification ×10.)

Maxillary Pneumatization

When all of these biomechanical principles are combined, the best explanation for pneumatization of the maxillary sinus is a biomechanical one: it is a result of disuse atrophy with endosteal (sinus floor) resorption caused by lack of occlusal function due to missing teeth. This explanation, previously thought to be a hypothesis, has been proven to be valid in both animal and clinical studies by Boyne (see chapter 1). In short, pneumatization is a phenomenon of the mechanostat, a result of disuse osteopenia, atrophy, and resorption with the net effect of enlarging the sinus cavity.

Nonmechanical Agents and Factors

Research reveals numerous nonmechanical factors that affect skeletal health, disease, and healing of bone grafts.[49–51] Other factors that surgeons might propose include the bone effects of prostaglandins,[52,53] intermittent use of parathyroid hormone,[54] bone morphogenetic protein,[55,56] other cytokines and growth factors,[49,57] electrical current and external capacitive fields,[58,59] and ultrasound treatment.[60] How these approaches accelerate bone graft healing and modeling remains uncertain.

Pharmaceuticals

The incorporation phase of graft healing depends heavily on nonmechanical factors that promote cellular proliferation, migration, differentiation, and function of osteoblasts. These processes involve various growth factors, agents that affect gene expression, cellular adhesion, cellular-intercellular matrix interactions, apoptosis, and so forth. This problem falls mainly in the domain of cell and molecular biology[3] and provides an attractive target for "designer" drugs[61] or gene therapy (see chapter 31).

Bone strain and nonmechanical agents control graft replacement and modeling activities,[9,10] so even in completely unloaded grafts some replacement and modeling occurs while the remodeling mechanism proceeds to remove the entire graft. But both mechanisms provide essential mechanical functions in graft healing, and they depend on graft strains to guide and determine end points.[62] This means agents that increase responsiveness to modeling or BMU-based remodeling to strains will enhance those functions and hence graft success.

Some hormones, such as growth hormones, have such effects in adolescents, but in aged adults the effect is usually less.[63] Intermittent administration of parathyroid hormone can create new formation drifts of lamellar bone,[54,64] while some prostaglandins can stimulate woven bone formation.[53,65] This suggests such agents might enhance the modeling phase of graft healing. Little research has concerned them so far.

Timing the administration of such agents could be important.[6,9,10,66] For example, agents that improve cellular proliferation and differentiation should be most helpful early in the incorporation phase and less helpful near its end or in the replacement and modeling phases. Agents that enhance the responsiveness of modeling and remodeling to mechanical strains should provide little help early in the incorporation phase because those two activities would not begin working then. Such agents should work better after the replacement and modeling phases of healing begin.

What causes most failed RAPs remains a mystery. Excessive strain, malnutrition, and osteomalacia impair all phases of bone graft healing. Other factors that impair it include severe cardiac, hepatic, renal, or pulmonary failure; diabetes; and osteopetrosis.[67] In many if not most aging adults, a gradual decline in the responsiveness of bone's biologic mechanisms to appropriate stimuli seems to occur.[2,68-70] This adversely affects bone graft success. Until agents are developed that can correct this mechanism, surgeons and patients must learn to live with and try to make allowances for it.

Agents that impair the remodeling and modeling of a graft include X-radiation[71]; bisphosphonates[36]; drugs used to treat rheumatoid arthritis, malignancies, and organ transplant rejection[72]; and some NSAIDs.[13,73]

Conclusion

The biologic mechanisms that model and remodel bone, heal fractures, and incorporate bone grafts rely on nonmechanical factors to function properly. However, mechanical factors guide these biologic mechanisms in time and anatomic space. Nonmechanical factors help or hinder bone healing, but they do not replace the biologic mechanisms (since nonmechanical agents would otherwise normalize bone strength and mass in congenitally paralyzed limbs). Although knowledge of cellular- and molecular-biologic factors involved in bone physiology and healing has increased dramatically, how those factors exactly affect bone's biologic response to strain and other mechanical factors remains a mystery. Accordingly, future research is needed to study these phenomena.

BOX 3-1 Glossary

bone "mass": The amount of bone tissue, often estimated by absorptiometry, preferably viewed as volume minus the marrow cavity. It does not mean *gravimetric mass*, as used in physics. Bone mass provides an unreliable index of bone strength because it does not account for the contribution of bone architecture.[74] In this chapter, mass refers to absorptiometry.

BMU: Basic multicellular unit of bone remodeling. In approximately 4 months, and in a biologically coupled *activation → resorption → formation* (ARF) sequence, it turns over about 0.05 mm^3 of bone in humans. When it makes less bone than it resorbs (its disuse mode), this tends to remove bone, usually next to marrow. Adult humans may create about 3 million new BMUs annually and about a million function at any moment in the whole skeleton.[6]

disuse: When typical peak bone strain downshifts into the remodeling threshold region shown in Fig 3-3, disuse mode occurs for a bone or bone graft. In such situations disuse-mode remodeling usually removes local bone. For bone, disuse is the relationship between bone strength and its usual loads. The resulting strains and the remodeling threshold provide the criteria that recognize disuse. Very small loads can cause enough strain in that threshold region in a healing bone graft to avoid disuse resorption.

drift: See *modeling*.

MESm: Minimum effective strain range (or equivalent stimulus) for switching on mechanically controlled bone modeling drifts.[6,28] An operational concept, the center of this genetically determined "modeling threshold" probably lies near 1,000 microstrain in most adults (equivalent to about 20 MPa), which could be viewed as its set point. Its value currently causes some debate.[22] Nonmechanical agents, drugs, disease, age, race, and species might modify its value.

MESp: Minimum effective strain range for bone's operational microdamage threshold. Under parallel-grain loading it should center near 3,000 microstrain (equivalent to about 60 MPa). Its value for across-grain loading remains unknown at present.[6,22,24]

MESr: Minimum effective strain range (or equivalent stimulus) for mechanically controlled BMU-based remodeling.[23] Above it conservation-mode remodeling turns on to prevent net bone loss. Where strains stay below the MESr, disuse-mode remodeling turns on to cause net bone loss. Another operational concept, the center of this genetically determined threshold range would lie near 50 to 100 microstrain (equivalent to about 2 MPa), which could be viewed as its set point.[34,75] Nonmechanical agents, drugs, disease, age, race, and species might modify its value.

modeling: Producing functionally purposeful sizes and shapes to skeletal organs. Mostly independent resorption and formation modeling drifts do it in bones and bone grafts. Modeling drifts mainly determine outside bone diameter, cortical thickness, and the upper limit of bone strength.[15] Remodeling determines the lower limit of bone strength.

osteopenia: Less bone than usual for most healthy people of the same age, height, sex, and race. Its definition still involves problems and opinions this chapter does not discuss.

remodeling: Turnover of bone in small packets by basic multicellular units that reduce or stabilize the size of the bone or bone graft. While drifts and BMUs create and use what seem to be the same kinds of osteoblasts and osteoclasts to do their work,[15] in different parts of the same bone at the same time, osteoblasts and osteoclasts in drifts and BMUs act and respond differently even oppositely to many influences.[30] In remodeling's disuse mode, BMU creations increase and BMUs make less bone than they resorb. In conservation mode, BMU creations usually decrease and resorption and formation in completed BMUs tend to equalize.

remodeling space: Each BMU makes a temporary hole in bone or on a bone surface. The sum of all such holes equals the remodeling space, which can vary from about 3% to occasionally more than 30% of a bone's volume.[76] Due to surface-to-volume ratio effects, its value in trabecular bone usually exceeds the value in compact bone.

resorption: Different meanings of this term in the literature cause some confusion. Some authors use it to mean net bone loss, and in that sense discuss "antiresorption agents."[17] Others use it to mean bone resorption by osteoclasts, and refer to net losses of bone as such and separately. In this chapter, it means resorption by osteoclasts.[6,15] In that sense few true antiresorption agents exist, and they do not include estrogen or presently known and studied biphosphonates, which instead are "antiremodeling agents" that decrease BMU creations. Because of the ARF sequence, this reduces global resorption, and then formation, both about equally.[77,78] This could impair the replacement phase of bone graft healing and does impair

BOX 3-1 Glossary (cont)

microdamage repair, as some biphosphonates do. Where bone mass increases, modeling did it, not osteoblasts alone; where bone mass decreases, disuse-mode remodeling did it, not osteoclasts alone.

strain: The deformation or change in dimensions and/or shape caused by a load on any structure or structural material. Special gauges measure bone strains in the laboratory and in vivo. Load always causes strain, even if very small. In biomechanics, strain is often expressed in microstrain units, where 1,000 microstrain in compression would shorten a bone by 0.1% of its original length, 10,000 microstrain would shorten it by 1% of that length, and 100,000 microstrain would shorten it by 10% of that length (and break it).[8,24]

stress: The elastic resistance of the intermolecular bonds in a material being stretched by strain. Loads cause strains, which then cause stress. Three principal strains and stresses include tension, compression, and shear. Stress cannot be measured directly but must be calculated from other information that often includes strain. The stress-strain curve of bone is not linear. The material is stiffer at small loads than at large ones.

ultimate strength: The load or strain that, when applied once, usually fractures a bone. The fracture strength of normal lamellar bone is about 25,000 microstrain (CV about 0.3), which corresponds to a change in length of 2.5%, ie, from 100.0% to 97.5% of its original length under compression or to 102.5% of it under tension. That fracture strain corresponds to an ultimate or fracture stress of about 17,000 psi or about 120 MPa.[8]

unit load: The part of the total load on a bone carried by 1 mm^2, 1 cm^2, or 1 in^2 of its cross section or surface to cause corresponding principal strain and stress. The unit load (w) equals the total load (W) divided by the cross section area (A) of the bone carrying it ($w = W/A$). The unit compression load usually equals the unit compression stress. In ordinary discourse, people often equate them, which can lead to the false idea that stress causes strain.

vital biomechanics: A subfield of general biomechanics that concerns how and why biologic mechanisms respond to mechanical usage and lads, and other physical stimuli, to adapt structural tissues and organs to their usual mechanical usage to make them mechanically competent and then keep them so for life.

woven bone: Also known as *primary bone*, *primitive bone*, and *reactive bone*. At the tissue level, woven bone lacks the "grain" that characterizes lamellar bone. In the body, if it carries no load, it is slowly removed. If it does carry loads, lamellar bone slowly replaces it.

References

1. Habal MB, Reddi AH (eds). Bone Grafting—From Basic Science to Clinical Application. New York: Saunders, 1992.
2. Buckwalter JA, Mow VC, Trumble TE. Restoration of injured or degenerated articular cartilage. J Am Acad Orthop Surg 1994;2:192–201.
3. Goodman S, Aspenberg P, Song Y. The effects of intermittent micromotion versus polymer particles on tissue ingrowth: Experiment using the micromotion chamber implanted in rabbits. J Appl Biomater 1994;5:117–123.
4. Gowen M (ed). Cytokines and Bone Metabolism. Boca Raton, FL: CRC, 1992.
5. Kenwright J, Goodship AE. Controlled mechanical stimulation in the treatment of tibial fractures. Clin Orthop Rel Res 1989;241:36–47.
6. Frost HM. Introduction to a New Skeletal Physiology, vols I and II. Pueblo, CO: Pajaro Group, 1995.
7. Frost HM. Intermediary Organization of the Skeleton, vols I and II. Boca Raton, FL: CRC, 1986.
8. Martin RB, Burr DB. Structure, Function and Adaptation of Compact Bone. New York: Raven, 1989.
9. Frost HM. The biology of fracture healing. Part I. Clin Orthop Rel Res 1989;248:283–293.
10. Frost HM. The biology of fracture healing. Part II. Clin Orthop Rel Res 1989;248:294–309.
11. Woodard JC. Morphology of fracture nonunion and osteomyelitis. Vet Clin North Am 1991;21:813–844.
12. Altman RD, Latta LL, Keer R, Renfree K, Hornicek FJ, Banovac K. Effect of nonsteroidal anti-inflammatory drugs on fracture healing: A laboratory study in rats. J Orthop Trauma 1995;9:392–400.
13. Mei-Ling H, Je-Kan C, Gwo-Jaw W. Anti-inflammatory drug effects on bone repair and remodeling in rabbits. Clin Orthop Rel Res 1995;313:270–278.
14. Burr DB, Martin RB. Errors in bone remodeling: Toward a unified theory of metabolic bone disease. Am J Anat 1989;186:186–216.

In Memorium: Harold M. Frost, MD (1921–2004)

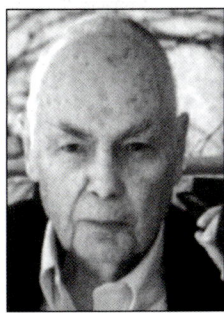

Before this edition went to press, Harold Frost passed away. Those of us who practice dental implantology owe a great debt to Dr Frost. The influence of his ideas on the fields of bone biology and orthopedic science, which includes restorative dentistry, is impossible to measure. Below is a partial list of his contributions:

- Development of the techniques to make quantitative measurements on nondecalcified bone sections and the invention of bone histomorphometry
- Use of the 11th rib biopsy for diagnosis of metabolic bone disease
- Discovery of the basic multicellular unit as the key effector of bone metabolism
- Experimental demonstration that estrogens reduce bone formation
- Histologic demonstration of microcracks in human bone biopsies
- Basic theories for bone growth plate adaptation to mechanical loading
- The "mechanostat theory" of bone adaptation to mechanical effects
- The Utah Paradigm of bone physiology
- Muscle-bone relationship

Dr Webster Jee, his mentor at the University of Utah for 30 years, paid eloquent tribute to Dr Frost,* which he concluded as follows:

There are few clinician scientists that have had such a profound impact on a scientific discipline as has Harold Frost. He has advanced the basic science of skeletal biology and used it to improve clinical diagnosis and treatment. It is impossible to overestimate his influence and contributions to the field of skeletal biology. He has molded the thoughts of a generation, in areas as widely divergent as orthopaedics, endocrinology, rheumatology, clinical medicine, anatomy, physiology, orthodontics, anthropology and bioengineering. It is not an overstatement to say that he has been the most influential theoretician in skeletal biology in this century.

With fond remembrance, we in dentistry strongly concur; the dental and medical professions will truly miss him.

*Tribute to Harold M. Frost, MD. J Musculoskel Neuronal Interact 2004;4:348.

15. Jee WSS. The skeletal tissues. In: Weiss L (ed). Cell and Tissue Biology. A Textbook of Histology. Baltimore: Urban and Schwartzenberg, 1989:211–259.
16. Evans RA. Is there a need for whole body physiology? Bone Miner 1987;2:243–244.
17. Rodan GA. Bone mass homeostasis and bisphosphonate action. Bone 1997;20:1–4.
18. Mundy GR. Regulation of bone formation by bone morphogenetic proteins and other growth factors. Clin Orthop Rel Res 1996;324:24–28.
19. Polanyi M. Life's irreducible structure. Science 1968;160:1308–1312.
20. Skerry TM. Perspectives: Mechanical loading and bone. What sort of exercise is beneficial to the skeleton? Bone 1997;20:179–181.
21. Burr DB, Forwood MR, Fyrhie DP, Martin RB, Schaffler MB, Turner CH. Bone microdamage and skeletal fragility in osteoporotic and stress fractures. J Bone Miner Res 1997;12:6–15.
22. Kimmel DB. A paradigm for skeletal strength homeostasis. J Bone Miner Res 1993;8(suppl 2):515–522.
23. Takahashi HE (ed). Spinal Disorders and Growth and Aging. Tokyo: Springer, 1995.
24. Pattin CA, Caler WE, Carter DR. Cyclic mechanical property degradation during fatigue loading of cortical bone. J Biomech 1996;29:69–79.
25. Frost HM. Perspectives on artificial joint design. J Long-term Effects Med Implants 1992;2:9–35.
26. Forwood MR, Turner CH. Response of rat tibiae to incremental loading: A quantum concept for bone formation. Bone 1994;15:603–609.
27. Jee WSS (ed). Proceedings of the International Conference on Animal Models in the Prevention and Treatment of Osteopenia. Bone 1995;17(suppl):1–466.
28. Heinonen A, Sievanen H, Kannus P, Oja P, Vuori I. Effects of unilateral strength training and detraining on bone mineral mass and estimated mechanical characteristics of the upper limb bones in young women. J Bone Miner Res 1995;11:490–501.
29. Kannus P, Sievanen H, Vuori I. Physical loading, exercise and bone. Bone 1996;18(suppl 1):1–3.
30. Schönau E (ed). Paediatric Osteology. New Trends and Diagnostic Possibilities. Amsterdam: Elsevier Science, 1996.
31. Turner CH, Forwood MR, Rho J, Yoshikawa T. Mechanical loading thresholds for lamellar and woven bone formation. J Bone Miner Res 1994;9:87–97.

32. Nunamaker DM, Butterweck DM, Provost MP. Fatigue fractures in thoroughbred race horses: Relationship with age, peak bone strain and running. J Orthop Res 1990;8:604–611.
33. Frost HM. Structural adaptations to mechanical usage (SATMU). 1. Redefining Wolff's Law: The bone modeling problem. Anat Rec 1990;226:403–413.
34. Frost HM. Wolff's Law and bone's structural adaptations to mechanical usage: An overview for clinicians. Angle Orthod 1994;64:187–212.
35. Mori S, Burr DB. Increased intracortical remodeling following fatigue damage. Bone 1993;14:103–109.
36. Fleisch H. Bisphosphonates in Bone Disease. From the Laboratory to the Patient. London: Parthenon, 1995:5–176.
37. Shane E, Epstein S. Immunosuppressive therapy and the skeleton. Trends Endocrinol Metab 1994;5:169–175.
38. Aspenberg P, Goodman SB, Wang JJ-S. Influence of callus deformation time. Clin Orthop Rel Res 1996;322:253–261.
39. Blenman PR, Carter DR, Beaupre GS. Role of mechanical loading in the progressive ossification of a fracture callus. J Orthop Res 1989;7:398–407.
40. Carter DR, Blenman PR, Beaupre GS. Correlations between mechanical stress history and tissue differentiation in initial fracture healing. J Orthop Res 1988;6:736–748.
41. Hanafusa S, Matsusue Y, Yasunaga T, et al. Biodegradable plate fixation of rabbit femoral shaft osteotomies. Clin Orthop Rel Res 1995;315:262–271.
42. Karlsson M, Johnell O, Obrant K. Bone mineral density in weight lifters. Calcif Tissue Int 1993;52:212–215.
43. Nilsson BE, Andersson SM, Hardtrup T, Westlin NE. Ballet dancing and weight lifting—Effects on BMC. AJR Am J Roentgenol 1978;131:541–542.
44. Beaupre GS, Orr TE, Carter DR. An appproach for time-dependent bone modeling and remodeling—Theoretical development. J Orthop Res 1990;8:651–661.
45. Burr DB, Milgrom C, Fyrhie D, et al. In vivo measurement of human tibial strains during vigorous activity. Bone 1995;18:405–410.
46. Forwood MR, Turner CH. Skeletal adaptations to mechanical usage: Results from tibial loading studies in rats. Bone 1995;17(suppl):197–205.
47. Turner CH, Forwood MR. Bone adaptation to mechanical forces in the rat tibia. In: Odgaard A, Weinans H (eds). Bone Structure and Remodeling. London: World Scientific, 1995:65–78.
48. Frost HM. Perspectives: Bone's mechanical usage windows. Bone Miner 1992;19:257–271.
49. Bilezikian JP, Raisz LG, Rodan GA. Principles of Bone Biology. Orlando, FL: Academic, 1996.
50. Favus MJ (ed). Primer on the Metabolic Bone Diseases and Disorders of Mineral Metabolism, ed 3. New York: Lippincott-Raven, 1996.
51. Shore EM, Kaplan FS. Molecular biology for the clinician. Part I. General principles. Clin Orthop Rel Res 1994;306:264–283.
52. Akamine T, Jee WSS, Ke HZ, Lin BY. Prostaglandin E2 prevents bone loss and adds extra bone to immobilized distal femoral metaphysis in female rats. Bone 1992;13:11–22.
53. Jee WSS, Mori X, Li X, Chan S. Prostaglandin E2 enhances cortical bone mass and activates intracortical bone remodeling in intact and ovariectomized female rats. Bone 1990;11:253–266.
54. Takahashi HE, Tanizawa T, Hori M, Uzawa T. Effect of intermittent administration of human parathyroid hormone (1-34) on experimental osteopenia of rats induced by ovariectomy. In: Jee WSS (ed). The Rat Model for Bone Biology Studies. Cells Mater 1991;(suppl 1):113–118.
55. Reddi AH. Bone morphogenetic proteins, bone marrow stromal cells, and mesenchymal cells. Maureen Owen revisited. Clin Orthop Rel Res 1995;313:115–119.
56. Urist MR. The first three decades of bone morphogenetic protein research. Osteologie 1995;4:207–223.
57. Goldring SR, Goldring MB. Cytokines and skeletal physiology. Clin Orthop Rel Res 1996;324:13–23.
58. Brighton CT, Shaman P, Heppenstall RB, Esterhai JL, Pollack SR, Friedenberg ZB. Tibial nonunion treated with direct current, capacitive coupling, or bone graft. Clin Orthop Rel Res 1995;321:223–234.
59. Sharrard WJW. A double-blind trial of pulsed electromagnetic fields for delayed union of tibial fractures. J Bone Joint Surg 1990;72B:347–355.
60. Heckman JD, Ryaby JP, McCabe J, Frey JJ, Kilcoyne RF. Acceleration of tibial fracture-healing by non-invasive, low intensity pulsed ultrasound. J Bone Joint Surg 1994;76A:26–34.
61. Economides AN, Ravetch JV, Yancopoulos GD, Stahl N. Designer cytokines: Targeting actions to cells of choice. Science 1995;270:1351–1353.
62. Harter LV, Hruska KA, Duncan RL. Human osteoblast-like cells respond to mechanical strain with increased bone matrix protein production independent of hormonal regulation. Endocrinology 1995;136:528–535.
63. Meling TR, Nylen ES. Growth hormone deficiency in adults: A review. Am J Med Sci 1996;311:153–166.
64. Hori M, Uzawa T, Morita L, Noda T, Takahashi H, Inoue J. Effect of human parathyroid hormone (PTH[1-34]) on experimental osteopenia of rats induced by ovariectomy. Bone Miner 1988;3:193–199.
65. High WB. Effects of orally administered prostaglandin on cortical bone turnover in dogs: A histomorphometric study. Bone 1988;8:363–373.
66. Bak B, Jorgensen PH, Andreassen TT. The stimulating effect of growth hormone on fracture healing is dependent on onset and duration of administration. Clin Orthop Rel Res 1991;264:295–299.
67. de Palma L, Tulli A, Macccauro G, Sabetta SP, del Torto M. Fracture callus in osteopetrosis. Clin Orthop Rel Res 1994;308:85–89.
68. Bergman RJ, Gazit D, Kahn AJ, Gruber H, McDougall S, Hahn TJ. Age-related changes in osteogenic stem cells in mice. J Bone Miner Res 1996;11:568–577.
69. Stanulis-Praeger BM. Cellular senescence revisited: A review. Mech Aging Dev 1989;38:1–48.
70. Quarto R, Thomas D, Liang CT. Bone progenitor cell deficits and the age-associated decline in bone repair activity. Calcif Tissue Int 1995;56:123–129.

71. Pelker RR, Friedlander GE, Panjabi MM, Kapp D, Doganis A. Radiation induced alterations of fracture healing biomechanics. J Orthop Res 1984;2:275–282.
72. Landmann J, Renner N, Gachter A, Thiel G, Harder F. Cyclosporin and osteonecrosis of the femoral head. J Bone Joint Surg 1987;69A:331–340.
73. Gebuhr P, Wilbek H, Soelberg M. Naproxen for 8 days can prevent heterotopic ossification after hip arthroplasty. Clin Orthop Rel Res 1995;314:166–169.
74. Ferreti JL. Perspectives of pQCT technology associated to biomechanical studies in skeletal research employing rat models. Bone 1995;17(suppl):353–364.
75. Frost HM. Bone development during childhood: Insights from a new paradigm. In: Schönau E (ed). Paediatric Osteology. New Trends and Developments in Diagnostics and Therapy. Amsterdam: Elsevier Science, 1996:3–39.
76. Recker RR (ed). Bone Histomorphometry. Techniques and Interpretation. Boca Raton, FL: CRC Press, 1983.
77. Baumann BD, Wronski TJ. Response of cortical bone to antiresorptive agents and parathyroid hormone in aged ovariectomized rats. Bone 1995;16:247–253.
78. Ma YF, Jee WSS, Chen YY, Gasser J, Ke HZ, Li XJ, Kimmel DB. Partial maintenance of extracancellous bone mass by antiresorptive agents after discontinuation of human parathyroid hormone (1-38) in right hindlimb immobilization rats. J Bone Miner Res 1995;10:1726–1734.

chapter 4
Indications for and Classification of Sinus Bone Grafts

Carl E. Misch, DDS, MDS
Matteo Chiapasco, MD
Ole T. Jensen, DDS, MS

The posterior maxilla presents many unique and challenging conditions for the implant dentist. Several proven and predictable treatment modalities have been developed in recent years, including sinus grafts to increase height, onlay grafts to increase alveolar width, and improved approaches for placing implants in low-density bone.[1] More than any other treatment modality, however, the sinus graft has revolutionized posterior dental restoration. This chapter describes indications for the sinus graft and classifications of specific posterior maxillary morphologies.

Indications for the Sinus Graft

Local conditions of the edentulous alveolar ridge, such as loss of alveolar bone height as a result of periodontal disease prior to tooth loss, can make implant placement unfavorable. Distal furcation of the maxillary molar frequently leads to bone loss because of facial or palatal inaccessibility for hygiene purposes. Because it is narrow, it is also difficult to curettage the furca to eliminate calculus. Consequently, periodontal disease progresses, and the resulting loss of bone height leads to tooth loss.

The posterior maxilla has a thin facial plate, and the underlying trabecular bone (type 3 or 4) has a low mineral content. Loss of maxillary posterior teeth results in decreased bone width at the expense of the labial plate. Because of this, the width of the posterior maxilla decreases more rapidly than other regions of the jaws.[2] This resorption phenomenon is accelerated by the loss of vascularization of the alveolar bone and the initial type 3 or 4 trabecular bone. Even if it decreases by 60%, however, the residual ridge is wide enough in the posterior maxilla for root form implants. Progressive resorption shifts the alveolar crest toward the palate at the expense of bone width.[3] The posterior maxilla continues to atrophy until the entire alveolus is ablated to basal bone. The buccal cusp of the final restoration must cantilever facially to satisfy esthetic requirements at the expense of biomechanics in moderately to severely atrophic ridges (Fig 4-1).[4]

Pneumatization

The maxillary sinus maintains its overall size while the teeth remain in function, but it expands when posterior teeth are lost.[1] The antrum expands both inferiorly and laterally, potentially invading the canine region and even the lateral piriform. After the loss of teeth, the amount of available bone in the posterior maxilla is greatly reduced. This phenomenon is likely the result of atrophy caused by reduced bone strain from occlusal function. Implants placed beneath the *ungrafted* sinus floor are known to stimulate increased bone formation at the sinus floor.

chapter 4
Indications for and Classification of Sinus Bone Grafts

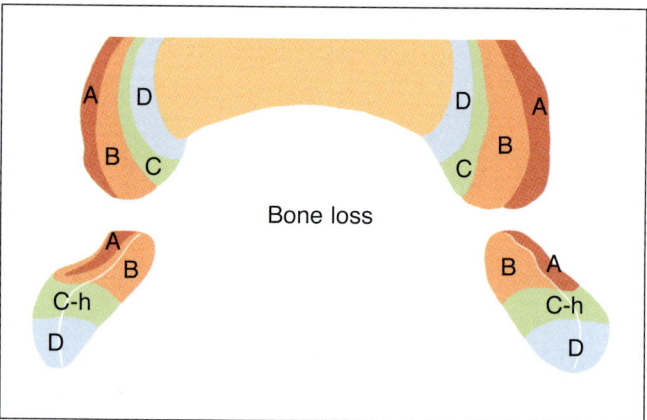

Fig 4-1 Maxillary posterior bone volume generally narrows in width toward the palate (divisions A and B). The ridge then resorbs in height (divisions C and D). Mandibular posterior bone shifts toward the lingual (divisions A and B), then decreases in height (divisions C and D) while shifting toward the facial. As a consequence, the mandibular ridge widens and the maxillary arch narrows in the moderate to severe resorption states.

A major criterion for successful implant treatment is availability of bone. A limited review of the literature reveals that implants 10 mm or less in height have a 16% lower survival rate than implants greater than 10 mm in height.[5] Therefore, height of bone is a consideration for predictable implant therapy. Because of periodontal disease, tooth loss, and sinus expansion, there is often less than 10 mm of bone between the alveolar ridge crest and the floor of the maxillary sinus. In these patients, a phenomenon known as *pneumatic trifurcation* is often observed, whereby the sinus dips down between the roots nearly to the furcation in the first molar area. Removal of the tooth leaves 4 to 5 mm of bone as a result of this anatomic sinus peculiarity. Limited vertical dimension compounds the problem of the medialized ridge position and compromised alveolar width. As a result, long-term prognosis is guarded unless these findings are addressed.

Poor bone density

As a general rule, the quality of bone in the posterior maxilla is poorer than in any other intraoral region.[6] The bone density of the maxilla is often 5 to 10 times lower than that of the anterior mandible.[7] Bone mineral density directly influences the amount of contact between the implant and the bone surface, which transmits load to bone.[8] Bone-implant contact is lowest in D4 bone. Strain pattern spreads farther toward the apex of the implant in poor-density bone than in dense bone.[9] When strain is excessive, bone loss in trabecular bone occurs along the entire implant body instead of only crestally, as occurs in dense bone. Type 4 (D4) bone also has the greatest biomechanical elastic modulus disparity to that of titanium under load.[7] Strategies to increase bone-implant contact, both surgically and by modification of implant topography, are being developed.

Bone mineral density is critically important for implant survival under load.[6] Implants are at greatest risk of failure under conditions of poor mineralization. A literature review of clinical studies published from 1981 to 2001 reveals that when implants are placed in the poorest bone mineral density, survival is reduced by an average of 16%,[5] with some reports as low as 40%.[10]

Deficient osseous structure jeopardizes not only initial implant stability but also load-bearing capacity. Absence of cortex on the ridge crest compromises implant stability, and since the labial cortical plate is usually quite thin and the ridge is relatively wide, it does little to improve stability. Without lateral cortical bone contact to stabilize the implant, initial stabilization in type 4 bone is often compromised.

Strong occlusal forces

Occlusal forces in the posterior region are greater than in the anterior region of the mouth by as much as a factor of five.[11] Maximum bite force in the anterior region ranges from 241 to 345 Pa. The bite force in the molar region of a dentate individual ranges from 1,378 to 1,723 Pa.[12] Natural maxillary molars have 200% more surface area as well as a significantly wider diameter than premolars,[1] and both of these factors reduce bone strain. Following the natural tooth model, implant support should be greater in the posterior molar region than in any other area of the mouth.[1] In addition, the posterior maxilla frequently opposes natural teeth or implant-supported restorations, contributing greater force to soft tissue–borne restorations. Therefore, decreased bone quantity and quality as well as increased bite forces should be considered in the treatment of this region of the mouth.

Implant Treatment Planning for the Posterior Maxilla

Implant size

The maxillary posterior teeth have the largest diameter, the greatest number of roots, and the largest root surface area of any of the natural dentition. All of these biomechanical strategies help the body to conserve energy (ie, reduce bone strain, sustain greater force to lower-density bone, etc). Implant treatment planning should simulate the function of the natural dentition. Because strain occurs primarily at the crest, implants are designed to minimize unfavorable biomechanical load.[13] Using wide-diameter implants is an effective means to disperse surface load at the crestal region. While implants of at least 4.0-mm diameter are generally recommended, a 5.0-mm implant provides a load-bearing advantage in the molar region.

The length of implants used in sinus grafts is generally an empirical choice.[14] In general, threaded root form implants should be at least 12 mm in length when placed in bone of poor density, as in grafted bone (see chapter 12). Implants of this size usually provide adequate bone-implant contact to dissipate the loads applied to the prosthesis. Rangert has shown that most of the load occurs at the crestal threads of an implant and that length is not as critical as crestal osseointegration. Therefore, surgeons must determine the crestal bone-healing capacity of a bone graft–directed implant in advance. For this reason, implants of less than 10 mm in length are generally not advocated.

Number of implants

Increasing the number of implants is an excellent means of decreasing strain to trabecular bone.[15] Until a more precise method of appraising implant load bearing is devised, one implant for each missing tooth is recommended to support a fixed prosthesis in the posterior maxilla. To further reduce bone strain, implants are generally splinted together. If strain is magnified by parafunction in the molar region and implant diameter cannot be increased, placing two implants for each missing molar is suggested.

Implant design

Surface roughness increases the surface area for osseointegration. A threaded implant has 30% to 200% more surface area than a cylindrical implant. Although threaded implants are more difficult to place, their use in low-density bone is strongly recommended. Biomechanical features of thread design (ie, thread pitch, shape, and depth) further influence the amount of surface area available.[13]

Contraindications for Implant Treatment in the Posterior Maxilla

A key to long-term success of implant therapy in the posterior maxilla is the presence of an adequate number of anterior teeth or implants. It is a rule in traditional prosthetics that if the canine and two adjacent teeth are missing, a fixed prosthesis is contraindicated.[16] This is because the length of the span results in 27 times the metal flexure resulting from a single pontic span. The amount and direction of the force at the canine region increases to such an extent that a fixed prosthesis should not be considered, regardless of the number of teeth that are splinted together. Therefore, when (a) both premolars, or (b) the first premolar and the lateral incisor, or (c) the lateral and central incisors are missing, along with the canine, a fixed restoration is contraindicated. A removable prosthesis that has no movement under function is considered a fixed prosthesis in terms of the number and position of the implants. Therefore, the treatment plan should provide for maintenance or restoration of healthy anterior teeth or placement of root form implants. Before posterior implants are considered, a healthy natural tooth or implant abutment is required in the canine region of the quadrant.

Crown height space should also be evaluated prior to implant placement. When the occlusal plane has been properly positioned, the crown height space should be greater than 8 mm.[4] If less than 8 mm is available, excess tissue can be removed via gingivoplasty; otherwise, osteoplasty or vertical impaction osteotomy of the alveolar process is indicated to restore interocclusal space.

Indications for and Classification of Sinus Bone Grafts

TABLE 4-1 Healing requirements for treatment options—Misch Classification

Treatment options	Residual bone height (mm)	Treatment procedures	Healing time (mos)
1	> 12	Division A implant placement	Implant osseointegration: 4–6
2	10–12	Sinus graft; simultaneous division A implant placement	Implant osseointegration: 6–8
3	5–10	Lateral wall approach sinus graft; delayed division A implant placement	Graft consolidation: 2–4 Implant osseointegration: 4–8*
4	> 5	Lateral wall approach sinus graft; delayed division A implant placement	Graft consolidation: 6–10 Implant osseointegration: 4–10*

*Evaluate at implant placement.

Abnormal intraoral conditions can compromise the outcome of sinus grafting procedures and jeopardize the survival of the implants. Dental contraindications to sinus grafting include inadequate oral hygiene, untreated periodontal disease of the residual dentition, severe malocclusion, and severe clenching or bruxism.

Misch Classification of the Posterior Maxilla

A sinus bone morphology classification published in 1987 by Misch and Judy described bone resorption patterns in edentulous ridges (see Fig 4-1).[3,17] According to this classification, an alveolar ridge with adequate bone for implant stability has the following dimensions: > 5 mm in width, > 7 mm in length, > 12 mm in height, and angulation of < 30 degrees to the occlusal load. A minimum residual width of 5 mm is required to support a 4-mm-diameter implant. The dimensions of a division B edentulous ridge are 2.5 to 5 mm in width, 7 mm in mesiodistal length, > 12 mm in height, and angulation to occlusal load of < 20 degrees. This decreased width in all jaw locations primarily occurs from the facial medial. Division C-w ridges consist of 0 to 2.5 mm in width and 10 to 12 mm in height. A C-h ridge is inadequate in height (< 10 mm) and has a crown height space to bone ratio of > 1:1. In division D, severe atrophy with significant height loss is present (a crown height to remaining bone ratio > 5:1).

This classification was based on treatment options available at the time it was created (Table 4-1)[4,18] and depended very much on the amount of bone height available between the floor of the antrum and the crest of the residual ridge as it related to ideal implant locations (Fig 4-2a). Each protocol suggested the surgical approach, the type of bone graft material to use, and a timetable for healing to take place prior to prosthetic reconstruction. In 1988, Cawood and Howell classified the edentulous posterior maxilla, emphasizing gradations of bone loss and relative or progressive pneumatization of the maxillary sinus.[19]

In 1999, Misch modified his 1987 classification to include the lateral dimension of the sinus cavity and used this dimension to modify the healing period protocol, since smaller-width sinuses (0 to 10 mm) form bone faster than larger-width (> 15 mm) sinuses.[4]

Option 1: Conventional implant placement

The first treatment option requires the presence of sufficient bone height to permit placement of endosteal implants following standard surgical protocol (Fig 4-2b).

Option 2: Sinus augmentation

The second option requires 10 to 12 mm of vertical bone (Fig 4-2c). Vertical bone for improved implant survival (division A) is developed via an osteotome technique through the alveolar crest.[20,21] The osteotomy is performed approximately 1 to 2 mm below the floor of the sinus using a flat-end osteotome firmly tapped 2 to 3 mm beyond the prepared implant osteotomy (see chapter 22). A greenstick upfracture of the sinus floor elevates the bone

Fig 4-2a Misch developed four surgical treatment categories for the posterior maxilla based on the amount of bone between the residual crest of the ridge and the floor of the maxillary antrum. (Reprinted with permission from Misch.[18])

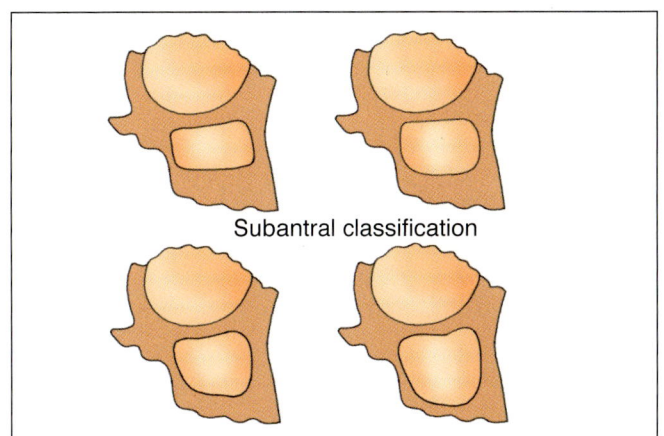

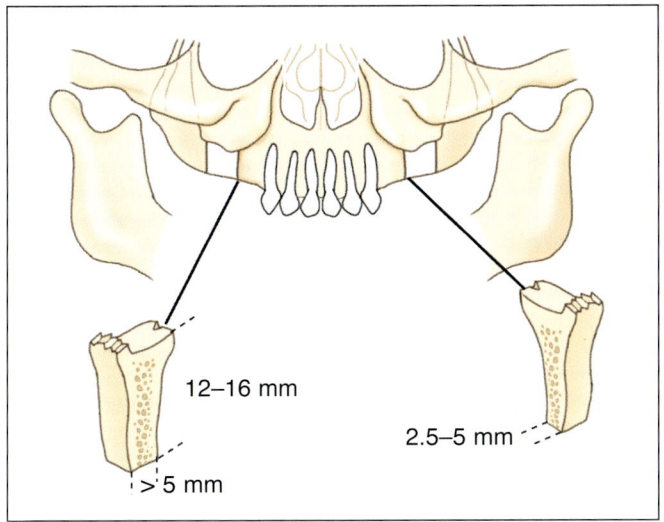

Fig 4-2b Option 1. More than 12 mm of bone below the floor of the maxillary sinus offers adequate height for an implant-supported prosthesis. When the crestal ridge is greater than 5 mm (division A), an implant may be placed without augmentation *(left)*. A crestal ridge that is less than 5 mm wide requires augmentation, ridge splitting, and/or ridge expansion prior to implant placement *(right)*.

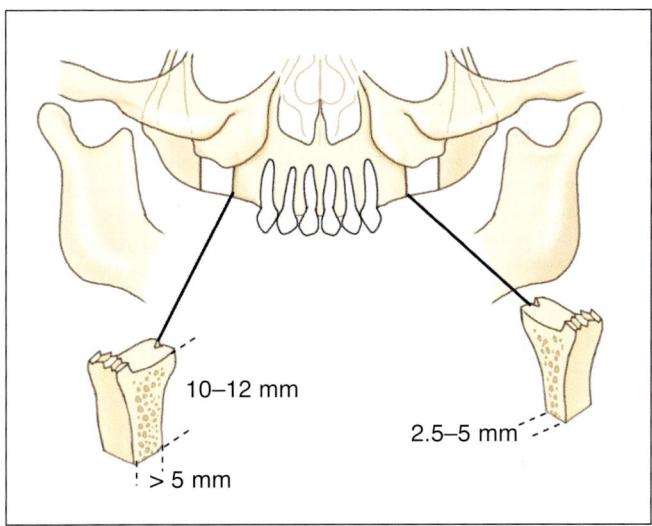

Fig 4-2c Option 2. When 10 to 12 mm of bone is present between the maxillary sinus floor and the crest of the ridge, the surgical approach may include sinus bone augmentation through the implant osteotomy, accompanied by implant placement.

and sinus membrane above the blunt end of the osteotome. A longer implant is then placed into the osteotomy, extending into the sinus cavity 2 to 3 mm beyond the available bone. It is not necessary to place bone graft material with so slight an elevation.

The success of sinus bone augmentation that is accomplished through the implant site cannot be confirmed at the time of implant placement.[4] Four to six months later, radiographic evidence of bone growth at the sinus floor demonstrates successful augmentation. Sinus perforation during the osteotome technique or implant placement will prevent bone formation from occurring. However, even if no bone forms around the apical portion of the implant, the cortical-like bone lining of the sinus engages the implant in the apical third region and improves implant rigidity and stress transfer to the bone-implant interface.

When alveolar width is insufficient (ie, division B or division C-w), onlay bone grafts are used to gain width either at the time of sinus elevation or after a healing delay (see chapter 21).

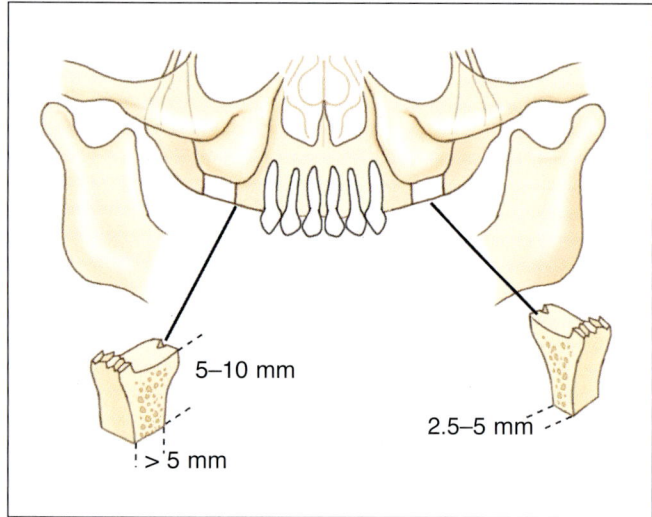 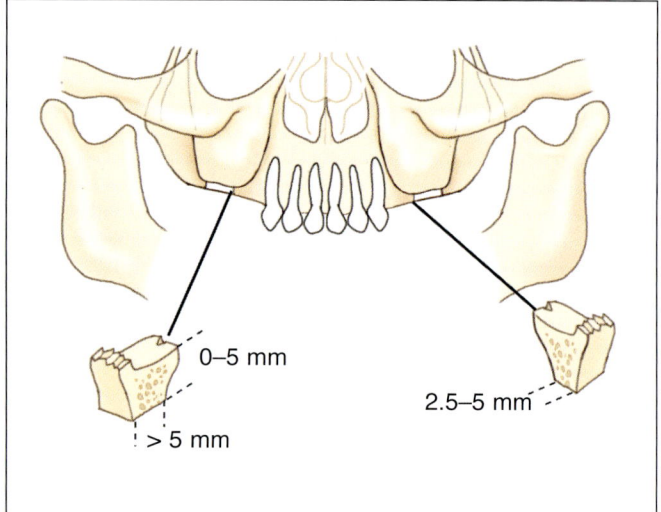

Fig 4-2d Option 3. When the remaining vertical bone height is 5 to 10 mm, a sinus graft is warranted to augment the residual bone. Dental implants may be placed under ideal conditions, either simultaneously or several months later to ensure that no sinus infection occurs postsurgery.

Fig 4-2e Option 4. Less than 5 mm of bone between the cortical floor and crest of the ridge requires sinus grafting prior to implant placement. When the crestal region is less than 5 mm in width (right), the ridge width should also be augmented.

Option 3: Sinus graft and immediate or delayed implant placement

When a minimum of 5 mm of vertical bone is present between the antral floor and the crest (Fig 4-2d), a third approach to the maxillary posterior edentulous region is indicated. A lateral approach to sinus augmentation is combined with onlay grafting when the original ridge width is narrow. If the ridge is adequate, the implant is placed at the same time as the sinus augmentation.[21–23] When implant stability is questionable, a delayed approach is recommended (see chapter 5).

A review of the literature on sinus grafts and simultaneous implant placement revealed success rates ranging from 75% to 97%.[24] Implants are lost most often because of postoperative complications such as infections. The infection rate is approximately 3% higher when implants are placed in conjunction with a sinus graft than when implants are placed in native bone.[21] When infection occurs, a bacterial smear layer forms over the implant surface, dramatically compromising the conditions necessary for osseointegration. The presence of an implant within the bone graft makes treatment of the infection more difficult. It is prudent to delay implant placement until the graft has consolidated in patients who are susceptible to infection, such as smokers and patients with poorly controlled diabetes. In addition, delayed implant placement into a healed graft allows the surgeon to assess bone quantity and quality at the same time. The delayed approach fixates the implant more rigidly than is possible during immediate placement because the apical portion of the implant engages mature bone graft.

The surgeon also is able to assess the availability of vertical bone when a delayed approach is used, avoiding inadvertent antral placement of the implants in "under-augmented" or resorbed sinus grafts. Upon re-entry to a sinus graft, it is not unusual to observe a craterlike bone defect at the lateral access window with attendant soft tissue invagination. This finding may relate to how densely the graft was placed or to the use of a barrier membrane (see chapters 14 and 19). If the implant is already in place in a poorly consolidated sinus graft, it may be difficult to remove nonossified tissues and accurately assess osseointegration. If possible, soft tissue is curetted and the site is re-grafted. Consideration should be given to removing an implant that is only partially integrated. The healing time for an implant placed into grafted bone depends on the type of graft materials used as well as host healing capacity.

Bone graft healing is related in part to the transantral dimension (medial to lateral wall). If this dimension is small (0 to 5 mm), healing time is optimal; if medium (5 to 15 mm), healing time is prolonged; if large (greater than 15 mm), healing time may be extended since graft material is further away from the endosteal blood supply. The suggested healing time after implant placement for these morphologies is 4, 6, and 8 months, respectively. In addition, a wide-flat sinus morphology suggests the use of autologous bone as the primary sinus graft material (see chapters 12 and 13).

Option 4: Delayed implant placement

When alveolar ridge height is 4 mm or less, a delayed approach is advocated (Fig 4-2e) (see chapter 5). At about 3 to 4 mm, the host bone is insufficient to provide implant stability at the time of sinus augmentation, and implant placement should be delayed. This option depends on minimal host bone, thus the need for greater graft volume. A compromised osseous bed, extensive pneumatization, and insufficient bone structure for primary implant stabilization require more time for bone graft consolidation prior to implant placement unless morphogenetic cell–based therapies are used (see chapters 25 and 30).

Regardless of the healing time before re-entry, the surgeon must consider sinus morphology, sinus depth (small, medium, or large), the amount of autologous bone in the graft, and overall graft volume when assessing the chances for success. The design of the implant, as in any region, depends on the amount and the morphology of available bone and the prosthesis that is planned.

In a staged approach, the bone graft is evaluated again at implant placement and after at least 4 additional months have elapsed for bone graft remodeling before prosthodontic reconstruction.

In 1998, Jensen[25] developed a similar classification based on a 10-mm (rather than a 12-mm) implant, which suggests a confluence of ideas from clinicians working independently.

Chiapasco Classification of the Posterior Maxilla

In 2003, Chiapasco modified existing sinus classifications with the aim of correlating morphology with current surgical reconstructive protocols.[26] He observed that implant placement in the residual bone of the posterior maxilla generally becomes less predictable when the absolute height of the residual alveolar ridge is less than 8 mm, regardless of the cause (sinus pneumatization or vertical alveolar resorption or a combination of both factors). Therefore, he evaluates and classifies the atrophic posterior maxilla not only by absolute residual bone height, but also by available width, intrasinus morphology, and the intermaxillary relationship, since the sinus-grafting procedures represent only one part of the reconstructive effort to restore orthoalveolar form.

His classification is based on three variables: width and height of the residual alveolus, and inter-ridge relation.[27–31] Evaluation of the horizontal and vertical relationship of the maxilla and mandible (and not only of residual bone volumes) is important to prevent construction of nonaxial prosthetic solutions (ie, long vertical crown height or unfavorable "crossbite" occlusion). These three variables are used to define nine types (classes A to I) of sinus–posterior maxillary–alveolar morphologies according to their treatment needs. Classes A to D address height and width, and the remaining classes define crown height space.

Class A

- Residual alveolar ridge height of 4 to 8 mm
- Residual alveolar width of at least 5 mm (ie, absence of significant horizontal resorption and maintenance of acceptable horizontal intermaxillary relationship)
- Absence of vertical resorption of the alveolar ridge with maintenance of acceptable vertical intermaxillary relationship

Suggested surgical protocol:
A. Sinus elevation with osteotome technique
B. Sinus elevation via lateral approach

Class B

- Residual alveolar ridge height of 4 to 8 mm
- Residual alveolar ridge width of less than 5 mm (ie, presence of horizontal resorption and unfavorable horizontal intermaxillary relationship)
- Absence of vertical resorption of the alveolar ridge with maintenance of acceptable vertical interarch distance

Suggested surgical protocol:
A. Sinus elevation and lateral bone grafting
B. Sinus elevation and guided bone regeneration

chapter 4 | Indications for and Classification of Sinus Bone Grafts

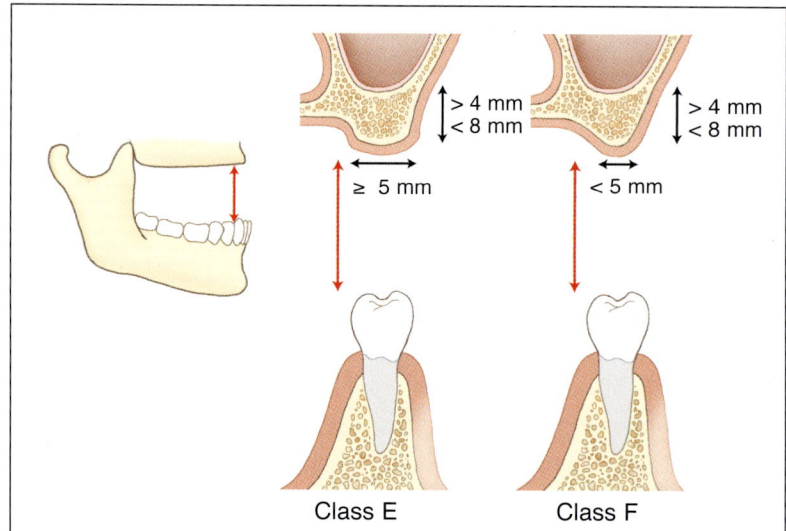

Fig 4-3a Class E: Increased crown height space with 4 to 8 mm of bone below the antrum and 5 mm or more of crestal bone width. Class F: Increased crown height space with 4 to 8 mm of bone below the antrum and less than 5 mm width of bone on the crest. (Reprinted from Chiapasco and Romeo[32] with permission.)

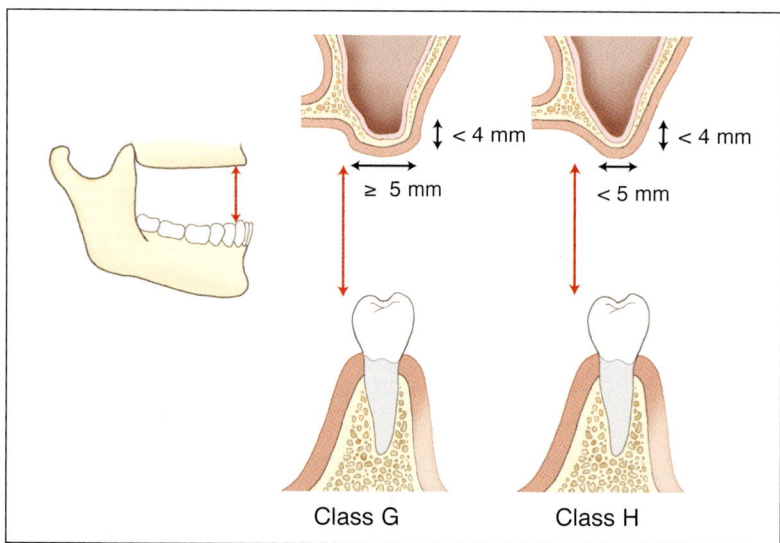

Fig 4-3b Class G: Increased crown height space with less than 4 mm of bone below the antrum and 5 mm or more of bone on the crest. Class H: Increased crown height space with less than 4 mm of bone below the antrum and less than 5 mm of bone in width on the crest. (Reprinted from Chiapasco and Romeo[32] with permission.)

Class C

- Residual alveolar ridge height of less than 4 mm
- Residual alveolar ridge width of at least 5 mm (ie, absence of significant horizontal resorption with maintenance of acceptable horizontal intermaxillary relationship)
- Absence of vertical resorption of the alveolar ridge with maintenance of acceptable vertical interarch distance

Suggested surgical protocol:
A. Sinus elevation via lateral approach

Class D

- Residual alveolar ridge height of less than 4 mm
- Residual alveolar ridge width of less than 5 mm (ie, presence of horizontal resorption and unfavorable horizontal intermaxillary relationship)
- Absence of vertical resorption of the alveolar ridge with maintenance of acceptable vertical interarch distance

Suggested surgical protocol:
A. Sinus elevation via lateral approach with lateral bone grafting
B. Sinus elevation and guided bone regeneration

Class E

- Same characteristics as class A except with increased crown height space (Fig 4-3a)

48

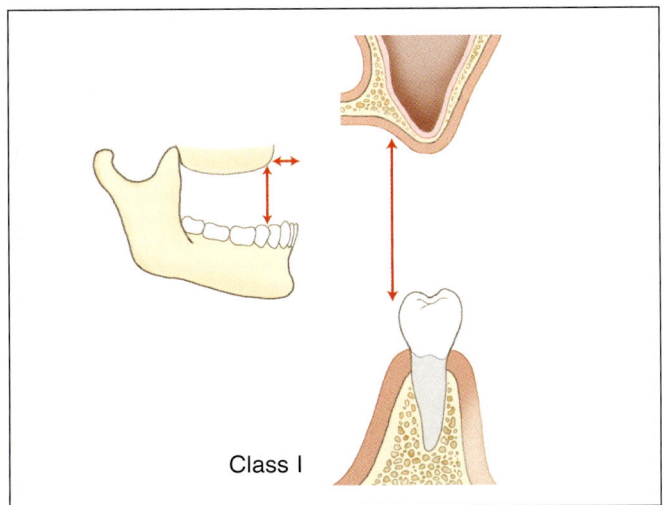

Fig 4-3c Class I: Three-dimensional atrophy of the edentulous maxilla with increased crown height space. (Reprinted from Chiapasco and Romeo[32] with permission.)

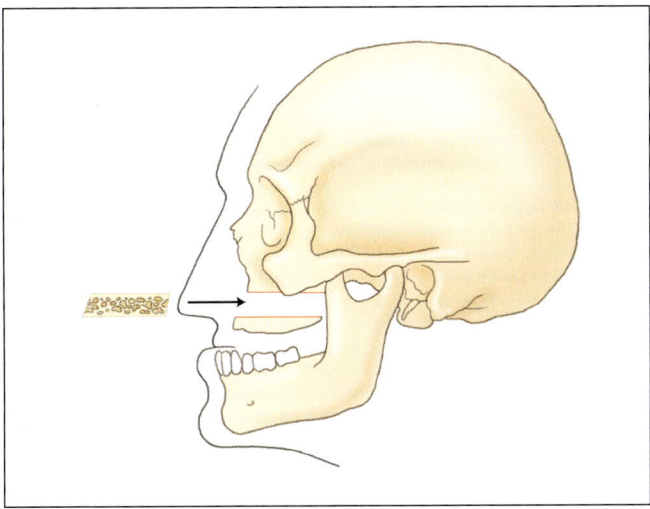

Fig 4-3d Le Fort I osteotomy with downward and forward repositioning of the maxilla and interpositional bone grafts. (Reprinted from Chiapasco and Romeo[32] with permission.)

Suggested surgical protocol:
A. Vertical onlay grafts with autogenous bone block
B. Interpositional alveolar bone graft (see chapter 24)
C. Vertical guided bone regeneration
D. Vertical distraction osteogenesis

The sinus graft procedure is associated with one of these procedures, but only if correction of the vertical intermaxillary discrepancy is insufficient to obtain adequate bone volume for implant placement.

Class F

- Same characteristics as class B except with increased vertical crown height space (see Fig 4-3a)

Suggested surgical protocol:
A. Simultaneous vertical and horizontal onlay grafts with autogenous bone blocks
B. Interpositional bone graft without sinus grafting
C. Simultaneous vertical and horizontal guided bone regeneration

Vertical distraction osteogenesis is not indicated because the technique does not correct the horizontal defect.

Class G

- Same characteristics as class C except with increased vertical crown height space (Fig 4-3b)

Suggested surgical protocol:
A. Sinus graft via a lateral approach combined with vertical autogenous block onlay graft
B. Sinus graft with vertical guided bone regeneration

Class H

- Same characteristics as class D except with increased vertical crown height space (see Fig 4-3b)

Suggested surgical protocol:
A. Sinus graft via a lateral approach with simultaneous vertical and horizontal onlay block grafts
B. Sinus graft with simultaneous vertical and horizontal guided bone regeneration

Class I

- Severe tridimensional atrophy of the edentulous maxilla to basal bone with increased vertical crown implant space, horizontal resorption, sagittal intermaxillary discrepancy with maxillary retrognathism, and flat maxillary morphology (Fig 4-3c)

Suggested surgical protocol[33–36]:
A. Le Fort I osteotomy with advancement and interpositional autogenous bone graft (Fig 4-3d)
B. Reconstruction with revascularized free flap (fibula free flap)

The Le Fort I osteotomy is combined with lateral and anterior bone onlay grafts to improve the width of the atrophic residual ridge (see chapter 20).

The free flap alternative is more complex and surgically demanding than the Le Fort I osteotomy. It requires harvesting a bone transplant with a vascular pedicle that must be anastomosed to cervical vessels through an extraoral approach. Therefore, this procedure is generally reserved for tumor resections or cases of such extreme atrophy that maxillary basal bone is essentially absent. Free flaps may also be indicated when there is poor quality and quantity of oral mucosa covering the residual bone of the maxilla from previous failed reconstruction attempts with bone grafts or irradiated tissues; bisphosphonate lesions; or odd antral defects in which free flaps are indicated.

Conclusion

Sinus grafting has been demonstrated to be a safe and predictable procedure for the correction of the atrophic edentulous maxilla, whether it is accomplished alone or in conjunction with other reconstructive procedures, such as bone grafts, guided bone regeneration, or distraction osteogenesis.

Disuse remodeling of the sinus and posterior maxillary morphology following tooth loss suggests various treatment options based on site classification. When approached and managed properly, these techniques lead not only to implant survival but also to restoration of interarch orthoalveolar form and function.

References

1. Misch CE. Treatment planning for edentulous maxillary posterior region. In: Misch CE (ed). Contemporary Implant Dentistry. St Louis: Mosby, 1993:241–255.
2. Pietrokovski J. The bony residual ridge in man. J Prosthet Dent 1975;34:456–462.
3. Misch CE. Divisions of available bone in implant dentistry. Int J Oral Maxillofac Implants 1990;7:9–17.
4. Misch CE. Treatment planning for edentulous posterior maxilla. In: Misch CE (ed). Contemporary Implant Dentistry, ed 2. St Louis: Mosby, 1999:193–204.
5. Goodacre JC, Bernal G, Riringcharassaeng K, Kan JY. Clinical complications with implants and implant prostheses. J Prosthet Dent 2003;2:121–132.
6. Misch CE. Bone character: Second vital implant criterion. Dent Today 1988;7:39–40.
7. Misch CE, Qu Z, Bidez MW. Mechanical properties of trabecular bone in the human mandible: Implications for dental implant treatment planning and surgical placement. J Oral Maxillofac Surg 1999;57:700–706.
8. Misch CE. Density of bone: Effect on treatment plans, surgical approach, healing and progressive loading. Int J Oral Implantol 1990;6:23–31.
9. Misch CE. Bone density. In: Misch CE (ed). Contemporary Implant Dentistry. St Louis: Mosby, 1993:241–255.
10. Jaffin RA, Berman CL. The excessive loss of Brånemark fixtures in Type IV bone: A 5-year analysis. J Periodontol 1991;62:2–4.
11. Scott I, Ash MM Jr. A six-channel intra-oral transmitter for measuring occlusal forces. J Prosthet Dent 1966;16:56.
12. Anderson DJ. Measurements of stress in mastication. J Dent Res 1958;35:644–671.
13. Misch CE, Bidez MW. A scientific rationale for dental implant design. In: Misch CE (ed). Contemporary Implant Dentistry, ed 2. St Louis: Mosby, 1999:329–343.
14. Misch CE. Divisions of available bone. In: Misch CE (ed). Contemporary Implant Dentistry, ed 2. St Louis: Mosby, 1999:89–107.
15. Bidez MW, Misch CE. Force transfer in implant dentistry: Basic concepts and principles. Oral Implantol 1992;18:264–274.
16. Shillingburg HE, Hobo S, Whitsett LD. Fundamentals of Fixed Prosthodontics. Chicago: Quintessence, 1997.
17. Misch CE, Judy KW. Classification of the partially edentulous arches for implant dentistry. Int J Oral Implantol 1987;4:7–12.
18. Misch CE. Maxillary sinus augmentation for endosteal implants: Organized alternative treatment plans. Int J Oral Implantol 1987;4:49–58.
19. Cawood JI, Howell R. A classification of the edentulous jaws. Int J Oral Maxillofac Surg 1988;17:232–236.
20. Tatum OH. Maxillary and sinus implant reconstruction. Dent Clin North Am 1986;30:107–119.
21. Tatum OH, Lebowitz MS, Tatum CA, et al. Sinus augmentation: Rationale, development, long term results. NY State Dent J 1993;(May):43–48.
22. Wood RM, Moore DL. Grafting of the maxillary sinus with intraorally harvested autogenous bone prior to implant placement. Int J Oral Maxillofac Implants 1988;3:209–214.
23. Blomqvist JE, Alberius P, Isaksson S. Retrospective analysis of one stage maxillary sinus augmentation with endosseous implants. Int J Oral Maxillofac Implants 1996;11:512–521.
24. Jensen OT (ed). The Sinus Bone Graft. Chicago: Quintessence, 1999.
25. Jensen OT, Leonard BS, Block MS, Iacono VJ. Report of the Sinus Consensus Conference of 1996. Int J Oral Maxillofac Implants 1998;13(suppl):11–30.
26. Chiapasco M. Tecniche ricostruttive con innesti e/o osteotomie. In: Chiapasco M, Romeo E (eds). Riabilitazione Implanto-Protesica Dei Casi Complessi. Torino: UTET, 2003:225–303.
27. Jensen J, Sindet-Pedersen S, Oliver AJ. Varying treatment strategies for reconstruction of maxillary atrophy with implants: Results in 98 patients. J Oral Maxillofac Surg 1994;52:210–216.

28. Chiapasco M, Romeo E, Vogel G. Vertical distraction osteogenesis of edentulous ridges for improvement of oral implant positioning: A clinical report of preliminary results. Int J Oral Maxillofac Implants 2001;16:43–51.
29. Chiapasco M, Consolo U, Bianchi A, Ronchi P. Alveolar distraction osteogenesis for the correction of vertically deficient edentulous ridges: A multicenter prospective study on humans. Int J Oral Maxillofac Implants 2004;19:399–407.
30. Chiapasco M, Ferrieri G, Rossi A, Senna A, Accardi S. Rialzo del seno mascellare a scopo implantologico. Implantologia Orale 2001;2:22–46.
31. Chiapasco M, Ronchi P. Sinus lift and endosseous implants: Preliminary surgical and prosthetic results. Eur J Prosthodont Restorative Dent 1994;3:15–21.
32. Chiapasco M, Romeo E, eds. Riabilitazione Implanto-Protesica Dei Casi Complessi. Torino: UTET, 2003.
33. Chiapasco M, Gatti C. Immediate loading of dental implants placed in revascularized fibula free flaps: A clinical report on two consecutive patients. Int J Oral Maxillofac Implants 2004;19:906–912.
34. Stoelinga PJW, Slagter AP, Brouns JJA. Rehabilitation of patients with severe (Class VI) maxillary resorption using Le Fort I osteotomy, interposed bone grafts, and endosteal implants: 1–8 years follow-up on a two-stage procedure. Int J Oral Maxillofac Surg 2000;29:188–193.
35. Nocini PF, De Santis G, Bedogni A, Chiarini L. Simultaneous bimaxillary alveolar ridge augmentation by a single free fibular transfer: A case report. J Craniomaxillofac Surg 2002;30:46–53.
36. Sailer HF. A new method of inserting endosseous implants in totally atrophic maxillae. J Craniomaxillofac Surg 1989;17:299–305.

chapter 5
Sinus Floor Augmentation: Simultaneous Versus Delayed Implant Placement

Ronald M. Achong, DMD, MD
Michael S. Block, DMD

Implant therapy in the posterior maxilla constitutes a challenging clinical situation. Alveolar bone resorption and pneumatization of the sinus cavity reduce the amount of alveolar bone necessary to maintain a predictable implant-supported prosthesis. This problem can be overcome by grafting the maxillary sinus floor to provide sufficient quantity of bone for placement of endosteal implants to support prosthetic reconstruction. This chapter presents the indications and contraindications for simultaneous implant placement into the bone-grafted sinus.

Tatum was the first clinician to suggest a crestal approach for sinus floor elevation and placement of submerged implants.[1] The technique, used in thin residual crestal bone, involved an upfracture into the sinus using a socket-forming instrument. A bone graft was placed beneath the tented sinus membrane. Later, a modified Caldwell-Luc procedure was developed in which the lateral sinus wall was infractured and the wall was used to help elevate the sinus membrane. Autogenous bone was then placed into the area. In 1980, Boyne reported a similar surgical procedure and demonstrated bone formation after placement of autogenous iliac marrow.[2] He suggested a horizontal incision starting from the canine fossa and extending posteriorly at a level 6 mm superior to the attached mucosa. A 1-cm-diameter antrostomy was made in the lateral sinus wall. Implants were placed 3 months after bone grafting. Since then, a variety of techniques have been described for augmenting the maxillary sinus floor.

Two general procedures for sinus elevation for dental implant placement are currently in use: a two-stage technique using a lateral window approach, and a one-stage technique using a lateral or a lateral from a crest approach.[3–6] The decision to use a one- or two-stage technique is made based on the amount of bone present at the alveolar crest and other case-specific considerations to be discussed in this chapter.

Sinus Augmentation and Delayed Implant Placement

Sinus augmentation with delayed implant placement has been performed for more than 20 years.[7,8] A review of the literature shows that delayed implant placement is more likely used in cases that have minimal available bone as opposed to simultaneous placement in cases that have a greater residual crestal bone height.[9–12] The Academy of Osseointegration Sinus Consensus Conference Failure Analysis Section reported that simultaneous placement in the severely atrophic maxilla (ie, in less than 2 mm of bone) is more prone to implant loss than a delayed technique unless blocks of bone are used to stabilize the implants.

In 1990, Jensen et al rehabilitated severely atrophic maxillae using bilateral sinus bone grafting and delayed

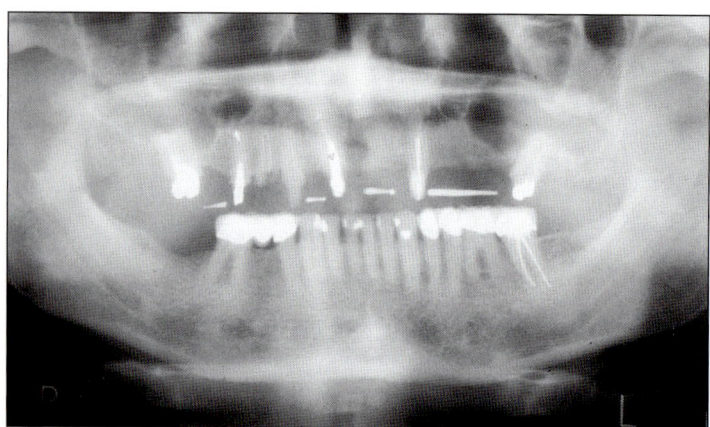

Fig 5-1a Preoperative panoramic radiograph.

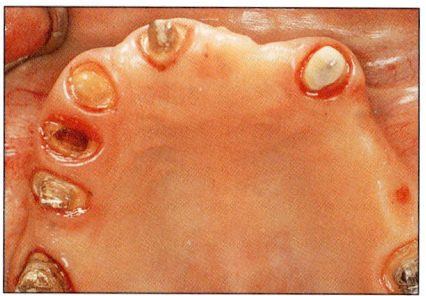

Fig 5-1b Occlusal view of maxilla prior to the sinus grafting procedure.

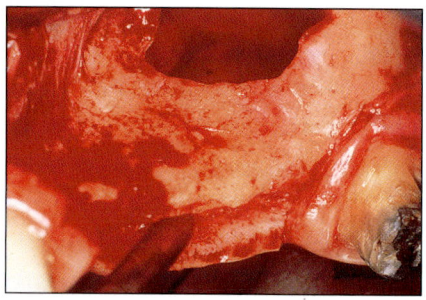

Fig 5-1c An incision is made over the crest with vertical release. The lateral wall of the maxilla has been rotated medially in preparation for the sinus graft.

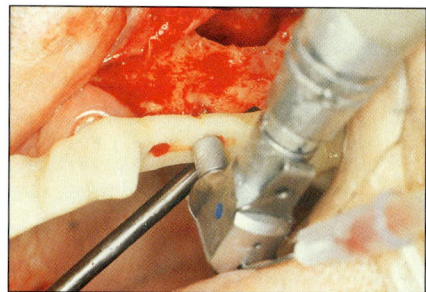

Fig 5-1d Because the patient has more than 3 mm of crestal bone, the template is placed and the implant sites are prepared.

placement of dental implants 4 months later.[9] Nine of the 36 implants placed in the grafted bone failed. In 1991, Hall and McKenna performed 44 maxillary sinus elevations in 22 patients using particulate bone and cancellous marrow with delayed implant placement.[10] Though the sinus floor was less than 3 mm thick, a 90% implant success rate was observed after 5 years of follow-up. In 2002, Hallman et al evaluated the survival rate of implants placed in delayed fashion into 30 maxillary sinuses augmented with a mixture of 80% bovine hydroxyapatite and 20% autogenous bone mixed with fibrin glue.[11] The mean alveolar bone height was 3.8 mm. After 6 months of primary healing, 108 implants were placed and followed for 1 year. Implant survival rate was 90.7%. Dimensional change of the bone grafts was also evaluated. A mean decrease of 1.4 mm (< 10%) in the height of the bone grafts was found after 1 year, which is statistically significant ($p < .001$). In 2004, Hallman and Nordin retrospectively evaluated a mixture of bovine hydroxyapatite and fibrin glue as grafting material using a delayed placement with nonsubmerged implants after graft consolidation.[12] A total of 71 maxillary sinuses were augmented and the grafts allowed to consolidate for 8 months. A total of 218 solid titanium screw-type implants were placed, and a mean of 10 weeks of healing was allowed before loading. In this study, there was a 94.5% implant survival rate after 20 months of occlusal function.

Sinus Augmentation and Simultaneous Implant Placement

Simultaneously with grafting procedures, Tatum placed implants via both lateral and crestal approaches.[1] In the latter, a "socket former" was used to establish the implant position, and greenstick fracture of the sinus floor was accomplished by hand tapping in a vertical direction. Summers[13] later described a similar technique using tapered osteotomes with increasing diameters. Adjacent bone is compressed by pushing and tapping as the sinus mem-

Sinus Augmentation and Simultaneous Implant Placement

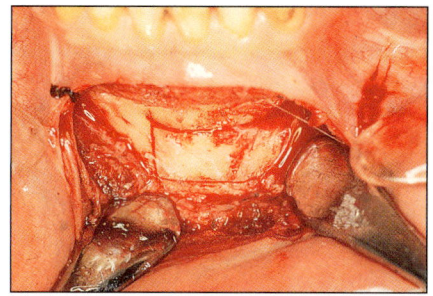

Fig 5-1e The chin is approached through a vestibular incision, and a sagittal saw is used to outline the cortex, which is then removed.

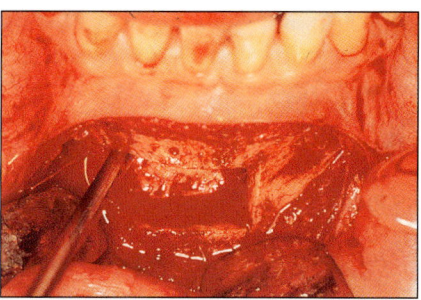

Fig 5-1f Cancellous bone is harvested from the chin.

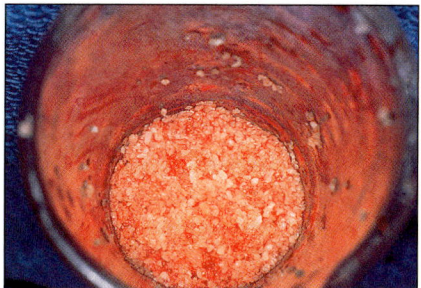

Fig 5-1g The cancellous bone is particulated and combined with an equal volume of demineralized bone.

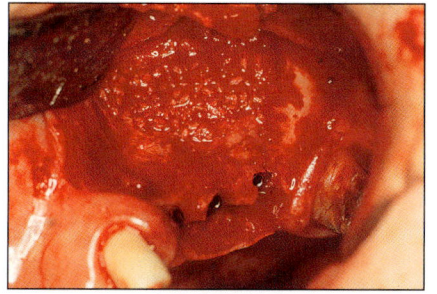

Fig 5-1h The bone is placed in the sinus with the membrane elevated. The implants are placed, and additional bone is placed over the implants and the thin alveolar ridge.

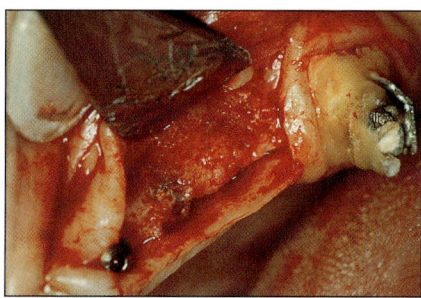

Fig 5-1i Six months later, a crestal incision bisecting the keratinized gingiva is used to expose the implants.

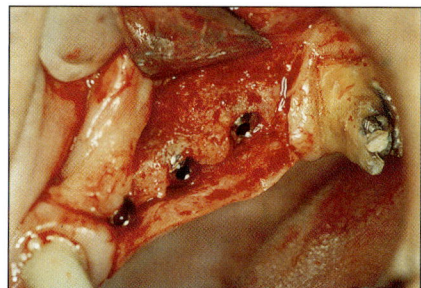

Fig 5-1j A rongeur forceps is used to expose the implants, which were covered with healing bone.

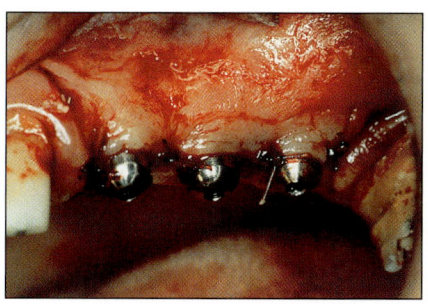

Fig 5-1k The gingiva is sutured around temporary healing abutments.

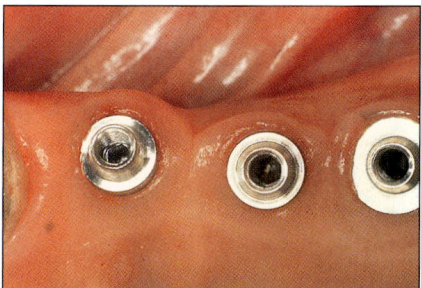

Fig 5-1l Occlusal view of the tissue around the implants.

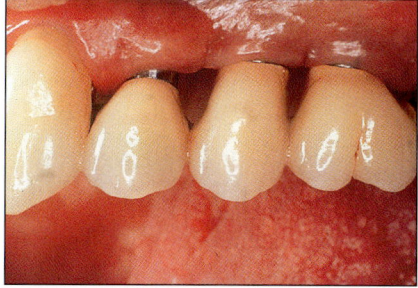

Fig 5-1m Lateral view of the implant-supported restoration. (Prosthetics by Dr Gerard Chiche, New Orleans, Louisiana.)

brane is elevated. Bone is conserved by the osteotome technique because no drilling is done. Summers added autogenous, allogeneic, or xenogenic bone and compacted the elevated sinus[13] (see chapter 22). Elevation of the sinus floor 4 to 5 mm was reported for this one-stage implant technique. Summers followed 143 press-fit submerged implants for 18 months of loading and reported a success rate of 96%.[13]

In the Sinus Consensus Conference,[14] the survival rate of implants placed simultaneously with a bone graft into the maxillary sinus was compared with the survival rate of those placed 6 to 9 months after sinus augmentation (Fig 5-1). Of the 785 implants in the simultaneous group, 133 had failed after 5 years for an overall success rate of 85.8%. However, this outcome was not statistically significant ($p < .001$). A confounding variable was found when

Chapter 5: Sinus Floor Augmentation: Simultaneous Versus Delayed Implant Placement

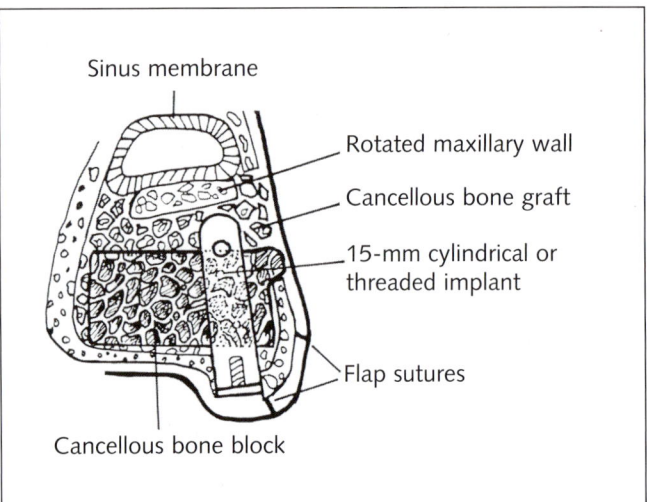

Fig 5-2a Method for treating the following patient, who has less than 1 mm of alveolar bone height. A block of bone will be used to support implants placed simultaneously with the graft.

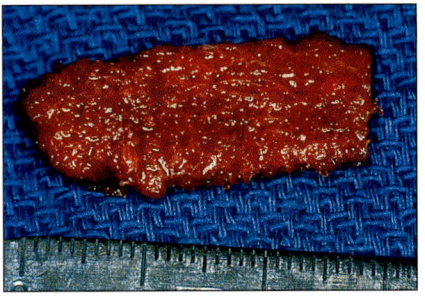

Fig 5-2b Cancellous bone harvested from the iliac crest.

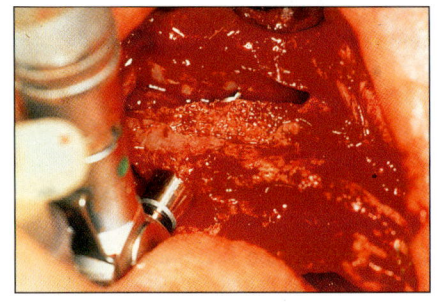

Fig 5-2c The cancellous bone is placed into the sinus after the lateral wall of the maxilla and the sinus membrane have been elevated. After placement of the cancellous bone block, the implant sites are prepared in a customary manner.

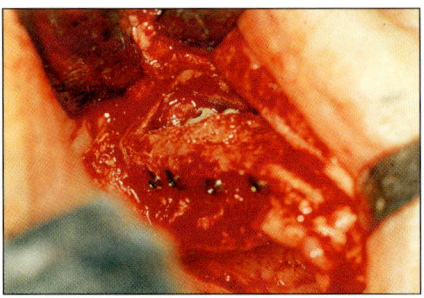

Fig 5-2d The graft and implants are in place. Additional cancellous bone was placed to cover the superior portion of the implants and fill in voids.

the surface of the implant in the simultaneous cases was rough, or coated with hydroxyapatite, which improved the rate of success in contrast to a machined surface. Despite these added variables, when all simultaneous cases were compared with all delayed approaches, a better success rate was found with a delayed approach.

When comparing simultaneous grafting to implant placement with delayed approaches, the length of the delay also was found to be a factor. A delay of 4 to 8 months compared with a delay of greater than 8 months demonstrated a much better success rate after 8 months with a 3-year survival rate of 97%. The shorter 4- to 8-month delay yielded a 3-year success rate of 84%.[14] These results suggest a clinical protocol for implant staging related to graft material selection.

Another comparison analyzed by the Sinus Consensus Conference was particulate versus block forms of graft material (Figs 5-2 and 5-3). Most of the blocks were obtained from the iliac crest, whereas particulate autogenous bone was harvested from the hip or jaw. There was minimal difference found between the form of the graft (particulate or block) and the final result. There was decreased success associated with use of the simultaneous block compared to the delayed block placement. However, because only a small number of blocks were available to the Consensus Conference, and because these block grafts tended to be used when there was very limited residual alveolar bone, the results may be biased to a more difficult bone mass scenario.

Failure analysis at the conference indicated that the initial thickness of residual alveolar bone is an important fac-

Fig 5-2e Lateral cephalogram showing the parallel placement of the implants.

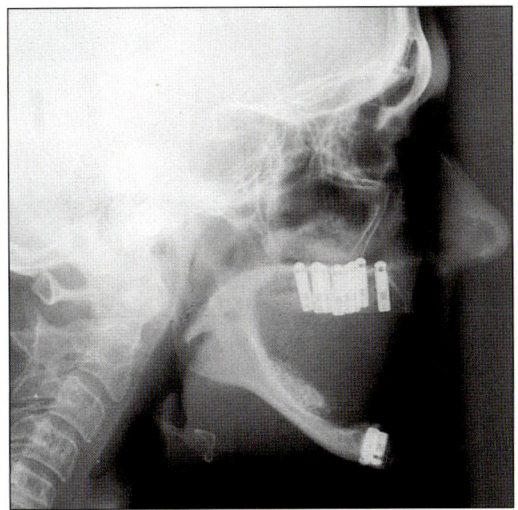

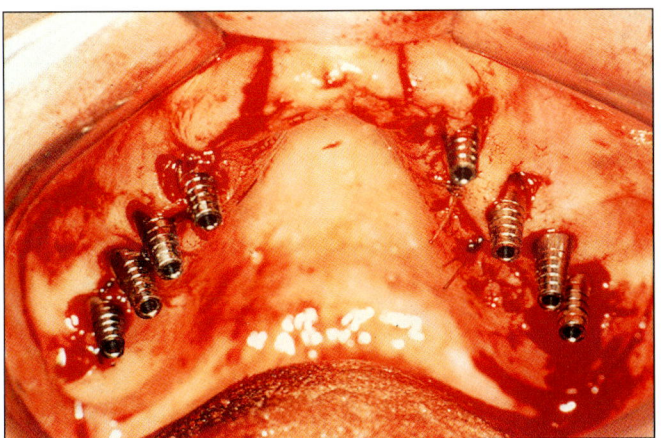

Fig 5-2f After 6 months, the implants are exposed and abutments are placed.

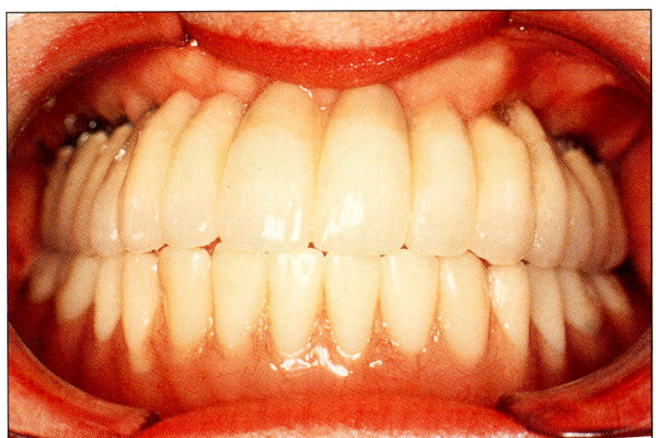

Fig 5-2g Fixed restoration in place. (Prosthetics by Dr Larry McMillen, Metairie, Louisiana.)

tor when considering treatment method. In a thin alveolus, implants are not adequately stabilized unless block bone is used to mechanically prevent implant mobility. Therefore, most clinicians use a guideline of a minimum thickness of remaining bone to determine the bone graft and treatment plan. Implants are placed simultaneously or by a two-stage delayed approach based on bone availability.

Based on empirical observations, a one-stage procedure with simultaneous grafting and implant placement is not performed unless at least 4 mm of alveolar bone is available to stabilize implants.[3] Less than 4 mm is considered insufficient endosteum to mechanically maintain the implants, and a two-stage procedure is recommended.[3] Though clinicians still cannot agree on an absolute bone mass minimum for simultaneous placement, a two-stage procedure is performed by experienced implant surgeons when there is a risk for implant displacement during the healing phase (Box 5-1).

The key to determining if the procedure should be performed in one stage or two is the ability of the surgeon to place a fixed dental implant. The distance between the threads of most threaded dental implants ranges from 0.65 to 0.80 mm. Therefore, in order to engage three threads, one must have at least 2.5 mm of bone, and for five threads, about 4 mm of bone. Most clinicians would prefer to have more than a few threads engaged in bone for a simultaneous sinus graft procedure. The 4- to 5-mm level is often suggested as a minimum by experienced sinus graft surgeons. In the end, it is a judgment call and should be based on surgical experience.[3]

chapter 5 Sinus Floor Augmentation: Simultaneous Versus Delayed Implant Placement

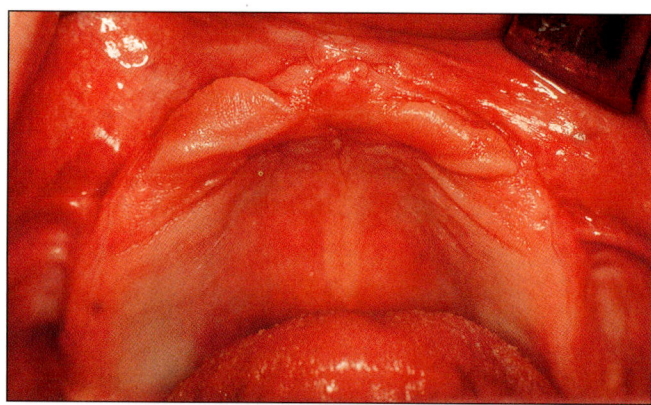

Fig 5-3a Maxilla of a patient who was unable to wear his maxillary denture and chew hard food comfortably. His physical examination revealed flabby anterior maxillary soft tissue and severe maxillary atrophy.

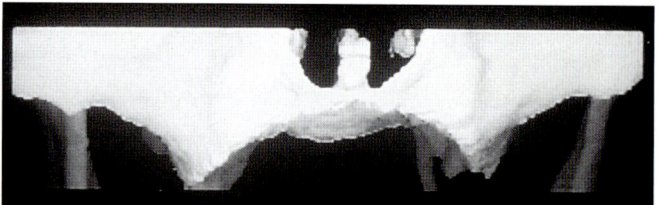

Fig 5-3b Three-dimensional reconstructed computerized tomography (CT) scan (Columbia Scientific Software) demonstrating severe anterior maxillary resorption, consistent with his opposing anterior mandibular intact dentition.

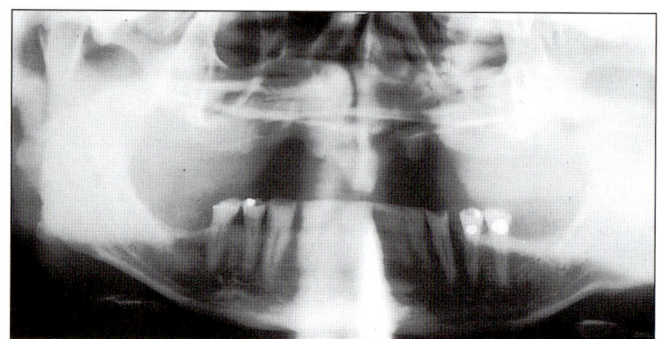

Fig 5-3c Panoramic radiograph showing the intact anterior mandibular teeth without posterior occlusion, resulting in severe anterior maxillary atrophy.

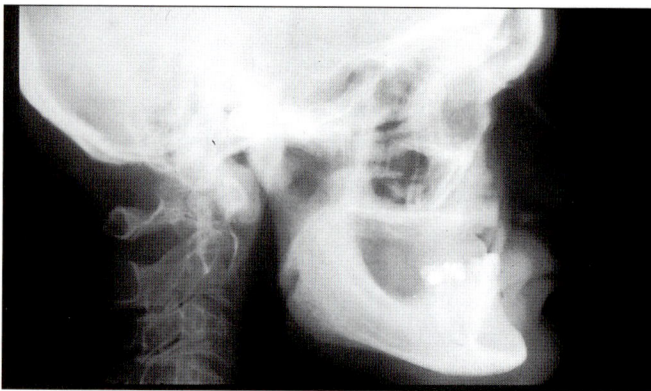

Fig 5-3d Lateral cephalogram showing the closed vertical dimension and flat occlusal plane.

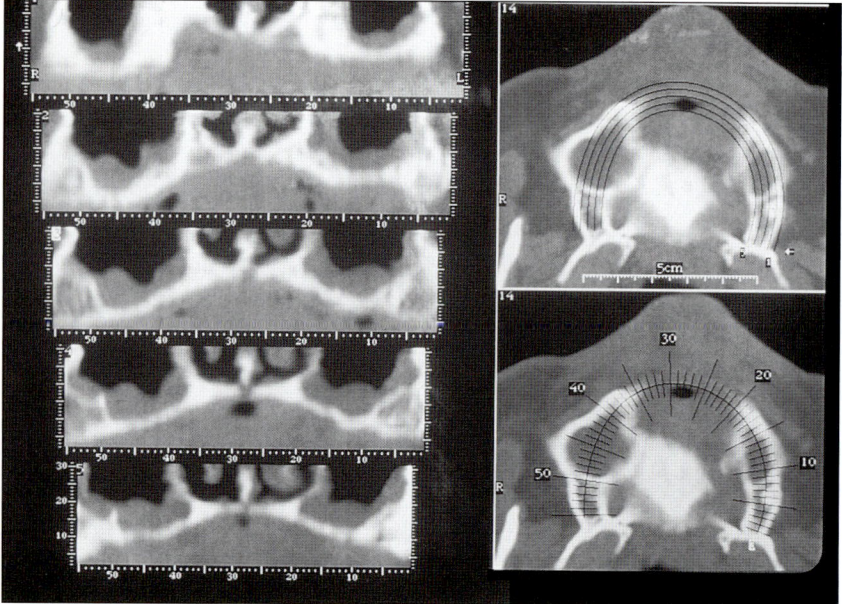

Fig 5-3e Reconstructed panoramic views showing the posterior and anterior severe maxillary atrophy. Without a bone graft, bone is insufficient for placement of implants in the maxilla.

Sinus Augmentation and Simultaneous Implant Placement

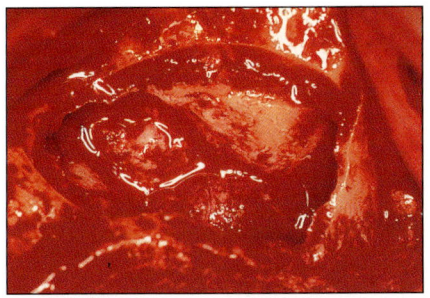

Fig 5-3f Bilaterally, the lateral wall of the maxilla is rotated medially with elevation of the sinus membrane.

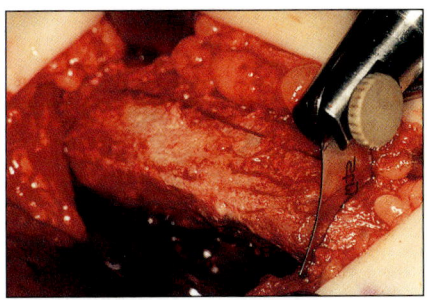

Fig 5-3g Corticocancellous blocks are harvested from the anterior iliac crest.

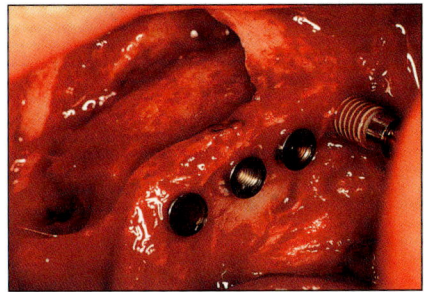

Fig 5-3h The bone blocks are trimmed to fit within the sinus and retained with hydroxyapatite-coated threaded implants.

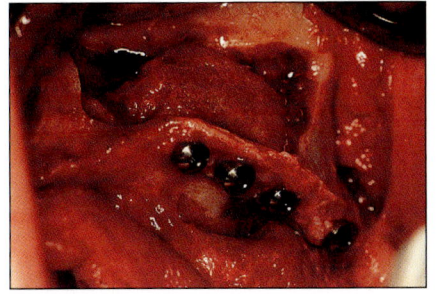

Fig 5-3i Four implants are placed into each graft on both sides of the maxilla.

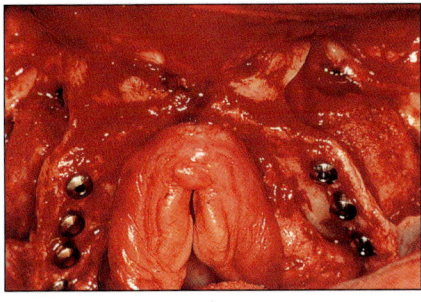

Fig 5-3j After the sinus grafts are completed, the anterior maxillary defect is examined.

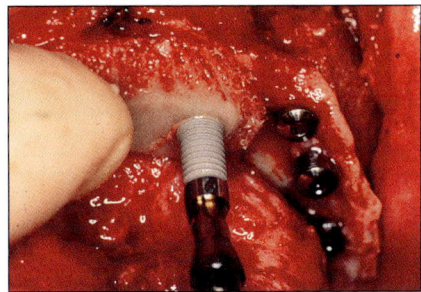

Fig 5-3k A block of bone is screw retained to the anterior maxilla, using two hydroxyapatite-coated threaded implants.

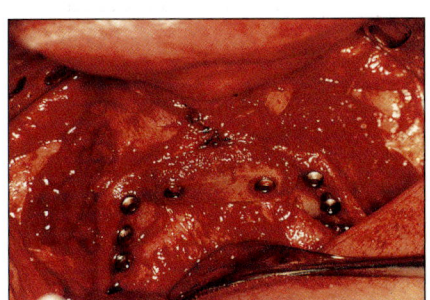

Fig 5-3l The reconstruction is completed.

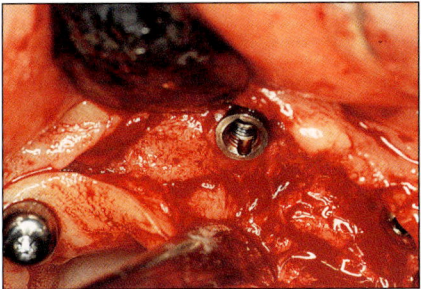

Fig 5-3m After 6 months, excellent bone is present over the anterior implants placed in the onlay bone graft.

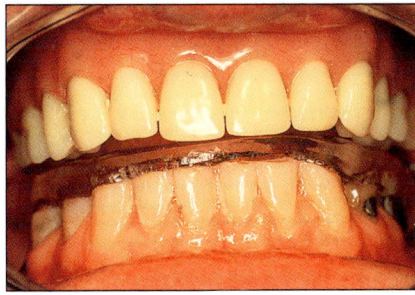

Fig 5-3n Spark-erosion prosthesis was made over the implants, and the vertical dimension of occlusion was increased gradually with a splint when a new mandibular prosthesis was made. (Prosthetics by Dr Israel Finger, New Orleans, Louisiana.)

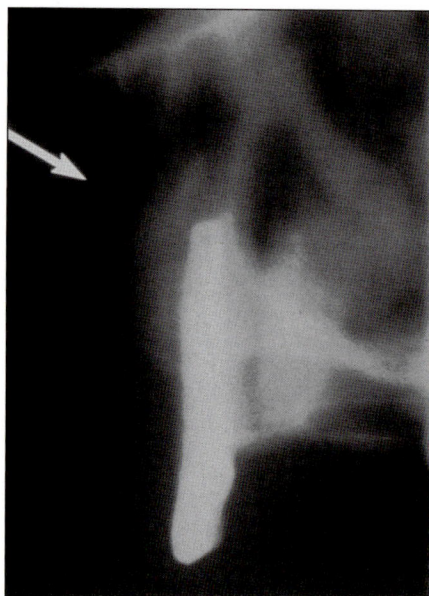 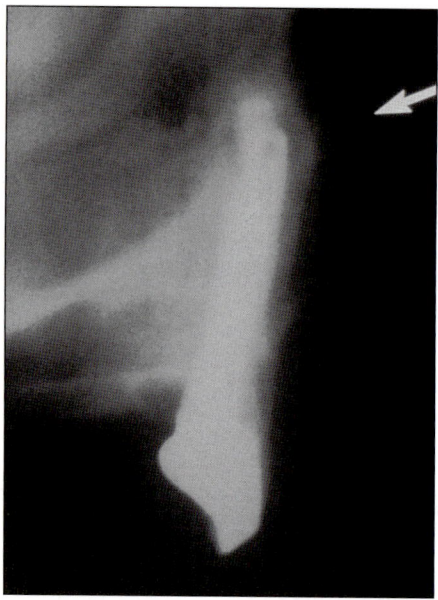

Fig 5-3o Five-year follow-up complex-motion tomogram of implants. *(Left)* Left posterior. *(Right)* Right posterior. *Arrows* indicate bone at apical region of implants.

BOX 5-1 Is there a minimum residual bone height for simultaneous implants and bone grafting?

There is no minimal bone height required for implant placement; rather, it is a question of implant stability sufficient for bone modeling leading to early osseointegration. Osseointegration in itself is dependent on many factors, and modeling and remodeling capacity of the bone graft is determined by a host of different physiologic factors.

From a biomechanical viewpoint, however, the question may be divided into two: *(a)* What residual bone height is required for the implant to remain stable *during* bone healing? And *(b)* what *healing time* is required before implant loading is possible?

Implant Stability
If type 3 bone is present and the cortex is approximately 1 mm, the rest of the bone height will not substantially contribute to the initial implant stability. This conclusion is based on clinical experience and is supported by FE-analysis.[15] If there is delayed loading, an insertion torque of less than 30 Ncm is sufficient for stable healing. If there is only 0.5 mm of residual bone height, but a fixed block bone graft is used in the sinus floor implant, anchorage will likely proceed to osseointegration.

Sufficient implant anchorage, not bone height, is the key factor with regard to osseointegration. Bone volume and density are relevant as implant procedure criteria when estimating load-bearing capacity for immediate function, but they are not as important for initial stability.

Healing Time
Before loading, bone remodeling is needed to increase the load-bearing capacity, which is the purpose of the grafting procedure. The remodeling is among other matters dependent on the bone vascularity and the implant surface, but not specifically on the initial stability when the implant is not loaded. The required healing time is dictated by how much increase in load-bearing capacity is wanted and the time sequences for the bone remodeling and formation to take place. In general, for loading of implants simultaneously placed in autograft, 4 months is minimum (see chapter 7). Cell-based therapies hold promise to reduce this to 2 to 3 months (see chapter 30).

In conclusion, there is no specific bone height limit for simultaneous implant placement and bone grafting. Practically speaking, the surgical requirement is to stabilize the implant one way or another so that osseointegration can take place.

Bo Rangert, Franck Renouard, Paulo Maló

Influence of Implant Surface and Graft Material on Success Rates

In 1989, Kent and Block presented a modified lateral maxillary wall infracture technique for sinus floor elevation and simultaneous placement of hydroxyapatite-coated implants.[16] Eighteen sinus augmentation procedures using iliac cancellous bone with placement of 54 implants were performed. The implants were restored 4 to 6 months later. No failures were noted over a 4-year follow-up period. To date, numerous studies have been published on simultaneous implant placement into augmented maxillary sinuses using various bone graft materials and implant surfaces. In 1999, Khoury reported on 216 sinus graft procedures in 216 patients.[17] The initial bone height at the implant site was between 1 and 5 mm. The maxillary sinus was augmented with block bone grafts harvested from the retromolar, ramus, or symphysis areas of the mandible. Implants were placed to stabilize the block grafts to the maxillary sinus floor and left to heal for 9 months. The average follow-up period was 49 months with a 94% implant success rate.

In 1997, Daelemans et al reported a similar success rate of 93.4% for the single-stage procedure.[18] In their study, 121 implants were placed in 44 maxillary sinuses augmented with corticocancellous iliac bone. The implants were uncovered 6 months later. Pretreatment alveolar bone height was less than 5 mm.

In 1999, Peleg et al assessed the efficacy of performing a one-stage procedure in patients whose available alveolar bone height in the posterior maxilla was between 3 and 5 mm prior to grafting: 3 mm in 23 patients, 4 mm in 18 patients, and 5 mm in 22 patients.[19] Using the modified Caldwell-Luc technique, the maxillary sinus was augmented with symphyseal and demineralized freeze-dried bone combined in a 1:1 ratio. Hydroxyapatite-coated dental implants, ranging in length from 13 to 15 mm, were placed and allowed to integrate. In all, 160 implants were placed in 63 grafted sinuses. A 100% success rate of both the implants and the prostheses was reported after a 4-year follow-up. Peleg et al reported a second study using a similar protocol, but the alveolar bone height was only 1 to 2 mm.[20] Fifty-five hydroxyapatite-coated dental implants were placed in 20 grafted sinuses. All implants osseointegrated successfully. No implants were lost after loading in a 26-month follow-up. In 2004, Hatano et al reported long-term maintenance of sinus graft height with simultaneous placement of implants in sinuses with 4 to 6 mm of alveolar bone height available for implant stabilization.[21]

Block et al[22] reported on bone maintenance 5 to 10 years after sinus grafting with simultaneous implant placement. After 70 implants were evaluated in 31 patients, the authors concluded that autogenous bone grafts are maintained after loading. Allograft adversely affects long-term bone levels in the implant apical region, but this was not clinically significant. In a simultaneous study by Block and Kent, the cumulative survival rate of the implants was 94.2%, and all of the implant losses occured within 3 years of placement.[23] After 2 to 3 years, the grafted sinus floor remodels to become level with or slightly below the implant apex. This relationship is maintained over the long term (Figs 5-4 and 5-5).[22]

Though individual studies involving simultaneous placement of implants in grafted maxillary sinuses report implant success rates comparable to those achieved in a delayed approach, studies that directly compare simultaneous with delayed implant placement report variable success rates. Valentini and Abensur[24] studied the survival rate of titanium plasma spray-coated cylindrical and machined screw-type implants placed in sinuses grafted exclusively with anorganic bovine bone. Twenty-seven implants were placed simultaneously during xenografting for a success rate of 92.6%. The delayed placement protocol yielded 98% success. Implant survival rates were similar for cylindrical and screw-type implants.

Wannfors et al[25] compared one- and two-stage sinus inlay bone grafting and implant placement after 1 year in function. Forty patients were evenly randomized to groups of one- or two-stage sinus inlay cortical iliac bone block grafts. The bone graft was allowed to consolidate for 6 months. The one-stage protocol had a reported success rate of 85.5% for 76 implants placed. The two-stage protocol had a 90.5% success rate for 74 implants placed. The maxillary sinus residual bone ranged from 2 to 7 mm. The study concluded that the risk of implant failure in grafted areas for one-stage patients was greater than that for two-stage patients.

Stricker et al reported placing Straumann implants with sandblasted, large-grit, acid-etched (SLA) surfaces into maxillary sinuses augmented with cancellous iliac crest autogenous bone grafts.[26] Forty-eight implants were

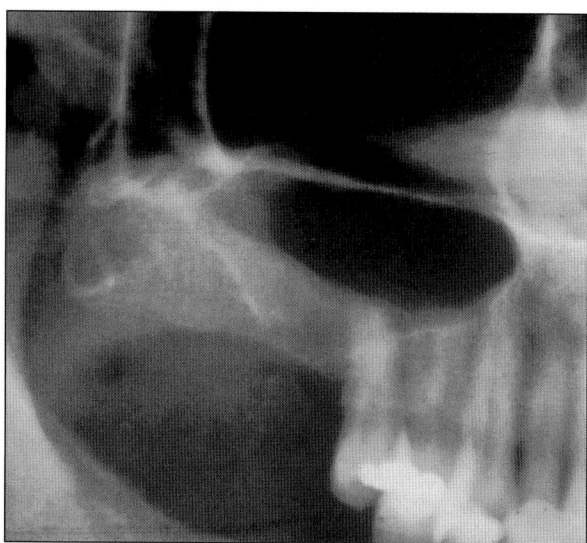

Fig 5-4a Preoperatve panoramic radiograph of a patient prior to receiving a sinus graft composed of maxillary tuberosity bone combined 1:1 by volume with demineralized bone particles.

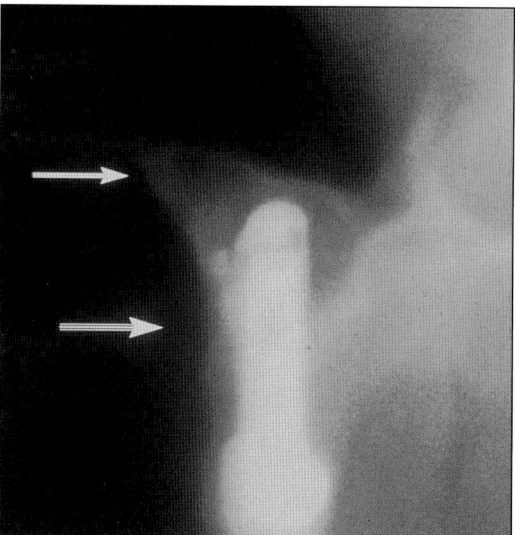

Fig 5-4b Seven-year postrestoration complex-motion tomogram showing maintenance of bone placed in the sinus. Apical bone level, *upper arrow*; original bone level, *lower arrow*.

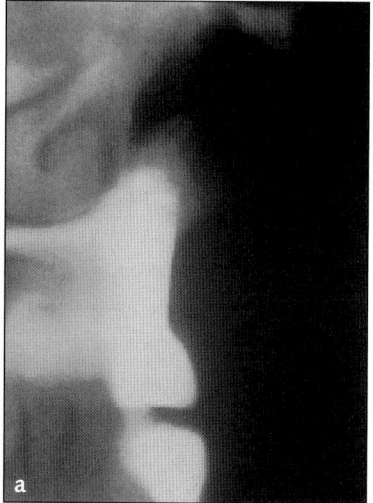
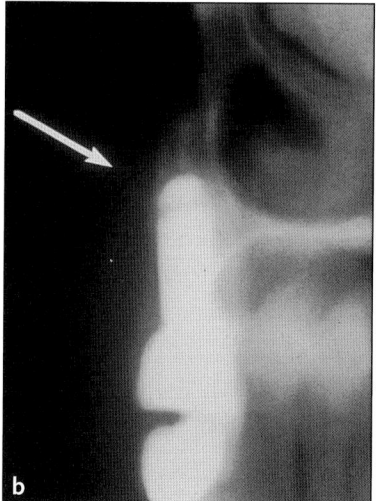

Figs 5-5a and 5-5b Ten-year postrestoration tomograms of implants placed simultaneously with iliac crest cancellous bone particles. *Arrow* points to bone at apical region of implant on left side.

placed simultaneously with sinus floor augmentation. Alveolar bone height was 5 mm or greater. One hundred thirty-five implants were placed in a staged procedure. The healing period for both groups was 4 months. The overall 2-year implant survival rate was 99.5%, and the success rate for both the one- and two-stage procedures was similar. Of the 183 implants placed, only 1 implant failed.

TABLE 5-1 Survival rate of implants classified by pretreatment bone height

Alveolar bone height	No. of implants	No. surviving	Survival rate (%)
4 mm or less	14	12	85.7
5 to 6 mm	50	48	96.0
7 mm or greater	110	106	96.4

TABLE 5-2 Survival rate of implants classified by shape and surface

Shape/surface	No. of implants	No. surviving	Survival rate (%)
Standard screw	45	42	93.3
TPS screw	35	34	97.1
HA screw	6	6	100
TPS cylinder	88	84	95.5

TPS, titanium plasma-sprayed; HA, hydroxyapatite

TABLE 5-3 Failure rate of implants classified by residual bone height

Residual bone height	No. of implants	Failures No.	Failures Percentage
4 mm or less	15	4	26.7
5 to 6 mm	78	4	5.1
7 mm or greater	183	10	5.5

Sinus Augmentation with Simultaneous Implant Placement

A less invasive alternative for sinus floor elevation with concurrent grafting and immediate implant placement was introduced by Summers in 1994.[13] This technique has gained widespread acceptance. In 1999, Rosen et al performed a retrospective clinical evaluation of patients consecutively treated from multiple centers.[27] Intruding bone graft onto the sinus floor using an osteotome, 174 implants were placed simultaneously. Implants from various manufacturers were both screw and cylinder shaped with machined, titanium plasma-sprayed, or hydroxyapatite-coated surfaces. The material used to augment the sinuses included autografts, allografts, and xenografts, alone or in combination. The results of the study are summarized in Tables 5-1 and 5-2.

A total of 166 implants, loaded a minimum of 6 months, had an overall survival rate of 94.7%. The average period of implant loading was 20.2 months, and the range was 6 to 66 months. The survival rate of implants was 96% or higher when pretreatment bone height was 5 mm or more and dropped to 85.7% when pretreatment bone height was 4 mm or less (see Table 5-1). A summary of survival rates for the various implant types is shown in Table 5-2. All types of implants had a survival rate of 93% or better. The authors concluded that the most important factor influencing implant survival was the amount of pre-existing bone height. The choices of bone graft material and implant surface or shape had a lesser influence on implant survival (see chapter 18).

In 2004, Toffler presented the results of osteotome-mediated sinus floor elevation using autogenous and xenograft bone and a variety of screw-type implants.[28] The mean residual bone height of 7.1 mm was relatively high, with a range of 3 to 10 mm. The results are presented in Table 5-3. The overall survival rate for 276 im-

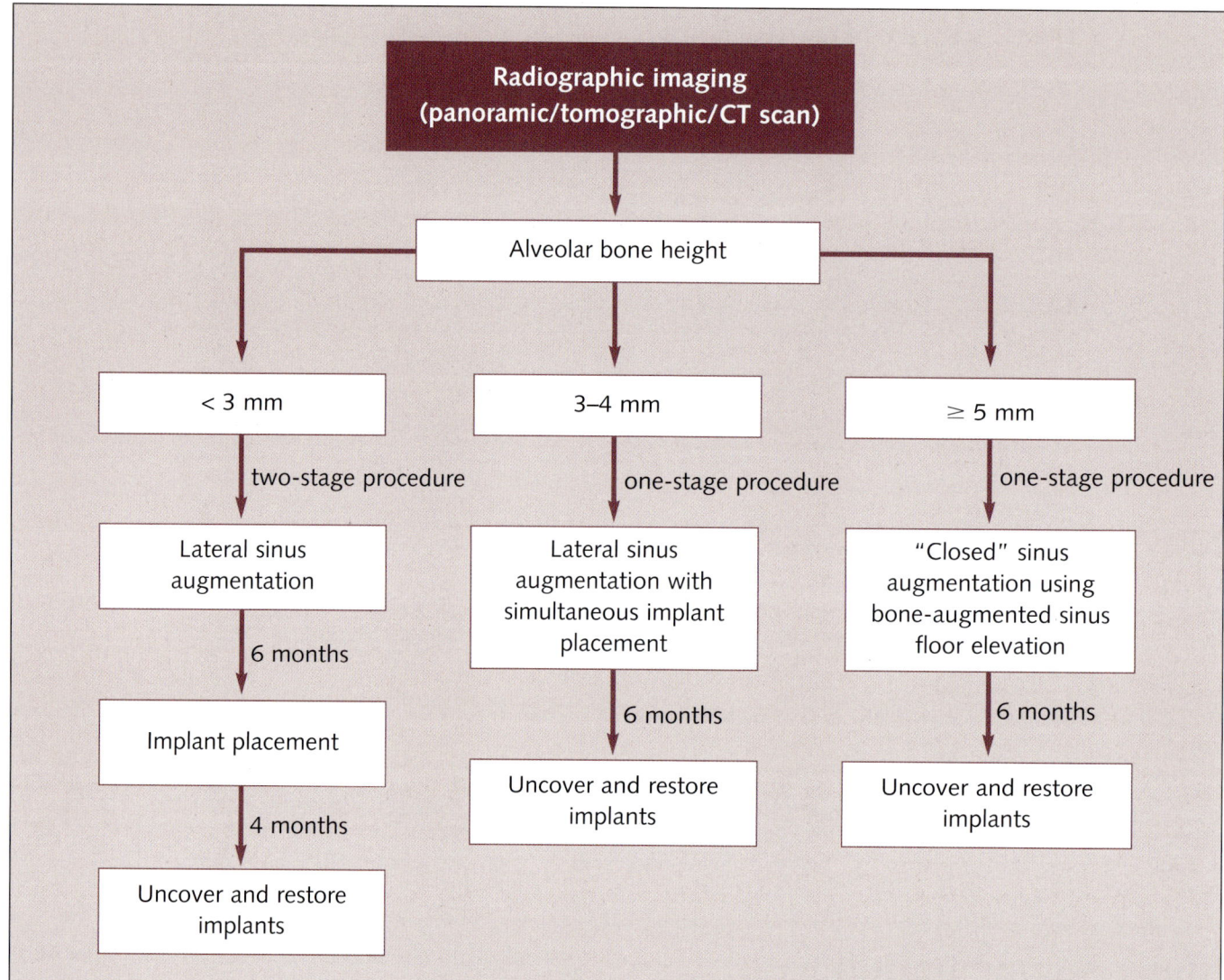

Fig 5-6 Treatment-planning flow chart. This flow chart draws on the experience of international surgeons who have developed a nuanced approach to bone and instrumentation, bone graft handling, and dental implant placement. While 3 mm of residual bone appears to be the critical threshold that determines the departure path for simultaneous implant treatment, the question of how much bone is needed to stabilize implants remains controversial. Screw-threaded implant torque values (fixation) increase as greater amounts of bone integrate with more screw threads. At 4 mm, there is a precipitous increase in insertion torque and, by inference, fixation. The bone mineral content (type 1 or 2) is a factor as well.

The fixation of an implant is dynamic, not static, and involves two biomechanical thresholds: early fixation, which is achieved at placement thrust of structural mechanics, and early *biologic* fixation, which occurs about 3 to 4 weeks later, during the demineralization phase of bone healing. Should fixation be lost by demineralization, implant mobility will prevent the early osseointegration that occurs at 5 to 6 weeks.

Surgeons must learn to deal with biologic and mechanical limitations. The experienced surgeon will occasionally depart from the formulaic approach and shift to the right side of the flow chart. When fixation appears dubious, regardless of the quality of pneumatized bone, it is advisable to delay sinus bone grafting. In this way, the highest degree of success is achieved.

Nevertheless, published data speak volumes. Simultaneous placement in very compromised settings of only a few millimeters of residual bone, combined with autogenous bone grafting, is just as successful statistically as delayed placement protocols.

| TABLE 5-4 Comparison of three approaches to sinus bone grafting ||||
Method	Advantages	Disadvantages
Two-step lateral antrostomy	Placement in augmented site with dense bone quality Controlled sinus elevation over broad area	Time intensive Longer treatment time Some increase in risk of sinus membrane perforation
One-step lateral antrostomy	Reduced treatment period	Primary implant stability may be problematic Technically more difficult Increased risk of implant failure
Osteotome technique	Less invasive Reduced treatment period Shorter healing time Implant site–specific augmentation	No visibility of elevation; tears may not be detected Possible endodontic injury to an adjacent tooth Elevation limited

plants placed simultaneously was 93.5% after an average period of 27.9 months.

A residual bone height of 5 mm or greater had a 94.7% success rate. With a residual bone height of 4 mm or less, the survival rate dropped to 73.3%. The primary determinant of implant survival was the pretreatment height of the residual alveolus. Implant type and proportion of autogenous graft to xenograft had a much weaker discernible influence on implant survival.

Zitzmann and Scharer compared three of the described methods for sinus elevation: (1) a two-step lateral antrostomy procedure, (2) a one-step lateral antrostomy procedure, and (3) the osteotome technique with a crestal approach.[4] A total of 79 implants were placed. When residual bone height was less than or equal to 4 mm, the two-step procedure was performed; residual bone heights of 4 to 6 mm were treated with a one-step lateral antrostomy; and residual bone heights greater than 6 mm were treated with the osteotome technique. The success rate for the osteotome technique was 95% over the 30-month study period; no failures occurred in any site treated by lateral antrostomy. The authors conclude that the osteotome technique is recommended when more than 6 mm of residual bone is present.

The resulting bone height after sinus augmentation also was investigated by Zitzmann and Scharer.[4] The gain in bone height was comparable for the one-step (median = 10 mm) and two-step (median = 12.7 mm) lateral approaches. These sites exhibited a significantly greater increase in bone height ($p < .001$) than the sites treated by osteotome (mean = 3.5 mm).

Based on a review of the literature, the criteria for deciding which method to use in any given situation are summarized in Fig 5-6. This flow chart facilitates treatment planning for placement of implants with regard to available bone using a delayed or simultaneous approach. The flow chart assumes adequate alveolar ridge width for implant placement. Radiographs determine the height of the pretreatment alveolar bone. For an alveolar ridge height of less than 3 mm, a two-stage protocol is recommended. The sinus is augmented with bone grafting and allowed to consolidate for 6 months. Implants are then placed and allowed to integrate for 4 months before being uncovered and restored. If residual bone height is 3 mm or greater, then a one-stage procedure is suggested. Simultaneous placement of implants in conjunction with sinus augmentation via a lateral window can be performed with residual bone heights of 3 to 4 mm. A healing period of 6 months is allowed before restoration of the implants. A so-called closed sinus elevation with bone grafting using osteotomes can be performed successfully in residual bone heights greater than or equal to 5 mm and the implants restored 6 months later.

Recommendations Based on Literature Review and Surgeon Experience

When should a one-stage procedure be performed, and when should a two-stage be performed (Table 5-4)? The ultimate answer to this question is based on a case-by-case analysis of several factors, each contributing to the final treatment plan.

Perhaps the most important question is: What is the thickness of the residual alveolar bone? If it is less than 3 mm and autogenous iliac blocks will not be harvested, then a staged procedure is indicated. In cases where there is a thickness of bone between 3 and 5 mm, the source of the bone graft becomes important in determining if a staged or a simultaneous approach is indicated. If allograft or xenograft is the primary graft material, then a staged procedure is indicated. If at least 50% of the graft is autogenous bone, especially bone marrow with viable osteoblasts, then a one-stage procedure can be performed. A bone thickness of 5 to 8 mm can be treated simultaneous with implant placement using either a lateral wall or a transalveolar approach. A two-stage procedure is performed if allograft or xenograft is the primary graft material.

Acknowledgments

Bo Rangert, Franck Renouard, and Paul Maló contributed to this chapter.

References

1. Tatum H. Maxillary and sinus implant reconstructions. Dent Clin North Am 1986;30:207–229.
2. Boyne PJ, James RA. Grafting of the maxillary sinus floor with autogenous marrow and bone. J Oral Surg 1980;38:613–616.
3. Loannidou E, Dean J. Osteotome sinus floor elevation and simultaneous, non-submerged implant placement: Case report and literature review. J Periodontol 2000;71:1613–1619.
4. Zitzman N, Scharer P. Sinus elevation procedures in the resorbed posterior maxilla: Comparison of the crestal and lateral approaches. Oral Surg Oral Med Oral Pathol Oral Radiol Endod 1998;85:8–17.
5. Wallace SS, Froum SJ. Effect of maxillary sinus augmentation on the survival of endosseous dental implants. A systematic review. Ann Periodontol 2003;8:328–343.
6. McCarthy C, Patel R, Wragg P, Brook I. Sinus augmentation bone grafts for the provision of dental implants: Report of clinical outcome. Int J Oral Maxillofac Implants 2003;18:377–382.
7. Tong D, Rioux K, Drangsholt M, Beirne O. A review of survival rates for implants placed in grafted maxillary sinuses using meta-analysis. Int J Oral Maxillofac Implants 1998;13:175–182.
8. Tolman DE. Reconstructive procedures with endosseous implants in grafted bone: A review of the literature. Int J Oral Maxillofac Implants 1995;10:275–294.
9. Jensen J, Krantz-Simonsen E, Sindet-Pedersen S. Reconstruction of the severely resorbed maxilla with bone grafting and osseointegrated implants: A preliminary report. J Oral Maxillofac Surg 1990;48:27–32.
10. Hall HD, McKenna SJ. Bone graft of the maxillary sinus floor for Brånemark implants. Oral Maxillofac Surg Clin North Am 1991;3:869–875.
11. Hallmann M, Hedin M, Sennerby L, Lundgren S. A prospective 1-year clinical and radiographic study of implants placed after maxillary sinus floor augmentation with bovine hydroxyapatite and autogenous bone. J Oral Maxillofac Surg 2002;60:277–284.
12. Hallman M, Nordin T. Sinus floor elevation with bovine hydroxyapatite mixed with fibrin glue and later placement of nonsubmerged implants: A retrospective study in 50 patients. Int J Oral Maxillofac Implants 2004;19:222–227.
13. Summers RB. The osteotome technique: Part 3—Less invasive methods of elevating the sinus floor. Compend Contin Educ Dent 1994;15:698–708.
14. Jensen OT, Shulman LB, Block MS, Iacono VJ. Report of the Sinus Consensus Conference of 1996. Int J Oral Maxillofac Implants 1998;13(suppl):11–31.
15. Pierrisnard L, Renouard F, Renault P, Barquins M. Influence of implant length and bicortical anchorage on implant stress distribution. Clin Implant Dent Relat Res 2003;5:254–262.
16. Kent J, Block M. Simultaneous maxillary sinus floor bone grafting and placement of hydroxylapatite-coated implants. J Oral Maxillofac Surg 1989;47:238–242.
17. Khoury F. Augmentation of the sinus floor with mandibular bone block and simultaneous implantation: 6-year clinical investigation. Int J Oral Maxillofac Implants 1999;14:557–564.
18. Daelemans P, Hermans M, Godet F, Malavez C. Autologous bone graft to augment the maxillary sinus in conjunction with immediate endosseous implants: A retrospective study up to 5 years. Int J Periodontics Restorative Dent 1997;17:27–39.
19. Peleg M, Mazor Z, Garg AK. Augmentation grafting of the maxillary sinus and simultaneous implant placement in patients with 3 to 5 mm of residual alveolar bone height. Int J Oral Maxillofac Implants 1999;14:549–556.
20. Peleg M, Mazor Z, Chaushu G, Garg AK. Sinus floor augmentation with simultaneous implant placement in the severely atrophic maxilla. J Periodontol 1998;69:1397–1403.
21. Hatano N, Shimizu Y, Ooya K. A clinical long-term radiographic evaluation of graft height changes after maxillary sinus floor augmentation with a 2:1 autogenous bone/xenograft mixture and simultaneous placement of dental implants. Clin Oral Implants Res 2004;15:339–345.
22. Block MS, Kent JN, Kallukaran FU, Thunthy K, Weinberg R. Bone maintenance 5 to 10 years after sinus grafting. J Oral Maxillofac Surg 1998;56:706–714.
23. Block MS, Kent JN. Part I: Sinus augmentation for dental implants. J Oral Maxillofac Surg 1997;55:1281–1286.
24. Valentini P, Abensur DJ. Maxillary sinus grafting with anorganic bovine bone: A clinical report of long-term results. Int J Oral Maxillofac Implants 2003;18:556–560.
25. Wannfors K, Johansson B, Hallman M, Strandkvist T. A prospective randomized study of 1- and 2-stage sinus inlay bone grafts: 1-year follow up. Int J Oral Maxillofac Implants 2000;15:725–632.
26. Stricker A, Voss P, Gutwald R, Schramm A, Schmelzeisen R. Maxillary sinus floor augmentation with autogenous bone grafts to enable placement of SLA-surfaced implants: Preliminary results after 15–40 months. Clin Oral Implants Res 2003;14:207–212.
27. Rosen PS, Summers R, Mellado JR, et al. The bone-added osteotome sinus floor elevation technique: Multi-center retrospective report of consecutively treated patients. Int J Oral Maxillofac Implants 1999;14:853–858.
28. Toffler M. Osteotome-mediated sinus floor elevation: A clinical report. Int J Oral Maxillofac Implants 2004;19:266–273.

chapter 6
Sinus Floor Augmentation at the Time of Tooth Removal

Paul A. Fugazzotto, DDS
Ole T. Jensen, DDS, MS

With the advent of osseointegration, tooth removal procedures may be modified to take advantage of what can be described as *root replacement technology*. Tooth removal and implant placement may proceed simultaneously in incisor, canine, and premolar sites. This approach generally cannot be used in molar sites,[1] especially maxillary first and second molar sites, however, because they frequently involve some of the sinus floor within the trifurcation. Typically following tooth removal and healing, bone height is approximately 5 mm. This type of bone deficiency can be avoided through treatment performed *at the time of extraction* using an interradicular bone intrusion osteotomy.[2,3]

Interradicular Bone Intrusion Osteotomy Technique

When a sufficient quantity (ie, 4 to 5 mm) of interradicular bone is present immediately after tooth removal, a standard osteotome is used to free the central portion (Fig 6-1). Next, a round osteotome is used to upfracture and intrude the bone fragment (and sinus floor) superiorly onto the sinus floor. The intruded bone fragment, which typically measures 4 or 5 mm in dimension, is wedged beneath the sinus membrane. The socket wound effectively extends superior to the sinus floor. The socket should be left to heal for 4 months without a barrier membrane or a bone graft. Providing there is no buccal wall dehiscence, the socket will most likely heal to near-ideal buccolingual morphology with greater vertical osseous dimension. Endoscopic studies have shown that the sinus floor can consistently be elevated 4 to 5 mm without perforation.[4] If a sinus perforation does occur, collagen or oxidized cellulose can be placed so as to occlude the osteotomy site.

When interradicular bone intrusion grafts heal, they generally add about 5 mm to the available bone height (Figs 6-2a to 6-2c). If the height is still inadequate at the time of implant placement, a second intrusion may be accomplished as part of the implant placement procedure, again without the need for bone grafting (see chapter 22). Note the bone-healing pattern in Fig 6-2d around the apex of the sinus-directed implant 1 year after it has been restored.

Chapter 6: Sinus Floor Augmentation at the Time of Tooth Removal

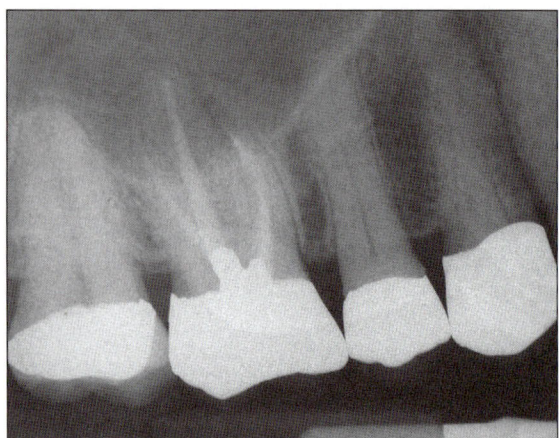

Fig 6-1a Maxillary first molar with interradicular sinus pneumatization.

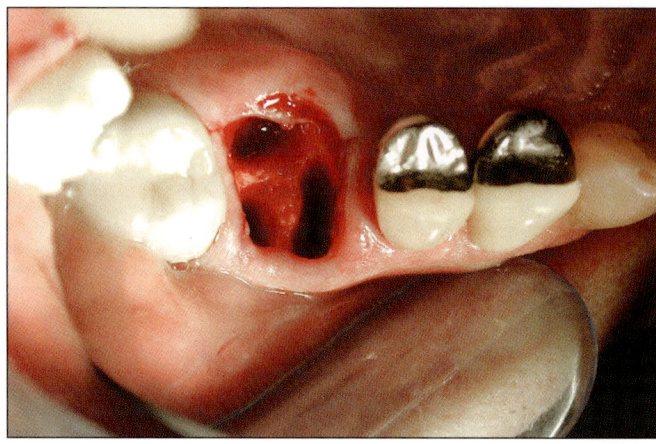

Fig 6-1b Extraction of maxillary first molar reveals the presence of interradicular bone. Because of a prominent interradicular sinus, there is insufficient vertical bone available for dental implant placement.

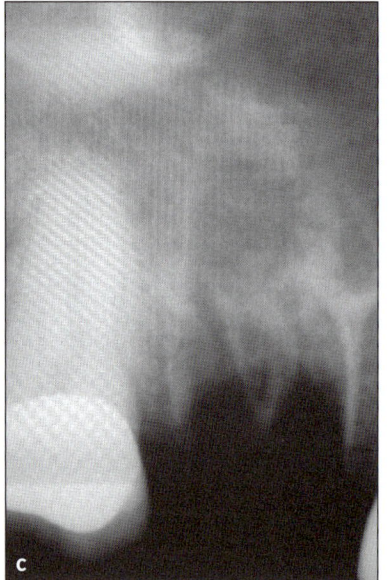

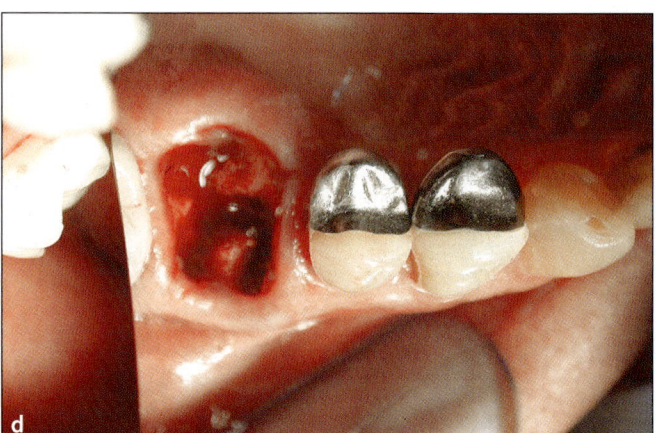

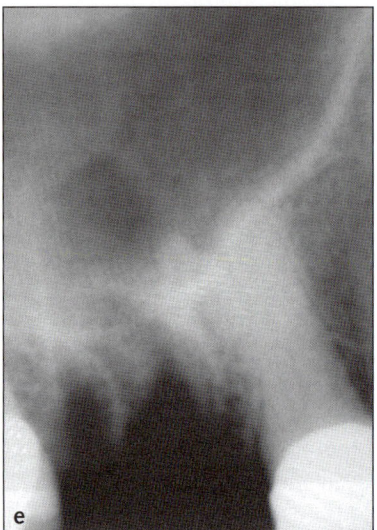

Fig 6-1c Postextraction radiograph confirming the presence of prominent interradicular bone.

Fig 6-1d Osteotome intrusion of bone fragment into the sinus.

Fig 6-1e Addition of 4 to 5 mm of vertical height following osteotome intrusion.

Fig 6-2a Maxillary first molar with minimal interradicular bone and a relatively low sinus.

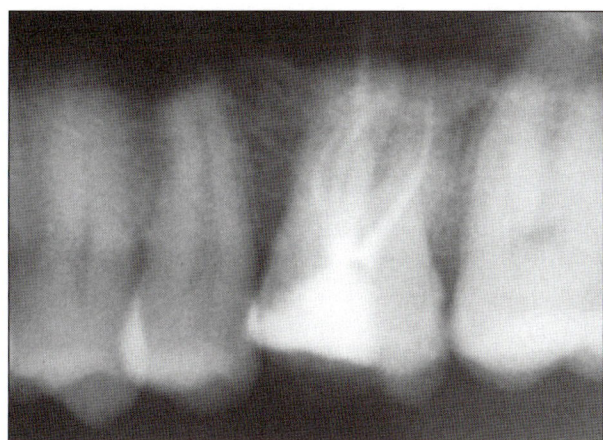

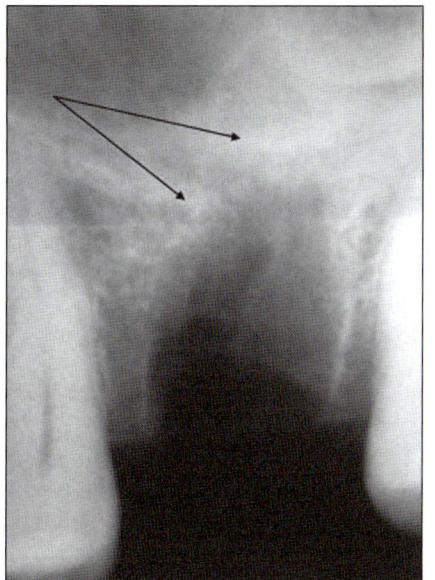

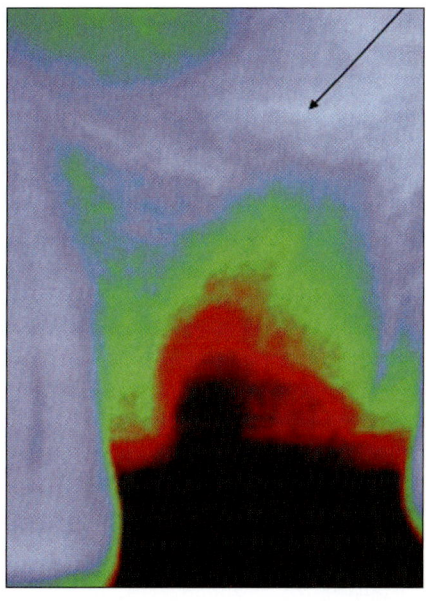

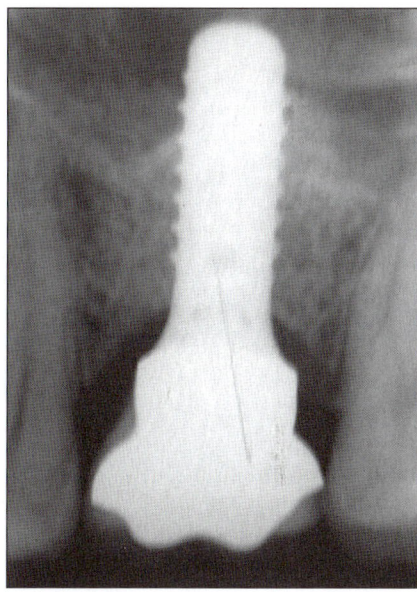

Fig 6-2b Postintrusion of sinus floor about 5 mm at time of tooth removal. *Arrows* indicate original and intruded sinus floor bone.

Fig 6-2c Colorized radiograph demonstrating elevation of sinus floor with bone fragment above *(arrow)*.

Fig 6-2d Final restoration of 12-mm-long implant placed entirely without extraneous bone graft in what appears to be a well-ossified site with stable vertical dimension.

The interradicular bone intrusion technique offers the advantage of completely avoiding extraneous bone graft (Fig 6-3). The procedure is simple to perform and very brief. Surgeons skilled with osteotomes generally accomplish the procedure without complication. If a more controlled approach is desired, the trephine technique (described below) may be used.

chapter 6 Sinus Floor Augmentation at the Time of Tooth Removal

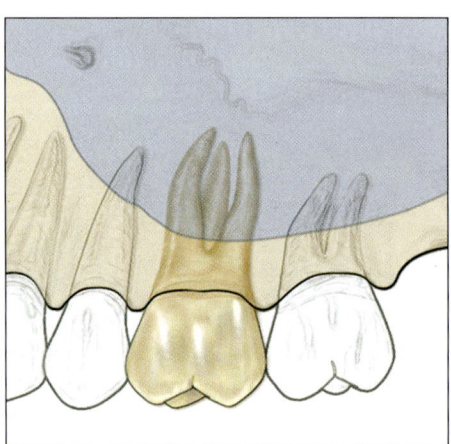

Fig 6-3a The maxillary first molar often has interradicular pneumatization.

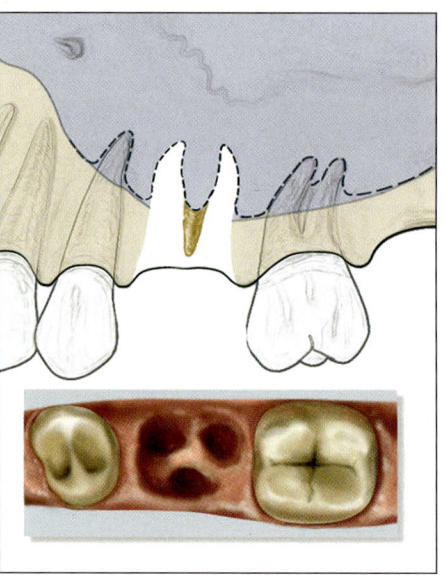

Fig 6-3b Interradicular bone illustrated with associated sinus membrane following tooth removal.

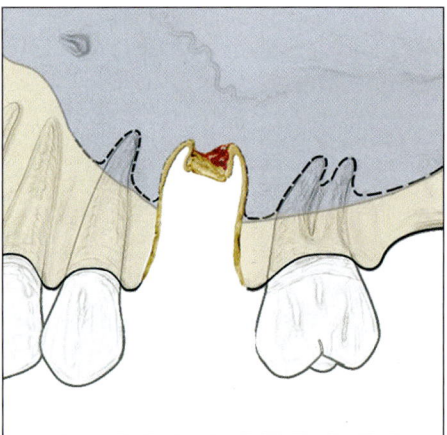

Fig 6-3c Intrusion of the central interradicular bone 3 to 5 mm.

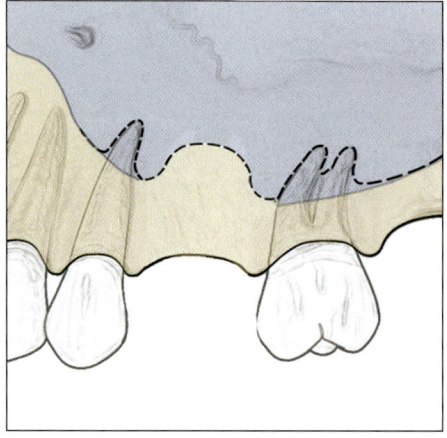

Fig 6-3d Healed osteotomy site with increased vertical dimension.

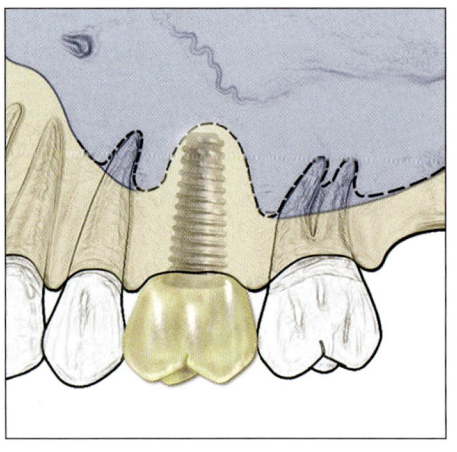

Fig 6-3e Increased bone allows for implant placement.

Sinus Augmentation and Maxillary Posterior Tooth Removal

Implants may osseointegrate successfully without the use of overlying membranes when placed into fresh extraction sockets, especially in the presence of small horizontal defects. However, this approach can result in buccolingual ridge collapse. Though often not significant in many cases, collapse of the buccolingual ridge may require soft tissue augmentation to maximize the esthetic outcome. In such cases, membranes can be used at the time of implant placement into fresh extraction sockets to minimize unavoidable extraction site remodeling.

To avoid buccolingual dimensional changes resulting from remodeling, a variety of treatment options are possible at the time of tooth removal, as follows:

I. Filling the extraction socket with particulate graft and covering with a membrane. This is especially valuable to consider when:
   - Implant placement is in a visible zone and buccal bone loss has occurred. While discussion of esthetics seems unusual for sinus-directed implants, some maxillary posterior teeth, such as premolars, may be quite visible.
   - Adequate fixation of the implant in the desired restorative position is not possible.
   - Implant placement is in a defect that is too wide to stabilize the implant in the desired restorative position, as in the case of molar extractions.
II. Particulate grafting plus implant placement after tooth removal to facilitate regeneration of alveolar bone as well as osseointegration of the implant.
III. Intrusion of the sinus floor at the apex of the extraction socket in conjunction with implant placement. Particulate graft and a membrane can be placed to facilitate regeneration.
IV. Combined buccal sinus augmentation of the extraction site with bone graft and membranes. This option is advocated for complex defects.
V. Lateral augmentation with simultaneous implant placement and bone graft regenerative procedures. This can be accomplished only if the implant can be fixated into available bone.

The use of various materials and techniques for augmenting extraction socket defects is well documented. Yet regeneration of bone in the extraction socket often does not adequately address all of the problems in the area being treated. Placement of an implant at the time of tooth removal is site specific. The minimum dimension necessary for implant placement must be determined first. Consideration of the alveolar morphology, which sometimes has an esthetic component, should follow. Therefore, predictable treatment must include options for both tooth and bone replacement.

A single-rooted premolar within the proximity of the sinus should be removed atraumatically and the defect debrided.[5] A two-rooted maxillary premolar may be hemisected and each root atraumatically extracted. Interradicular bone generally provides a stable base for osteotomy sinus floor intrusion. If some interdental bone is removed, it can be placed in sterile saline for future use.

Implant placement is carried out if adequate bone height is present. The osseous coagulum collected during osteotomy preparation is combined with interradicular bone and packed around the implant in the socket defect. Buccal or palatal extraction walls can be "swedged" by forcing adjacent bone up against the implant. No membrane is placed.

Trephine Sinus Intrusion Technique

If bone height is inadequate for placement of an implant, the floor of the sinus is intruded by applying a trephine technique followed by the use of an osteotome, and the implant is then placed (Fig 6-4). Particulate graft and swedging may be employed. Placement of a membrane is optional. Alternatively, the osteotome and trephine techniques are employed with particulate graft and then covered with a membrane. The area is re-entered 4 months later, at which time the implant is placed. If bone height is inadequate for sinus intrusion, a lateral approach to sinus augmentation is recommended. If nonautogenous grafting material is used, the area is re-entered 8 months later for implant placement.

chapter 6 Sinus Floor Augmentation at the Time of Tooth Removal

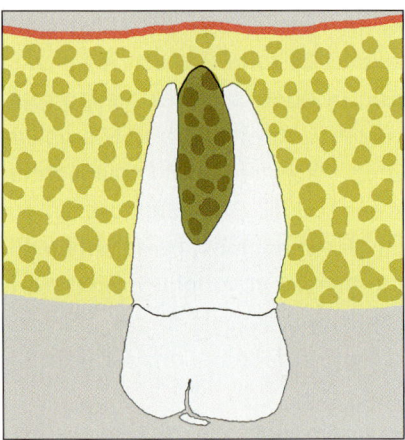

Fig 6-4a Hopeless maxillary molar will be removed.

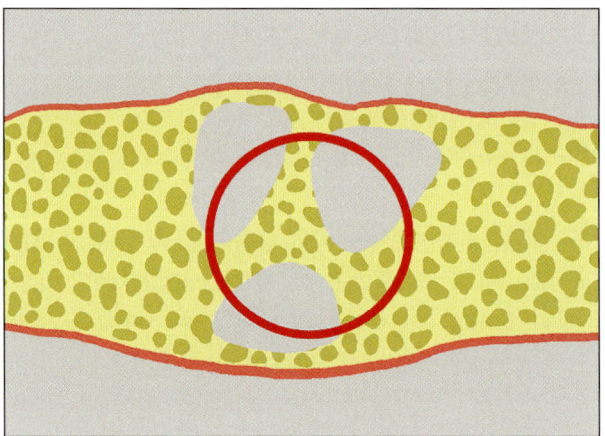

Fig 6-4b The trephine must be of adequate diameter to encompass the interradicular bone.

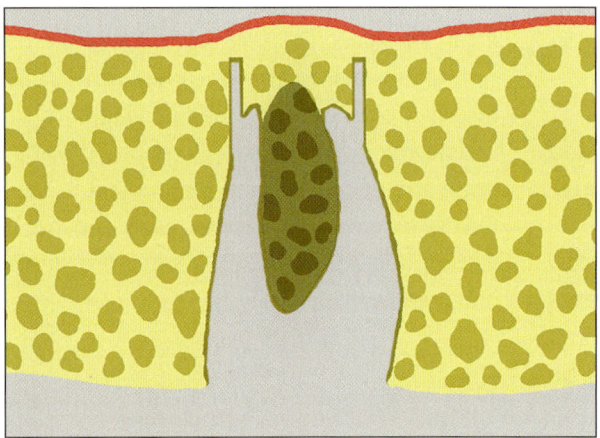

Fig 6-4c Preparation of an osteotomy to a depth 1 mm short of the sinus membrane.

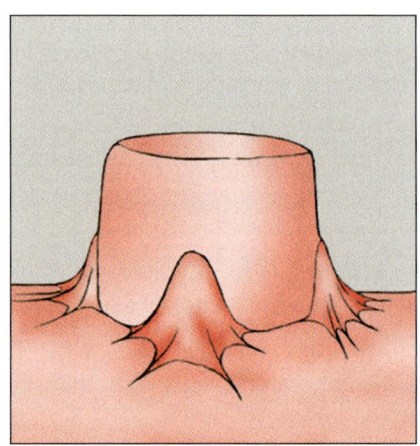

Fig 6-4d Intrasinus view of intruded bone core and elevated sinus membrane.

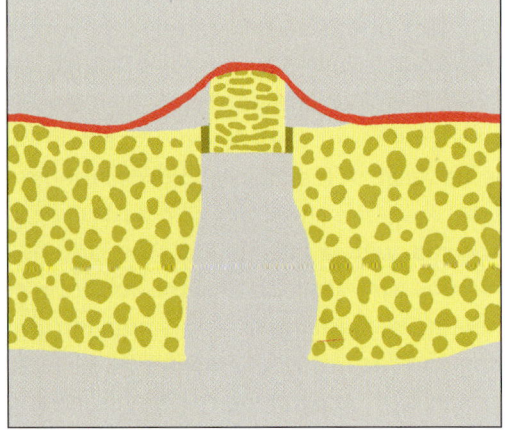

Fig 6-4e Intrusion of the bone core to a depth 1 mm less than that of the prepared osteotomy.

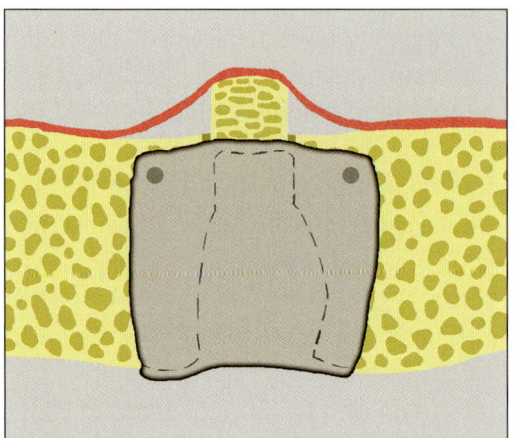

Fig 6-4f Placement of the particulate graft material and membrane.

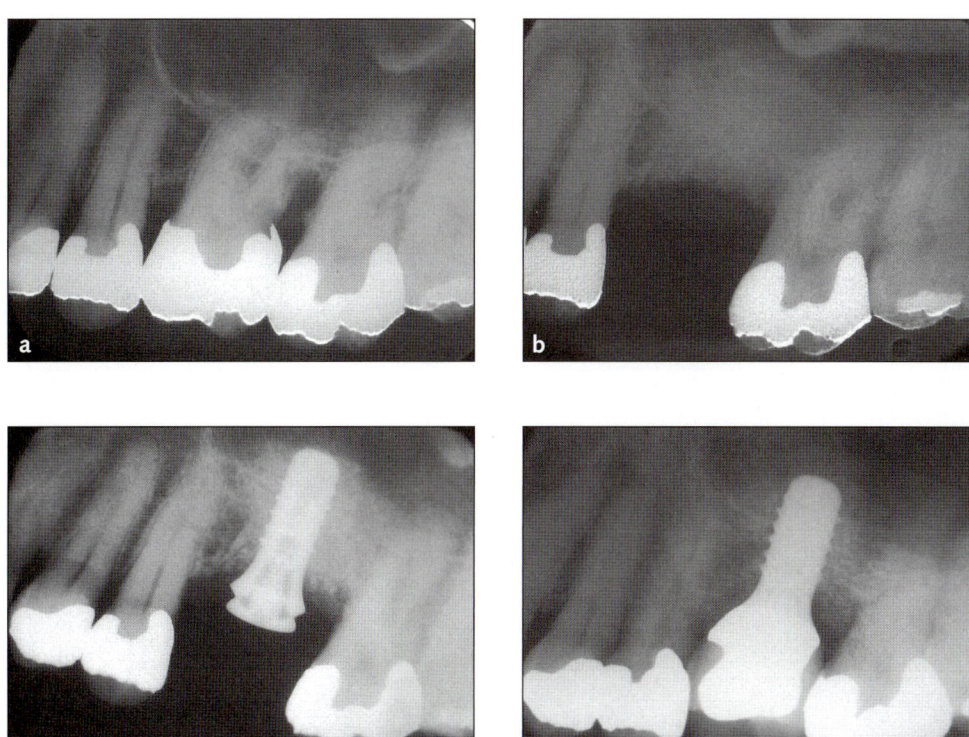

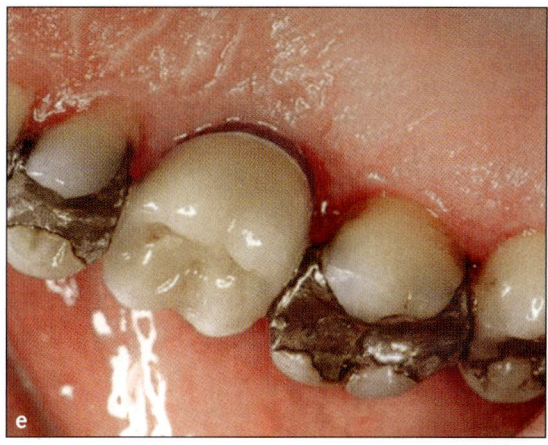

Fig 6-5a The maxillary first molar is to be extracted. The distal aspect of the buccal alveolar plate has been destroyed by periodontal disease. Note the compromised bone protecting the mesial furcation of the second molar.

Fig 6-5b The first molar is extracted, a bone core is intruded, and particulate material and a membrane are placed.

Fig 6-5c A Straumann implant with a 4.8-mm-wide body and a 6.5-mm-wide neck is placed in the augmented bone.

Fig 6-5d The implant is restored with a cemented crown.

Fig 6-5e Clinical view of the restored implant.

Sinus Floor Intrusion Following Molar Extraction

When primary stability can be obtained in a molar site, particulate graft and a secured membrane are used to promote alveolar bone regeneration. If bone height is inadequate for implant placement, which is more often the case, the trephine is employed to free the residual interradicular bone, which is then intruded into the sinus using a blunt osteotome.[6] Use of particulate graft material and a membrane beneath primary closed flaps is recommended. The area is re-entered 6 months after regeneration for implant placement (Figs 6-5 and 6-6). If bone height is inadequate to accomplish a trephine intrusion bone graft, a lateral window sinus augmentation procedure is performed, with simultaneous augmentation of the extraction socket.

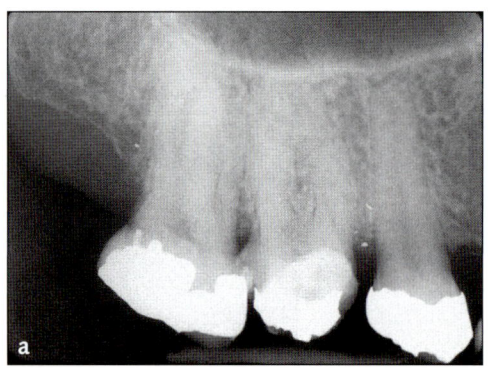
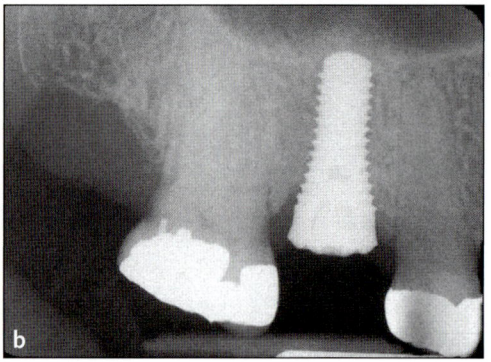
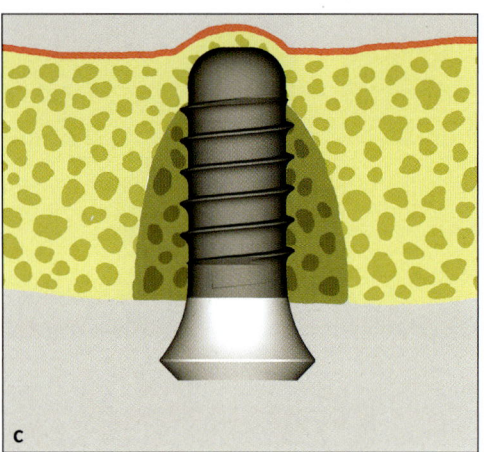

Fig 6-6a A first molar is to be extracted as a result of an intrafurcal fracture. Although the radiograph seems to indicate a paucity of interradicular bone, adequate bone is present for manipulation and simultaneous implant placement.

Fig 6-6b A 10-mm-long TE implant (Straumann) has been placed and bone has regenerated around the implant.

Fig 6-6c Illustrated view after sequential widening of the osteotomy with osteotomes to the appropriate width for the planned implant.

Conclusion

Interradicular bone in postextraction sockets of maxillary molars can be used to augment the sites for future implant placement. Using osteotomes, the interradicular bone is released and intruded, thus providing up to 5 mm of additional vertical bone after healing. The technique simplifies sinus augmentation for the placement of implants in the molar region.

References

1. Fugazzotto PA. Implant placement in maxillary first premolar fresh extraction sockets: Description of technique and report of preliminary results. J Periodontol 2002;73:669–674.
2. Fugazzotto PA. The modified trephine/osteotome sinus augmentation technique: Technical considerations and discussion of indications. Implant Dent 2001;10:259–264.
3. Simsek B, Simsek S. Evaluation of success rates of immediate and delayed implants after tooth extraction. Chin Med J 2003; 8:1216–1219.
4. Engelke W, Deckwer I. Endoscopically controlled sinus floor augmentation. A preliminary report. Clin Oral Implants Res 1997;8: 527–531.
5. Fugazzotto PA. Simplified technique for immediate implant insertion into maxillary first premolar extraction sockets: Report of technique and preliminary results. Implant Dent 2002;11:79–82.
6. Fugazzotto PA. Sinus floor augmentation of the maxillary molar extraction socket: A modified technique to increase bone height. Int J Oral Maxillofac Implants 1999;14:536–542.

chapter 7
Prosthetic Management of the Sinus Graft Patient

Ira D. Zinner, DDS, MSD
Stanley A. Small, DDS
Lloyd S. Landa, DDS, MSD

A team approach is essential for successful treatment of the sinus graft patient. To create a favorable prognosis, the prosthodontist, surgeon, and dental technician must be involved in the diagnosis, final insertion, and postinsertion maintenance of the prosthesis. Each member of the team should understand the long-term goals of treatment as well as how to manage a prosthetic or surgical failure. The prosthodontist directs the team, since implant placement depends on subsequent prosthetic care.

Diagnosis and Treatment Planning

A cursory diagnosis invites a less-than-favorable prognosis. For a comprehensive diagnosis, intraoral radiographs, a panoramic radiograph, and computerized tomography (CT) scans of the maxilla are necessary. Next, a critical clinical examination of the patient, followed by a careful assessment of the patient's expectations, will help the prosthodontist determine the feasibility of treatment.[1,2]

If the patient is an acceptable candidate for a sinus graft, maxillary and mandibular diagnostic casts are fabricated and then mounted on an articulator to verify the maxillomandibular relationship. The diagnostic casts are duplicated, and one set is used to create a diagnostic waxup that will help determine the prospective plane of occlusion, occlusal scheme, and esthetics. If acceptable, an impression of the waxup is made, and another set of casts is fabricated. These casts are used to create a surgical template and a provisional prosthesis and to aid in the creation of both the second-stage screw-retained provisional prosthesis and the definitive prosthesis. Therefore, this waxup creates the template for the restoration of the sinus-grafted maxilla. Prior to construction of the surgical template, a consultation with the surgical member of the team is needed to determine whether buccal grooves (ie, drilled 2-mm-diameter holes) or stent tubes will be used for implant placement. An open buccal surface usually provides more room for the surgical sinus augmentation procedure.[3] Grooves are preferable to stent tubes because they give the surgeon more favorable access to the surgical site.[4]

In general, one implant is planned for each missing tooth, either in the sinus-grafted site or in the adjacent residual bone. Cantilevers are generally not recommended.[5] Because maxillary bone is not as dense as mandibular bone, torquing stresses from cantilevers during function may cause screw loosening or breakage and unwanted bending moments on the implants, leading to implant loss.

Important diagnostic considerations

Buccal bone loss

Loss of buccal bone commonly follows the loss of maxillary posterior teeth. Because the direction of bone loss is generally both palatal and vertical, the prognosis may be compromised if buccal as well as occlusal bone augmentation is not performed (see chapter 21). Loss of the buccal width of bone can result in a buccal cantilever that places undue torquing stresses on the implants and often serves as a food trap. In addition, when implants are palatally placed, the arch form is narrowed, crowding the tongue space and often resulting in speech problems as well as an esthetic compromise. To reduce torquing moments, a crossbite must be created to direct occlusal forces within the long axes of the implants.

To avoid these problems, hard tissue augmentation of the ridge crest with lateral veneer bone grafting can be combined with sinus augmentation in a staged surgical procedure. The bone grafting is performed and allowed to heal prior to implant placement. After 4 months, implants may be placed in their optimum positions as determined by the diagnostic waxup, CT scan evaluation, and surgical template.

Advanced vertical bone loss

Advanced vertical bone loss of the posterior maxillary ridge requires placement of a crestal bone graft prior to or in conjunction with sinus augmentation. This will prevent an unfavorable crown-to-implant ratio, which can reduce implant longevity. Placement of the vertical bone graft can be determined by the diagnostic workup. When a crestal bone graft is needed, the surgical phase of treatment is staged.

Bruxism

The surgical placement of a sinus graft and implants in a patient with severe bruxism can result in significant problems. The Sinus Consensus Conference[6] identified bruxism as a major cause of implant loss. Management of bruxism patients involves placement of implants that are wider and longer than average as well as a greater number of implants. Implants should be submerged, and the patient should refrain from wearing a provisional prosthesis. In addition, it is advisable to allow a longer period of healing between implant placement and uncovering.

At the second-stage surgery, a screw-retained metal and acrylic resin provisional prosthesis is placed, sometimes for up to 1 year, to allow time for the graft to mature and to ensure osseointegration. If one or more implants fails, it is easier to replace them surgically with the provisional in place. The definitive prosthesis should employ a gold framework with acrylic resin occlusal veneering for shock absorption in a harmonious occlusal scheme.[7–9] When anterior implants are not an option because of lack of bone height, the use of a bar-retained overdenture rather than a fixed-detachable prosthesis is advised. In addition, an occlusal nightguard should be worn by bruxism patients when feasible.

First-Stage Provisional Prosthesis

Removable partial denture

Provisional removable partial dentures are used to replace posterior teeth (ie, those distal to the canine).[3,10] For optimum stability and cross-arch transmission of occlusal forces, the removable partial denture should be fabricated from a cobalt–chrome alloy metal, and the retaining system should include shallow occlusal or incisal rests as well as retaining and bracing arms. A combination clasp system, in which the buccal clasp arm of wrought gold is soldered to the minor connector on the proximal zone, provides stress relief and also permits easy adaptation and subsequent adjustment of the retainer system to abutment teeth.

The removable partial denture requires relief over the edentulous ridge in areas of implant placement. It should be fabricated prior to surgery. Because the prosthesis is to be worn for at least 9 months, it must be durable and permit relining with tissue treatment materials, such as Hydro-cast (Sultan Chemists), and/or soft acrylic resin liners. Following first-stage surgery, it is refitted, and the tissue treatment material is replaced weekly until the surgical site is healed, when a more durable soft liner is placed.

Pressure from the transitional removable prosthesis may result in micromovement of poorly fixed implants and ultimately in implant loss. Thus, the patient should be informed prior to surgery that the removable prosthesis may not be worn for the first 3 weeks following implant surgery. At the time of insertion, the denture flange must be kept away from grafted areas.

It was reported at the Sinus Consensus Conference that most of the implants placed in sinus grafts that were lost occurred during the first year.[6] Two possible contributory causes may be premature insertion of a removable partial denture and the use of an all-acrylic resin removable partial denture with wrought buccal clasp arms and no occlusal or incisal rests. This type of appliance does not provide cross-arch stabilization to maintain the prosthesis in a stable position. Likewise, inadequate relief of the denture base or improper use of soft liners may contribute to adverse loading. To avoid loss of the bone graft and precariously fixed implants, a complete provisional maxillary denture should not be refitted and reinserted until the surgical areas are completely healed, which is usually 3 weeks postsurgery. When implant fixation is secure and lateral grafting is minimal, the provisional denture can be placed the day of surgery, provided that there is adequate relief for the surgical sites.

Fixed prosthesis

With as few as four teeth strategically located in the maxillary arch, a cast metal framework and an acrylic resin–veneered provisional fixed prosthesis can be fabricated.[1,10,11] If the remaining teeth are to be retained, full-coverage restorations are prepared and a provisional prosthesis is cemented into place. When teeth are not to be retained after implant restoration, cast metal retainers with occlusal rests are waxed and cast without tooth preparation. If there are no posterior teeth remaining, the provisional fixed prosthesis can incorporate cantilevered pontics. To reduce torquing on the abutment teeth, pontics should not be placed in occlusion and their occlusal table should be narrow buccolingually.

The provisional fixed prosthesis is inserted on the day of sinus augmentation and implant placement because it will place no mucosal load on the surgical sites. This restoration allows the patient to return to function and resume a normal lifestyle with the smallest degree of emotional trauma.

Abutment selection

Generally, three or four implants will be placed into a sinus graft. The authors prefer to use conical abutments, which increase the surface area coverage of the gold cylinder over the abutment head, thus reducing torquing forces.[11] To use a conical abutment, at least 7.5 mm of occlusogingival height is required. If less space is available, then a standard 3-mm-high abutment or a multiunit (4.5-mm-high) abutment should be selected. Use of a direct connection to the implant[12] is not recommended because of problems related to screw retrievability following the fracture of a prosthetic or abutment screw. If the prosthetic screw breaks, it is easier to change an abutment screw if the prosthetic screw cannot be unscrewed from its receptacle in the abutment screw. Cementation of the prosthesis also is not recommended due to the lack of retrievability and predictability. When functional and parafunctional forces of occlusion cause an abutment screw to bend or fracture, a retrievable restoration is easily repaired. Retrievable fixed partial dentures are also needed to maintain the acrylic occlusal veneers.

Second-Stage Provisional Prosthesis

Following implant uncovering and abutment installation, a screw-retained fixed-detachable prosthesis is fabricated.[1,3] This second-stage prosthesis is fabricated as soon as it is feasible following installation of the preselected abutments; it permits loading of the grafting material and surrounding residual alveolar bone without going directly to the final restoration. Provisional loading allows the graft and native alveolar bone to remodel in response to bone strains transmitted through loading. Because early implant integration may not be strong, "progressive" loading through the use of a screw-retained, metal-reinforced, acrylic resin–veneered prosthesis allows time for maturation of the graft as it adapts to the adjacent alveolar bone.

Tatum[13] believes that the length of time required for progressive loading depends on the type, particle size, and height of the graft, and on the length of the implant. According to Misch,[14] "each step of the progressive loading process is allowed sufficient time for the bone to respond to the increased stimulation. Ideally, woven bone transforms into load bearing lamellar bone, along with an increase in the percentage of bone at the implant interface." Binon and Sullivan[15] have stated that "the use of a resilient shock-absorbing acrylic resin provisional restoration limits stress wave and shock transfer to the implant, enhancing the desired gradual trabecular reorientation."

Despite the controversy surrounding the concept of provisional loading, the clinician should know that the occlusion on a provisional prosthesis should load in a vertical direction, reducing lateral force and minimizing unwanted torquing forces on implants.

Fabrication technique

The screw-retained provisional prosthesis usually is fabricated on the day of implant uncovering and abutment installation. Tapered transfer copings are screwed into place in the transmucosal abutments, and a full-arch impression is made. Because sutures are usually placed after uncovering, screw-secured impression copings and an overall elastomeric impression, which can tear sutures open, are not used.

Abutment analogs are screwed onto the transfer copings, and a die stone cast is poured. After separation, the maxillary and mandibular casts are mounted to verify maxillomandibular relation. Provisional titanium cylinders are selected for the abutments and screwed on the abutment replicas. The metal cylinders are luted together with autopolymerizing acrylic resin, allowed to set on the cast, and tried intraorally to verify accuracy of the impression. When a misfit of the components is observed, it is corrected intraorally.

The heights of the metal channels of these transitional cylinders are reduced to achieve a correct occlusal relationship. Metal provisional cylinders should contact the opposing dentition at a centric occlusal position. The cylinders are sandblasted, painted with opaque, and air dried. Polyethylene fibers, a stainless steel wire, a titanium bar, or a cast-metal reinforcement is applied to add rigidity to the acrylic resin–veneered provisional prosthesis.

When all necessary modifications have been made, the prosthesis is waxed and processed with heat-cured acrylic resin to a preselected shade. To avoid the need for flasking and deflasking, which may mar the gingival portions of the metal provisional cylinders, a heat- and pressure-curing machine (Ivomat, Ivoclar/Vivadent) can be used. The Ivomat machine requires the construction of facial and palatal indices of the waxup. After setup and separation, the wax is boiled off the cast and provisional cylinders. A separating medium is painted onto the gypsum cast and index. The metal reinforcement is secured in place with autopolymerizing acrylic resin. Monomer and polymer are painted around the cylinders to the required contour, then slightly overbuilt.

When the glossy appearance of the acrylic resin has faded, the indices are replaced, and the entire assembly is cured. After cooling, the acrylic resin material is carved and any additions of the acrylic resin are cured in the Ivomat. The restoration is refined, the screw access channels are cleaned of debris, and the fit is verified on the cast. If the fit is accurate and has not distorted during fabrication, then the occlusion is evaluated and altered where necessary. The provisional prosthesis is then polished and inserted into the patient's mouth, where occlusion is verified.

The restoration is evaluated using a so-called one-screw test, where one screw is inserted and tightened in the anteriormost or posteriormost cylinder. At this time, all the provisional cylinders must fit accurately without a seating error. If it does not fit, the prosthesis is sectioned and re-attached intraorally with autopolymerizing resin.

Once the resin has set, the restoration is removed and reinforced with nonflexible metal. At this time, the occlusal table should be narrowed, the centric occlusal contacts verified, and eccentric contacts minimized to avoid torquing forces on the implants—all strategies to concentrate occlusal forces in a vertical direction.

The provisional prosthesis is worn for at least 6 months. When the anterior implant(s) are in ungrafted alveolar bone and the posterior implants are in the sinus graft, the definitive prosthesis is constructed approximately 6 months after placement of the second-stage provisional prosthesis. If the prosthesis is supported only by implants placed in graft material, the provisional restoration is worn for about 1 year prior to fabrication of the definitive prosthesis to allow time for maturation of the graft.

The advantages of a second-stage screw-retained provisional prosthesis are that it:

1. Acts as a template for the definitive prosthesis
2. Allows the patient to wear a fixed prosthesis after second-stage surgery
3. Allows the patient to learn how to function with and maintain a screw-retained fixed-detachable prosthesis
4. Can be altered after soft tissue healing when exposed metal mars esthetics and the abutments can be changed
5. Is retained by the patient after completion of the definitive prosthesis, and may be used if alterations to the final prosthesis are ever required.

Definitive Prosthesis

The definitive prosthesis is a fixed-detachable screw-retained restoration, usually constructed from type IV gold alloy with a heat-cured acrylic resin veneer.[3,10,11] For shock absorption, acrylic resin occlusal surfaces may be employed to reduce forces on the underlying graft and implants.[7,8]

Acrylic resin occlusal surfaces are used when less than 5 mm of residual bone remained beneath the sinus before the grafting procedure was performed. With 5 mm or more residual bone beneath the sinus, gold occlusal surfaces are used.

A preferred implant design is one that has an external hex head,[16] which allows a manufactured abutment with antirotational capacity to be secured to the implant with an abutment screw and facilitates fabrication of a prosthesis retained by a gold retaining screw. The advantages of the gold retaining screw are its retrievability and its ability to break rather than torque the implants if overloaded.

Fabrication technique

Tapered impression copings are screwed into place, and a hydrocolloid impression is made. The impression copings are removed from the mouth and screwed to their analogs, and a die stone cast is poured. The casts are mounted on a semi-adjustable articulator to verify maxillomandibular relation.

Prefabricated gold-palladium cylinders are screwed into place on brass analogs. The use of manufactured gold cylinders ensures optimal fit between the gingival portion of the cylinder and the abutment head. Steel waxing pins secure the gold cylinders, and autopolymerizing acrylic resin joins all the gold cylinders together.

To verify the impression, this assembly is tried in the mouth by placment of a single gold screw into the anteriormost cylinder. If the gold cylinders do not fit the abutment heads accurately, the resin splint is sectioned, the gold cylinders are screwed into place, and the splint is reattached intraorally.

After the resin has set, the splinted gold cylinders are removed, and the analogs in the master cast are altered to their proper position. At this time, the intraoral abutments and their replicas in the cast are in the same position. Waxing pins are shortened to proper occlusal contact, and a new groove is cut for a straight-slotted screwdriver. The design of the gold framework includes a high palatal wall short of the occlusal, a short buccal waxup, and a gingival gold finishing line to allow room for the buccal and occlusal acrylic resin veneering material. The screw-access channels are waxed into occlusal contact.

The completed waxup is sectioned to allow for individual casting of each gold cylinder. Ten-gauge sprues are attached to the lingual surfaces of the waxup. A separating medium such as Nicrobraz (Wall Colmonoy) is painted into and around the gold cylinders to prevent their loss from casting errors. If spillage of gold alloy into the gold cylinders occurs, it can be removed with a scalpel blade. The waxup is invested, cast with a type IV gold alloy, and then divested.

The screw-access channels are sandblasted and then cleaned with a safe-ended, straight-fluted milling bur known as an E cutter (Brasseler). Steel protection caps are screwed into place before refinement of the castings by rotary instrumentation to prevent damage to the manufactured gold cylinders. The framework castings should fit the analogs on the cast before they are tried in the patient's mouth.

At the intraoral try-in, the parts of the cast prosthesis framework are secured with gold retaining screws. These fit more accurately than waxing pins, which may have debris on them and also may interfere with occlusal evaluation and adjustment. Right-angled radiographs are taken to evaluate the fit of the component parts. An intraoral soldering index using autopolymerizing acrylic resin and/or a buccal plaster index is taken of the castings. Once set, the entire assembly is removed, and a soldering verification cast is created using new analogs and gold prosthetic screws. Once the investment is set, the prosthesis is soldered.

After cleaning, the framework is verified by placing one gold retaining screw in the anteriormost or posteriormost cylinder.[3,4] At this time, all of the gold cylinders must fit accurately. If there is an error, a new soldering index is taken. After setting and removal from the cast, the parts are invested, soldered, and retried on the cast. Once the fit of the prosthesis has been verified using a one-screw test and laboratory inspection, the framework is evaluated intraorally. Right-angled radiographs are taken using the one-screw test as well as clinical verification.

To protect the gold cylinders and screw-access channels during the soldering procedure as well as to maintain the parts in place to reduce movement, brass analogs are secured with steel waxing pins. Then the index, with the prosthesis, steel pins, and analogs, is invested for soldering. A soldering index cast is then created by fixing analogs to the gold cylinders with gold screws after removal of the framework from the mouth. Fast-setting die stone is mixed and placed in a small plastic form, and the framework, with the soldering index and analog, is placed in the form. Only the analogs are placed in the stone. Once the stone is set, the gold screws are removed, and the assembly is removed from the analogs.

Chapter 7: Prosthetic Management of the Sinus Graft Patient

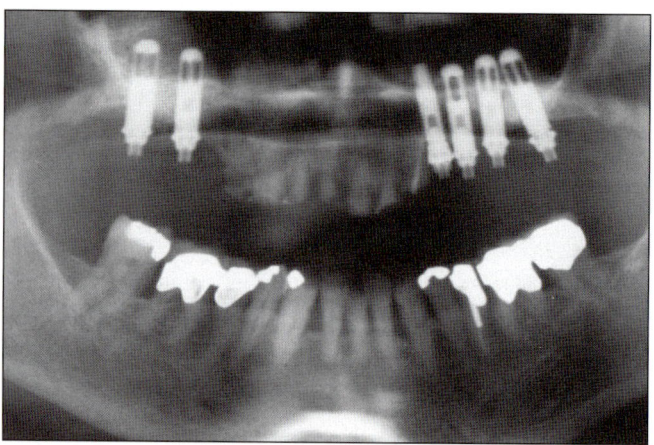

Fig 7-1a Case 1. Panoramic radiograph of a maxillary bilateral sinus graft following second-stage surgery and installation of 1-mm conical abutments. In this case, provisional screw-retained metal and acrylic resin prostheses were fabricated and inserted. After a 3- to 4-month healing period, cast gold screw-retained prostheses with acrylic resin veneers were fabricated. A cast gold bar was then waxed, cast, and soldered to the posterior prostheses, and acrylic resin veneers were prepared for the anterior teeth.

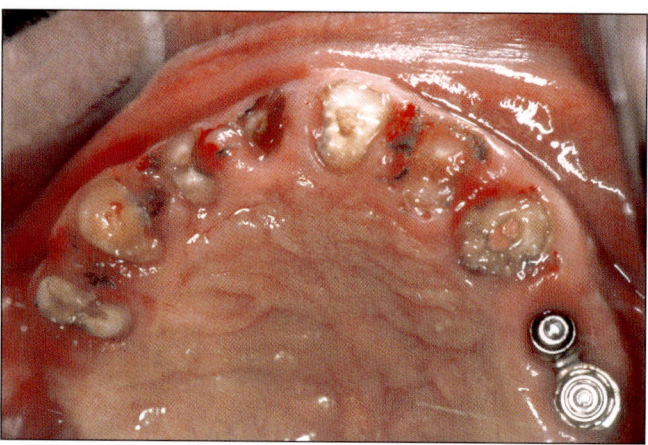

Fig 7-1b The maxillary anterior teeth were reduced to the gingival margins and the prosthesis was inserted. The teeth were then removed, and implants were placed. The prosthesis was inserted after completion of surgery.

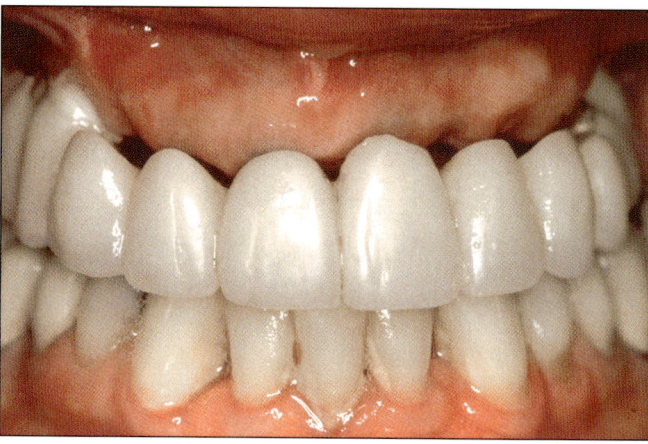

Fig 7-1c Prosthesis in place 1 week after surgery. The patient will wear the prosthesis until the implants are uncovered.

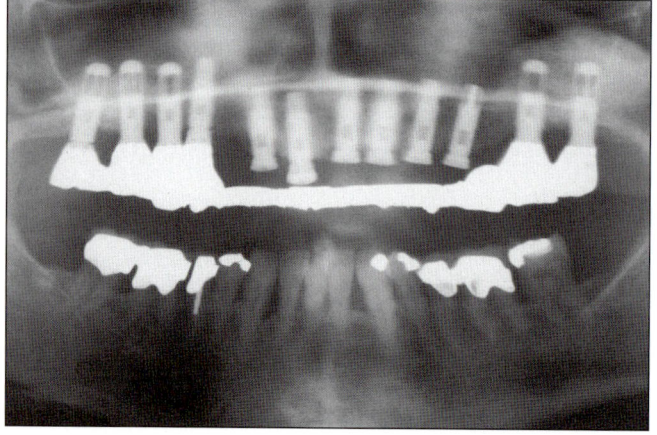

Fig 7-1d Panoramic radiograph following surgical placement of maxillary anterior implants and the gold and acrylic resin–veneered prosthesis.

The indexed framework is invested and soldered. After soldering and divesting, the assembly is verified on the soldering cast and then tried intraorally.

The centric occlusal contacts and contours of the restoration are evaluated. The gold screws are removed, and steel waxing pins are inserted into each screw-access channel. An elastomeric impression is made.

Definitive Prosthesis

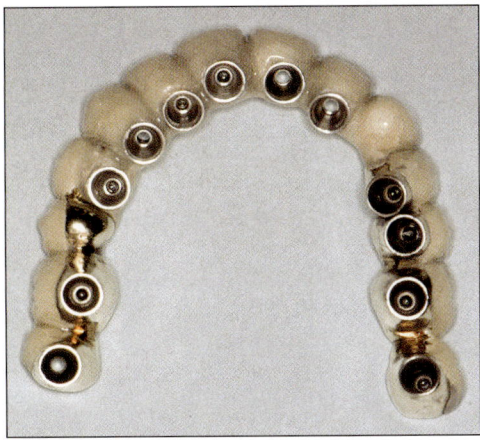

Fig 7-1e After 6 months, the anterior implants were uncovered, conical abutments were installed, and the anterior implants were loaded with a screw-retained metal and acrylic section attached to the posterior gold and acrylic–veneered prosthesis.

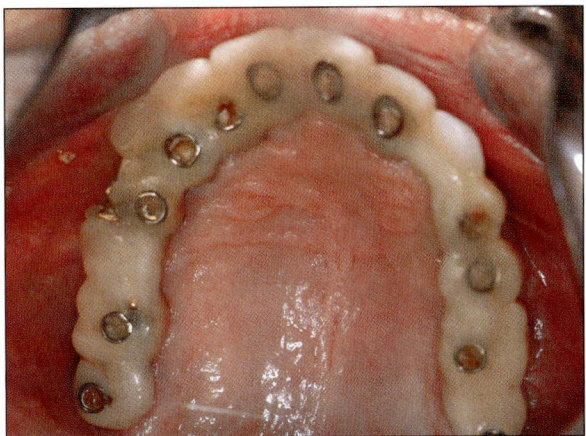

Fig 7-1f Acrylic resin with fabricated metal provisional cylinders inserted during fabrication of the gold and acrylic resin definitive prosthesis.

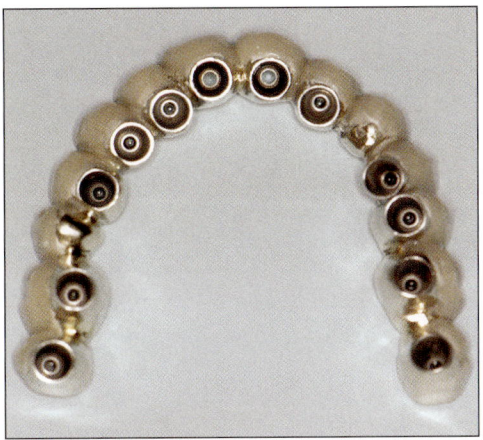
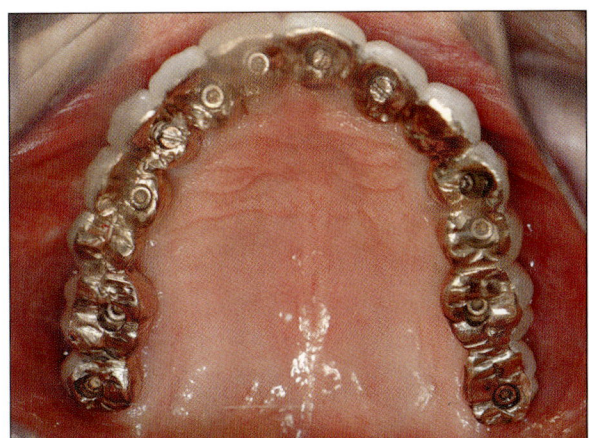

Figs 7-1g and 7-1h Gingival and occlusal views of the definitive screw-retained prosthesis.

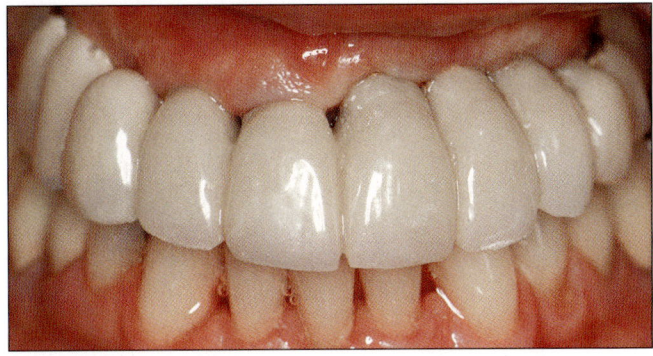

Fig 7-1i Facial view of the definitive prosthesis.

Analogs are screwed to the gold cylinders, and silicone soft tissue casting material is syringed around the gingival area of the prosthesis. The impression is then boxed and poured. After it has set, the cast is mounted on the articulator to verified maxillomandibular relation. The gold framework is refined and polished, and occlusal contacts are verified. The acrylic resin veneer is then processed and the occlusion refined (Figs 7-1a to 7-1i). A harmonious occlusal scheme, both at the intra-arch and at the inter-arch, is established.

81

Chapter 7: Prosthetic Management of the Sinus Graft Patient

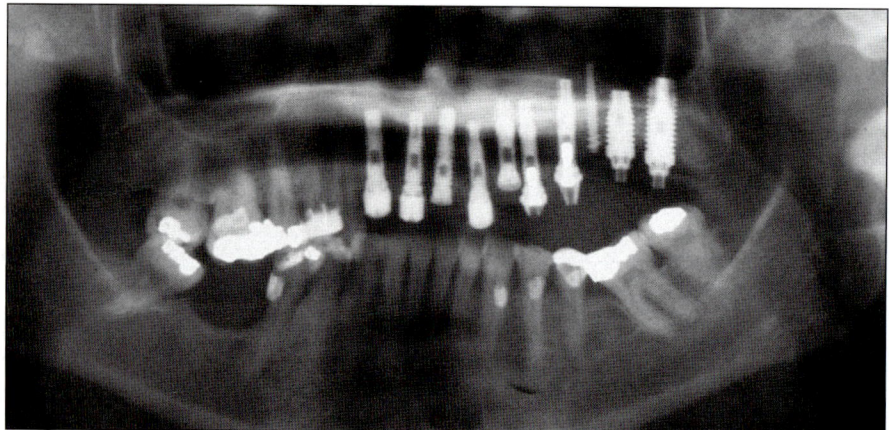

Fig 7-2a Case 2. Panoramic radiograph following implant uncovering and installation of conical abutments posteriorly and 17-degree multi-unit angulated abutments (Nobel Biocare) anteriorly. Provisional implants were placed to support a cemented provisional prosthesis. The provisional implant placed in the left maxilla integrated and had to be reduced to the level of the bone.

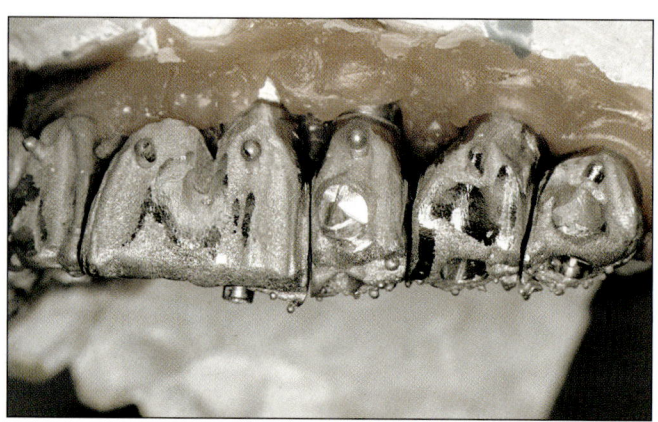

Fig 7-2b Buccal view of ceramometal casting fitted on the soft tissue cast. Each implant casting was cast and fitted separately. Intraoral soldering indices were used for assembly.

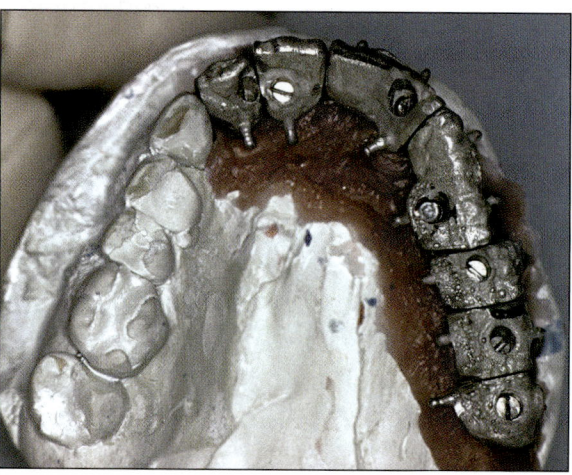

Fig 7-2c Occlusal view of ceramometal castings made of 52% gold and palladium alloy without silver.

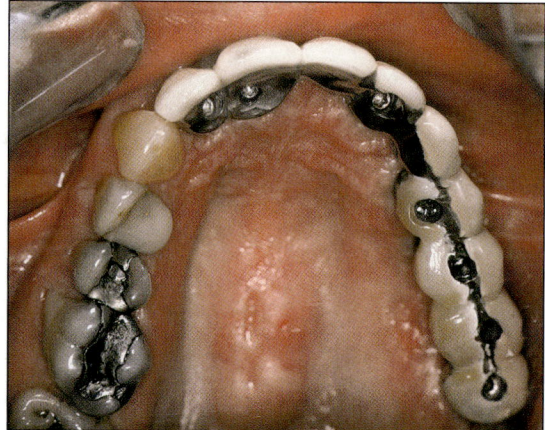

Fig 7-2d Intraoral view of maxillary anterior and left posterior prosthesis. The posterior portion of the prosthesis was fabricated with porcelain veneering on the buccal aspect and a heat-cured acrylic resin veneering on the occlusal and palatal aspects. The occlusobuccal metal delineates the buccal porcelain veneers from the occlusal acrylic resin. The gold screw access channels contact the opposing dentition.

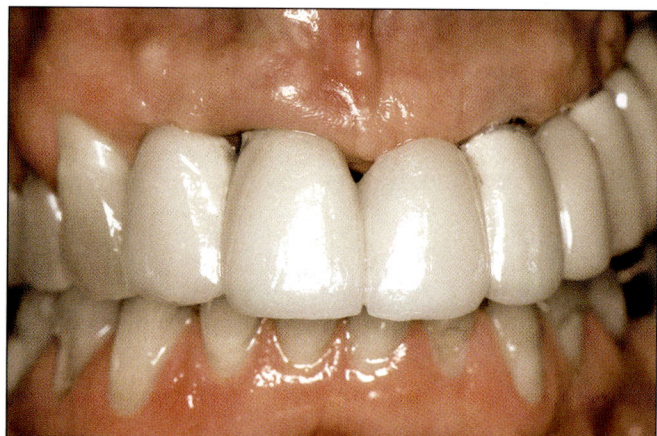

Fig 7-2e Facial view of the definitive prosthesis.

Fig 7-3a Case 3. Panoramic radiograph following bilateral sinus grafting and implant placement. One implant was lost in the left second molar area. The patient had inadequate maxillary bone for anterior implant placement, which was probably related to her history of Crohn disease requiring high-dose cortisone treatment.

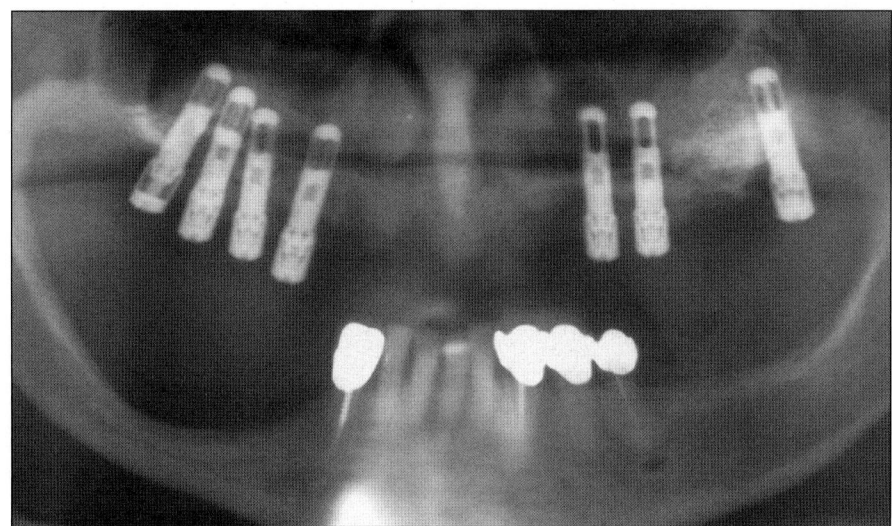

Alternative fabrication techniques

Acrylic resin–porcelain veneers

An alternative method that can be used to create the definitive prosthesis uses multiple-unit gold cylinders with a combination of acrylic resin and porcelain veneers.[17] The positions of the gold cylinders are verified intraorally. The framework is waxed with an occlusal ridge between the screw-access channels and the buccal veneer. Mechanical retention is added occlusally and palatally. The retention terminates at the occlusal ridge.

The waxup is sectioned, sprued, and invested with a phosphate bonding. Castings of gold–palladium alloy are made, cooled, and fitted to the cast. They are then tried intraorally, and a solder index is obtained. The castings are invested and soldered with the appropriate ceramometal solder, and the assembly is evaluated on the soldering verification cast using a one-screw test. After the fit is evaluated on this cast, the framework is evaluated intraorally using the one-screw test, clinical evaluation, and right-angle radiographs. If the fit is accurate, a second complete-arch impression is made and a soft tissue cast is poured.

The portion of the casting facial to the occlusal ridge of gold is baked with porcelain veneer. This is evaluated intraorally for contour, shade, and facial appearance. Occlusal contacts are verified, and the occlusal and palatal surfaces are heat-cured in the Ivomat in acrylic resin of the same shade (Figs 7-2a to 7-2e). This technique uses acrylic resin occlusally for shock absorption while optimizing the esthetic result.

Porcelain-fused-to-gold materials

A third method for fabricating a screw-retained fixed prosthesis employs porcelain-fused-to-gold materials.[18,19] Multiple-unit gold cylinders are used to overcome distortions of metal during the baking of the porcelain veneers. Problems can result from the increased impact forces generated by the porcelain veneering material. No long-term studies have been published on the use of this material to restore an implant placed in a sinus graft.

Removable bar prosthesis

An additional method for a completely edentulous maxilla utilizes a removable bar type of definitive prosthesis.[20–22] This is employed to improve patient function, comfort, and hygiene. If the anterior maxilla is allowed to remain without implants because of the advanced alveolar bone resorption, a removable appliance will reduce stress on the graft and posterior implants and improve the esthetic result. Bilateral sinus grafts with three or four implants in each graft site are performed with either a one- or two-stage surgical procedure, depending on residual available bone.

A Dolder, Ackermann, or milled bar is usually employed. If the length and width of the implants placed into the sinus grafts are sufficient and at least six are in place, a milled bar with or without spark-erosion plus the retaining devices is commonly used. The milled bar is less resilient and less tissue-borne than the other types of bar prostheses. Usually less than a full palate major connector is utilized. The bar strategy is basically a solution to the presence of an extensive anterior cantilever (Figs 7-3a to 7-3f).

chapter 7 Prosthetic Management of the Sinus Graft Patient

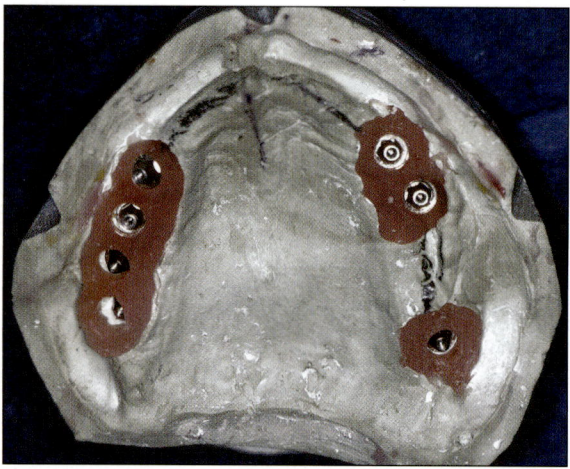

Fig 7-3b Maxillary soft tissue cast with conical abutment replicas.

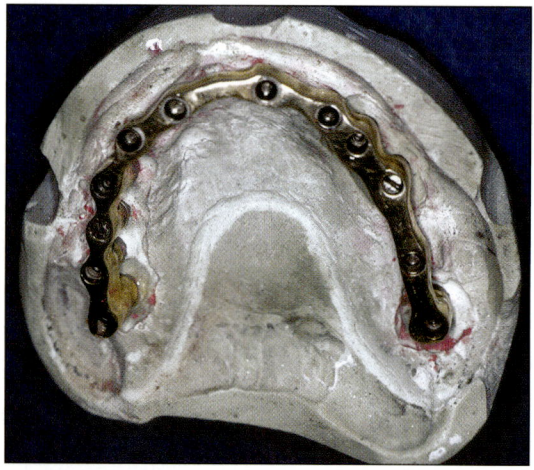

Fig 7-3c Assembled bar on the maxillary cast. Ceka-Revax (Preat) retentive devices were used for the overdenture.

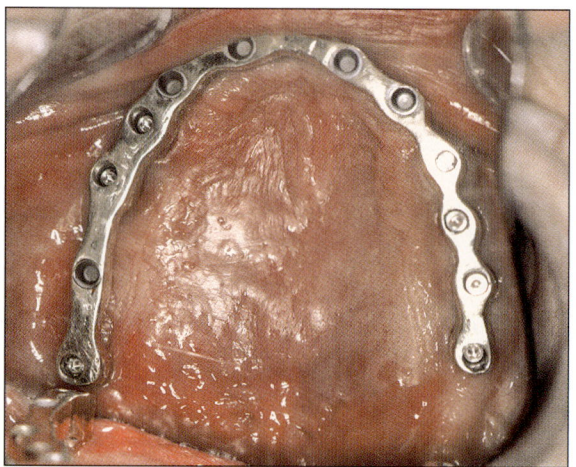

Fig 7-3d Assembled bar prior to insertion of the overdenture. Vertical bitewing radiographs verified the fit of the gold cylinders to the abutments.

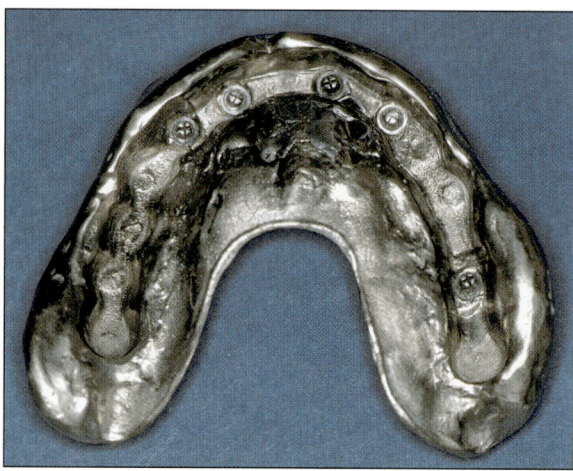

Fig 7-3e Superstructure overdenture retained with Ceka-Revax devices. Type IV gold alloy was used for the overdenture casting. All denture borders were fabricated in gold alloy.

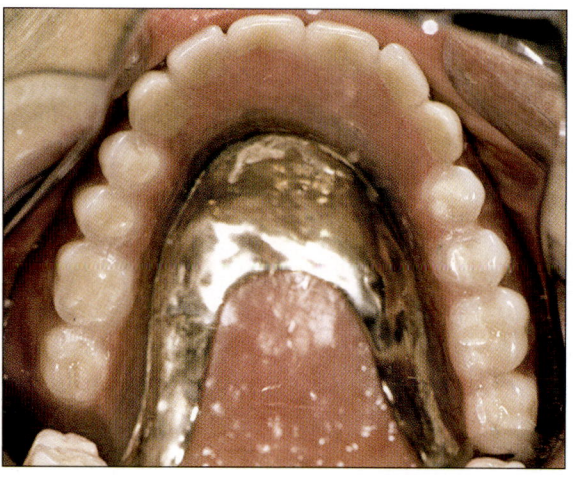

Fig 7-3f Completed maxillary overdenture in situ.

References

1. Zinner ID, Small SA. Maxillary sinus grafts and prosthetic management. In: Zinner ID, Panno FV, Small SA, Landa LS. Implant Dentistry: From Failure to Success. Chicago: Quintessence, 2004:33–49, 61–80, 99–115.
2. Bain CA, Moy PK. The association between the failure of dental implants and cigarette smoking. Int J Oral Maxillofac Implants 1993;8:609–615.
3. Zinner ID, Small SA. Sinus-lift graft: Using the maxillary sinuses to support implants. J Am Dent Assoc 1996;127:51–57.
4. Spiekermann H. Implantology. New York: Thieme, 1995:88, 214, 230.
5. Small SA, Zinner ID, Panno FV, Shapiro HJ, Stein JI. Augmenting the maxillary sinus for implants: Report of 27 patients. Int J Oral Maxillofac Implants 1993;8:523–528.
6. Jensen O, Shulman LB, Block MS, Iacono VJ. Report of the Sinus Graft Consensus Conference of 1996. Int J Maxillofac Implants 1998;13(Suppl):11–45.
7. Skalak RS. Biomechanical considerations in osseointegrated prostheses. J Prosthet Dent 1983;49:843–848.
8. Skalak R. Aspects of biomechanical considerations. In: Brånemark P-I, Zarb GA, Albrektsson T (eds). Tissue-Integrated Prostheses: Osseointegration in Clinical Dentistry. Chicago: Quintessence, 1985:117–128.
9. Gracis SE, Nicholls JI, Chalupnik JD, Yuodelis RA. Shock-absorbing behavior of five restorative materials used on implants. Int J Prosthodont 1991;4:282–291.
10. Zinner ID, Small SA, Panno FV, Pines MS. Provisional and definitive prostheses following sinus lift and augmentation procedures. Implant Dent 1994;3:24–28.
11. Zinner ID. Provisional and definitive sinus lift prosthodontics. Presented at the International College of Prosthodontists Biennial Meeting, San Diego, 1995.
12. Binon PP. Evaluation of machining accuracy and consistency of selected implants, standard abutments and laboratory analogues. Int J Prosthodont 1995;8:162–178.
13. Tatum H Jr. Maxillary and sinus implant reconstructions. Dent Clin North Am 1986;30:207–229.
14. Misch CE. Density of bone: Effect on treatment plans, surgical approach, healing and progressive bone loading. Int J Oral Implantol 1990;6(2):23–31.
15. Binon PP, Sullivan DY. Provisional fixed restorations technique for osseointegrated implants. J Calif Dent Assoc 1990;18(1):23–30.
16. Lazzara RJ. Restorative advantages of the coronally hexed implant. Compend Contin Educ Dent 1991;12:924–930.
17. Fredrickson EJ, Stevens PJ, Gress ML. Implant Prosthodontics, Clinical and Laboratory Procedures. St Louis: Mosby, 1995:84–113.
18. Davis DM, Rimrott R, Zarb GA. Studies on frameworks for osseointegrated prostheses. Part 2. The effect of adding acrylic resin or porcelain to form the occlusal superstructure. Int J Oral Maxillofac Implants 1988;3:275–280.
19. Naert I, Quirynen M, van Steenberghe D, Darius P. A six-year prosthodontic study of 509 consecutively inserted implants for the treatment of partial edentulism. J Prosthet Dent 1992;67:236–245.
20. Enquist B, Bergendal T, Kallus T, Linden U. A retrospective multicenter evaluation of osseointegrated implants supporting overdentures. Int J Oral Maxillofac Implants 1988;3:129–134.
21. Block MS, Kent JN, Finger IM. Use of the integral implant for overdenture stabilization. Int J Oral Maxillofac Implants 1990;5:140–147.
22. Finger IM, Block MS, Salinas TJ. Treatment of a resorbed maxilla with sinus grafting, implants, and a spark erosion overdenture: A clinical report. Implant Dent 1992;1:150–153.

chapter 8
Contraindications for Sinus Graft Procedures

Matteo Chiapasco, MD
Joel L. Rosenlicht, DMD
Salvatore L. Ruggiero, DMD, MD
Ronald E. Schneider, DDS

Rehabilitation of partially and completely edentulous patients with dental implants has become a commonplace procedure with reliable long-term results.[1-8] In some patients, however, local conditions of the edentulous alveolar ridges may be unfavorable for implant placement. The posterior edentulous maxilla, in particular, often presents a challenge as a result of alveolar ridge resorption and/or maxillary sinus pneumatization, which lead to bone loss (Figs 8-1a and 8-1b). Moreover, low-quality residual bone can compromise final results. Grafting of the maxillary sinus to overcome these problems has become a popular procedure (Figs 8-1c and 8-1d).[9-21]

The maxillary sinus graft procedure is a well-established technique for increasing bone volume in preparation for implant placement. When executed properly on the appropriate patient, this surgical procedure is one of the most successful bone-grafting procedures performed today. Numerous studies of maxillary sinus grafting, both prospective and retrospective, report long-term success, which is remarkable given the wide assortment of graft materials being used.

As with any surgical procedure, a number of potential complications of sinus floor augmentation may interfere with the normal function of the sinus. It is important to understand maxillary sinus function and how it is affected by the sinus graft procedure. There are limits to this treatment modality. Medical and surgical risk factors should always be addressed before a decision is made to proceed with surgery. Risks and benefits are important and should be considered and discussed with the patient.

The maxilla comprises a variety of anatomic structures, including the maxillary sinus, lateral nasal wall, pterygoid plates, associated vasculature, and teeth. Understanding these structures and their functions is a prerequisite to the sinus bone graft.[22] The maxillary sinus is lined with flattened, pseudostratified, ciliated epithelium composed of basal cells, goblet cells (which synthesize and discharge glycoprotein-containing mucus), seromucinous glands, and ciliated columnar cells. The ciliated epithelium clears sinus fluid that is evacuated by antigravitational movement. The natural ostium allows drainage of sinus fluid through the middle meatus of the nose, which is located cranially. Mucociliary clearance, in physiologic health, spreads from the sinus floor in a starlike pattern, ascends the sinus walls, and passes through the ostium.[23-25]

Proper function of the maxillary sinus depends on a delicate balance between mucus production, transport by ciliated epithelium, sinus ventilation, and sustainable drainage through the ostium. In addition, there are communicating ethmoid and frontal sinuses that affect the maxillary sinus if they are unhealthy or chronically inflamed. These conditions can arise unilaterally or bilaterally. Any factor interfering with one of these functions will compromise maxillary sinus health. A grafting procedure generally does not interfere with sinus function when performed on a healthy sinus[26-31]; however, when performed on an unhealthy sinus, the same procedure will contribute to fluid stagnation and bacterial overgrowth, leading to an exacerbated sinusitis. Moreover, the presence of space-occupying masses such as polyps, tumors, and hyperplastic

chapter 8 Contraindications for Sinus Graft Procedures

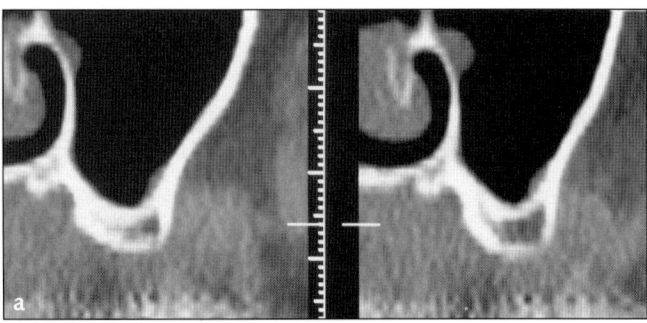

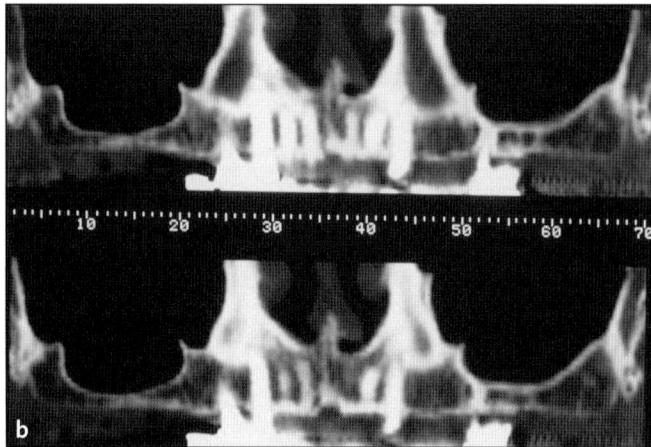

Figs 8-1a and 8-1b Pneumatized maxillary sinus showing no evidence of pathology.

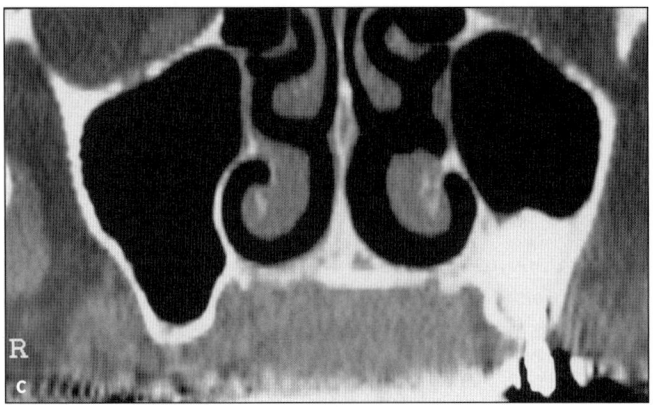

Fig 8-1c No adverse effects visible following sinus grafting and implant placement.

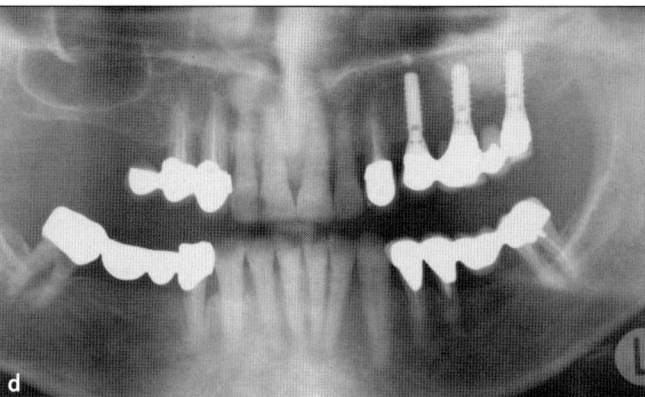

Fig 8-1d Definitive implant-borne prosthesis placed in grafted maxillary sinus.

mucosa represent obstacles to the elevation of the sinus mucosa. Pre-existing local pathologic conditions represent relative or absolute contraindications to the sinus graft procedure and therefore must be carefully scrutinized before surgery.

Sinus-grafting procedures are performed to enable implant placement and rehabilitation with implant-supported prostheses. Therefore, all intraoral contraindications for the placement of dental implants must be considered as well.

Finally, as with all surgical procedures, the systemic medical health of the patient must be evaluated. All patients who undergo sinus surgical procedures should receive a thorough medical evaluation. The degree and type of surgery, type of anesthesia, and general health of the patient are all critical factors that must be reviewed to establish candidacy.

Local Contraindications

Local contraindications fall into two main groups: *(1)* potentially reversible (relative); and *(2)* irreversible (absolute). The first group includes pathologies that, if not treated, contraindicate sinus grafting. The second group includes pathologies that, even after surgical management, leave irreversible dysfunction of the osteomeatal complex.

Potentially reversible, relative contraindications to sinus grafting

Some anatomic and/or structural alterations of the nasomaxillary complex may interfere with normal ventilation and mucociliary clearance of the maxillary sinus. Compen-

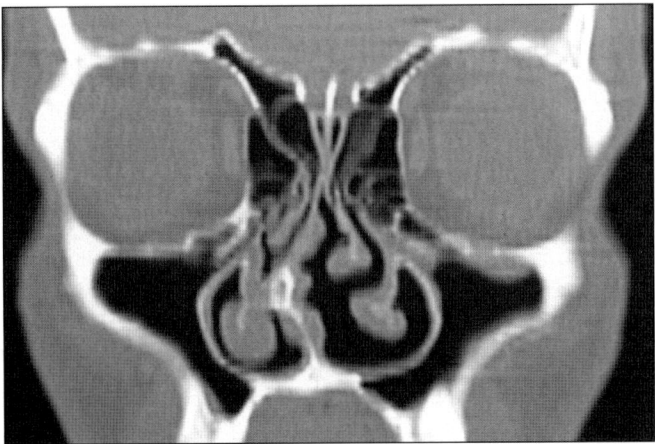

Fig 8-2 Deviated septum.

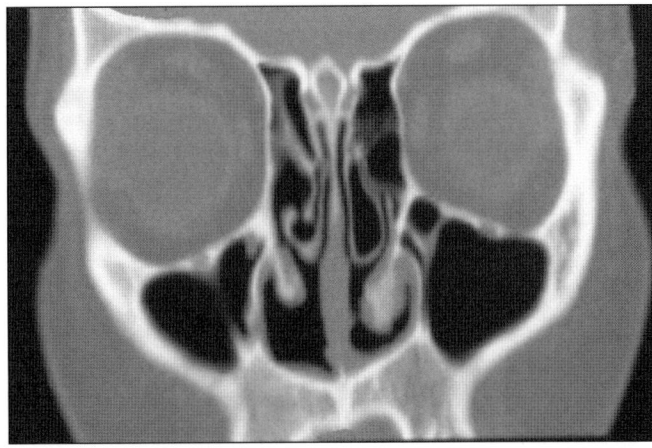

Fig 8-3 Concha bullosa.

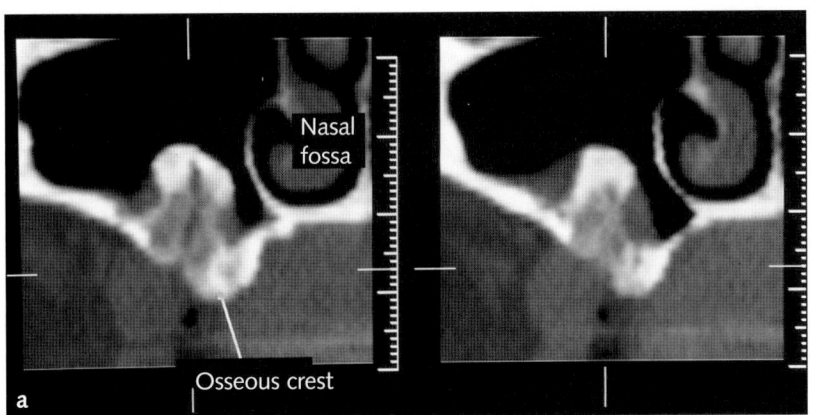
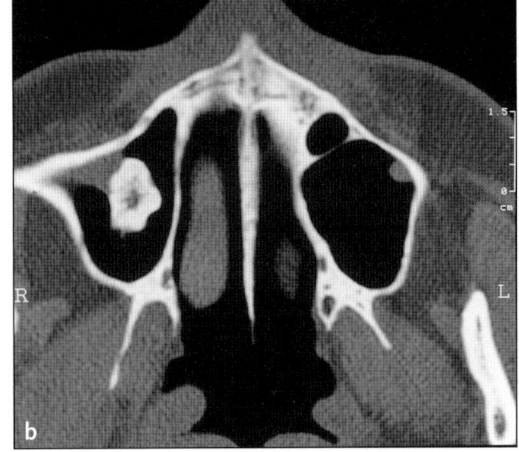

Figs 8-4a and 8-4b Intrasinusal osteoma of the maxillary sinus.

sation may occur over time, leaving such abnormal conditions clinically silent or with only mild to moderate, sometimes intermittent, symptoms. Sinus-grafting procedures in this setting decompensate a compromised sinus, causing mucus stasis, suprainfection, and subacute sinusitis. The elevation of the sinus floor and/or modification of sinus anatomy may on occasion lead to better sinus drainage in the presence of mild sinus membrane dysfunction. But in general, alterations in function of the maxillary sinus membrane and the osteomeatal complex should be identified and treated *before* sinus grafting is performed. It is imperative that patients undergo thorough radiographic evaluation to identify underlying sinus pathology and anatomic disturbance. Computerized tomography (CT) scans, plain film radiographs, and patient history are part of the comprehensive workup of the patient. Positive radiographic findings include:

1. Narrowing of the osteomeatal complex due to a deviated septum (Fig 8-2); abnormal morphology of the middle turbinate; enlargement of air cells within the middle turbinate, known as *concha bullosa* (Fig 8-3); enlargement of an air cell in the roof of the sinus (Haller cell); medial or lateral rotation of the uncinate process; enlargement of the bulla ethmoidale with narrowing of the uncinate process; or post-traumatic or postsurgical scarring
2. Benign tumors of the nasomaxillary complex such as papillomas, schwannomas, osteomas, polyps, or mucus retention cysts (Figs 8-4 and 8-5)

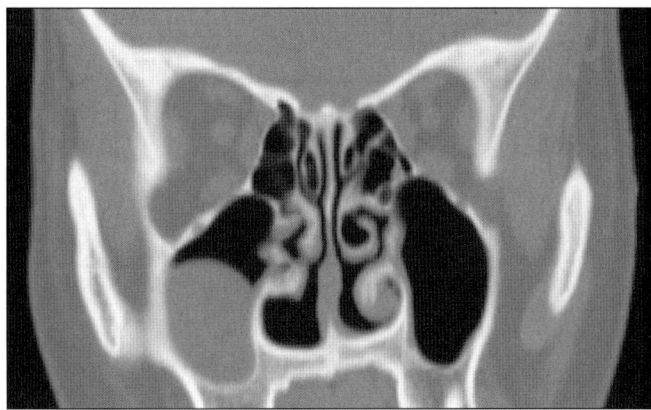

Fig 8-5 Mucus retention cyst.

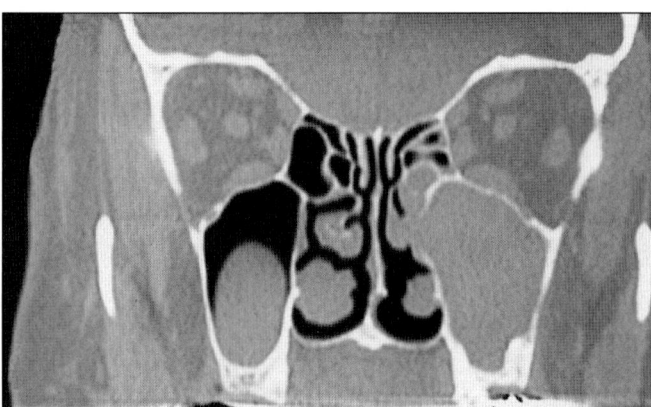

Fig 8-6 Bacterial sinusitis of the left maxillary sinus and mucus retention cyst on the right sinus.

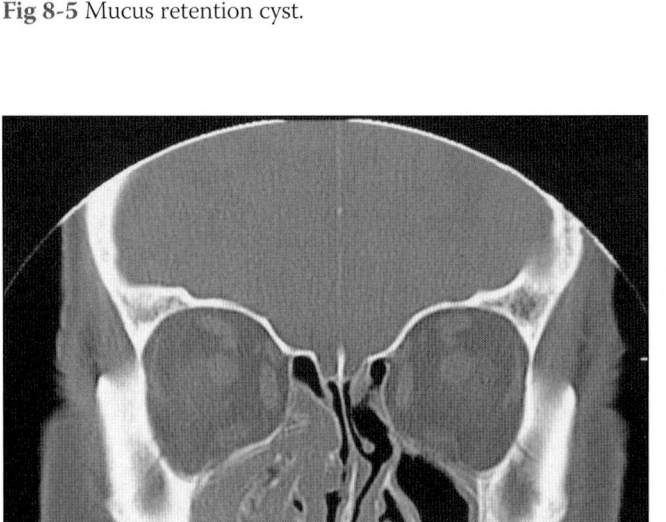

Fig 8-7 Micotic sinusitis caused by intrasinusal foreign body.

3. Viral, bacterial, and micotic rhinosinusitis (Figs 8-6 and 8-7); allergic sinusitis; sinusitis caused by intrasinusal foreign bodies; or odontogenic sinusitis originating from necrotic teeth of the lateral-posterior maxilla
4. Malignancy of the nasomaxillary region (Fig 8-8)

Treatment of the offending etiology (eg, endodontic treatment of necrotic teeth, medical or surgical therapy of sinusitis, removal of tumors or polyps) must eradicate the pathologic condition prior to sinus graft augmentation. Resolution of a compromised sinus is accomplished by functional endoscopic sinus surgery. This approach corrects anatomic or structural alterations of the nasomaxillary complex and removes pathologic sinus tissue that is otherwise not susceptible to medical management.[25,32] After functional endoscopic sinus surgery, if radiographic and/or endoscopic evidence demonstrates resolution of the pre-existing pathology, it is possible to perform a sinus graft procedure.

Local Contraindications

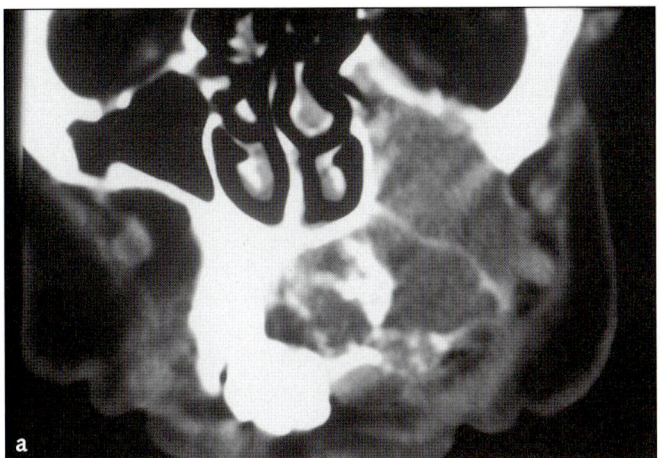

Fig 8-8a Large ameloblastoma of the maxilla.

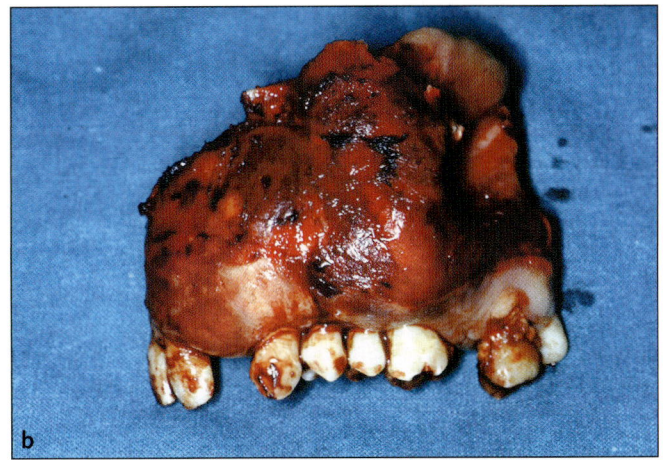

Fig 8-8b View of resected tumor.

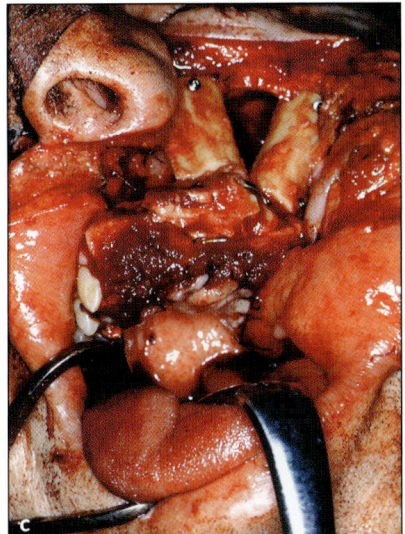

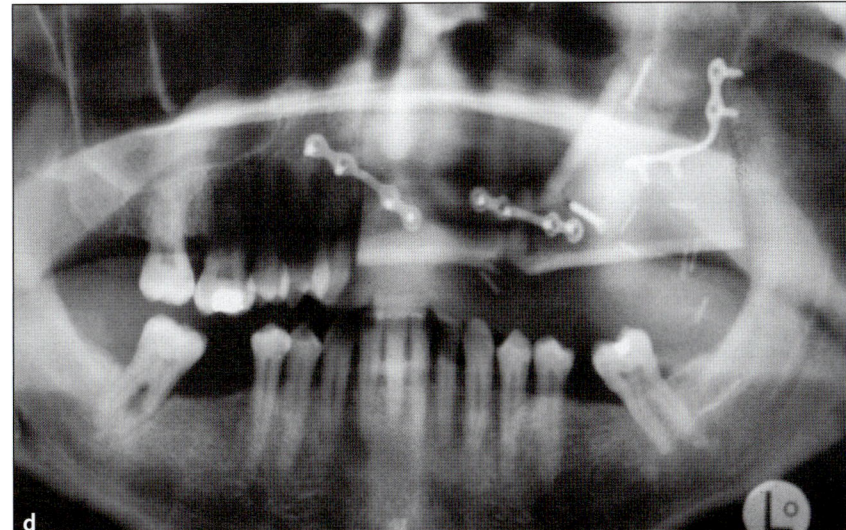

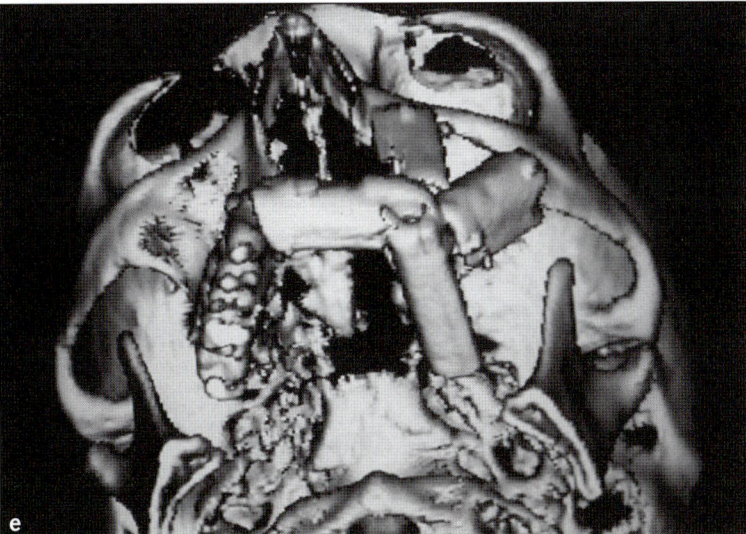

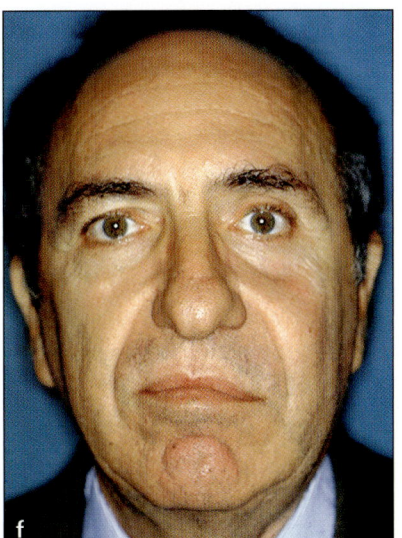

Figs 8-8c to 8-8f Despite adequate reconstruction of the resected maxilla and acceptable face morphology, sinus function is permanently compromised. (Surgery by Dr M. Chiapasco and Prof R. Brusati, Milan, Italy.)

Irreversible, absolute contraindications to sinus grafting

Some anatomic and/or structural alterations or pathologies of the nasomaxillary complex may represent absolute contraindications to the sinus graft procedure. These include:

1. Severe (noncorrectable) deformities of the maxillary sinus
2. Scarred and hypofunctional sinus mucosa following trauma or previous operation
3. Radiotherapy of the head and neck area (radiation dose above 45 Gy[60])
4. Chronic recurrent sinusitis, with or without polyposis, that disrupts mucociliary clearance and is unresponsive to medical or surgical treatment
5. Local expression of a systemic granulomatous disease such as Wegener granulomatosis or midline idiopathic granuloma
6. Sarcoidosis
7. Benign but locally aggressive tumor (eg, ameloblastoma, myxoma, desmoplastic fibroma, inverted papilloma)
8. Malignant tumor, both primary and metastatic, deriving from epithelial, connective, or odontogenic tissues (eg, squamous cell carcinoma, esthesioneuroblastoma, adenoid cystic carcinoma, adenocarcinoma, sarcoma). These tumors may require extensive resection and may permanently disturb mucociliary function.[32]

Intraoral Contraindications

Abnormal intraoral conditions may compromise the sinus-grafting procedure and/or survival of dental implants placed into the grafted sinuses. These contraindications are similar to those reported in non–sinus-directed implant locations and include the following:

1. Grossly inadequate oral hygiene or inability to perform or maintain appropriate oral hygiene
2. Untreated periodontal disease of adjacent dentition
3. Gross malocclusion and insufficient freeway space for restoration
4. Severe pathologic parafunctional habit (clenching or bruxism)
5. Fulminant mucosal disease (desquamative mucosal disease, erosive lichen planus)
6. Severe xerostomia

General Medical Conditions of Concern

Compromised general health may represent a relative or absolute contraindication to sinus grafting. Generally speaking, systemic pathoses, such as increased risk for myocardial infarction, hypertensive crisis, or sudden hypoglycemia, may proscribe surgical intervention. The sinus graft procedure should be avoided in patients with compromised healing, such as patients with uncontrolled diabetes, immunocompromised patients, or patients on antitumoral chemotherapy. The following conditions, unless treated and under control with the patient's complete understanding of the risks, generally contraindicate the sinus graft procedure:

1. Chronic renal disease
2. Chronic liver disease
3. Uncontrolled diabetes
4. Uncontrolled hypertension
5. Hemophilia or treatment with anticoagulant therapy
6. Metabolic bone disorders
7. Uncontrolled thyroid disorders
8. Uncontrolled adrenal disorders
9. Immunocompromise, including HIV
10. Steroid treatment at the time of the sinus graft procedure
11. Pregnancy

General surgical contraindications include:

1. Chemotherapy for the treatment of malignant tumors at the time of the sinus graft procedure
2. Radiotherapy
3. Drug or alcohol abuse
4. Heavy smoking
5. Physical or psychiatric handicaps
6. Patient noncompliance

It is beyond the objectives of this chapter to correlate each systemic pathology with the effects it may have on the outcome of oral surgery procedures such as sinus grafting. Therefore, only selected aspects will be addressed in this section.

Myocardial infarction

A history of myocardial infarction, particularly recent infarction (within the previous 6 months), may represent a contraindication. With the exclusion of recent myocardial infarction, after thorough analysis of ventricular function, compromised patients should be treated in a hospital setting. Generally, elective surgery should be delayed 6 months after infarction. Stable medical management and medical clearance for the sinus graft procedure should be obtained.

A critical factor of concern in a patient with a history of myocardial infarction is the severity of myocardial ischemia, ventricular irritability, and ventricular ejection fraction. It is imperative that elective dental procedures be delayed 6 months after infarction. Close communication with the patient's treating physician is strongly recommended to avoid inordinate medical risk.[33]

Other cardiac pathologies

Patients with cardiac prosthetic valves, a history of subacute bacterial endocarditis, congenital malformation, rheumatic heart disease, sequelae of vascular surgery, cardiomyopathy, or vascular disease with regurgitation may be treated with sinus grafting, but they require antibiotic prophylaxis.[34] Patients with an isolated nongrafted septal defect, mitral valve prolapse without regurgitation, functional murmur, or cardiac pacemaker, and those who have undergone coronary bypass are treated without antibiotic prophylaxis.

Anticoagulant therapy

Patients who take anticoagulants may undergo a sinus graft procedure, but only after authorization of the patient's treating physician to verify coagulation status.[35,36] Discontinuing anticoagulants is no longer considered absolutely necessary if the INR value is within an acceptable range. Many patients today self-administer aspirin or holistic vitamin therapy. These can significantly affect bleeding time and coagulation. Discontinuing these medications at least 1 week prior to surgery is appropriate.

Radiotherapy

Radiotherapy in the head and neck area will affect the outcome of bone grafting and survival of dental implants. Irradiation produces both early and late tissue damage. The early effects involve the soft tissues, leading to xerostomia and mucositis. The late effects include hypocellularity, hypovascularity, and endothelial hypoxia, involving both hard and soft tissues. Radiation tissue damage compromises bone regeneration and graft incorporation and increases the likelihood of wound dehiscence.[37] Because of impaired vascularity, hard and soft tissues offer less resistance to surgical trauma, which can lead to osteoradionecrosis.[37,38] Modifying factors include the interval of time between the end of radiation and surgery, the radiation fractionation, the radiation source, and the total dose of radiation. A higher complication rate occurs when superfractionation rather than standard fractionation is delivered.[39,40] Complications are more commonly observed at doses above 65 Gy but rarely seen at doses below 48 Gy.[41]

Definitive data are lacking on the question of whether a prolonged interval is needed between radiation and implant placement or bone-grafting procedures. Some authors[37,42] advocate an extended waiting period between irradiation and rehabilitation surgery in order to avoid complications, recommending at least 12 months prior to implant placement.[43–45] Hyperbaric oxygen therapy may also be helpful in reducing the risk of radionecrosis or failure of bone incorporation.[42,45–50] In general, irradiated patients who undergo open-flap osseous surgery should be treated with extreme caution.[46,51,52]

Chemotherapy

Patients who undergo chemotherapy for cancer treatment present with immunosuppression, myelosuppression, and oral tissue cytotoxicity. These conditions manifest as mucositis, xerostomia, heightened risk of infection, mucosal ulceration, or hemorrhage. There is a paucity of information concerning the direct effect of chemotherapy on sinus bone grafting and implant placement. Available data are controversial. A retrospective study by Wolfaardt et al (1996)[53] showed that the rate of implant loss for patients who had received chemotherapy was 21.9%. However, other authors report no negative influence of chemotherapy on the osseointegration process.[54–56]

A conservative approach is to delay implant placement or grafting procedures until 3 months after chemotherapy so that the hematopoietic response can return to within normal limits. The patient must have physician clearance for the procedure and must understand the added risk should the disease recur and additional chemotherapy be required. Patients with bone grafts and implants that are already in place, who then undergo chemotherapy, seem to do well. However, the risk of infection, negative tissue response, and so forth is increased.

Due to the relevant side effects of chemotherapy and the insufficient information concerning its effects on sinus-grafting procedures, extreme caution is suggested when treating these patients. Current chemotherapy (in particular, high-dose chemotherapy) for malignant tumors represents an absolute contraindication for sinus-grafting procedures. Moreover, these patients generally present with active malignancies and an uncertain prognosis, a further contraindication for an elective surgical procedure. Low-dose chemotherapy or a history of previous chemotherapy with an acceptable general health condition may represent only a relative contraindication. In these cases, contacting the treating oncologist and ascertaining the status of the patient's immune system is suggested. The patient's white blood cell count and platelet status must be determined before surgery. In general, surgical procedures may be performed if the granulocyte count is above 2,000/mm^3 and the platelet count is above 40,000/mm^3.[57]

Any potential source of oral infection, such as plaque, calculus, or dental disease, must be identified and eliminated prior to surgery. Chlorhexidine mouthrinse and antibiotic prophylaxis are advisable prior to starting the sinus-grafting procedure.

Bisphosphonate therapy

Bisphosphonates are nonmetabolized analogs of pyrophosphate that localize to bone and inhibit osteoclast function. Following infusion, bisphosphonates bind avidly to exposed bone mineral around resorbing osteoclasts, resulting in high levels of bisphosphonate in the resorption lacunae. Since bisphosphonates are not metabolized, high concentrations are maintained within bone for a long time. Bisphosphonates are internalized by the osteoclast, causing disruption of osteoclast-mediated bone resorption. This results in markedly decreased osteoclast-mediated lysis of bone. The efficacy of these agents in reducing bone pain, hypercalcemia, and skeletal complications has been extensively documented in patients with metastatic breast cancer and multiple myeloma. Bisphosphonates are considered by most oncologists to be standard treatment in patients with clinical or radiographic evidence of metastases. Pamidronate (Aredia, Novartis) is a second-generation bisphosphonate that is administered intravenously every 3 to 4 weeks at a dose of 90 mg, primarily in patients with multiple myeloma. Zoledronic acid (Zometa, Novartis), a third-generation bisphosphonate, was recently approved for patients with metastatic breast cancer, multiple myeloma, hypercalcemia of malignancy, Paget disease of bone, and documented bone metastases from any solid tumor (eg, prostate cancer, lung cancer). Compared to pamidronate, zoledronic acid is significantly more potent and much more effective in controlling hypercalcemia of malignancy and reducing the overall number of skeletal complications.

There has been growing awareness of compromised jawbone healing in patients receiving bisphosphonate therapy. Based on several reports in the literature, it appears that the pathogenesis of this process is most consistent with a defect in jawbone healing and/or localized vascular insufficiency.[58–61] Hypothetically, the mechanism by which bisphosphonates can have this effect may be related to their effect on osteoclasts. With significant impairment of osteoclast function, normal bone turnover and resorption are inhibited. This could result in decreased new bone formation and diminished capillary ingrowth. Bisphosphonates have also demonstrated effects unrelated to osteoclast inhibition. Pamidronate was reported to significantly depress bone blood flow in rats.[62,63] The mechanism of this effect may be attributable to a complex interaction of pamidronate with growth hormone and insulin-like growth factor I, both of which are thought to play a role in the regulation of blood circulation in bones. In a recent study, bisphosphonates were shown to inhibit endothelial cell function in vitro and in vivo.[64] Cells treated with bisphosphonates demonstrated decreased proliferation, an increased rate of apoptosis, and a decrease in capillary tube formation.[65] Bisphosphonates have also demonstrated antiangiogenic properties due to their ability to significantly decrease circulating levels of vascular endothelial growth factor (VEGF, a potent angiogenic factor) in breast cancer patients with bone metastases.[66] Furthermore, these bisphosphonate properties could explain the apparent ischemic changes noted in the affected patients' jawbones.

Typical signs and symptoms include pain, soft tissue swelling and infection, loosening of teeth, and exposed bone, which may occur spontaneously or, more commonly, at a site of jawbone trauma (eg, an extraction site). These lesions may remain asymptomatic for many weeks or months and may only be recognized by the presence of pain or exposed bone in the oral cavity (Fig 8-9). Chronic maxillary sinusitis secondary to necrotic bone and an oroantral fistula are possible manifestations in patients

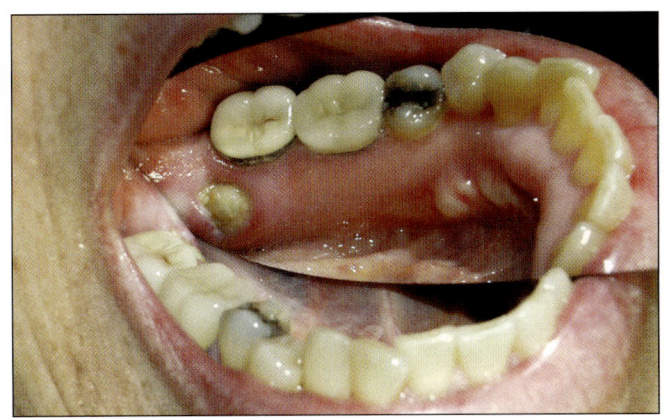

Fig 8-9 Soft tissue swelling and exposed bone in a patient undergoing treatment with bisphosphonate therapy.

with posterior maxillary involvement. If osteonecrosis is suspected, panoramic and tomographic imaging may be performed to rule out other etiologies. However, a thorough intraoral clinical exam, coupled with radiographs, is the most effective way to establish the diagnosis.

The apparent selective involvement of the maxilla and mandible may be a reflection of the unique environment of the oral cavity. Typically, healing of an open bony wound (eg, extraction socket) in the presence of normal oral microflora occurs quickly and without infection. However, when the vascular supply or the healing potential of the mandible or maxilla is compromised either by radiation therapy or some other agent(s), then minor injury or disease in these sites is much more likely to progress to widespread necrosis and osteomyelitis.

Management of patients with bisphosphonate-related osteonecrosis is extremely difficult. Surgical debridement has not been effective in eradicating the necrotic bone, and hyperbaric oxygen therapy has not been uniformly effective in limiting the progression of this process. It is difficult to obtain a surgical margin with viable bleeding bone. Therefore, surgical treatment should be avoided in most cases. Areas of necrotic bone that are a constant source of soft tissue irritation should be removed without exposing additional bone. However, it is likely that the margin of the debridement will remain exposed. Symptomatic patients with pathologic mandibular fractures may require a segmental resection with a continuity defect and immediate reconstruction with a rigid plate. Reconstruction of these patients with free or vascularized bone is not feasible given the likelihood that necrotic bone will be present or develop at the resection margin. Most patients with limited areas of exposed bone can be managed with irrigations and antibiotic therapy that is tailored to the culture and sensitivity data. Cessation of bisphosphonate treatment has not had a major impact on the osteonecrosis.

Although it is difficult to assess a patient's risk of developing this complication, patients who are receiving intravenous bisphosphonates or who have established sites of necrotic bone are more likely to develop a problem following any type of dentoalveolar surgery. Although patients with a history of osteoporosis who are receiving the less potent oral bisphosphonates alendronate (Fosamax, Merck) or risedronate (Actonel, Proctor & Gamble) are probably at a reduced risk of developing these problems, compromised bone healing and osteonecrosis have been reported in these patients as well.[58,59] Dental implant failures attributable to oral bisphosphonate therapy also have been reported in patients with osteoporosis.[60] It is clear from the current information that the short- and long-term effects of bisphosphonates on dental implant osseointegration and alveolar bone healing need to be studied further. Until such time, clinicians should be aware of the potential for delayed wound healing and osteonecrosis in these patients.

Smoking

Among factors that negatively affect the outcome of sinus grafting, smoking plays a prominent role. Overall, the failure rate of bone grafts placed in the posterior maxilla is up to 10% greater in smokers than in nonsmokers.[20,67] Smoking is known to be associated with an increased susceptibility to allergy and infections because it interferes with ciliary function and secretory immunity of the nasorespiratory tract. In the maxillary sinus, this may affect immune exclusion and suppression because both surface immunoglobulin A (sIgA) and sIgM responses are reduced, whereas IgE responses are increased.[68] Smoking disturbs bone graft healing because it reduces local blood flow by increasing peripheral resistance and platelet aggregation. By-product chemicals such as hydrogen cyanide and carbon monoxide inhibit wound healing, as does nicotine, which inhibits cellular proliferation. Tobacco may interfere directly with osteoblastic function, and there is a strong correlation of decreased bone formation in smokers, leading to a significant reduction of bone mineral content. Bone mineral density is reduced two to six times in the chronic smoker.[67–76] Overall, tobacco results in poor bone quality and poor healing capacity due to vascular and osteoblastic dysfunction.

Although smokers may be treated with sinus-grafting procedures, smoking represents a relative contraindication because of the risk of wound dehiscence, graft infection and/or resorption, and a 10% reduced probability of osseointegration. Patients who are smokers should be instructed to refrain from smoking for 15 to 30 days prior to surgery (to allow nicotine to clear systemically) and for 4 to 6 weeks after surgery. Moreover, smokers should sign a waiver that clearly explains the increased risk related to smoking. Patients who smoke more than 15 cigarettes per day are considered to be at risk for bone graft and implant failure in both the short and long term.

Osteoporosis

The concern that patients with osteoporosis are at an increased risk for dental implant failure is based on the assumption that the impaired bone metabolism in other areas of the skeleton affects the mandible or maxilla in a similar manner. However, whether there is a relationship between osteoporosis and decreased oral bone mass or density is controversial.[77–79] It is difficult to assess bone quality and quantity in the mandible and maxilla with the same specificity as the rest of the skeleton. Osteoporosis studies frequently involve small numbers of subjects, and measurements of bone loss are not uniformly defined (eg, the terms *bone mass* and *bone density* are often used interchangeably).[80–83]

The popular assumption that the impaired bone metabolism of osteoporosis can affect osseointegration of dental implants[80] has not been found to be true. Careful studies of bone remodeling reveal that it is not a uniform process: remodeling differs from one bone to another, from cortical to trabecular bone, and from one trabecular bone site to another.[81] Trabecular bone is much more likely to be affected by metabolic changes of the skeleton than is cortical bone. For this reason, the maxilla, which is largely trabecular bone, is more susceptible to rapid bone turnover from trauma, inflammation, atrophy, or high metabolic states than the mandible, which is primarily cortical bone.[84]

Osteoporotic fractures heal normally, suggesting that the osseous repair process in patients with osteoporosis is fundamentally sound. This further suggests that the bone modeling and remodeling processes following implant placement into osteoporotic bone will not differ substantially from that of a healthy patient.[85]

There is controversy in the literature, in both clinical and experimental studies, regarding the survival rate of implants placed into osteoporotic bone.[83,86–89] Both human trials and animal studies indicate that implant therapy is generally successful in osteoporotic bone. No study to date has proven an association between implant failure and osteoporosis.[90] Therefore, the available data do not contraindicate sinus grafting for patients with osteoporosis.

Considerations for the osteoporotic patient include:

1. Prior to sinus grafting, the osteoporotic patient should undergo a comprehensive assessment, including endocrinologic, orthopedic, and, if necessary, obstetric examination. A therapeutic regimen of physiologic doses of vitamin D (from 400 to 800 IU/day) and calcium (1,500 mg/day) is recommended. Calcitonin, which inhibits bone resorption and alters calcium metabolism, may be prescribed. Patients with osteoporosis should continue this regimen throughout the healing period following grafting procedures.[91] Smoking significantly increases the overall risk for demineralization and subsequent failure of osseointegration in patients with osteoporosis.

2. In patients with insufficient alveolar bone, such as highly pneumatized sinuses, implant sites should be augmented prior to implant placement to increase bone support. Simultaneous implant and grafting procedures should be avoided.

3. A clinical evaluation of bone density should be performed at the time of implant placement to reduce the risk of implant instability. Osteoporosis may prevent biomechanical fixation of osseointegrating implants (see chapter 27). An implant design that will ensure primary stability in osteoporotic bone of reduced density is preferred. Assessment of the bone quality at the time of the grafting and/or implant procedure may be aided by a careful analysis of radiographs (especially CT scans or radiofrequency analysis), which provide more informa-

tion about implant failure expectation than peripheral dual-energy x-ray absorptiometry of the radius or ulna.
4. At present there is no basis for advocating immediate loading of dental implants to enhance osteogenesis in osteoporotic bone.[92]

Diabetes

Diabetes is associated with a wide range of systemic complications such as retinopathy, micro- and macrovascular disease, altered wound healing, and susceptibility to infection. In the oral cavity, diabetes is associated with xerostomia, increased levels of salivary glucose, and an increased incidence of periodontal disease. In particular, the risk of developing periodontitis is significantly higher in patients with diabetes than in nondiabetic patients. This increased susceptibility may be due to a compromised host defense system (exemplified by decreased chemotaxis and phagocytosis, as well as decreased bactericidal action of polymorphonuclear neutrophil leukocytes). In addition, microvascular disease adversely affects the blood supply and contributes to a higher susceptibility to infection.[83]

Regarding the impact of diabetes on the healing response to endosseous implants, studies using animal models have shown significantly reduced bone-implant contact compared to nondiabetic controls.[93] Although the total bone-implant contact is lower in diabetic than in nondiabetic animals, osseointegration is primarily reduced in trabecular bone, whereas no difference was shown in cortical bone.[94] This finding indicates that although the healing process in animals with uncontrolled diabetes is impaired, osseointegration will occur especially in the mandible. In the maxilla (and hence in bone-grafted sinuses) where trabecular bone predominates, one would expect an increased risk for implant failure.

Several studies have specifically addressed the failure rate of dental implants in the diabetic patient,[75,83,91,95–98] but little information is available for diabetes and the sinus graft procedure.[99]

Definitive guidelines about implant treatment for diabetic patients have not been established,[75,83,91,95–99] but studies do indicate that diabetes must remain a relative contraindication to implant placement. Although a majority of the published studies are concerned with the influence of diabetes on dental implants rather than on sinus bone grafting, the following guidelines should be considered:

1. Good metabolic control of diabetic patients is recommended. When implants are placed in patients with well-controlled diabetes, successful osseointegration is the same as in the general population.[101] Patients who do not demonstrate strict metabolic control should be metabolically optimized before reconstructive procedures are attempted.
2. There is general agreement in advocating the use of antibiotic prophylaxis in diabetic patients; the use of chlorhexidine mouth rinse is also recommended to reduce oral bacterial count.[91,102–105]

Alcohol abuse

Alcohol abuse produces a variety of deleterious systemic effects, including decreased liver function, cardiomyopathies, anemias, and neurologic events. Although no definitive guidelines have been established, the degree of alcohol abuse may suggest either a relative or an absolute contraindication.[106] Patients who abuse alcohol frequently present with poor oral hygiene and noncompliance,[91] which reduces the prospect for a favorable prognosis of sinus-directed implants.

Thyroid disorders

Surgical concerns related to a patient with hypothyroidism are a decreased metabolic rate and significant potential for hypotension. The most common causes of hypothyroidism are Hashimoto thyroiditis, idiopathic hypothyroidism, and surgical or radiation treatment to the thyroid. Patients with hyperthyroidism need to be carefully watched for thyroid storm, which is a life-threatening condition. The most common causes of hyperthyroidism are Graves disease, toxic nodular goiter, and subacute thyroiditis. Medical clearance and careful medical follow-up are strongly recommended.

Adrenal disorders

Although less common than the preceding medical problems, adrenal disorders raise significant concerns for elective treatment. Risks associated with adrenal disorders include shock, dehydration, abdominal pain, nausea, and vomiting. All these events need to be carefully monitored in patients with any history of adrenal disease and in those whose disease is suppressed by steroid therapy. Steroid supplementation is recommended prophylactically; following is the most common regimen:

1. Hydrocortisone sodium succinate, 100 mg intravenously, available in operating room
2. Hydrocortisone, 50 mg intravenously, every 6 hours for the first 24 hours
3. Hydrocortisone, 25 mg intravenously, every 6 hours for 3 to 5 days postoperatively.

If the postoperative course is complicated by fever or hypotension, the hydrocortisone dose must be increased.

Summary

Sinus bone grafting for gaining bone mass in the atrophic edentulous maxilla has been demonstrated to be both safe and predictable. The modifications of sinus morphology by sinus membrane elevation and bone grafting do not jeopardize sinus function unless there is pre-existing sinus pathology. Sinus graft failure is generally avoided by careful preoperative clinical and radiographic examination to optimize the chance for success. Otolaryngologic procedures, such as functional endoscopic surgery, resolve most sinus pathology so that sinus grafts can be accomplished. Overall, the contraindications to sinus grafting must be based on sound clinical judgment with particular emphasis placed on healthy sinus function and systemic vigor.

Absolute and relative contraindications for the sinus bone graft procedure take into account systemic manifestations of disease as well as local pathophysiology. The experienced surgeon will confer with medical colleagues and defer treatment until optimal medical management is possible and general operative risk is low.

References

1. Albrektsson T, Zarb G, Worthington P, Eriksson RA. The long-term efficacy of currently used dental implants: A review and proposed criteria of success. Int J Oral Maxillofac Implants 1986;1:11–25.
2. Adell R, Eriksson B, Lekholm U, Brånemark P-I, Jemt T. A long-term follow-up study of osseointegrated implants in the treatment of totally edentulous jaws. Int J Oral Maxillofac Implants 1990;5:347–359.
3. Lekholm U, van Steenberghe D, Herrmann I, et al. Osseointegrated implants in the treatment of partially edentulous jaws: A prospective 5-year multicenter study. Int J Oral Maxillofac Implants 1994;9:627–635.
4. Lindquist LW, Carlsson GE, Jemt TA. A prospective 15-year follow-up study of mandibular fixed prostheses supported by osseointegrated implants. Clinical results and marginal bone loss. Clin Oral Implants Res 1996;7:329–336.
5. Buser D, Mericske-Stern R, Bernard JP, Behneke A, et al. Long-term evaluation of non-submerged ITI implants. Part I: 8-year life table analysis of a prospective multicenter study with 2,359 implants. Clin Oral Implants Res 1997;8:161–172.
6. Arvidson K, Bystedt H, Frykholm A, von Konow L, Lothigius E. Five-year prospective follow-up report of Astra Tech Implant System in the treatment of edentulous mandibles. Clin Oral Implants Res 1998;9:225–234.
7. Weber HP, Crohin CC, Fiorellini JP. A 5-year prospective clinical and radiographic study of non-submerged dental implants. Clin Oral Implants Res 2000;11:144–153.
8. Leonhardt A, Grondahl K, Bergstrom C, Lekholm U. Long-term follow-up of osseointegrated titanium implants using clinical, radiographic and microbiological parameters. Clin Oral Implants Res 2000;13:127–132.
9. Boyne PJ, James RA. Grafting of the maxillary sinus floor with autogenous marrow and bone. J Oral Surg 1980;38:613–616.
10. Tatum H. Maxillary and sinus implant reconstruction. Dent Clin North Am 1986;30:107–119.
11. Smiler DG, Holmes RE. Sinus lift procedure using porous hydroxylapatite: A preliminary clinical report. J Oral Implantol 1987;13:2–14.
12. Chanavaz M. Maxillary sinus: Anatomy, physiology, surgery and bone grafting relating to implantology—Eleven years of clinical experience (1979-1990). J Oral Implantol 1990;16:199–209.
13. Tidwell JK, Blijdorp PA, Stoelinga PJW, Brouns JB, Hinderks F. Composite grafting of the maxillary sinus for placement of endosteal implants. Int J Oral Maxillofac Surg 1992;21:204–209.
14. Loukota RA, Isaksson SG, Linner EL, Blomqvist JE. A technique for inserting endoosseous implants in the atrophic maxilla in a single stage procedure. Br J Oral Maxillofac Surg 1992;30:46–49.
15. Smiler DG, Johnson PW, Lozada JL, et al. Sinus lift grafts and endosseous implants: Treatment of the atrophic posterior maxilla. Dent Clin North Am 1992;36:151–186.
16. Summers RB: Maxillary implant surgery: The osteotome technique. Compend Cont Educ Dent 1994;15:152–162.
17. Jensen J, Sindet-Petersen S, Oliver AJ. Varying treatment strategies for reconstruction of maxillary atrophy with implants: Results in 98 patients. J Oral Maxillofac Surg 1994;52:210–216.
18. Chiapasco M, Ronchi P. Sinus lift and endosseous implants: Preliminary surgical and prosthetic results. Eur J Prosthodont Rest Dent 1994;3:15–21.
19. Blomqvist JE, Alberius P, Isaksson S. Retrospective analysis of one-stage maxillary sinus augmentation with endosseous implants. Int J Oral Maxillofac Implants 1996;11:512–521.
20. Jensen OT, Leonard BS, Block MS, Iacono VJ. Report of the Sinus Consensus Conference of 1996. Int J Oral Maxillofac Implants 1998;13(suppl):11–30.

21. Valentini P, Abensur DJ. Maxillary sinus grafting with anorganic bovine bone: A clinical report of long-term results. Int J Oral Maxillofac Implants 2003;18:556–560.
22. Chanavez M. Maxillary sinus. Anatomy, physiology, surgery, and bone grafting relating to implantology—Eleven years of clinical experience (1979-1990). J Oral Implantol 1990;16:199–209.
23. Takahashi R. The formation of the human paranasal sinuses. Acta Otolaryngol 1984;408:1–28.
24. Stammberger H. History of rhinology: Anatomy of the paranasal sinuses. Rhinology 1989;27:197–210.
25. Kennedy DW, Zinreich SJ. Endoscopic sinus surgery. In: Paparella MM, Shumrick DA, Gluckman JL, Meyerhoff WL (eds). Otolaryngology, vol 3. Philadelphia: Saunders, 1991:1861–1872.
26. Regev E, Smith RA, Perrot DH, Pogrel MA. Maxillary sinus complications related to endosseous implants. Int J Oral Maxillofac Implants 1995;10:451–461.
27. Timmenga NM, Raghoebar GM, Boering G, van Weissenbruch R. Maxillary sinus function after sinus lifts for the insertion of dental implants. J Oral Maxillofac Surg 1997;55:936–939.
28. Zimbler MS, Lebowitz RA, Glickman R. Antral augmentation osseointegration and sinusitis: The otolaryngologist perspective. Am J Rhinol 1998;12:311–316.
29. Watelet JB, Van Cauwenberge P. Applied anatomy and physiology of the nose and paranasal sinuses. Allergy 1999;54:14–25.
30. Peleg M, Chaushu G, Mazor Z, et al. Radiological findings of the post-sinusitis lift maxillary sinus: A computerized tomography follow-up. Periodontol 1999;70:1564–1573.
31. Van den Berg JP, Ten Bruggenkate CM, Disch FJ, Tuinzing DB. Anatomical aspects of sinus floor elevations. Clin Oral Implants Res 2000;11:256–265.
32. Sambataro G, Mantovani M, Scotti A. Rialzo del seno mascellare e implicazioni sulle sue funzioni. In: Chiapasco M, Romeo E (eds). La riabilitazione implanto-protesica nei casi complessi. Torino, Italy: UTET, 2003:292–298.
33. Goldman L. Cardiac risks and complications of noncardiac surgery. Ann Intern Med 1983;98:504–513.
34. Dajani A, Bisno AL, Chung KS, et al. Prevention of bacterial endocarditis. Recommendations by the American Heart Association. JAMA 1990;264:2419–2422.
35. Goldman L, Caldera DL, Nussbaum SR, et al. Multifactorial index of cardiac risk in noncardiac surgical procedures. N Engl J Med 1977;297:845–850.
36. Cygan R, Watzkin H. Stopping and restarting medications in the perioperative period. J Gen Intern Med 1987;2:270.
37. Marx RE, Johnson RP. Studies in the radiobiology of osteoradionecrosis and their clinical significance. Oral Surg Oral Med Oral Pathol 1987;64:379–390.
38. Epstein JB, Wong FLW, Stevenson-Moore P. Osteoradionecrosis: Clinical experience and a proposal for classification. J Oral Maxillofac Surg 1987;45:104–110.
39. Nguyen TD, Panis X, Froissart D, Legros M, Coninx P, Loirette M. Analysis of late complications after rapid hyperfractionated radiotherapy in advanced head and neck cancers. Int J Radiat Oncol Biol Physics 1988;14:23–25.
40. Widmark G, Sagne S, Heikel P. Osteoradionecrosis of the jaws. Int J Oral Maxillofac Surg 1989;18:302–306.
41. Murray CG, Herson J, Daly TE, Zimmerman S. Radiation necrosis of the mandible: A 10 year study. I. Factors influencing the onset of necrosis. Int J Radiat Oncol Biol Physics 1980;6:543–548.
42. Granstromm G, Bergstrom K, Tjellstrom A, Brånemark P-I. A detailed analysis of titanium implants lost in irradiated tissue. Int J Oral Maxillofac Implants 1994;9:653–662.
43. Jacobsson MG, Jonsson AK, Albrektsson TO, Turesson IE. Short- and long-term effects of irradiation on bone regeneration. Plast Reconstr Surg 1985;76:841–848.
44. Ueda M, Kaneda T, Takahashi H. Effect of hyperbaric oxygen therapy on osseointegration of titanium implants in irradiated bone: A preliminary report. Int J Oral Maxillofac Implants 1993;8:41–44.
45. Watzinger F, Ewers R, Henninger A, Sudasch G, Babka A, Woelf G. Endosteal implants in the irradiated lower jaw. J Craniomaxillofac Surg 1996;24:237–244.
46. Jisander S, Grenthe B, Alberius P. Dental implant survival in the irradiated jaw: A preliminary report. Int J Oral Maxillofac Implants 1997;12:643–648.
47. Ali A, Patton DW, El-Sharkawi AM, Davies J. Implant rehabilitation of irradiated jaws: A preliminary report. Int J Oral Maxillofac Implants 1997;12:523–526.
48. Ekert SE, Desjardins RP, Keller E, Tolman DA. Endosseous implants in an irradiated tissue bed. J Prosthet Dent 1996;76:45–49.
49. Niimi A, Ueda M, Keller EE, Worthington P. Experience with osseointegrated implants placed in irradiated tissues in Japan and in the United States. Int J Oral Maxillofac Implants 1998;13:407–411.
50. Andersson G, Andreasson L, Bjelkengren G. Oral implant rehabilitation in irradiated patients without adjunctive hyperbaric oxygen. Int J Oral Maxillofac Implants 1998;13:647–654.
51. Asikainen P, Klemetti E, Kotilainen R, et al. Osseointegration of dental implants in bone irradiated with 40, 50, or 60 Gy doses. An experimental study with beagle dogs. Clin Oral Implants Res 1998;9:20–25.
52. Chiapasco M. Implants for patients with maxillofacial defects and following irradiation. In: Lang NL, Lang T, Karring T, Lindhe J (eds). Proceedings of the 3rd European Workshop on Periodontology. Chicago: Quintessence, 1999:557–607.
53. Wolfaardt JF, Granstrom G, Friberg B, Jha N, Tjellstrom A. A retrospective study on effects of chemotherapy on osseointegration. J Facial Somato Prosthet 1996;2:99–107.
54. McDonald AR, Pogrel MA, Sharnna A. Effects of chemotherapy on osseointegration of implants: A case report. J Oral Implantol 1998;24:11–13.
55. Ihara K, Coto M, Miyahra A, Toyota J, Katsuki T. Multicenter experience with maxillary prostheses supported by Brånemark implants: A clinical report. Int J Oral Maxillofac Implants 1998;13:531–538.
56. van Steenberghe D, Quirynen M, Molly L, Jacobs R. Impact of systemic diseases and medication on osseointegration. Periodontol 2000 2003;33:163–171.
57. DePaola LG, Peterson DE, Overholser CD, et al. Dental care for patients receiving chemotherapy. J Am Dent Assoc 1996;112:198–203.

58. Ruggiero SL, Mehrotra B, Rosenberg TJ, Engroff SL. Osteonecrosis of the jaws associated with the use of bisphosphonates: A review of 63 cases. J Oral Maxillofac Surg 2004;62:527–534.
59. Marx RE. Pamidronate (Aredia) and zolendronate (Zometa) induced avascular necrosis of the jaws: A growing epidemic. J Oral Maxillofac Surg 2003;61:1115–1117.
60. Bagan JV, Murillo J, Jimenez Y, et al. Avascular jaw osteonecrosis in association with cancer chemotherapy: Series of 10 cases. J Oral Pathol Med 2005;34:120–123.
61. Migliorati CA. Bisphosphonates and oral cavity avascular bone necrosis. J Clin Oncol 2003;21:4253–4254.
62. Kapitola J, Zak J, Lacinova Z, Justova V. Effect of growth hormone and pamidronate on bone blood flow, bone mineral and IGF-I levels in the rat. Physiol Res 2000;49(suppl1):S101–S106.
63. Kapitola J, Zak J. Effect of pamidronate on bone blood flow in oophorectomized rats. Physiol Res 1998;47:237–240.
64. Fournier P, Boissier S, Filleur S, et al. Bisphosphonates inhibit angiogenesis in vitro and testosterone-stimulated vascular regrowth in the ventral prostate in castrated rats. Cancer Res 2002;62:6538–6544.
65. Santini D, Vincenzi B, Avvisati G, et al. Pamidronate induces modifications of circulating angiogenic factors in cancer patients. Clin Cancer Res 2002;8:1080–1084.
66. Starck WJ, Epker BN. Failure of osseointegrated dental implants after diphosphonate therapy for osteoporosis: A case report. Int J Oral Maxillofac Implants 1995;10:74–78.
67. Bain CA, Moy PR. The association between the failure of dental implants and cigarette smoking. Int J Oral Maxillofac Implants 1993;8:609–615.
68. Barton JR, Riad MA, Gaze MN, Maran Ferguson A. Mucosal immunodeficiency in smokers and patients with epithelial head and neck tumors. GUT 1990;31:378–382.
69. Mosely LH, Finseth F, Goody M. Nicotine and its effects on wound healing. J Plast Reconstr Surg 1978;61:570–576.
70. Wittbjer J, Palmer B, Rohlin M, Thorngren KG. Osteogenic activity in composite grafts of demineralized compact bone and marrow. Clin Orthop Relat Res 1983;173:229–238.
71. Davis JW, Davis RE. Acute effect of tobacco cigarette smoking on the platelet aggregate ratio. Am J Med Sci 1979;278:139–143.
72. Hawkins RI. Smoking, platelets and thrombosis. Nature 1972;236:450–452.
73. Broulik PD, Jarab J. The effect of chronic nicotine administration on bone mineral content in mice. Horm Metab Res 1993;25:219–221.
74. Daftari TK, Whitesides TE, Heller JG, et al. Nicotine on the revascularization of bone graft. An experimental study in rabbits. Spine 1994;19:904–911.
75. Nolan J, Jenkins RA, Kurihara K, Schultz R. The acute effects of cigarette smoke exposure on experimental skin flaps. Plast Reconstr Surg 1985;75:544–551.
76. Forrest CR, Pang CY, Lindsay WK. Detrimental effect of nicotine on skin flap viability and blood flow in random skin flap operation on rats and pigs. Surg Forrim 1985;36:611–613.
77. Kribbs PJ. Comparison of mandibular bone in normal and osteoporotic women. J Prosthet Dent 1990;63:218–222.
78. Birkenfeld L, Yemini M, Kase NG, Birkenfeld A. Menopause-related oral alveolar bone resorption: A review of relatively unexplored consequences of estrogen deficiency. Menopause 1999;6:129–133.
79. Payne JB, Reinhardty RA, Nummikoski PV, Patil KD. Longitudinal alveolar bone loss in postmenopausal osteoporotic/osteopenic women. Osteoporosis Int 1999;10:34–40.
80. Mori H, Manabe M, Kurachi Y, Nagumo M. Osseointegration of dental implants in rabbit bone with low mineral density. J Oral Maxillofac Surg 1997;55:351–362.
81. Heersche JN, Bellows CG, Ishida Y. The decrease in bone mass associated with aging and menopause. J Prosthet Dent 1998;79:14–16.
82. Hildebolt CF. Osteoporosis and oral bone loss. Dentomaxillofac Radiol 1997;26:3–15.
83. Beikler T, Flemming TF. Implants in the medically compromised patient. Crit Rev Oral Biol Med 2003;14:305–316.
84. Roberts WE, Simmons KE, Garetto LP, DeCastro RA. Bone physiology and metabolism in dental implantology: Risk factors for osteoporosis and other metabolic bone diseases. Implant Dent 1992;1:11–21.
85. Dao TT, Anderson JD, Zarb GA. Is osteoporosis a risk factor for osseointegration of dental implants?. Int J Oral Maxillofac Implants 1993;8:137–144.
86. Fujimoto T, Niimi A, Sawai T, Ueda M. Effects of steroid-induced osteoporosis on osseointegration of titanium implants. Int J Oral Maxillofac Implants 1998;13:183–189.
87. Nasu M, Amano Y, Kurita A, Yosue T. Osseointegration in implant-embedded mandible in rats fed calcium-deficient diet: A radiological study. Oral Dis 1998;4:84–89.
88. Blomqvist JE, Alberius P, Isaksson S, Linde A, Hansson BG. Factors in implant integration failure after bone grafting: An osteometric and endocrinologic matched analysis. Int J Oral Maxillofac Surg 1996;25:63–68.
89. August M, Chung K, Chang Y, Glowacki J. Influence of estrogen status on endosseous implant osseointegration. J Oral Maxillofac Surg 2001;59:1285–1289.
90. van Steenberghe D, Jacobs R, Desnyder M, Maffei G, Quirynen M. The relative impact of local and endogenous patient-related factors on implant failure up to the abutment stage. Clin Oral Implants Res 2002;13:617–622.
91. Balshi TJ, Wolfinger GJ. Management of the posterior maxilla in the compromised patient: Historical, current, and future perspectives. Periodontol 2000 2003;33:67–81.
92. Cooper LF. Systemic effects of alveolar bone mass and implications in dental therapy. Periodontol 2000 2000;23:103–109.
93. Nevins ML, Karimbux NY, Weber HP, Giannobile WV, Fiorellini JP. Wound healing around endosseous implants in experimental diabetes. Int J Oral Maxillofac Implants 1998;13:620–629.
94. Iyama S, Takeshita F, Ayukawa Y, Kido MA, Suetsugu T, Tanaka T. A study of the regional distribution of bone formed around hydroxylapatite implants in the tibiae of streptozotocin-induced dietetic rats using multiple fluorescent labeling and confocal laser scanning microscopy. J Periodontol 1997;68:1169–1175.

95. Smith RA, Berger R, Dodson TB. Risk factors associated with dental implants in healthy and medically compromised patients. Int J Oral Maxillofac Implants 1992;7:367–372.
96. Kapur KK, Garrett NR, Hamada MO, et al. A randomized clinical trial comparing the efficacy of mandibular implant-supported overdentures and conventional dentures in diabetic patients. Part I: Methodology and clinical outcomes. J Prosthet Dent 1998;79:555–569.
97. Fiorellini JP, Chen PK, Nevins MI, Nevins ML. A retrospective study of dental implants in diabetic patients. Int J Periodontics Restorative Dent 2000;20:366–373.
98. Peled M, Ardekian L, Tagger-Green N, Gutmacher Z, Matchtei EE. Dental implants in patients with type 2 diabetes mellitus: A clinical study. Implant Dent 2003;12:116–122.
99. Farzad P, Andersson L, Nyberg J. Dental implant treatment in diabetic patients. Implant Dentistry 2002;11:262–267.
100. Shernoff AF, Coldwell JA, Bingham SF. Implants for type II diabetic patients: Interim report. VA implants in diabetes study group. Implant Dent 1994;3:183–185.
101. Proceedings of the 1996 World Workshop in Periodontics 1996. Consensus Report: Implant therapy II. Ann Periodontol 1996; 1:816–820.
102. Sbordone L, Barone A, Ramaglia L, Ciaglia RN, Iacono VJ. Antimicrobial susceptibility of periodontopathic bacteria associated with failing implants. J Periodontol 1995;66:69–74.
103. Dent CD, Olson JW, Farish SE, et al. The influence of preoperative antibiotics on success of endosseous implants up to and including stage II surgery: A study of 2,641 implants. J Oral Maxillofac Surg 1997;55:19–24.
104. Blanchaert RH. Implants in the medically challanged patient. Dent Clin North Am 1998;42:35–45.
105. Morris HF, Ochi S, Winkler S. Implant survival in patients with type 2 diabetes: Placement to 36 months. Ann Periodontol 2000;5:157–165.
106. Rosenlicht JL. Indications and contraindications for sinus grafting. In: Jensen OT (ed). The Sinus Bone Graft. Chicago: Quintessence, 1999:7–15.

chapter 9
Complications of Maxillary Sinus Augmentation

Michael A. Pikos, DDS

Grafting of the maxillary sinus has become a highly predictable surgical technique for site development and implant reconstruction.[1-7] Excellent success rates have been reported for sinus grafting and implant placement in both one- and two-stage protocols.[8-13] Despite its predictability and the high success rates achieved with this augmentation technique, however, complications do occur.

Preoperative Assessment

As with any surgical procedure, careful patient selection will maximize predictability and success. Absolute contraindications to sinus grafting include acute sinusitis, allergic rhinitis, acute exacerbation of chronic sinusitis, any systemic medical condition affecting bone metabolism, immunosuppression, and the presence of maxillary sinus neoplasms, among others (see chapter 8). In addition, the presence of odontogenic, periapical, or radicular cysts in the proximity of the maxillary sinus should be addressed prior to grafting. Smoking is considered both a relative and an absolute contraindication.

Relative contraindications to sinus grafting include some medical conditions that, if not controlled, may result in a compromised surgical outcome. The presence of mucus cysts in the maxillary sinus generally can be ignored, but they are considered by some surgeons to represent a relative contraindication to surgery. Opinion is divided on whether this pathology should be treated prior to[15,16] or simultaneous with[17] maxillary sinus augmentation.

Smoking is considered to be an absolute contraindication by some; Small et al[14] reported infection in 2 (of 45) patients who were smokers after they received sinus grafts consisting of a combination of freeze-dried bone and hydroxyapatite. Whereas Levin et al[18] found no significant influence of smoking on sinus graft procedures (n = 79) in patients followed over an 8-year period, other clinicians disagree. Kan et al[19] found a significantly higher cumulative implant success rate in nonsmokers (82.7%) than in smokers (65.3%). They concluded that cigarette smoking is detrimental to the success rate of osseointegrated implants in grafted maxillary sinuses regardless of the amount of cigarette consumption. Olson et al,[20] who followed 120 implants placed into 45 augmented maxillary sinuses for up to 71 months, concluded that failures seemed to be associated with smoking. The present author limits to less than one pack per day, assuming no medical contraindications to surgery in general, for smokers who wish to receive sinus graft surgery. In addition, the patient must refrain from smoking on the day of surgery and for the first 4 days following surgery (see chapter 8).

chapter 9 — Complications of Maxillary Sinus Augmentation

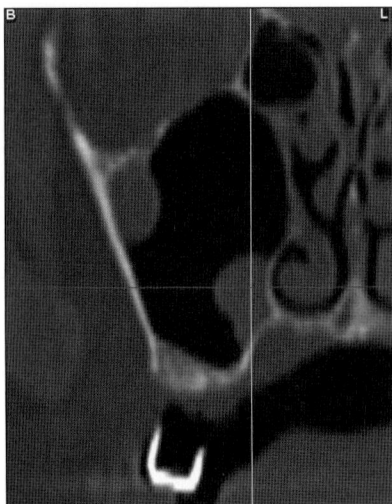

Fig 9-1 Pseudocysts in right maxillary sinus.

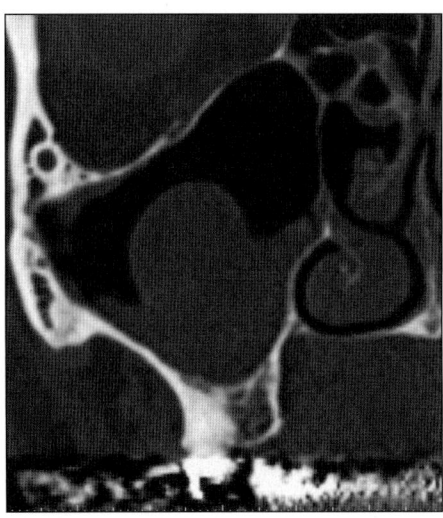

Fig 9-2 Mucus retention cyst in right maxillary sinus.

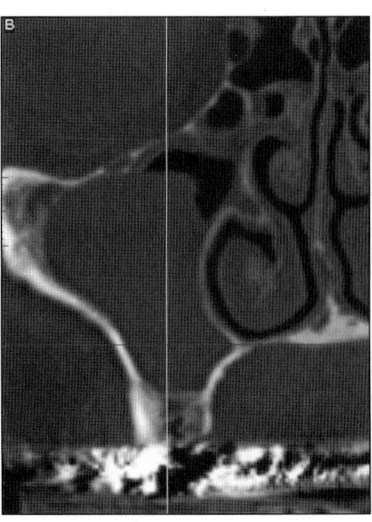

Fig 9-3 Mucocele in right maxillary sinus.

Patient evaluation for posterior maxillary implant reconstruction must include conventional record taking as well as a thorough history and clinical evaluation of the maxillary sinus. Articulated study casts, plain film radiographs, and computerized tomography (CT) scanning reveal ridge anatomy, interarch relationships, and saliant anatomic information in preparation for optimal implant selection and placement.

A physical examination of the maxillary sinus evaluates the infraorbital, lateral nasal, and superior labial areas of the face for tenderness to palpation, swelling, asymmetry, or ecchymosis. Nasal congestion, discharge, and/or the presence of epistaxis are also evaluated. Acute, allergic, and chronic sinusitis may be diagnosed on the basis of patient history and clinical evaluation. The symptomatology is generally nonspecific and includes allergic rhinitis. The patient usually presents with throbbing pain of the maxillary sinus area, headaches and swelling, and erythema overlying the infraorbital area. Although chronic sinusitis is an infection of long duration (greater than 3 months), symptoms are similar to those of acute sinusitis except in milder form. Symptomatic chronic sinusitis as well as acute and allergic sinusitis must be treated prior to sinus graft surgery. All of these disease entities share a bacterial etiology that results in a pathogenesis associated with obstruction of the osteomeatal complex.[21] The blockage of normal mucous flow from the middle meatus into the posterior nasal pharynx can result in infection of the sinus graft. These patients must be treated with antibiotics, steroids, and in some cases surgery to establish a new sinus ostium prior to grafting.

Preoperative evaluation for pathology of the maxillary sinus should include plain film radiography and CT scans. Although generally not considered mandatory, CT scanning prior to sinus grafting may be advisable. For evaluating disease of the nose and paranasal sinuses[22] and for detecting both benign and malignant neoplasms of the maxillary sinus, CT remains the modality of choice. In addition, it reveals periapical, radicular, and odontogenic cysts that extend into the sinus, which may be missed with conventional radiography. Osteomeatal complex patency, especially in the presence of mucus cysts, also is important to assess presurgically via CT imaging.

A variety of mucus cysts can be found in the maxillary sinus.[23] Pseudocysts (Fig 9-1) and mucus retention cysts (Fig 9-2) contribute to mucosal thickening and can occlude the osteomeatal complex after membrane elevation, resulting in infection of the graft. Mucoceles (Fig 9-3) typically are expansile, destructive lesions resulting from blockage of the ostium and/or trauma and can cause extensive bony wall erosion. In general, patients presenting with symptoms of acute sinusitis, chronic sinusitis, allergic rhinitis, neoplasms, and cysts should undergo further evaluation prior to sinus graft surgery. Pseudocysts, mucus retention cysts, and mucoceles are often treated simultaneously with sinus grafting.

TABLE 9-1 Intraoperative, early-postoperative, and late-postoperative complications of maxillary sinus augmentation with identification of their most probable cause

Complication	Possible cause
Intraoperative	
Bleeding	Osteomeatal complex obstruction
Buccal flap tear	Inadequate graft fill
Infraorbital nerve injury	Alveolar ridge fracture
Membrane perforation	Damage to adjacent dentition
Early Postoperative	
Incision line opening	Acute infection
Bleeding	Graft loss (partial or complete)
Barrier membrane exposure	Implant failure
Infraorbital nerve paresthesia	Oroantral fistula
Late Postoperative	
Graft loss/failure	Soft tissue invasion over access window
Implant failure	Maxillary cyst
Oroantral fistula	Chronic sinus disease
Implant migration	Chronic infection
Inadequate graft fill sequelae	Chronic pain

Intraoperative Complications

A number of complications can occur during the sinus elevation surgery (Table 9-1). Bone bleeders from the bony window, as well as bleeding from the membrane itself, can easily be handled with cautery. Care must be taken to avoid laceration to the buccal flap, which can result in oroantral fistulae. Careful handling of the buccal flap with good surgical technique will prevent this potential complication. Injury to the infraorbital neurovascular bundle can result from dissection to free up the buccal flap for tension-free closure. It can also result from blunt trauma when a retractor is placed directly over the nerve bundle. This injury causes transient loss of sensation of the lateral nasal, infraorbital, and superior labial areas of the face. Prevention of these injuries requires careful surgical technique.

Membrane perforation (Fig 9-4) is the most common intraoperative complication associated with maxillary sinus augmentation. During the sinus graft procedure, the sinus membrane must be elevated superiorly, away from the bony floor and walls, to allow for grafting of the area beneath it. The sinus membrane is composed of pseudostratified, ciliated, cuboidal, or columnar epithelium with goblet cells and ranges in thickness from 0.3 to 0.8 mm.[24] Because it has very few elastic fibers, its elevation from the bony walls often presents a significant challenge. Ideally, the membrane is not perforated and will confine the graft to the space created between it and the bony floor. In practice, however, membrane perforation occurs 10% to 40% of the time during elevation.[16,17,25,26] Membrane perforation also may be found as a result of previous sinus surgery or caused during window osteotomy outline.

When perforation occurs intraoperatively, it is best to continue membrane elevation in a direction opposite that of the tear to prevent creation of a larger opening. Elevation should expose the bony floor as well as the anterior, posterior, and medial walls. Small tears (less than 5 mm) (Fig 9-5) can easily be resolved by placing a fast-resorbing collagen membrane (CollaTape, Zimmer Dental) over the opening. Large tears (Fig 9-6) along with total membrane perforation require the use of a more rigid collagen membrane of longer duration (BioMend, Zimmer Dental).[17] A large tear can result from the presence of a thin membrane or from overinstrumentation; sometimes it is made intentionally to remove existing pathology. When a relatively

Chapter 9: Complications of Maxillary Sinus Augmentation

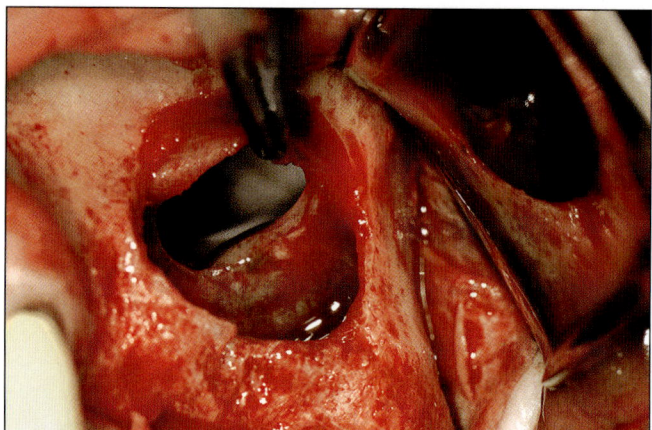

Fig 9-4 Membrane perforation of left maxillary sinus.

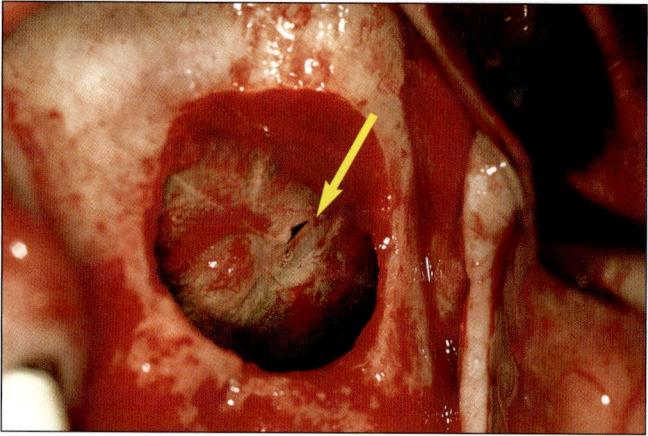

Fig 9-5 Small membrane tear *(arrow)* of left maxillary sinus. A tear of this size (< 5 mm) can be repaired with fast-resorbing collagen membrane (CollaTape).

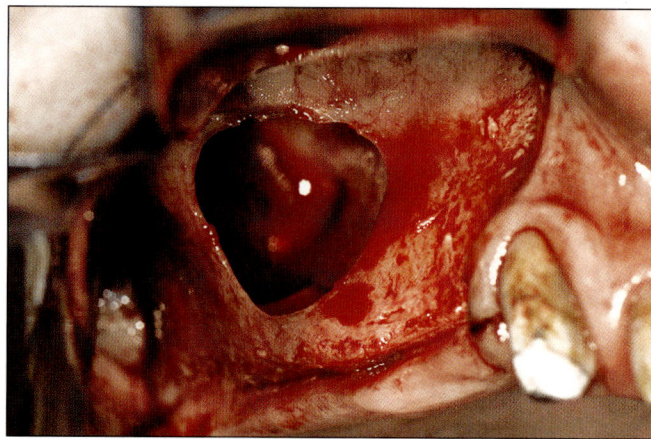

Fig 9-6 Large membrane tear of right maxillary sinus, which requires the use of a rigid collagen membrane (BioMend).

thin membrane (approximately 0.3 mm) is found, even meticulous attention to detail can result in total perforation. Most clinicians will abort the grafting procedure at this point and wait the 6 to 9 months often suggested for membrane regeneration.[15,27] The same risk applies when larger cysts and polyps are found to be symptomatic or have the potential to obstruct the osteomeatal complex upon membrane elevation. Re-entry of sinuses after a previously aborted procedure due to perforation or graft failure, pathology, or presence of a thin membrane are likely to be technically problematic in a second attempt at surgery (Fig 9-7a).

Even with loss of a large portion of the sinus membrane, it is not necessary to abort the graft surgery. Instead, a resorbable (6 to 8 weeks), biocompatible, hemostatic membrane (BioMend) can be used to create a superior barrier to confine the grafts (Figs 9-7b to 9-7h).[17] Depending on the mediolateral dimension of the sinus, this membrane can be used without fixation. The larger the mediolateral dimension, the greater the need for external tack fixation of the collagen membrane. In all these cases, patency of the osteomeatal complex must be verified presurgically via CT scan.

Because the incidence of infection increases with membrane perforation, it is best to avoid simultaneous sinus grafting and implant placement in the presence of a membrane tear.[16,28] A waiting period of at least 4 months is recommended for healing of the graft complex before placing implants. In general, membrane perforation can lead to short- and long-term complications as a result of bacterial contamination from the nasal sinus floor. Graft migration is one potential complication, evidenced by granules in the ostium and nasal pharynx. Mucosal inflammation secondary to sinus graft surgery can lead to obstruction of

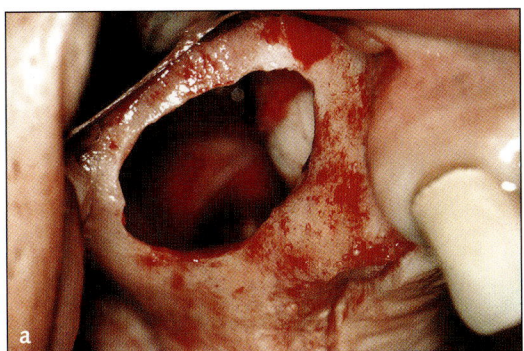 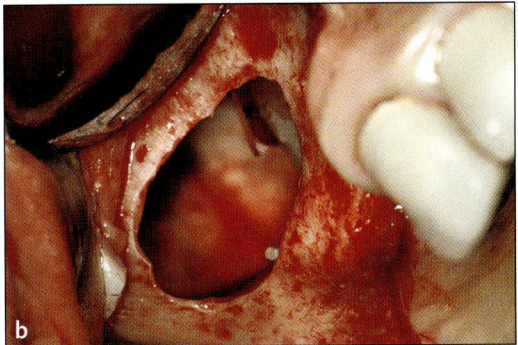

Figs 9-7a and 9-7b *(a)* Re-entry of right maxillary sinus 6 months after initial graft attempt was aborted because of complete membrane tear. Note complete lack of membrane formation. *(b)* Placement of moderately slow-resorbing collagen membrane into sinus to confine particulate graft.

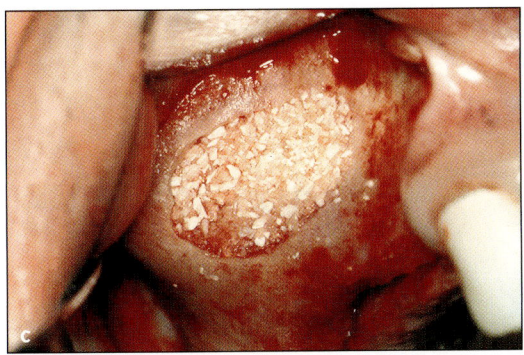 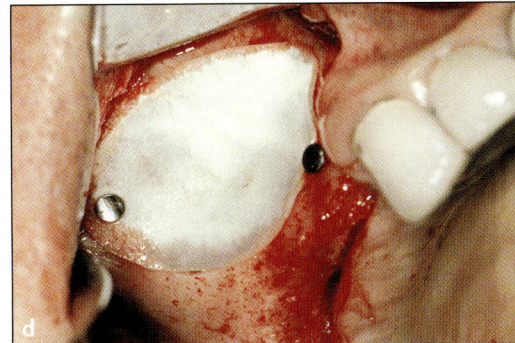

Figs 9-7c and 9-7d *(c)* Completion of grafting procedure after placement of collagen membrane into sinus. *(d)* Placement of slow-resorbing collagen membrane (BioMend Extend) over access window with tack fixation.

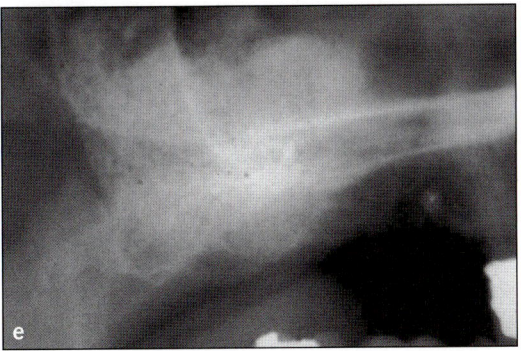 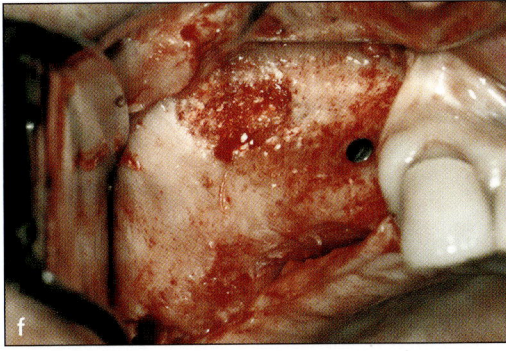

Figs 9-7e and 9-7f *(e)* Nine-month postgrafting radiograph with densely opaque outline indicating a well-incorporated graft. *(f)* Exposed right sinus graft at 9 months. Membrane fixation tacks are removed at the stage-one surgery.

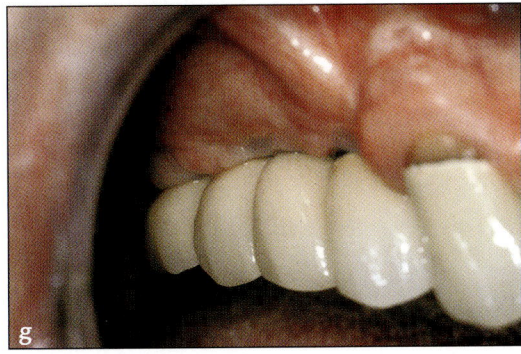 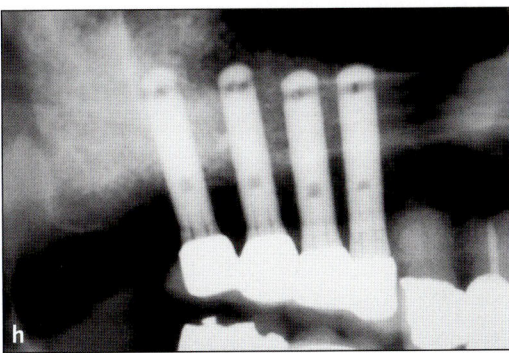

Figs 9-7g and 9-7h Four-unit fixed partial denture 3 years after functional loading.

chapter 9 | Complications of Maxillary Sinus Augmentation

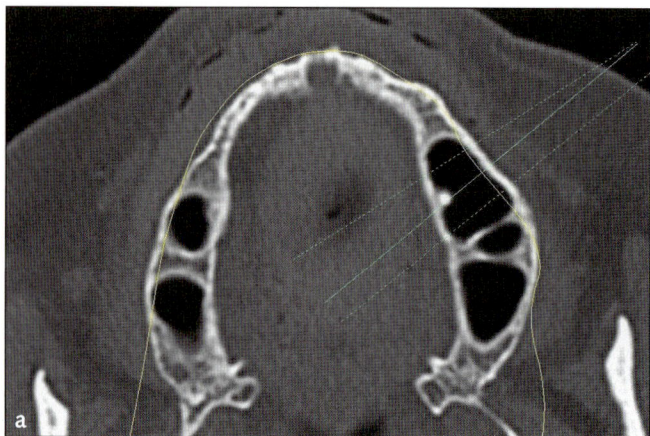 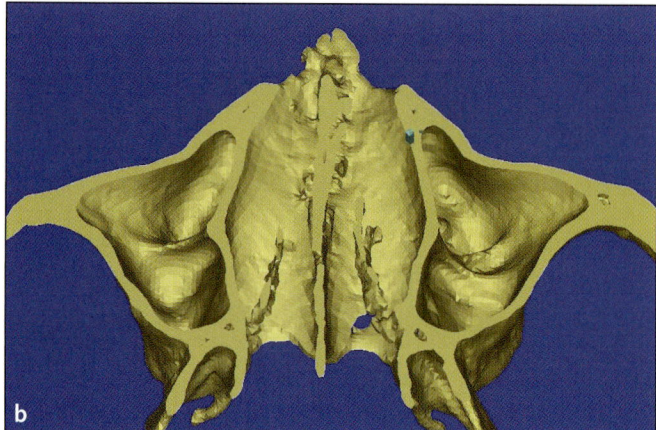

Figs 9-8a and 9-8b Bilateral septa in maxillary sinuses. *(a)* CT axial section; *(b)* Interactive CT three-dimensional reformatted virtual model.

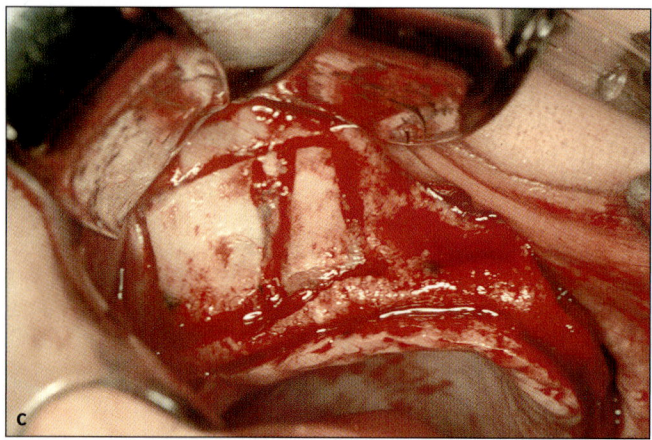 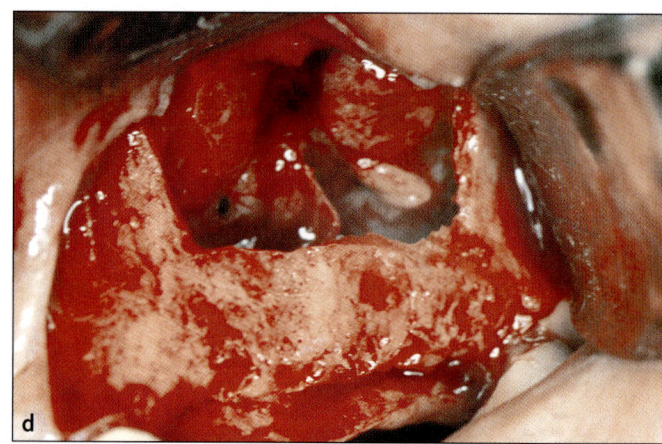

Fig 9-8c Bony window outlined to allow for creation of two windows due to the presence of a septum.

Fig 9-8d Access window created to accommodate midline septum. Note complete membrane perforation.

the osteomeatal complex, greatly increasing the potential for infection. In the report of the Sinus Consensus Conference of 1996,[28] analysis of failed sinus grafts demonstrated that 79 of 164 failures (48%) could be attributed to perioperative complications, and 38 (48%) of these were associated with sinus membrane perforations.

Some authors recommend using block rather than particulate grafts for all perforations greater than 5 mm.[29] Keller et al[30] assert that an intact membrane is not critical for the corticocancellous block grafting technique. Jensen et al[31] reported no infection in any patients treated with autograft despite a 35% incidence of membrane perforation.

The presence of septa in the maxillary sinus usually results in a higher incidence of perforation. Although septa can be seen on plain film, Ulm et al[32] reported that panoramic radiography led to a false diagnosis based on the positive or negative identification of antral septa in 21.3% of cases. For this reason, CT imaging is recommended for accurate identification of septa (Figs 9-8a and 9-8b). Both transillumination as well as instrument percussion of the window outline at time of surgery can be used to further identify septa. Typically, the membrane is thinner over the area of the septum, causing a tear upon elevation. Also, the lateral wall with the adjoining septum can perforate the membrane more easily upon rotation toward the medial wall. Modifying the window outline[33] by dividing the access window into two or even three areas (depending on the number of septa), thus creating additional vertical bone cuts (Figs 9-8c and 9-8d) will facilitate infracture of each window area separately.

Despite the problems associated with membrane perforation, septa do offer some advantages for sinus grafting.

First, they create more bony walls within the sinus and hence more bone surface availability for endosteal osteogenesis. Second, septa confine graft material more readily. Third, the base of the septum provides excellent bone stability for simultaneous implant placement.[16]

Osteomeatal complex obstruction can occur if excessive graft material is placed, which prevents normal mucous flow between the middle meatus and the nasal pharynx. Discretion in the quantity of graft material used is advised. Typically, the goal is to place graft material to a height of 20 to 25 mm from the sinus floor. Conversely, an insufficient quantity of graft material can preclude implant placement or longevity. The medial wall is a common area of insufficient grafting when membrane elevation away from it is incomplete. Another common area is the anterior wall, which is easy to forget. Grafting the anterior wall first is a habit many surgeons develop to prevent this problem.

Generally, it is a good practice to remove any compromised teeth in proximity to the sinus prior to augmentation to avoid the potential for bacterial contamination from the dentition and/or alveolar wall infracture. A 2- to 3-month postextraction healing period is recommended prior to grafting. Damage to adjacent teeth is rare and can be avoided by careful surgical technique. There have been no incidences reported of loss of adjacent tooth vitality as a result of sinus graft surgery.

Early-Postoperative Complications

Early complications are defined as those that occur within 7 to 10 days of surgery (see Table 9-1). Though uncommon, incision line opening can result in graft extravasation, infection, and even total graft failure. Conventional surgical principles for proper incision design, as well as appropriate suture material selection and technique, will prevent this problem. In addition, care must be exercised when placing a prosthesis. A complete maxillary denture can be placed immediately postsurgery if the buccal flange in the area of the graft is reduced and/or soft-lined. A partial denture, however, should be used only if it is acrylic-based to allow alteration for appropriate relief and to facilitate placement of a soft liner.

Bleeding of the original incision line is uncommon. Nasal bleeding also is unusual and can be treated with a cotton ball pressure pack as needed for hemostasis. Premature exposure of the membrane has been seen but is very unlikely unless there is total wound breakdown. When this occurs, the site is treated as indicated for graft failure. No reports of premature membrane exposure have been associated with the use of a resorbable collagen membrane.

Paresthesia of the lateral nasal, infraorbital, or superior labial areas of the face are caused by blunt retraction over the infraorbital neurovascular bundle. Typically this is transient (a few weeks) though occasionally relatively long lasting (several months). Care in positioning the buccal flap retractor anterior and posterior to the neurovascular bundle will prevent this complication.

Infection of the grafted sinus, although uncommon, is usually seen 3 to 7 days postsurgery. Despite presurgical antibiotic prophylaxis and good surgical technique, postoperative infection can occur, sometimes leading to total graft failure. Potential sequelae secondary to infection may involve a pansinusitis as well as infection spreading to the orbit, dura, or even the brain.[34] Other problems involve oroantral or oronasal fistulae that require further surgery for repair, and finally, graft incorporation compromise. For all of these reasons, an infected sinus graft must be treated aggressively.

Intraoral swelling over the grafted window area is the most common initial finding associated with infection. It is usually seen 1 week postsurgery, although it can occur as early as 3 days postsurgery. Antibiotic therapy, such as clindamycin (Cleocin, Pfizer) (600-mg loading dose and 300 mg four times per day) is recommended as an empiric drug of choice. Metronidazole (Flagyl, Pfizer) (500 mg three times per day) can also be added, especially for anaerobic coverage. Sometimes an infection is restricted to a local area and will respond to antibiotic therapy alone. In cases of persistent symptomatology, however, it is imperative to pursue aggressive treatment that includes incision and drainage. The graft should be re-entered via the original incision line. It may be tempting to make an incision in the area of the window, but this can result in an oroantral fistula. A full-thickness mucoperiosteal flap is reflected, allowing for direct visualization of the graft site. Aerobic and anaerobic culture and sensitivity, in addition to a gram stain, is recommended. If the infection is confined to a localized area, then local debridement is the appropriate therapy (Figs 9-9a to 9-9c). If infection has penetrated the entire graft, then removal of the entire graft and possibly of the sinus membrane is recommended (Figs 9-9d to 9-9g). If implants were placed simultaneous with the graft,

chapter 9 Complications of Maxillary Sinus Augmentation

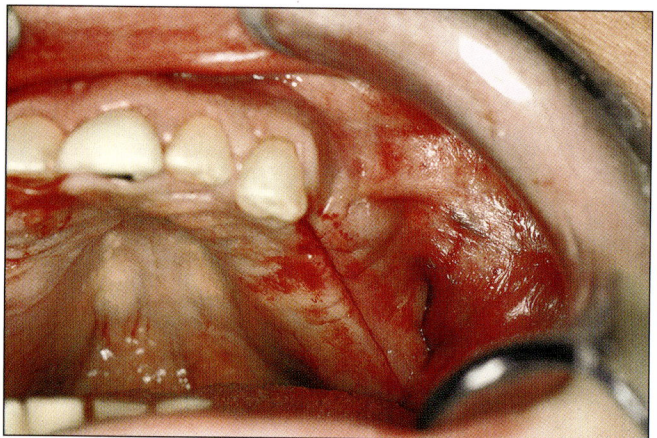

Fig 9-9a Left sinus graft infection 10 days postsurgery. Note ecchymosis of the mucosa over the access window area.

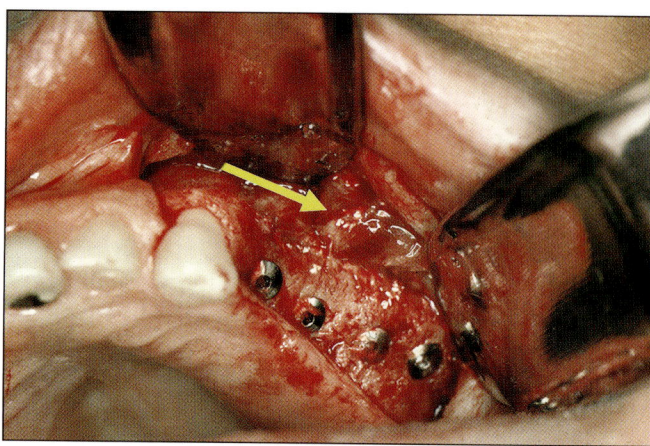

Fig 9-9b Full flap reflection of infected maxillary left sinus 10 days postsurgery. Note superficial area of infection *(arrow)*.

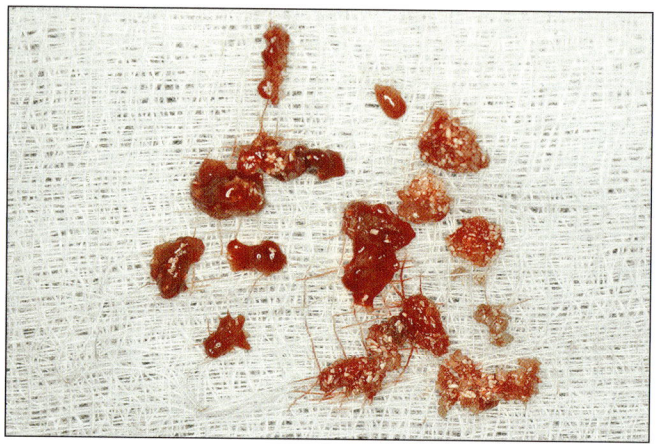

Fig 9-9c Particulate graft remnants after debridement of infected sinus.

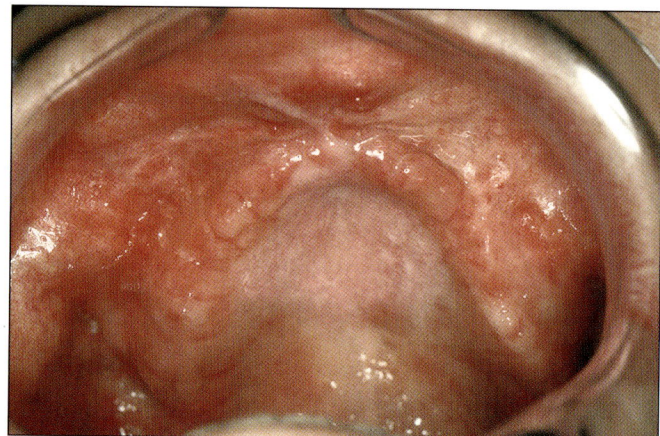

Fig 9-9d Ecchymosis of right buccal vestibule.

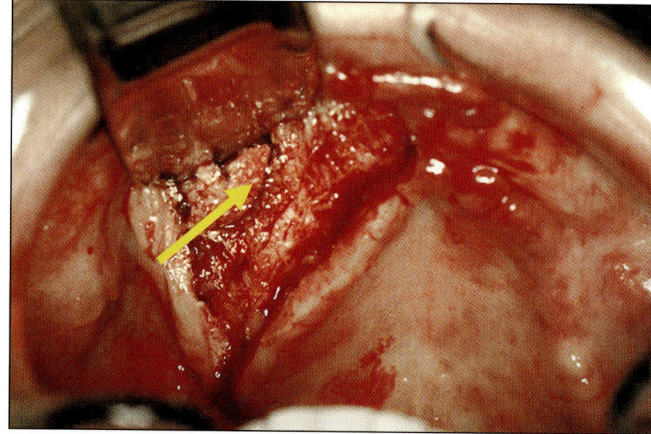

Fig 9-9e Full flap reflection along original incision. Note graft breakdown *(arrow)*.

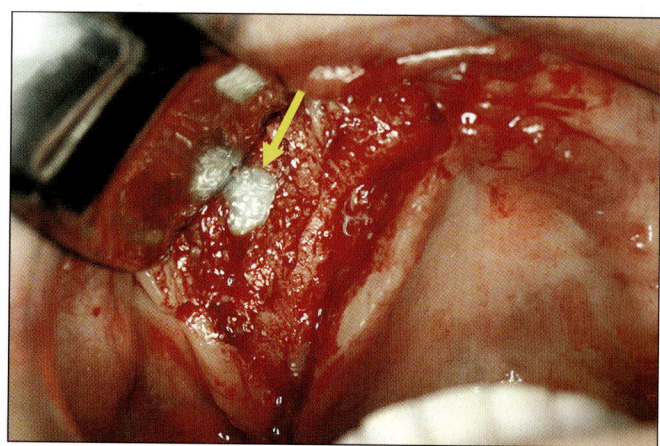

Fig 9-9f Purulent exudate *(arrow)*.

110

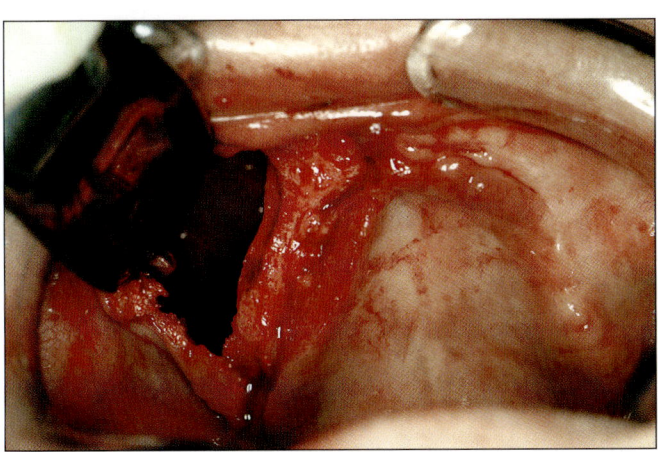

Fig 9-9g Complete graft and membrane removal from infected maxillary right sinus at 10 days.

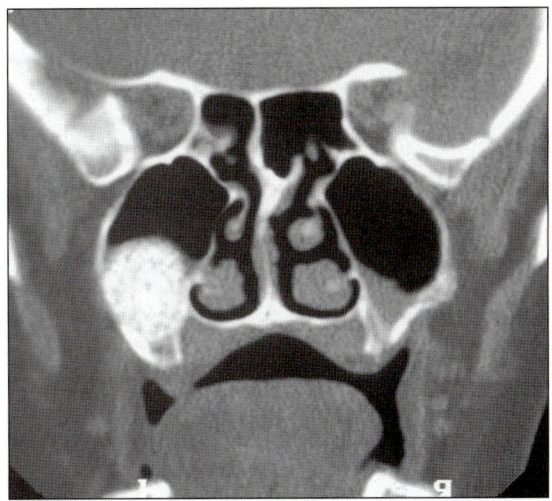

Fig 9-9h CT coronal view of maxillary sinuses 1 week after removal of right graft.

they also should be removed, and a long-acting collagen membrane should be placed over the window. A follow-up CT scan should be ordered to verify total graft removal and to evaluate osteomeatal complex patency (Fig 9-9h). Grafting can be redone 3 to 4 months later, assuming the sinus is again healthy.

Oroantral fistulae can occur as a result of sinus graft infection. If small, they often respond to antibiotic therapy and oral chlorhexidine gluconate rinses. Larger ones, however, can persist and may require surgical intervention.

Late-Postoperative Complications

Complications of maxillary sinus augmentation that occur more than 3 months postoperative are very uncommon (see Table 9-1). Most of these are seen at stage-one surgery when a two-stage approach is used. Graft infection can manifest as a dehiscence of the mucosa overlying the access window, resulting in partial graft loss (Fig 9-10a). Treatment of this condition involves antibiotic therapy, followed by incision and drainage using the original midcrestal incision with an anterior oblique release for full flap reflection (Figs 9-10b and 9-10c). As with treatment of immediate postoperative infections, it is important to obtain an aerobic and anaerobic culture and sensitivity, including a gram stain. Debridement of the infected graft should follow (Fig 9-10d). If no active infection is found, regrafting can be performed at this time. Otherwise, a re-entry graft can be accomplished 3 to 4 months later.

Total graft failure can also occur at this time, requiring complete removal of the graft, including membrane. Regrafting can be accomplished approximately 3 to 4 months later. If implants were placed in a one-stage approach, they also would be removed along with the graft.

An oroantral fistula can occur secondary to a late-infected graft (Fig 9-11), which would require closure by one of a variety of surgical procedures prior to regrafting.

Implant failure at stage-two surgery can result from lack of osseointegration. Implant migration, either early or late postoperative, can also be seen if there is inadequate bone volume and/or density for implant stabilization (Fig 9-12).

Another cause of stage-two implant failure is insufficient graft fill resulting from failure to elevate the membrane up to and including the medial wall. This can also occur if the recess adjoining the anterior wall is not grafted adequately. Treatment requires secondary grafting of the spaces.

Soft tissue invasion of the graft site can occur at stage-one surgery if a barrier membrane was not used to cover the access window (see chapter 19). A long-lasting collagen membrane with tack fixation will prevent this complication. Treatment involves regrafting the void after soft tissue debridement.

Development of an epithelial cyst of the maxillary sinus postsurgically has been associated with virtually every procedure that involves the sinus (Fig 9-13). This cyst, first

chapter 9 | Complications of Maxillary Sinus Augmentation

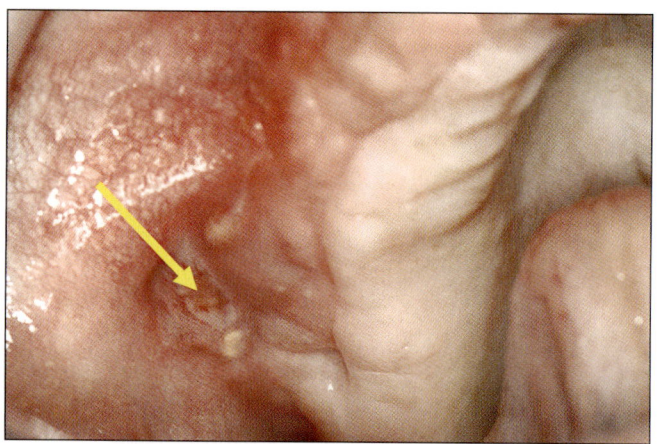

Fig 9-10a Right sinus graft infection at 3 months postsurgery. Note dehiscence over access window area *(arrow)*.

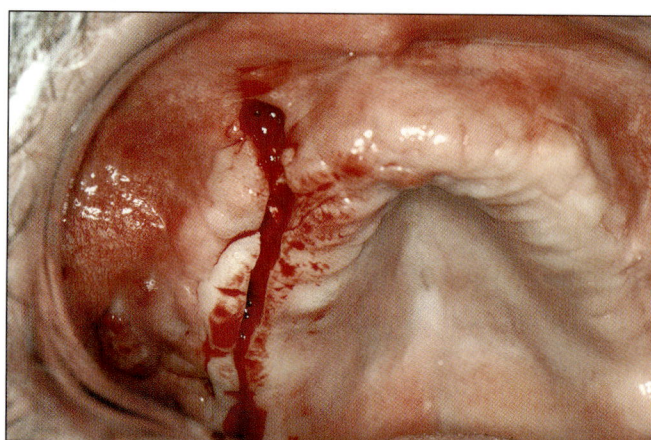

Fig 9-10b Midcrestal incision for graft removal with anterior oblique release.

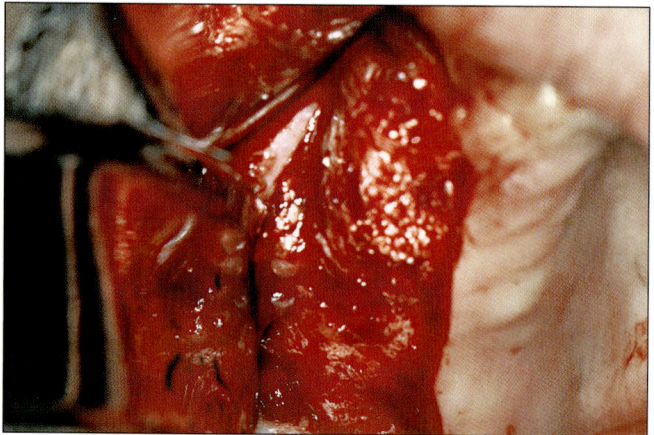

Fig 9-10c Initial access reveals breakdown of graft in central area of access window.

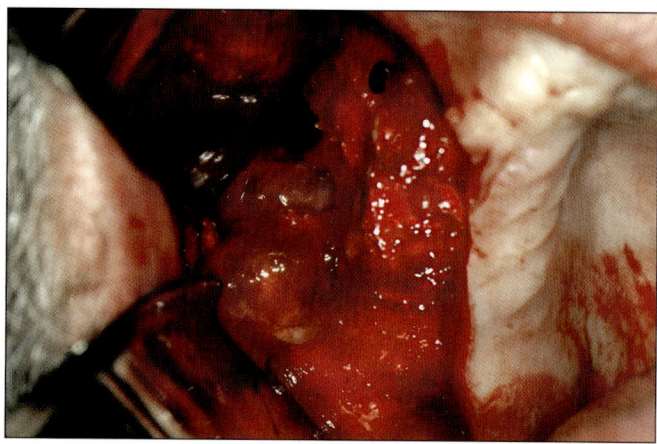

Fig 9-10d Removal of polyps and partially failed graft from right sinus 3 months postsurgery.

reported by Kubo in 1927,[35] is thought to derive from epithelial tissue tags that become entrapped during wound closure. This cyst has been referred to by a variety of names, including *postoperative maxillary cyst*,[36] *postoperative buccal cyst*,[37] *mucocele*,[38] and *postoperative paranasal cyst*.[39] Treatment consists of complete removal of the cyst with simultaneous bone grafting of the cyst cavity.

Chronic sinus disease seen preoperatively must be dealt with accordingly. Generally speaking, chronic sinus disease resulting in an excessively thickened membrane (Fig 9-14) may require membrane removal presurgically. These patients are more prone to have persistent disease. Timmenga et al[40] evaluated 45 patients with sinus grafts for sinus pathology 12 to 60 months after bone grafting using a questionnaire, conventional radiographic examination, and nasal endoscopy. Their results showed postoperative maxillary sinusitis in 2 of 5 patients with a predisposition for sinusitis but in none of the remaining 40 patients. Also, the occurrence of perforation was not related to the development of postoperative sinusitis in patients with healthy sinuses. They concluded that postoperative sinusitis appears to be limited to patients with a predisposition for this condition.

Chronic infection can occur secondary to an initial sinus graft infection, resulting in a persistent disease process refractory to conventional antibiotic treatment. This is especially true if a fungal infection is involved. These patients must be aggressively treated with intravenous drug therapy and surgical intervention. Finally, chronic pain can occur secondary to maxillary sinus augmentation, especially in the presence of implants. Although rare, this problem can be persistent and may require implant removal.

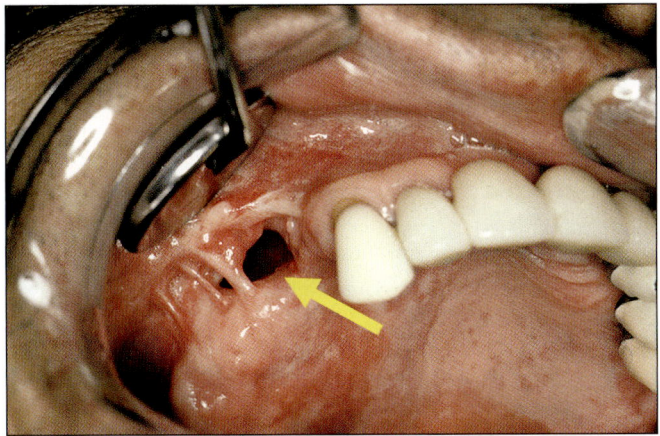

Fig 9-11 Oroantral fistula *(arrow)* of right maxillary sinus after sinus graft failure in a heavy smoker.

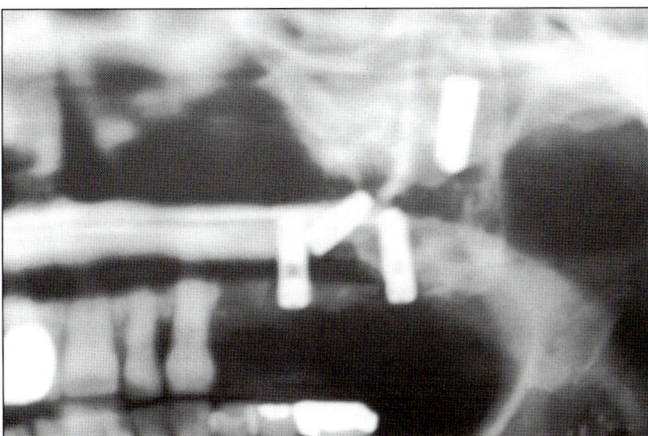

Fig 9-12 Implant migration within left maxillary sinus.

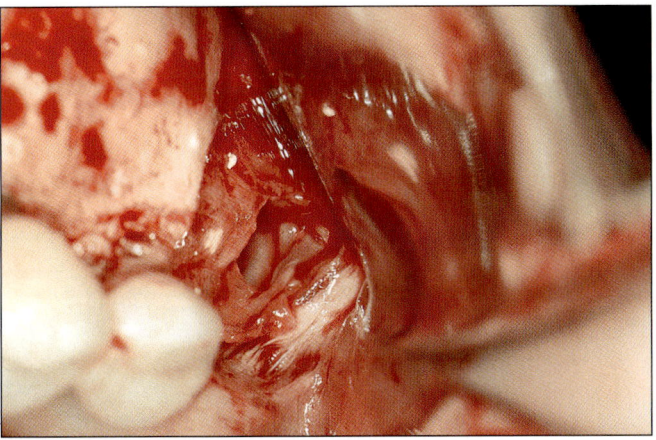

Fig 9-13 Epithelial cyst (Kubo cyst) of left maxillary sinus found 4 years after placement of the graft.

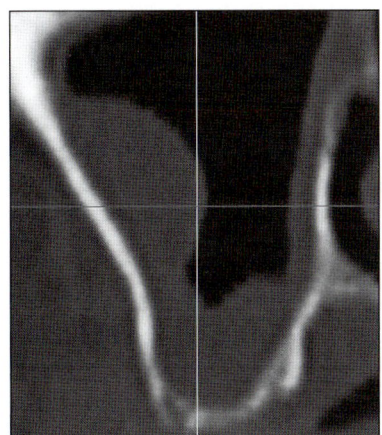

Fig 9-14 CT coronal section of right maxillary sinus. Note presence of thickened sinus membrane consistent with chronic sinusitis.

Summary

Maxillary sinus augmentation for implant reconstruction of the posterior maxilla is a predictable surgical procedure requiring the fulfillment of a number of criteria for optimal results. A methodical preoperative evaluation, including appropriate patient selection, is critical to the success of this surgery. Factors that must be analyzed include confirmation of a patent osteomeatal complex and healthy functioning paranasal sinuses. Good surgical technique is essential, including complication management. Implant failure, especially after several years in function, usually indicates inadequate treatment planning or poor maintenance rather than a problem with the graft itself.

The data presented at the Sinus Consensus Conference[28] confirm the high predictability of this procedure. Thirty-eight clinicians provided data on 1,007 sinus grafts that had 3,354 implants in function for at least 3 years. Long-term survival rates were in the 90% to 97% range. Autogenous bone or combinations of allografts, alloplasts, xenografts, and autogenous bone all yielded similar results.

Complications, although not commonly seen with sinus graft surgery, must be handled appropriately by the treating surgeon. When complications occur, treatment is usually successful if appropriate surgical and medical management is carried out. Well-treated complications will assure a highly predictable and successful long-term outcome.

References

1. Tatum H Jr. Maxillary and sinus implant reconstructions. Dent Clin North Am 1986;30:207–229.
2. Boyne PJ, James RA. Grafting of the maxillary sinus floor with autogenous marrow and bone. J Oral Surg 1980;38:613–616.
3. Misch CE. Maxillary sinus augmentation for endosteal implants: Organized alternative treatment plans. Int J Oral Implantol 1987;4:49–58.
4. Zinner ID, Small SA. Sinus-lift graft: Using the maxillary sinuses to support implants. J Am Dent Assoc 1996;127:51–57.
5. Tidwell JK, Blijdorp PA, Stoelinga PJW, Brouns JB, Hinderks F. Composite grafting of the maxillary sinus for placement of endosteal implants. A preliminary report of 48 patients. Int J Oral Maxillofac Surg 1992;21:204–209.
6. Triplett RG, Schow SR. Autologous bone grafts and endosseous implants: Complementary techniques. J Oral Maxillofac Surg 1996;54:486–494.
7. Smiler DG, Johnson PW, Lozada JL, et al. Sinus lift grafts and endosseous implants. Treatment of the atrophic posterior maxilla. Dent Clin North Am 1992;36:151–186.
8. Wheeler SL, Holmes RE, Calhoun CJ. Six-year clinical and histologic study of sinus-lift grafts. Int J Oral Maxillofac Implants 1996;11:26–34.
9. Block MS, Kent JN, Kallukaran FU, Thunthy K, Weinberg R. Bone maintenance 5 to 10 years after sinus grafting. J Oral Maxillofac Surg 1998;56:706–714.
10. Raghoebar GM, Brouwer TJ, Reintsema H, Van Oort RP. Augmentation of the maxillary sinus floor with autogenous bone for the placement of endosseous implants: A preliminary report. J Oral Maxillofac Surg 1993;51:1198–1203.
11. Keller EE, van Roekel NB, Desjardins RP, Tolman DE. Prosthetic-surgical reconstruction of the severely resorbed maxilla with iliac bone grafting and tissue-integrated prostheses. Int J Oral Maxillofac Implants 1987;2:155–165.
12. Peleg M, Mazor Z, Chaushu G, Garg AK. Sinus floor augmentation with simultaneous implant placement in the severely atrophic maxilla. J Periodontol 1998;69:1397–1403.
13. Wood RM, Moore DL. Grafting of the maxillary sinus with intraorally harvested autogenous bone prior to implant placement. Int J Oral Maxillofac Implants 1988;3:209–214.
14. Small SA, Zinner ID, Panno FV, Shapiro HJ, Stein JI. Augmenting the maxillary sinus for implants: Report of 27 patients. Int J Oral Maxillofac Implants 1993;8:523–528.
15. Ziccardi VB, Betts NJ. Complications of maxillary sinus augmentation. In: Jensen OT (ed). The Sinus Bone Graft. Chicago: Quintessence, 1999:201–208.
16. Misch CE. Contemporary Implant Dentistry, ed 2. St Louis: Mosby, 1999:469–495.
17. Pikos MA. Maxillary sinus membrane repair: Report of a technique for large perforations. Implant Dent 1999;8:29–33.
18. Levin L, Herzberg R, Dolev E, Schwartz-Arad D. Smoking and complications of onlay bone grafts and sinus lift operations. Int J Oral Maxillofac Implants 2004;19:369–373.
19. Kan JY, Rungcharassaeng K, Lozada JL, Goodacre CJ. Effects of smoking on implant success in grafted maxillary sinuses. J Prosthet Dent 1999;82:307–311.
20. Olson JW, Dent CD, Morris HF, Ochi S. Long-term assessment (5 to 71 months) of endosseous dental implants placed in the augmented maxillary sinus. Ann Periodontol 2000;5:152–156.
21. Stammberger H. Functional Endoscopic Sinus Surgery. St Louis: Mosby, 1991.
22. Marks SC. Nasal and Sinus Surgery. Philadelphia: Saunders, 2000:65–81.
23. Kudo K, et al. Clinicopathological study of postoperative maxillary cysts. J Jpn Stomatol Soc 1972;21:250–257.
24. Morgensen C, Tos M. Quantitative histology of the maxillary sinus. Rhinology 1977;15:129.
25. Block MS, Kent JN. Sinus augmentation for dental implants: The use of autogenous bone. J Oral Maxillofac Surg 1997;55:1281–1286.
26. Timmenga NM, Raghoebar GM, Boering G, van Weissenbruch R. Maxillary sinus function after sinus lifts for the insertion of dental implants. J Oral Maxillofac Surg 1997;55:936–939.
27. Tatum OH, Lebowitz MS, Tatum CA, Borgner RA. Sinus augmentation: Rationale, development, long-term results. NY State Dent J 1993;59:43–48.
28. Jensen OT, Shulman LB, Block MS, Iacono VJ. Report of the Sinus Consensus Conference of 1996. Int J Oral Maxillofac Implants 1998;13(suppl):11–45.
29. Triplett RG, Schow ST. Autologous bone grafts and endosseous implants: Complementary techniques. J Oral Maxillofac Surg 1996;54:486–494.
30. Keller EE, Eckert SE, Tolman DE. Maxillary antral and nasal one-stage inlay composite bone graft: Preliminary report on 30 recipient sites. J Oral Maxillofac Surg 1994;52:438–447.
31. Jensen J, Sindet-Pedersen S, Oliver AJ. Varying treatment strategies for reconstruction of maxillary atrophy with implants: Results in 98 patients. J Oral Maxillofac Surg 1994;52:210–216.
32. Ulm CW, Solar P, Gsellman B, Matehka M, Watzek G. The edentulous maxillary alveolar process in the region of the maxillary sinus—A study of physical dimension. Int J Oral Maxillofac Surg 1995;24:279–282.
33. Betts NJ, Miloro M. Modification of the sinus lift procedure for septa in the maxillary antrum. J Oral Maxillofac Surg 1994;52:332–333.
34. Smith D, Goycollea M, Meyerhoff WL. Fulminant odontogenic sinusitis. Ear Nose Throat J 1979;58:411.
35. Kubo I. A buccal cyst occurring after a radical operation of the maxillary sinus. Z Otol (Tokyo) 1927;33:896.
36. Kaneshiro S, Nakajima T, Yoshikawa Y, Iwasaki H, Tokiwa N. The postoperative maxillary cyst: A report of 71 cases. J Oral Surg 1981;39:191–198.
37. Nique T, Fonseca RJ, Upton LG, Scott R. Particulate allogeneic bone grafts into maxillary alveolar clefts in humans: A preliminary report. Int J Oral Maxillofac Surg 1987;45:386–392.
38. Mennig H. Zur Pathogenese der Kieferhohen Mucocelen. Arch Otorhinolaryngol 1956;169(suppl):465.
39. Tamura S. Study on the postoperative paranasal cyst. J Otolaryngol Jpn 1960;63:319.
40. Timmenga NM, Raghoebar GM, Boering G, van Weissenbruch R. Maxillary sinus function after sinus lifts for the insertion of dental implants. J Oral Maxillofac Surg 1997;55:936–939.

chapter 10
Sinus Reactions to Invasive Surgery

Chantal Malevez, MD, DDS

The atrophied edentulous maxilla represents a challenge for maxillofacial rehabilitation. Following tooth removal, bone resorption coupled with sinus pneumatization results in inadequate height for the placement of implants. In 1980,[1] Boyne used autogenous cancellous bone as a graft material, and today sinus grafting using a variety of biomaterials in preparation for oral implant placement has become standard treatment.

Despite improved understanding of biologic parameters[2] and well-documented use of various grafting materials, long-term follow-up is lacking.[3] Moreover, the reports of prospective randomized clinical trials[4] do not cover all aspects of success or failure as recommended by the Sinus Consensus Conference of 1996.[5]

A review of 831 articles on sinus grafting up to December 30, 2004, using the keywords *sinus graft*, *sinus floor elevation*, *bone grafting*, *sinus lifts*, *sinus inlay*, *dental implants*, and *osseointegration failures* resulted in 98 reports of sinus graft–related complications. Case reports of complications were included in the review when they were written by a clinician other than the surgeon who performed the sinus grafts. The other 733 articles did not focus on success or failure and therefore were excluded.

Potential Complications

It is often difficult to determine what is responsible for a complication: sinus health and/or anatomy, graft type, implant surface or length, bone quality, lack of osseointegration, prosthetic overload. Nonspecific findings[6] reported in this subset of publications included swelling, hematoma, purulent secretion from the incision, adjacent tooth sensitivity, and systemic fever. Specific findings were sinus congestion, hemoptysis, graft-induced sinusitis, cyst formation, and infection. Some reports of complications were not specific to the sinus graft procedure.

A healthy maxillary sinus is maintained in a bacteria-balanced environment through mucociliary action. This ensures effective transport to the ostium and inhibits colonization by microorganisms.[7] The sinus graft technique[8] invades the sinus to a sufficient degree to violate anatomic integrity and interfere with physiologic function, potentially creating complications such as infection, implant migration, and bone loss. Pre-existing conditions can alter sinus membrane furcation and impact incorporation of a sinus floor bone graft. Except a few prospective studies,[9–12] most of the reports barely mention medical history of the patient or significant antecedents of sinusitis. The lack of information on this subject, on the patient's use of tobacco, or on sinus impaction medicaments makes it difficult to establish success or failure criteria for sinus grafting.

Contraindications to sinus grafting include immune system disorders,[13] uncontrolled diabetes, smoking, ongoing chemotherapy, and chronic sinusitis, each of which jeopardizes the sinus elevation procedure. However, no scientific evidence available to date quantifies increased risk, and these parameters have not been systematically studied or examined by meta-analysis[14] (see chapter 8).

Most studies report the use of orthopantomographic evaluation as the only preoperative and postoperative examination of the sinus.[15] However, orthopantomographic evaluation is insufficient and often of inadequate

chapter 10 Sinus Reactions to Invasive Surgery

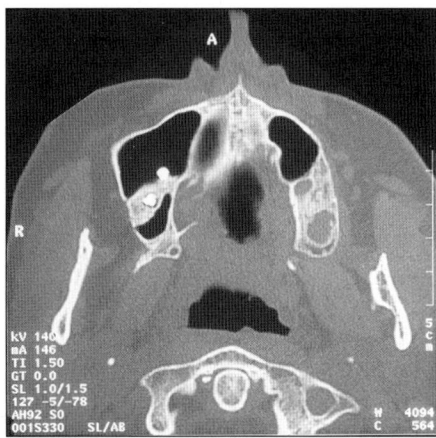

Fig 10-1a CT scan of left and right sinuses 2 years postloading and block bone grafting. Note sinusitis in left sinus.

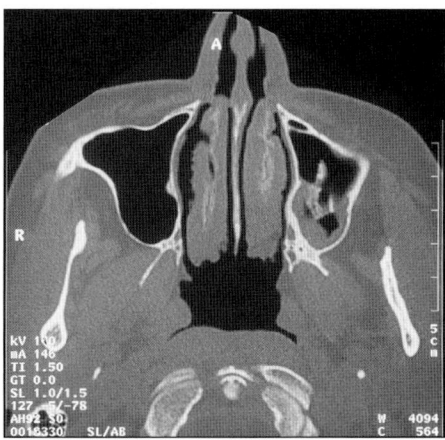

Fig 10-1b Two years later, left sinus shows bone graft extrusion and sinusitis, though without loss of implants.

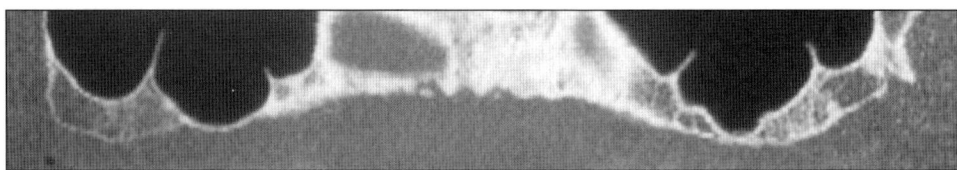

Fig 10-2 CT scan (Dentascan) lacking a view of the osteomeatal complex.

resolution[8]; two-dimensional volume change should not be established by deformed imaging. While some centers[16] advocate the use of lateral cephalograms or posteroanterior oblique radiographs to elucidate sinus pathology, the current standard of care for evaluating sinus health and morphology is computerized tomography (CT)[8] (Fig 10-1a).

For some cases in which CT scans are obtained, no information concerning the osteomeatal complex is reported.[17] For most cases, CT scans are obtained only after complications such as bone graft extrusion (Fig 10-1b) or oroantral fistula arise. Preoperative CT scans that are only at the dental level do not provide information about the osteomeatal complex or the complete volume of the sinus[17,18] (Fig 10-2). The patency of the osteomeatal complex and overall sinus health cannot be assessed.[19] The CT scan may suggest early intervention with prompt ventilation and drainage of an infected maxillary sinus to prevent loss of graft material and implants.[16,17] Excessive radiation of the patient must be considered, but the risk of obstruction or infection must also be considered. Preoperative CT scans aid not only in diagnosis of sinus ventilation and membrane health but also show postsurgical graft mass and consolidation and aid in detection of late complications[7] (Fig 10-3).

Preoperative sinus endoscopy[20] would help avoid complications when infraliminal sinusitis is detected.[17] Appraisal of sinus anatomy and middle meatus function by nasoendoscopy is useful in the diagnosis of subclinical sinusitis. When inflammation is present, the middle meatus is reduced and the thickness of an inflamed mucosal lining diminishes ventilation of the sinus.

The health of the sinus may be ascertained via endoscopic examination[20,21] before, during, and after sinus grafting. First, the endoscope may be used preoperatively to confirm positive radiologic or sonographic findings that exclude patients as candidates for a sinus graft. Second, endoscopic removal of polypoid mucosal lesions in the

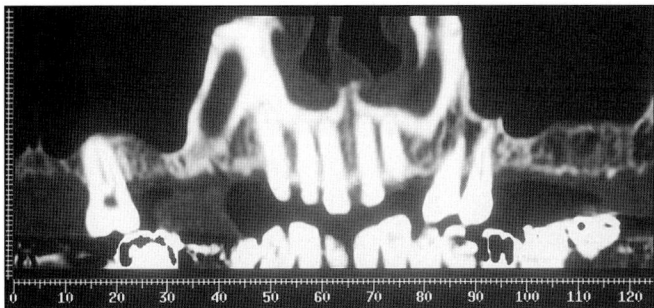
Fig 10-3a Preoperative CT scan prior to sinus graft procedure using bone harvested from the calvarium.

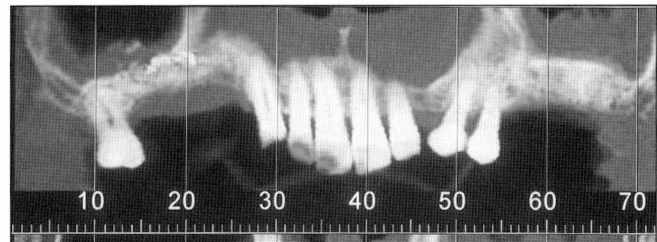
Fig 10-3b Postoperative CT scan taken 6 months later.

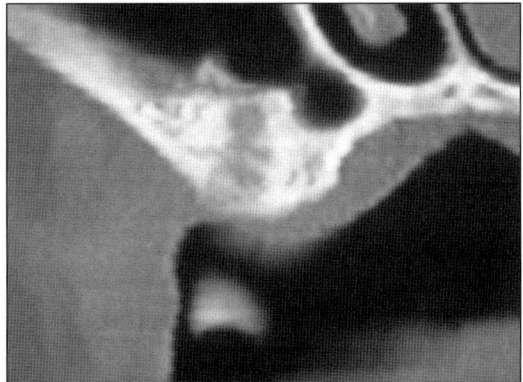
Fig 10-3c CT scan of right sinus showing lack of bone regeneration.

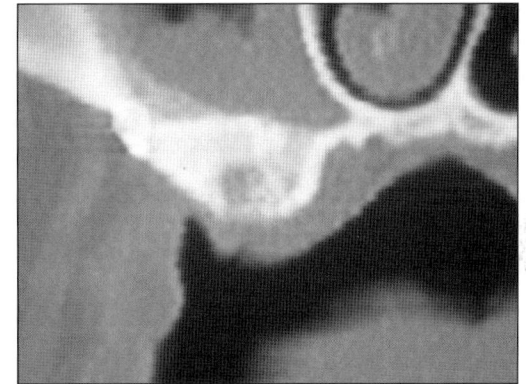
Fig 10-3d CT scan of left sinus showing lack of bone regeneration. The four implants were lost at the loading stage.

area will improve sinus graft healing. Timmenga et al[22] undertook a prospective clinical study of 17 patients analyzed via endoscopy; via light and electron microscopy; and via bacteriology, both prior to and 3 and 9 months after autogenous bone grafting. This well-documented study, the first of its kind in this field, confirmed that the sinus is not a sterile cavity, that the mucociliary membrane recovers completely 9 months after bone grafting, and that overall sinus bone grafting has minimal effect on sinus physiology. In another endoscopic prospective study, the osteotome technique was used, and the authors concluded that the sinus floor can be elevated 4 mm without perforation of the sinus membrane.[23–25] A recent animal study evaluated the health of the sinus membrane after osteotomy in goats[26] and concluded that the mucosa undergoes physiologic adaptation with a limited number of reconstructed glandular elements assessing the health of the modified mucosa. In humans,[27] endoscopy of healthy membranes without inflammation has been observed around sinus-perforating miniplates and screws.

The influence of smoking is controversial (see chapters 8 and 9). Some authors consider it a contraindication while others see no correlation between the success rate and smoking.[6,28–31] The reported success rate of sinus floor augmentation ranges from 75% to 93%.[20] Although some have reported 100% success, these are retrospective nonconsecutive studies.[14]

Another problem with case series[32] concerns the reporting of sinus graft failures. The success rate is then calculated based on implants placed without taking into account the two or three additional implants that could have been placed had the graft consolidated. Moreover, the gross underreporting of marginally failed sinus bone grafts certainly impacts the statistical analysis of bone graft success. At present, no correlation has been established between failure and sinus graft technique used (eg, lateral window, endoscopic, transalveolar osteotome, etc) or between failure and the type of graft material used (eg, autogenous bone from the ilium, tibia, chin, or calvarium; allograft; or alloplast).

Another underreported finding is the preoperative height of available bone and the length of the implants used. No CT scan data have been accompanied by before-and-after sinus graft imaging. Only panoramic radiographs have been available for meta-analysis.[33] Also, few follow-up studies of more than 3 years include data on complications and failures, and those that do[6,16,34] lack standardization or sufficient explanation of the failures.

Based on the recommendations of the Sinus Consensus Conference,[5] failure of sinus bone grafting should be based exclusively on the following criteria:

- Implant mobility
- Peri-implant radiolucency
- Implant-associated pain
- Implant-associated graft infection
- Bone loss cervical or apical to the implant
- Implants that could not be loaded, for whatever reason

Failure of sinus bone grafts by graft site was never addressed by the Sinus Consensus Conference; therefore, only indirect analysis of sinus-grafted bone was undertaken. Furthermore, sinuses that were grafted but never received oral implants were not included in the database.

Sinus Reactions to Bone Grafting

Membrane perforation

For many authors, membrane perforation is the most serious complication,[15,35,36] although its effect on the success of the graft is controversial (primarily because success is measured indirectly based on implant placement and not on graft persistence). Perforation can lead to infection as well as loss of the bone or bone substitute[17,19] and even loss of the entire graft. For this reason, many authors advocate the necessity of avoiding membrane perforation and propose a variety of solutions for confining the graft when it occurs, including the use of fibrin glue,[36,37] collagen,[35,38,39] suturing,[40] resorbable foil,[20] lamellar bone,[41] resorbable or nonresorbable barrier membrane,[42,43] metal crib, and so forth. The use of a balloon to expand the sinus membrane has been described as a technical strategy to avoid damaging the sinus membrane.[44] Others propose using block rather than particulate grafting for the same purpose.[45] Whatever method is chosen, if the rent is too large, the sinus graft procedure should be aborted until the membrane has had an opportunity to re-epithelialize.

Membrane perforation alone does not generate complications in most cases[16] unless it is large. Perforation without infection (35%) has been described.[5] Other studies that have focused on complications with long-term follow-up found no correlation between small perforations and subsequent complications.[6,34,46] The size or extent of perforation is the most important correlate, especially when a nonautogenous (marrow) graft is used. At present, however, no clear difference in success has been reported with regard to type of graft approach or grafting material used when there is damage to the sinus membrane.[47] The author uses corticospongious bone blocks harvested from the iliac crest and ignores incidental perforation of the sinus membrane.[48] In a series of 40 sinus grafts performed with immediate implant placement, no graft loss occurred with an implant failure rate of 6.6% over 4 years of follow-up. All implant losses occurred prior to loading with no apparent cause.

Sinusitis

Sinusitis is a common complication of sinus grafting.[15,19,49,50] One factor that predisposes to sinusitis is perforation of the sinus membrane. With delayed placement of implants, acute sinusitis risk is reduced as it relates to potential implant loss.[6,10,15,16,51,52] For this reason, many practitioners advocate a two-stage approach.

In an interesting analysis of sinus function following sinus elevation,[53] 45 patients who received 85 sinus bone grafts underwent evaluation by endoscopy, Water's view radiography, and questionnaire 12 to 60 months postsurgery. Of the 45 patients, only 5 were found to have sinusitis after sinus grafting. In the 5 patients, endoscopy revealed oversized turbinates and septal deviation. The results of this study clearly show that the incidence of sinusitis after bone grafting is low and is predominantly found in patients who are predisposed to sinusitis. One author[53] recommended nasoendoscopy in patients presenting with anatomic or functional disorders before sinus graft surgery.

Slight inflammation of the sinus membrane has been shown after placement of hydroxyapatite (HA) in a study on monkeys.[54,55] The study also showed increased lymphocytosis. These results suggest that sinusitis is infrequent as a complication of sinus graft procedure, although it has the potential to result in the loss of graft and implants.

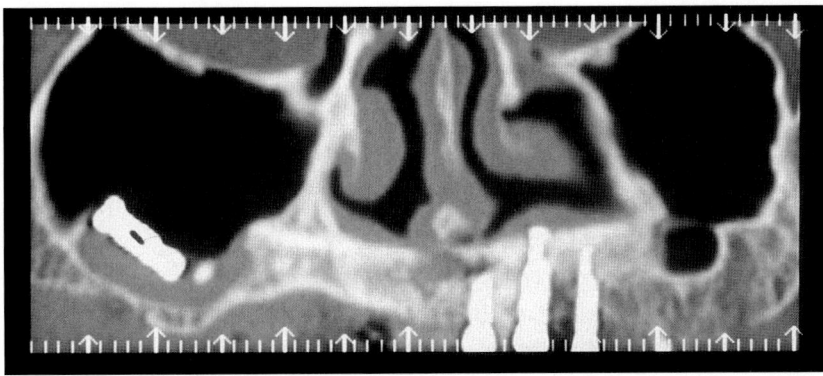

Fig 10-4 Implant migration following a two-stage technique (Le Fort I and interpositional bone grafting using calvarial bone). The implants were placed 6 months after bone grafting.

Other complications

Many other complications have been reported, including:

- Dehiscence of oral mucosa[30,45,56]
- Profuse bleeding during surgery[38,46,57]
- Implant migration[8] (Fig 10-4)
- Hematoma[6]
- Suture abscess[6]
- Adjacent tooth sensitivity[6,58]
- Loss of bone graft and late-term sequestration[8,16,59]

Loss of bone graft was found in 2.6% of 77 sinuses reconstructed with calvarial bone grafts using a two-stage procedure. The authors reported a 100% success rate in a retrospective study from 1992 to 2002.[57] Unfortunately, no CT scan data were reported, and no life table analysis was conducted. Complications at the graft site[57] included penetration into the cranial cavity (without further complication) in three patients.

For other authors, late-term complications included:

- Chronic infection[8,35,52,60,61]
- Oroantral fistula[8,16,57,62]
- Graft exposure[16,57,61]
- Separation of the graft from basal bone[60]
- Expulsion of the implant through the nose[8]
- Chronic pain[8,63]
- Aspergillosis[8,64]
- Wound dehiscency[16,52]
- Sinus cyst and scar tissue replacement of the graft[6,7,65,66]

One case report of an unexposed implant placed 9 years earlier and retrieved with associated tissues for histomorphometric evaluation demonstrated some bone and abundant connective tissue between graft particles and the HA-coated implant. Alteration of voice quality has been reported in only one patient.[67]

Loss of Implants

A high success rate of stable implants is, of course, the purpose of the sinus graft procedure. Analysis of 2,997 implants during the Sinus Consensus Conference showed 229 osseointegration failures.[5] No scientific consideration could be given to this retrospective data to draw any credible conclusion. Too many studies were conducted without real scientific protocols. Most of them were retrospective and nonconsecutive instead of prospective or randomized.

Loss of implants cannot be the sole criterion for determining the success of a sinus graft. The failure rate of implants placed without sinus elevation surgery, regardless of the type of graft used, is lower than that with sinus elevation surgery. Prospective studies[10,51,68,69] show success ranging from 61.2% to 89.5%. However, retrospective clinical studies[16,31,34,40,47,51,65,70–80] report similar results. Implants that are lost before loading indicate a failure of osseointegration. Nevertheless, implant survival of 80% to 90% is considered acceptable. A prospective clinical study[81] with 5 years of follow-up clearly demonstrated that implant failures were higher in grafted than in nongrafted areas, suggesting that the quality of bone in grafted areas is poorer than in nongrafted areas. A restorative study showed no significant differences in the prostheses of grafted and nongrafted patients.[11]

Loss of implants placed as part of the sinus elevation procedure remains inadequately explained. A randomized clinical trial that compared one-stage and two-stage techniques with iliac bone grafts[9] reported that the results of the two-stage approach were twice as good. Nonetheless, the success rate for sinus elevation using iliac bone grafting material is lower than the success rate for other materials after 1 year (see chapter 17).

Calvarial bone grafting combined with human recombinant tissue factor, platelet-rich plasma (PRP), and tetracycline in a prospective clinical trial of 18 patients with 25 grafted sinuses induced a high success rate[32] (90% for the graft and 91.3% for implant integration). However, 2 of the 25 sinuses were excluded due to focal infections, and for the other failures no explanation was offered for the loss of the implants.

Loss of implants due to failure of integration can lead to therapeutic problems as well as patient anxiety and discomfort.[80] One author compared patients who had lost a significant number of implants (43%) with those who had lost only one or two (6%) but could find no significant hematologic, osteometric, or anamnestic differences between the two groups.

Influence of implant surface

Surface roughness of an implant has a significant influence on its success in grafted bone. In a consecutive study,[82] 78 Brånemark machined implants were compared with the same number of Straumann sand-blasted, large-grit, acid-etched (SLA) implants, but the diameter of the implants varied and no distinction was made between disparate thread patterns. The authors reported an 81% success rate for the machined implants and a 98% success rate for the SLA implants, with no adverse sinus reactions. The study was not randomized, and CT evaluation was not conducted. However, more recent studies using implants with an oxidized surface placed into grafted areas reported survival rates of 98% to 99%.[83,84] In another study, 1 implant was lost without explanation[85] out of 27 implants placed using bioglass (BioGran, Implant Innovations Inc), autogenous bone, and an acid-etched titanium implant[80] (see chapter 18).

Periodontal disease

A 1997 study[86] found no correlation between periodontal disease and loss of implants placed in sinus grafted bone. Peri-implantitis[60,87] is the same in grafted and native bone.

Maintenance of Sinus Graft Height

Few studies evaluate the follow-up after the bone graft has been inserted in the sinus. In a study involving 191 patients with up to 10 years of follow-up,[88] the height of the composite graft (autograft-xenograft in a 2:1 ratio) was shown to decrease with time, particularly during the first 2- to 3-year period, displaying no significant change thereafter. Panoramic radiographs were used as the basis for the analysis.

Complications at the Donor Site

Many authors rationalize the use of bone substitutes based on the potential morbidity of bone harvesting. However, very few donor site complications have been reported. Common forms of morbidity associated with the iliac crest are hematoma, seroma, pain, discomfort, gait disturbances, and paresthesia.[16] Tibia bone harvesting rarely results in fracture of the tibial plateau; mandibular ramus bone harvesting has caused transient hypoesthesia of the labial gingiva and of inferior alveolar bone[16]; and the harvesting of calvarial bone has occasionally caused intracranial penetration with rents in the dura.[57]

Sinus Reactions to Zygomatic Implants

The zygomatic implant was developed by Brånemark[89] in the 1980s for rehabilitation of maxillary defects, primarily those resulting from ablative cancer surgery. The favorable results obtained with zygoma anchorage led to modification of the technique for use in the atrophic edentulous maxilla. Following the publication of a 1999 multicenter study involving 16 centers,[90] which reported a 98% implant survival rate after 1 year and a 97.1% rate after 3 years, the popularity of this relatively new procedure steadily rose.[91] Some authors reported 100% success.[92,93] The advantage of the zygomatic implant is that anchorage

Fig 10-5 Two-year follow-up view of patient rehabilitated with four standard and two zygomatic implants.

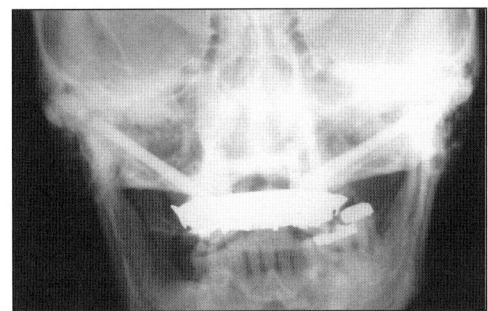

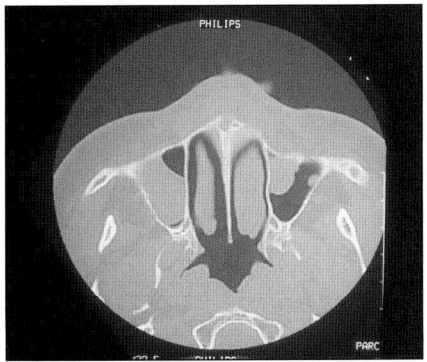

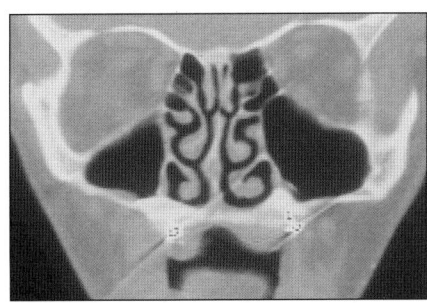

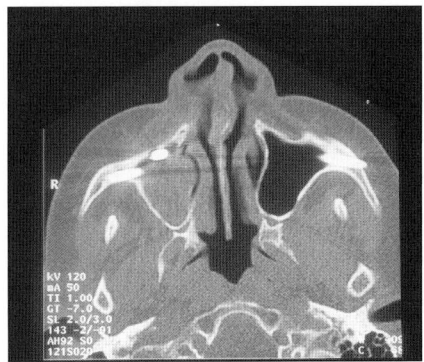

Fig 10-6a Presurgical radiographic view of patient with transitional sinusitis, which subsequently regressed, taken in 1999.

Fig 10-6b Calvarial bone grafting and delayed implant placement for treatment of severely atrophied maxilla (1999). There is no evidence of sinusitis. The five implants were subsequently lost.

Fig 10-6c CT scan taken in 2004 showing evidence of sinusitis in one sinus. Despite the earlier loss of five implants and the subsequent loss (3 years later) of the calvarial bone graft, the two zygomatic implants placed in 1997, along with an anterior iliac bone graft, have been retained and remain in good function.

(and hence osseointegration) is obtained at a site other than the maxilla.

Zygomatic bone is comparable in density to mandibular bone.[94,95] The surgical protocol necessitates initial penetration of the zygomatic implant through the sinus along the lateral wall (without damaging the sinus membrane) (see chapter 26). While maintaining the integrity of the sinus membrane is not controversial for the sinus graft procedure, it may not be relevant for the zygomatic implant. The use of a bone graft with zygomatic implants is inappropriate and counterintuitive. In an interesting endoscopic examination of the zygomatic trans-sinus implant,[96] no inflammation or signs of infection of the sinus membrane was demonstrated after more than 1 year of function.

Until now, few published papers have elucidated adverse sinus reactions around zygomatic implants. Those that have been described[93]—ie, sinusitis, hematomas, and fistulae—are similar to reactions observed in sinus-grafting procedures. Surprisingly, when sinusitis is a factor, it does not compromise the success of zygomatic implants. Sinus complications have been treated medically or by meatotomy when necessary. Demonstration of the excellent biomechanical advantage of the zygomatic implant is provided in Fig 10-5. A patient lost two bone grafts—including an iliac bone graft placed in 1997 together with two zygomatic and three conventional implants, and a calvarial bone graft with five implants and all conventional implants at least in part from bruxism over a 5-year period—but nevertheless retained her osseointegrated zygomatic implants that were placed in 1997 (Fig 10-6). Additional preoperative investigation as well as randomized trials are still needed to study the zygomatic implant.[97]

Zygomatic implants constitute a valuable addition to the surgeon's repertoire in the management of the compromised maxilla[87] and offer a viable alternative to sinus grafts or extensive onlay bone grafting. They provide a biomechanical advantage comparable to that of Le Fort I advancement combined with sinus grafting.

Conclusion

Sinus reactions sometimes occur after sinus surgery. Before entering the sinus cavity, thorough clinical and radiographic investigations must be routinely performed. The sinus graft is a well-documented procedure that has been used for more than 20 years with a high rate of success.

Zygomatic implants have been shown to cause minimal complications and have demonstrated a high success rate. The development of this new alternative to sinus grafting could shorten the surgical procedure, reduce costs, diminish the length of rehabilitation with the possibility of immediate function, and improve comfort and oral function for the patient.

Acknowledgment

The author thanks Mrs Maïté Stiévenart for researching and collecting the articles surveyed in this chapter.

References

1. Boyne PJ, James RA. Grafting of the maxillary sinus floor with autologous marrow and bone. J Oral Surg 1980;38:613–616.
2. Merkx MA, Maltha JC, Stoelinga PJ. Assessment of the value of anorganic bone additives in sinus floor augmentation: A review of clinical reports. Int J Oral Maxillofac Surg 2003;32:1–6.
3. Piatelli M, Favero AF, Scarano A, Orsini G, Piatello A. Bone reactions to anorganic bovine bone (Bio-Oss) used in sinus augmentation procedures: A histologic long-term reports of 20 cases in humans. Int J Oral Maxillofac Implants 1999;14:835–840.
4. Wallace SS, Froum SJ. Effect of maxillary sinus augmentation on the survival of endosseous dental implants. A systematic review. Ann Periodontol 2003;8:328–343.
5. Jensen OT. Treatment planning for sinus grafts. In: Jensen OT (ed). The Sinus Bone Graft. Chicago: Quintessence, 1999:49–68.
6. Schwartz-Arad D, Herzberg R, Dolev E. The prevalence of surgical complications of the sinus graft procedure and their impact on implant survival. J Periodontol 2004;75:511–516.
7. Lockhart R, Ceccaldi J, Bertrand JC. Postoperative maxillary cyst following sinus bone graft: Report of a case. Int J Oral Maxillofac Implants 2000;15:583–586.
8. Regev E, Smith RA, Perrott DH, Pogrel MA. Maxillary sinus complications related to endosseous implants. Int J Oral Maxillofac Implants 1995;10:451–461.
9. Wannfors K, Johansson B, Hallman M, Strandkvist T. A prospective randomized study of 1-and 2-stage sinus inlay bone grafts: 1-year follow-up. Int J Oral Maxillofac Implants 2000;15:625–632.
10. Kahnberg KE, Ekestubbe A, Grondahl K, et al. Sinus lifting procedure. I. One-stage surgery with bone transplant and implants. Clin Oral Implants Res 2001;12:479–487.
11. Smedberg JI, Johansson P, Ekenback D, Wannfors K. Implants and sinus-inlay graft in a 1-stage procedure in severely atrophied maxillae: Prosthodontic aspects in a 3-year follow-up study. Int J Oral Maxillofac Implants 2001;16:668–674.
12. Timmenga NM, Raghoebar GM, Liem RSB, van Weissenbruck R, Manson WL, Vissink A. Effects of maxillary sinus floor elevation surgery on maxillary sinus physiology. Eur J Oral Sci 2003;111:189–197.
13. Wheeler SL, Holmes RE, Calhoun CJ. Six-year clinical and histologic study of sinus-lift grafts. Int J Oral Maxillofac Implants 1996;11:26–34.
14. Van den Bergh JP, ten Bruggenkate CM, Krekeler G, Tuinzing DB. Sinus floor elevation and grafting with autogenous iliac crest bone. Clin Oral Implants Res 1998;9:429–435.
15. Tidwell JK, Blijdorp PA, Stoelinga PJW, Brouns JB, Hinderks F. Composite grafting of the maxillary sinus for placement of endosteal implants: A preliminary report of 48 patients. Int J Oral Maxillofac Surg 1992;21:204–209.
16. Raghoebar GM, Timmenga NM, Reintsema H, Stegenga B, Vissink A. Maxillary bone grafting for insertion of endosseous implants: Results after 12–124 months. Clin Oral Implants Res 2001;12:279–286.
17. Zimbler MS, Lebowitz RA, Glickman R, Brecht LE, Jacobs JB. Antral augmentation osseointegration and sinusitis: The otolaryngologist's perspective. Am J Rhinol 1998;12:311–316.
18. Szabo G, Suba Z, Hrabak K, Barabas J, Nemeth Z. Autogenous bone versus beta-tricalcium phosphate graft alone for bilateral sinus elevations (2–3–dimensional computed tomographic, histologic and histomorphometric evaluations): Preliminary results. Int J Oral Maxillofac Implants 2001;16:681–692.
19. Doud Galli SK, Lebowitz RA, Giacchi RJ, Glickman R, Jacobs JB. Chronic sinusitis complicating sinus lift surgery. Am J Rhinol 2001;15:181–186.
20. Wiltfang J, Schultze-Mosgau S, Merten HA, Kessler P, Ludwig A, Engelke W. Endoscopic and ultrasonographic evaluation of the maxillary sinus after combined sinus floor augmentation and implant insertion. Oral Surg Oral Med Oral Pathol Oral Radiol Endod 2000;89:288–291.
21. Grunenberg M, Gerlach KL. Clinical, radiographic and endoscopic evaluation of the maxilla sinus after maxillary osteotomy. Dtsch Z Mund Kiefer Gesichtschir 1990;14:202–205.

22. Timmenga NM, Raghoebar GM, van Weissenbruch R, Vissink A. Maxillary sinus floor elevation surgery. A clinical, radiographic and endoscopic evaluation. Clin Oral Implants Res 2003; 14:322–328.
23. Nkenke E, Schlegel A, Schultze-Mosgau S, Neukam FW, Wiltfang J. The endoscopically controlled osteotome sinus floor elevation: A preliminary prospective study. Int J Oral Maxillofac Implants 2002;17:557–566.
24. Engelke W, Deckwer I. Endoscopically controlled sinus floor augmentation. A preliminary report. Clin Oral Implants Res 1997;8:527–531.
25. Engelke W, Schwarzwaller W, Behnsen A, Jacobs HG. Subantroscopic laterobasal sinus floor augmentation (SALSA): An up-to-5-year clinical study. Int J Oral Maxillofac Implants 2003;18: 135–143.
26. Bravetti P, Membre H, Marchal L, Jankowski R. Histologic changes in the sinus membrane after maxillary sinus augmentation in goats. J Oral Maxillofac Surg 1998;56:1170–1176.
27. Berengo M, Sivolella S, Majzoub Z, Cordiolo G. Endoscopic evaluation of the bone-added osteotome sinus floor elevation procedure. J Oral Maxillofac Surg 2004;33:189–194.
28. Bergstrom J, Eliasson S, Preber H. Cigarette smoking and the periodontal bone loss. J Periodontol 1991;62:242–246.
29. Levin L, Herzberg R, Dolev E, Schwartz-Arad D. Smoking and complications of onlay bone grafts and sinus lift operations. Int J Oral Maxillofac Implants 2004;19:369–373.
30. Rosen PS, Summers R, Mellado JR, et al. The bone-added osteotome sinus floor elevation technique: Multicenter retrospective report of consecutively treated patients. Int J Oral Maxillofac Implants 1999;14:853–858.
31. Kan JY, Rungcharassaeng K, Kim J, Lozada JL, Goodacre CJ. Factors affecting the survival of implants placed in grafted maxillary sinuses: A clinical report. J Prosth Dent 2002;87:485–489.
32. Philippart P, Brasseur M, Hoyaux D, Pochet R. Human recombinant tissue factor, platelet-rich plasma, and tetracycline induce a high-quality human bone graft: A 5-year survey. Int J Oral Maxillofac Implants 2003;18:411–416.
33. Tong DC, Rioux K, Drangsholt M, Beirne OR. A review of survival rates for implants placed in grafted maxillary sinuses using meta-analysis. Int J Oral Maxillofac Implants 1998;13:175–182.
34. Keller EE, Eckert SE, Tolman DE. Maxillary antral nasal and nasal one-stage inlay composite bone graft: Preliminary report on 30 recipient sites. Int J Oral Maxillofac Surg 1994;52:438–447.
35. Smiler DG, Johnson PW, Lozada JL, et al. Sinus lift grafts and endosseous implants. Treatment of the atrophic posterior maxilla. Dent Clin North Am 1992;36:151–186.
36. Sullivan SM, Bulard RA, Meaders R, Patterson MK. The use of fibrin adhesive in sinus lift procedures. Oral Surg Oral Med Oral Pathol Oral Radiol Endod 1997;84:616–619.
37. Mazor Z, Peleg M, Gross M. Sinus augmentation for single tooth replacement in the posterior maxilla: A 3-year follow-up clinical report. Int J Oral Maxillofac Implants 1999;14:55–60.
38. Small SA, Zinner ID, Panno FV, Shapiro HJ, Stein JI. Augmenting the maxillary sinus for implants: Report of 127 patients. Int J Oral Maxillofac Implants 1993;8:523–528.
39. De Leonardis D, Pecora GE. Augmentation of the maxillary sinus with calcium sulphate: One-year clinical report from a prospective longitudinal study. Int J Oral Maxillofac Implants 1999;14:869–878.
40. Krekmanov L. A modified method of simultaneous bone grafting and placement of endosseous implants in the severely atrophic maxilla. Int J Oral Maxillofac Implants 1995;10:682–688.
41. Betts NJ, Miloro M. Modification of the sinus lift procedure for septa in the maxillary antrum. J Oral Maxillofac Surg 1994;52: 332–333.
42. Avera SP, Stampley WA, McAllister BS. Histologic and clinical observations of resorbable and nonresorbable barrier membranes used in maxillary sinus graft containment. Int J Oral Maxillofac Implants 1997;12:88–94.
43. Proussaefs P, Lozada J. Histologic evaluation of a 9-year-old hydroxyapatite-coated cylindric implant placed in conjunction with a subantral augmentation procedure: A case report. Int J Oral Maxillofac Implants 2001;16:737–741.
44. Muronoi M, Xu H, Shimizu Y, Ooya K. Simplified procedure for augmentation of the sinus floor using a haemostatic balloon. Br J Oral Maxillofac Surg 2003;41:120–121.
45. Jensen J, Sindet-Pedersen S. Autogenous mandibular bone grafts and osseointegrated implants for reconstruction of the severely atrophied maxilla: A preliminary report. J Oral Maxillofac Surg 1991;49:1277–1287.
46. Shlomi B, Horowitz I, Kahn A, Dobriyan A, Chaushu G. The effect of sinus membrane perforation and repair with Lambone on the outcome of the maxillary sinus floor augmentation: Radiographic assessment. Int J Oral Maxillofac Implants 2004; 19:559–562.
47. Jensen J, Sindet-Pedersen S, Oliver AJ. Varying treatment strategies for reconstruction of maxillary atrophy with implants: Results in 98 patients. J Oral Maxillofac Surg 1994;52:210–216.
48. Daelemans P, Hermans M, Godet F, Malevez C. Autologous bone graft to augment maxillary sinus in conjunction with immediate endosseous implants: A retrospective study up to 5 years. Int J Periodontics Restorative Dent 1997;17:27–39.
49. Bhatacharyya N. Bilateral chronic maxillary sinusitis after the sinus lift procedure. Am J Otolaryngol 1999;20:133–135.
50. Van den Bergh JP, ten Bruggenkate CM, Disch FJ, Tuinzing DB. Anatomical aspects of sinus floor elevations. Clin Oral Implants Res 2000;11:256–265.
51. Hallman M, Nordin T. Sinus floor augmentation with bovine hydroxyapatite mixed with fibrin glue and later placement of non-submerged implants: A retrospective study in 50 patients. Int J Oral Maxillofac Implants 2004;19:222–227.
52. McCarthy PF, Patel RR, Wragg PF, Brook IM. Sinus augmentation bone grafts for the provision of dental implants: Report of clinical outcome. Int J Oral Maxillofac Implants 2003;18:377–382.
53. Timmenga NM, Raghoebar GM, Boering G, Van Weissenbruch R. Maxillary sinus function after sinus lifts for insertion of dental implants. J Oral Maxillofac Surg 1997;55:936–939.

54. Quinones CR, Hurzeler MB, Schupbach P, et al. Maxillary sinus augmentation using different grafting materials and osseointegrated dental implants in monkeys. Part II. Evaluation of porous hydroxyapatite as a grafting material. Clin Oral Implants Res 1997;8:487–496.
55. Quinones CR, Hurzeler MB, Schupbach P, Arnold DR, Strub JR, Caffesse RG. Maxillary sinus augmentation using different grafting materials and dental implants in monkeys. Part IV. Evaluation of hydroxyapatite-coated implants. Clin Oral Implants Res 1997;8:497–505.
56. Raghoebar GM, Brouwer TJ, Reintsema H, Van Oort RP. Augmentation of the maxillary sinus floor with autogenous bone for the placement of endosseous implants: A preliminary report. J Oral Maxillofac Surg 1993;51:1198–1203; discussion 1203–1205.
57. Iturriaga MT, Ruiz CC. Maxillary sinus reconstruction with calvarium bone grafts and endosseous implants. J Oral Maxillofac Surg 2004;62:344–347.
58. Jensen J, Simenson EK, Sindet-Pedersen S. Reconstruction of severely resorbed maxilla with bone grafting and osseointegrated implants. J Oral Maxillofac Surg 1990;48:27–32.
59. Triplett RG, Schow SR. Autologous bone grafts and endosseous implants: Complementary techniques. J Oral Maxillofac Surg 1996;54:486–494.
60. Olson JW, Dent CD, Morris HF, Ochi S. Long-term assessment (5 to 71 months) of endosseous dental implants placed in the augmented maxillary sinus. Ann Periodontol 2000;5:152–156.
61. Cawood JL, Stoelinga PJW, Brouns JJA. Reconstruction of the severely resorbed (class VI) maxilla. Int J Oral Maxillofac Surg 1994;23:219–225.
62. Johansson B, Smedberg JI, Langley M, Embery G. Glycosaminoglycans in peri-implant sulcus fluid from implants placed in sinus-inlay bone grafts. Clin Oral Implants Res 2001;12:202–206.
63. Draft W. Facial neuralgia after Caldwell-Luc-Operation-Prophylaxis and therapy. Laryngol Rhinol Otol(stuttg) 1980;59:308–311.
64. De Foer C, Fossion E, Vaillant JM. Sinus Aspergillosis. J Craniomaxillofac Surg 1990;18:33–40.
65. Van den Bergh JP, ten Bruggenkate CM, Groeneveld HH, Burger EH, Tuinzing DB. Recombinant human bone morphogenetic protein-7 in maxillary sinus floor elevation surgery in 3 patients compared to autogenous bone grafts: A clinical pilot study. J Clin Periodontol 2000;27:627–636.
66. Misch CM, Misch CE, Resnik RR, Ismail YH, Appel B. Postoperative maxillary cyst associated with a maxillary sinus elevation procedure. A case report. J Oral Implantol 1991;17:432–437.
67. Tepper G, Haas R, Schneider B, et al. Effects of sinus lifting on voice quality. A prospective study and risk assessment. Clin Oral Implants Res 2003;14:767–774.
68. Yildirim M, Spiekermann H, Biesterfeld S, Edelhoff D. Maxillary sinus augmentation using xenogeneic bone substitute material Bio-Oss in combination with venous blood. A histologic and histomorphometric study in humans. Clin Oral Implants Res 2000;11:217–229.
69. Blomqvist JE, Alberius P, Isaksson S. Two-stage maxillary sinus reconstruction with endosseous implants: A prospective study. Int J Oral Maxillofac Implants 1998;13:758–766.
70. Isaksson S, Ekfeldt A, Alberius P, Blomqvist JE. Early results from reconstruction of severely atrophic (class VI) maxillas by immediate endosseous implants in conjunction with bone grafting and Le Fort I osteotomy. Int J Oral Maxillofac Surg 1993;22:144–148.
71. Nystrom E, Lundgren S, Gunne J, Nilson H. Interpositional bone grafting and LeFort I osteotomy for reconstruction of the atrophic edentulous maxilla. A two-stage technique. Int J Oral Maxillofac Surg 1997;26:423–427.
72. Lundgren S, Nystrom E, Nilson H, Gunne J, Lindhaven O. Bone grafting to the maxillary sinuses, nasal floor and anterior maxilla in the atrophic edentulous maxilla. A two-stage technique. Int J Oral Maxillofac Surg 1997;26:428–434.
73. Williamson RA. Rehabilitation of the resorbed maxilla and mandible using autogenous bone grafts and osseointegrated implants. Int J Oral Maxillofac Implants 1996;11:476–488.
74. Hallman M, Sennerby L, Lundgren S. A clinical and histologic evaluation of implant integration in the posterior maxilla after sinus floor augmentation with autogenous bone, bovine hydroxyapatite, or a 20:80 mixture. Int J Oral Maxillofac Implants 2002;17:635–643.
75. Laine J, Vahatalo K, Peltola J, Tammisalo T, Happonen RP. Rehabilitation of patients with congenital unrepaired cleft palate defects using free iliac crest bone grafts and dental implants. Int J Oral Maxillofac Implants 2002;17:573–580.
76. Jansma J, Raghoebar GM, Batenburg RH, Stellingsma C, van Oort RP. Bone grafting of cleft lip and palatal patients for placement of endosseous implants. Cleft Palate Craniofac J 1999;36:67–72.
77. Block MS, Kent JN. Sinus augmentation for dental implants: The use of autogenous bone. J Oral Maxillofac Surg 1997;55:1281–1286.
78. Rodriguez A, Anastassov GE, Lee H, Buchbinder D, Wettan H. Maxillary sinus augmentation with deproteinated bovine bone and platelet-rich plasma with simultaneous insertion of endosseous implants. J Oral Maxillofac Surg 2003;61:157–163.
79. Lekholm U, Wannfors K, Isaksson S, Adielsson B. Oral implants in combination with bone grafts. A 3-year retrospective multicenter study using the Brånemark implant system. Int J Oral Maxillofac Surg 1999;28:181–187.
80. Blomqvist JE, Alberius P, Isaksson S. Retrospective analysis of one-stage maxillary sinus augmentation with endosseous implants. Int J Oral Maxillofac Implants 1996;11:512–521.
81. Widmark G, Andersson B, Carlsson GE, Lindvall AM, Ivanoff CJ. Rehabilitation of patients with severely resorbed maxillae by means of implants with or without bone grafts: A 3- to 5-year follow-up clinical report. Int J Oral Maxillofac Implants 2001;16:73–79.
82. Pinholt EM. Brånemark and ITI dental implants in the human bone-graft maxilla: A comparative evaluation. Clin Oral Implants Res 2003;14:584–592.

83. Brechter M, Nilson H, Lundgren S. Oxidized titanium implants in reconstructive jaw surgery. Clin Implant Dent Rel Res 2005;7(suppl 1):S83–S87.
84. Langer L, Langer B, Mellonig JT. Safety and use of bone allograft for sinus grafting. In: Jensen OT (ed). The Sinus Bone Graft, ed 2. Chicago: Quintessence, 2006:183–200.
85. Cordioli G, Mazzocco C, Schepers E, Brugnolo E, Majzoub Z. Maxillary sinus floor augmentation using bioactive glass granules and autogenous bone with simultaneous implant placement. Clinical and histological findings. Clin Oral Implants Res 2001;12:270–278.
86. Ellegaard B, Kolsen-Petersen J, Baelum V. Implant therapy involving maxillary sinus lift in periodontal compromised patients. Clin Oral Implants Res 1997;8:305–315.
87. Buchmann R, Khoury F, Faust C, Lange D. Peri-implant conditions in periodontally compromised patients following maxillary sinus augmentation. A long-term post-therapy trial. Clin Oral Implant Res 1999;10:103–110.
88. Hatano N, Shimizu Y, Ooya K. A clinical long-term radiographic evaluation of graft height changes after maxillary sinus floor augmentation with a 2:1 autogenous bone/xenograft mixture and simultaneous placement of dental implants. Clin Oral Implants Res 2004;15:339–345.
89. Brånemark P-I, Grondahl K, Ohrnell LO, et al. Zygoma fixture in the management of advanced atrophy of the maxilla: Technique and long-term results. Scand J Plast Reconstr Surg Hand Surg 2004;38:70–85.
90. Hirsch JM, Ohrnell LO, Henry PJ, et al. A clinical evaluation of the zygoma fixture: One year of follow-up at 16 clinics. J Oral Maxillofac Surg 2004;62:22–29.
91. Brånemark P-I, Andreasson L, Chiapasco M, et al. Up to 3-year results from a multi-centre study of the zygomaticus implants. Clin Oral Implants Res 2004;15:xlvi.
92. Bedrossian E, Stumpel L III, Beckely M, Indersano T. The zygomatic implant: Preliminary data on treatment of severely resorbed maxillae. A clinical report. Int J Oral Maxillofac Implants 2002;17:861–865.
93. Malevez C, Abarca M, Durdu F, Daelemans P. Clinical outcome of 103 zygomatic implants. A 6–48 months follow-up study. Clin Oral Implants Res 2004;15:18–22.
94. Nkenke E, Schlegel A, Schultze-Mosgau S, Neukam FW, Wiltfang J. The endoscopically controlled osteotome sinus floor elevation: A preliminary prospective study. Int J Oral Maxillofac Implants 2002;17:557–566.
95. Nkenke E, Hahn M, Weinzierl K, Radespiel-Troger M, Neukam FW, Engelke K. Implant stability and histomorphometry: A correlation study in human cadavers using stepped cylinder implants. Clin Oral Implants Res 2003;14:601–609.
96. Petruson B. Sinuscopy in patients with titanium implants in the nose and sinuses. Scand J Plast Reconstr Surg Hand Surg 2004;38:86–93.
97. Esposito M, Worthington HV, Thomsen P, Coulthard P. Interventions for replacing missing teeth: Dental implants in zygomatic bone for the rehabilitation of the severely deficient edentulous maxilla. Cochrane Database Syst Rev 2003;CD004151.

Section 2

Graft Sources and Materials

chapter 11
Maxillofacial Donor Sites for Sinus Floor and Alveolar Reconstruction

Craig M. Misch, DDS, MDS, PA

During the early development of the sinus bone-grafting procedure in the 1970s, autologous bone alone was used to augment the posterior maxilla for dental implants. Based on favorable outcomes in other types of maxillofacial reconstruction, cancellous bone from the ilium was used to graft the sinus floor through a Caldwell-Luc approach.[1,2] Surgeons were knowledgeable about the biology, safety, and healing capabilities of autografts, but little was known about the ability of bone substitutes to help develop supporting bone around endosteal dental implants. Tricalcium phosphate was the first bone substitute used successfully in sinus grafts.[2] Over the years, allografts, alloplasts, and xenografts of many types have been used alone and in combination with autologous bone for sinus grafting. The 1996 Sinus Consensus Conference evaluated retrospective data on various graft materials and concluded that all of them seemed to perform well.[3] However, the data analysis did not factor in the amount of residual bone below the sinus. Bone substitutes have since been suggested for use in the posterior maxilla with modest resorption or sinus pneumatization. For the severely atrophic maxilla, autologous bone is still preferred and has been shown to provide very predictable results. The benefits of using autologous bone in sinus grafting also warrant its consideration for many other indications.

Advantages of Using Autologous Bone

The use of autologous bone in sinus grafts offers many advantages, especially when minimal bone remains below the sinus floor (Box 11-1).[4,5] Cancellous autologous bone grafts contain viable cells that proliferate and contribute to new bone growth.[6] Autologous bone grafts have bone morphogenetic proteins (BMPs), which are capable of inducing osteocompetent cells in the surrounding tissues to produce bone. They also contain other growth factors integral to the process of graft healing and incorporation. Cortical bone provides an osteoconductive scaffold for bone formation and is replaced by creeping substitution.[1] Several studies have reported increased bone formation when autologous bone is used alone or in combination with other graft materials in sinus grafts.[4,7-11] Froum et al[7] found a statistically significant increase in vital bone formation when as little as 20% autologous bone was added to bovine-derived grafts. The use of a barrier membrane over the sinus window has also been advocated to increase bone formation when bone substitutes are used,[12] whereas a membrane may not be necessary when a significant portion of the graft is autologous bone (see chapter 19).

BOX 11-1 Advantages of using autologous bone in sinus grafting

1. Increased bone formation
2. Shorter healing time requirements than for bone substitutes
3. Possibility for simultaneous lateral augmentation
4. Low operator costs
5. No risk of disease transmission

TABLE 11-1 Vital bone analysis of bovine hydroxyapatite combined with intraorally harvested particulate autograft and PRP in sinus bone grafts*

Patient	HA:Autograft	Healing period (mos)	Vital bone (%)
1	25:75	4	32
2	20:80	5	48
3	40:60	6	36
4	20:80	4	27
5	20:80	5	28
6	20:80	5	33
7	60:40	4	43
8	60:40	4	28
9	60:40	4	38
10	60:40	4	48

*From Misch and Krauser.[20] Histologic evaluation by Dr Michael Roher, University of Minnesota, Minneapolis, MN.

Healing of autologous bone grafts is faster compared with that of allografts, xenografts, and alloplasts, especially in larger pneumatized sinuses. This offers a significant advantage, since patients often object to extended treatment. The healing period for sinuses grafted with autologous bone can be as short as 3 to 4 months versus the 8 to 10 months often recommended for bone substitutes.[1,7,9,13–18] Adding autologous bone to other graft materials also can shorten healing times.[7,19] Froum et al[7] found a mean vital bone formation of 27.1% at 6 to 9 months after sinus grafting with 80% bovine hydroxyapatite and only 20% autogenous bone. Misch and Krauser[20] found an average of 36.5% vital bone at 4 to 6 months when autogenous bone was used in equal proportions with bovine hydroxyapatite (Table 11-1).

It is also beneficial to use autologous bone for sinus grafting when simultaneous onlay augmentation is desired. The posterior maxilla resorbs medially following tooth loss; this pattern of bone loss often results in an unfavorable ridge relationship with the opposing mandibular dentition. It is common for patients to require sinus bone grafting to increase the vertical bone dimension as well as onlay bone grafting to augment the alveolar ridge width and/or correct bone deficiencies in the posterior maxilla.

Autologous bone blocks may be harvested for sinus bone grafting and simultaneous residual ridge reconstruction. The healing period for the onlay block and sinus bone grafts will be comparable, allowing for earlier implant placement. This approach may be preferred over a staged reconstruction, where sinus grafting using bone substitutes is performed first and alveolar ridge augmentation with autologous block bone grafts is accomplished at a later date.[18] Using an autologous platelet concentrate with the autograft has been shown to provide further acceleration of graft incorporation (see chapter 25).[21,22] Autologous bone grafts not only heal faster than bone substitutes, but they also result in a better quality of regenerated bone. Histologic studies have shown greater bone formation and a higher percentage of bone-implant contact when autologous bone grafts are used compared with allografts.[11] Improved bone formation can allow for shorter implant healing periods compared to the use of bone substitutes. Immediate implant loading may be an option if adequate primary stability has been achieved.

Alveolar distraction can be used to transport a bony segment inferiorly beneath the sinus graft (see chapter 24). Osseous distraction for sinus grafting requires the use of autologous bone.[23] Studies on distraction through bone substitutes are lacking at this time.[24]

Indications for Using Autologous Bone Harvested from the Maxillofacial Region

The use of autologous bone should be considered when treating large, pneumatized sinuses. When minimal bone is present below the sinus floor, a staged approach to maxillary reconstruction is preferred. Bone substitutes may perform satisfactorily in these situations, but the healing time is lengthy. If a shorter treatment period is a priority, then the use of autologous bone is indicated. Some patients object to the idea of using cadaver or bovine tissue and prefer to use their own bone. As noted above, simultaneous ridge augmentation and sinus grafting can be accomplished more quickly with autogenous block bone. When retreating sinus bone graft failures, the use of autologous bone alone is strongly recommended.

The donor sites that can be used for harvesting bone for sinus bone grafting in the maxillofacial region include the maxillary tuberosity, zygomaticomaxillary buttress, zygoma, mandibular symphysis, mandibular body, and ramus, all of which are accessible intraorally. Bone may be removed in block sections, milled, or harvested in a particulate form. Bone can also be collected during implant osteotomies or alveoloplasty following tooth removal. The primary risk of harvesting autogenous bone is morbidity at the bone harvest site. However, intraoral donor sites are associated with minimal complications, and the many benefits of using autologous bone generally outweigh the risks.

Bone-Harvesting Procedures

Patient preparation

Sinus bone grafting with bone harvested from a maxillofacial site is typically performed in an office setting. Preoperative antibiotics and anti-inflammatory medications, such as dexamethasone and ibuprofen, are administered to the patient prior to surgery.[25] Antiseptic rinses and antisialologues reduce salivary contamination of the graft. The sinus recipient site is prepared prior to bone harvest. The sinus window is infractured and the mucosa is elevated to expose the internal bony walls. Any sinus membrane perforations or tears should be repaired with collagen membranes or fibrin. If the tears are very large, or if pathology is encountered, the clinician may consider aborting the procedure. Particulate bone substitutes should be introduced first to facilitate the mucosal elevation. This also allows the surgeon to assess the amount of autologous bone needed. The donor site is determined by the graft volume requirement. When mixed with a bone substitute, approximately 2 to 3 mL of particulate autologous bone is usually sufficient for a large sinus cavity. When grafting with autologous bone alone, 5 to 6 mL may be necessary. The autologous bone should be placed promptly into the prepared cavity. The recipient site is then sutured closed prior to closure of the donor site.

Maxillary tuberosity and buttress

Because it is located in the same surgical field as the sinus, the maxillary tuberosity should routinely be considered as a donor site when a lateral approach to sinus grafting is used.[7,26,27] Because of thick mucosa over the tuberosity, however, it is often difficult to assess the amount of bone that may be obtained. Therefore, a periapical or panoramic radiograph is used to assess available bone. In addition, computerized tomography (CT) scans of the maxillary sinus region allow for three-dimensional quantification of the area. Generally, about 2 mL of bone can be harvested from this area. The anatomic limits of the tuberosity bone harvesting site include the maxillary sinus, the pterygoid plates, the molar teeth, and the greater palatine canal. An incision is made along the ridge crest in the posterior maxilla and continued poste-

Chapter 11: Maxillofacial Donor Sites for Sinus Floor and Alveolar Reconstruction

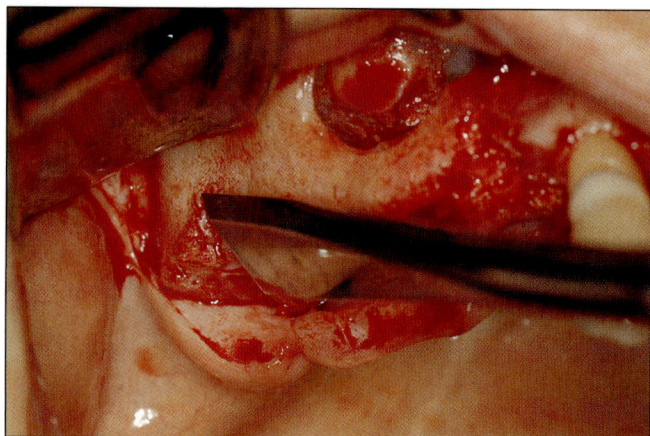

Fig 11-1 Harvesting of bone from the maxillary tuberosity using a chisel.

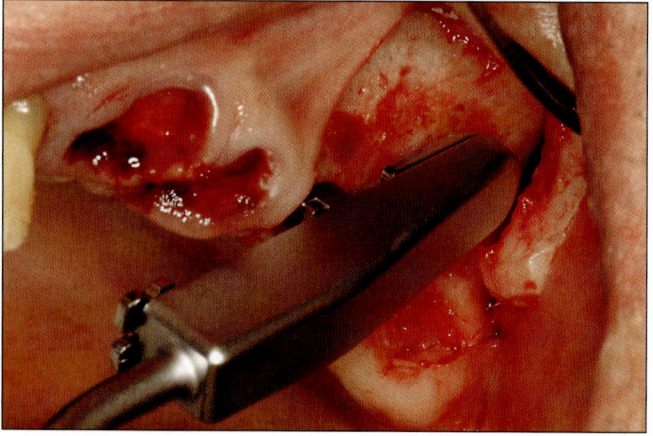

Fig 11-2a Harvesting of bone from the lateral maxilla and buttress region using a bone scraper device (Ebner Grafter).

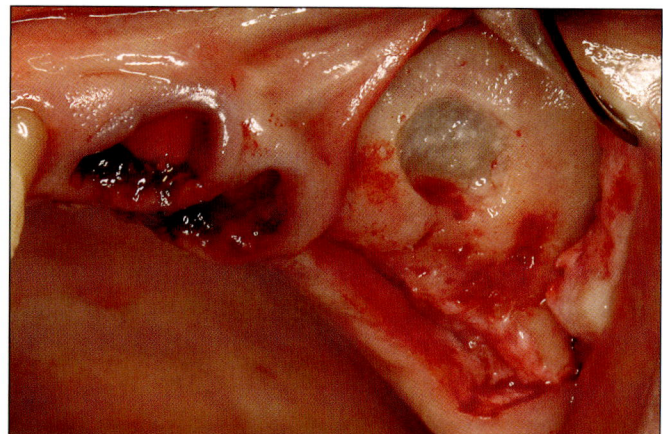

Fig 11-2b Exposure of sinus mucosa following bone scraping.

riorly over the tuberosity. A vertical releasing incision is made laterally. Mucoperiosteal reflection exposes the tuberosity, ridge crest, and lateral maxilla. The palatal tissue is elevated to reveal the entire tuberosity. Tuberosity bone is usually removed following reflection of the antral mucosa, which allows for more aggressive bone harvesting without concern for membrane perforation. The bone in the tuberosity area is porous. A chisel rather than a rongeur should be used to harvest the graft. The chisel edge should be kept slightly superficial to the maxilla to shave off pieces of tuberosity bone and prevent inadvertent sinus communication (Fig 11-1). A chisel can also be used along the posterior lateral maxilla to obtain a slice of cortical bone to place over the lateral sinus window.

A bone scraper (MX-Grafter or Ebner Grafter, Maxilon) may also be used to remove bone from the tuberosity area as well as from the lateral maxilla and the zygomaticomaxillary buttress region (Fig 11-2).[28] This is done prior to preparing the bony window for sinus access.

To harvest bone from the zygoma,[29] the mucoperiosteal flap used to gain access to the sinus is reflected higher to expose the inferior aspect of the zygoma. Just above the inferior border of the zygomatic rim, lateral from the maxillary sinus, cores or small blocks of bone are removed using a trephine bur or carbide fissure bur. The drill is kept parallel to the lateral maxilla, and penetration is limited to 12 to 14 mm to avoid the infratemporal fossa and orbital floor. Additional cancellous bone can sometimes be removed with a curette. Inadvertent sinus exposure is common and should not be cause for concern.[29]

Fig 11-3a Osteotomy performed with a sagittal saw for symphysis graft harvest.

Fig 11-3b Removal of a thick corticocancellous block bone graft.

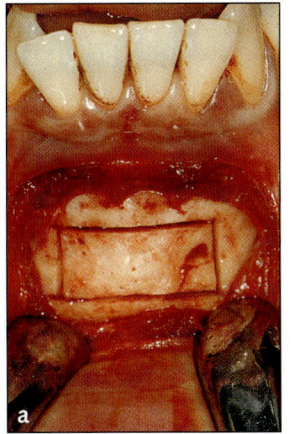
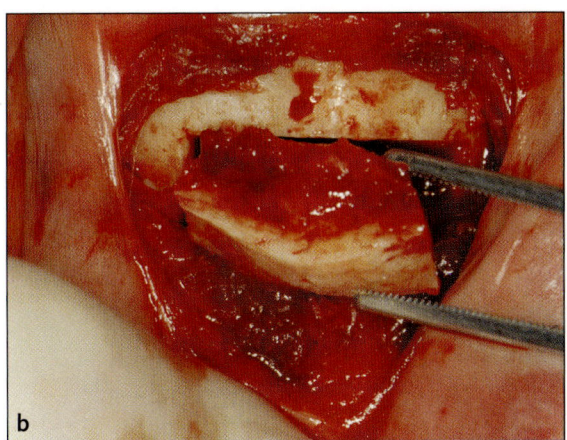

Mandibular symphysis

The symphysis of the mandible, which offers the greatest volume of intraoral bone, has been used extensively for sinus and onlay bone grafting in the maxilla.[30–35] The average interforaminal distance is approximately 5.0 cm, and the depth of the anterior mandible usually exceeds 1.0 cm.[36] A panoramic radiograph is used to evaluate the available bone in this donor site. A lateral cephalometric radiograph is also useful to determine the anteroposterior dimension of the anterior mandible. Periapical radiographs provide a more accurate measurement of the root lengths.

Ease of access is one of the main advantages of the symphysis region. Bilateral mandibular anesthetic blocks and local infiltration in the anterior mandible are accomplished by administering 2% lidocaine with 1:100,000 epinephrine. Exposure of the symphysis can be obtained through a sulcular or a vestibular incision. A vestibular approach allows easy access but produces more bleeding and intraoral scar formation. The vestibular incision is made in the mucosa distal to the canine teeth approximately 1 cm from the mucogingival junction. The sulcular approach may result in gingival recession and should not be used when mucogingival defects are present. A mucoperiosteal flap is reflected inferiorly to the inferior border of the mandible. Additional local anesthesia is often needed at the base of the mandible to block cervical innervation. Osteotomies should be at least 5 mm from the root apices and the mental foramina.[31,37,38] In most cases the inferior and lingual cortices of the mandible are left intact. The facial cortex is thick and the underlying cancellous bone is usually dense. Block bone grafts may be harvested using a carbide fissure bur (no. 557 or 701) or sagittal saw. Following an osteotomy through the outer cortex and into the cancellous bone, the graft is removed with an osteotome (Fig 11-3). The block bone may be used for sinus floor grafting or onlay grafting of the residual ridge. Alternatively, it may be particulated in a bone mill. Additional cancellous bone may be procured with a curette, chisel, rongeur, or trephine after the block is removed, but the volume is meager.[36] Following the removal of the block graft, hemostatic materials such as collagen or gelatin may be placed over the cancellous bone. When larger bone grafts are harvested, the donor site should be filled with a bone substitute such as resorbable hydroxyapatite to maintain facial contour.[31] Smaller or particulate bone grafts are procured using trephine burs, bone collection traps, or bone-scraping instruments (Fig 11-4).[28,39,40] Closure of the donor site is typically performed after sinus grafting to minimize the time between graft harvest and placement. The vestibular incision is closed in layers using resorbable sutures. Postoperative pressure dressings are placed over the chin to reduce edema, hematoma formation, and incision line opening.

The mandibular symphysis is associated with a higher incidence of postoperative complications compared with other maxillofacial donor sites.[34,41–43] Altered sensation of the anterior mandibular teeth is a relatively common complication following harvesting of bone blocks or trephine cores.[27,34,41–44] The contents of the incisive canal that innervate the teeth are disrupted during bone harvest. Patients describe dullness in sensation of the incisors, which usually resolves within 6 months. The need for endodontic treatment of anterior teeth is very rare. Neurosensory distur-

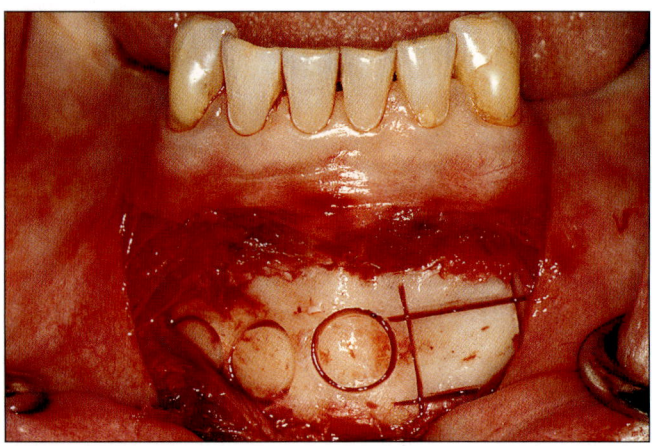

Fig 11-4a Osteotomies performed with a trephine bur and sagittal saw.

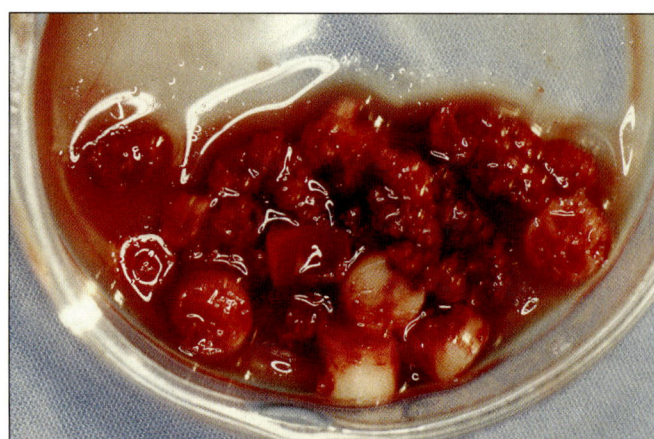

Fig 11-4b Bone cores harvested from the mandibular symphysis.

bances in the chin region also may be encountered, even when a sulcular approach is used.[41–43] The incidence of mental nerve paresthesia for symphysis graft patients has been found to be as high as 43%.[41] Meteorotropism of the chin has also been reported.[41] Although the vast majority of these nerve injuries resolve, they are nonetheless disconcerting to patients. It is prudent to discuss the possibility of temporary or permanent altered sensation of the teeth and chin prior to surgery. Although no postoperative alteration in soft tissue chin contour has been reported, patients are frequently concerned with the possible esthetic consequences of bone removal from this area.[41] Radiographic evidence of incomplete bony regeneration has been reported in elderly patients.[45] Filling the donor site with a resorbable bone substitute, such as allogeneic or bovine bone, can help alleviate the patient's concerns.[27] Ptosis of the chin can be prevented by avoiding the complete degloving of the mandible.[46]

Mandibular ramus

The posterior mandible is an excellent donor site for harvesting bone and offers several advantages over the symphysis.[13,34,43,47,48] Compared with the symphysis, the ramus area is associated with a much lower incidence of complications.[34,43] In addition, patients often express less concern about having bone removed from the ramus area. The masseter muscle provides soft tissue bulk, and augmentation of this donor site is unnecessary. Although neurosensory disturbances from bone harvest have not been encountered, the potential for damage to the inferior alveolar nerve must be recognized.

A panoramic radiograph is used to evaluate the bony anatomy of the ramus, external oblique ridge, and mandibular canal. A mandibular anesthetic block and buccal infiltration of the posterior mandible is accomplished by administering 2% lidocaine with 1:100,000 epinephrine. The incision design for access to this region depends on the type of graft harvested (block or particulate). When harvesting a block graft or trephine cores, the incision is similar to one used in third molar removal. A sulcular incision is made along the posterior teeth and continues posteriorly and lateral at a 45-degree angle from the distobuccal aspect of the second molar (or from the base of the retromolar pad if no molar is present). A mucoperiosteal flap is then reflected to expose the lateral ramus and body of the mandible. The masseter muscle may be reflected laterally with a specially designed retractor (Misch ramus retractor, Salvin Dental) to form a large open pocket. Additional local anesthesia is often required in this area to block cervical innervation. The limits of the ramus area are dictated by clinical access in addition to the coronoid process, molar teeth, and inferior alveolar canal. The average anteroposterior dimension of the mandibular ramus is 30 mm, with the lingula typically in the posterior third.[49]

To harvest a block bone graft, four osteotomies are made, one each to the external oblique, superior ramus, and anterior and inferior body of the mandible (Fig 11-5).[48] The cortical cuts are made with a carbide fissure bur (no. 557 or 701) in a straight handpiece or a saw under sterile

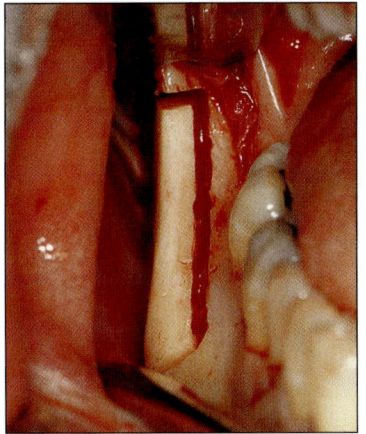

Fig 11-5 Osteotomies for block bone harvest from the mandibular ramus.

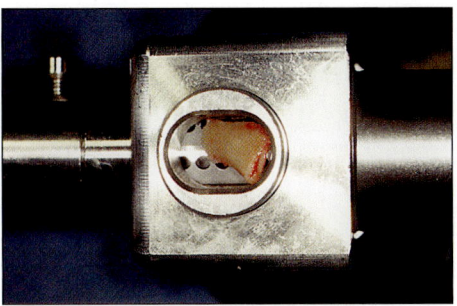

Fig 11-6a Cortical block graft placed into a bone mill.

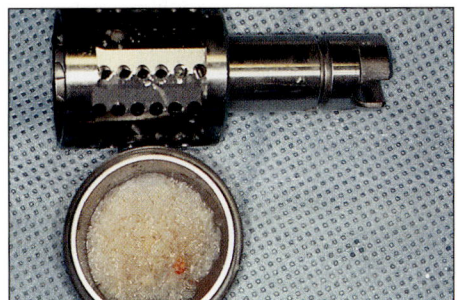

Fig 11-6b Cortical block graft particulated in the bone mill.

saline irrigation. The external oblique cut is made along the anterior border of the ramus approximately 4 to 6 mm medial to the external oblique ridge. This osteotomy can extend posterosuperiorly to the coronoid process and anteriorly to the first molar area, producing a graft of up to 40 mm in length. The superior ramus cut is made through the lateral cortex of the ramus and perpendicular to the external oblique cut. It may extend as far posteriorly on the ramus as the opposing lingula on the medial ramus. However, the length of this cut is typically about 10 mm. The anterior body cut will often extend over the path of the mandibular canal. Although the buccolingual position of the mandibular canal varies, the distance from the canal to the medial aspect of the buccal cortical plate (medullary bone thickness) has been found to be greatest at the distal half of the first molar (mean, 4.05 mm).[50] Therefore, the anterior body cut should be made in this area and not in the third molar region, where the canal is closer to the buccal surface. This anterior body cut is progressively deepened until bleeding from the underlying cancellous bone is observed. The inferior osteotomy is only a partial-thickness cut made with a round carbide bur (no. 8). It connects the superior ramus and anterior body cuts inferiorly. This osteotomy on the lateral aspect of the ramus parallels the external oblique cut and creates the base of the rectangular bone block. It extends only partially through the cortex and creates a line of fracture. The block graft is then removed with an osteotome wedged within the external oblique osteotomy. Care should be taken to parallel the chisel with the lateral surface of the mandible to limit the depth of penetration. An alternative technique is to insert an extraction elevator and pry the graft free. Because the inferior alveolar nerve may be exposed, this donor site is not augmented with bone substitutes. The incision is closed primarily with resorbable (chromic gut) sutures. A rectangular piece of bone, approximately 4 mm thick, may be harvested from the ramus. This morphology is well suited for veneer grafting to gain additional ridge width or may be particulated in a bone mill for sinus grafting (Fig 11-6).

Bone cores also may be harvested from the ramus and body of the mandible with a trephine bur.[51] The area surrounding the external oblique ridge is easily accessed. A 4- or 5-mm trephine bur can be used to drill through the outer cortex. Care should be taken to remain superior to the mandibular canal and limit penetration into the medullary cortex. The cores are fractured at their cancellous base with a thin elevator and removed. They can either be placed in toto along the sinus floor or particulated.

The posterior mandible is the preferred site for harvesting large amounts of particulate bone using a scraper device (Fig 11-7).[24] Generally, about 4 mL of particulate bone may be harvested from this area. There is minimal morbidity associated with harvesting bone from the cortical surface with a scraper blade. The initial incision for this approach is made in the buccal vestibule and is similar to one used in sagittal split osteotomies. It is made just lateral to the external oblique ridge and extends the length of the molar regions. This incision design requires minimal time to reflect the flap to gain access to the mandible and is easy to close. A larger area of mandibular exposure allows

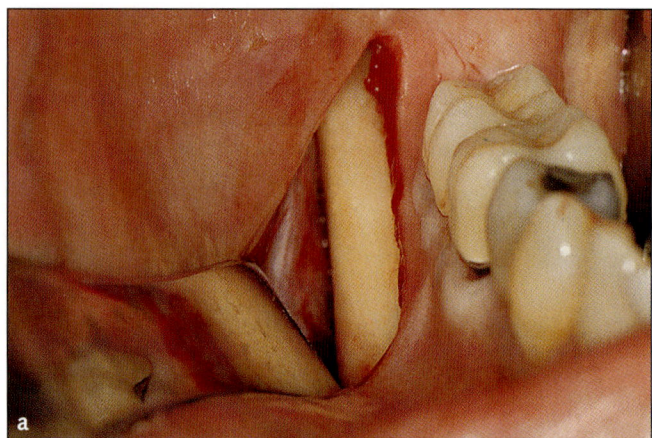
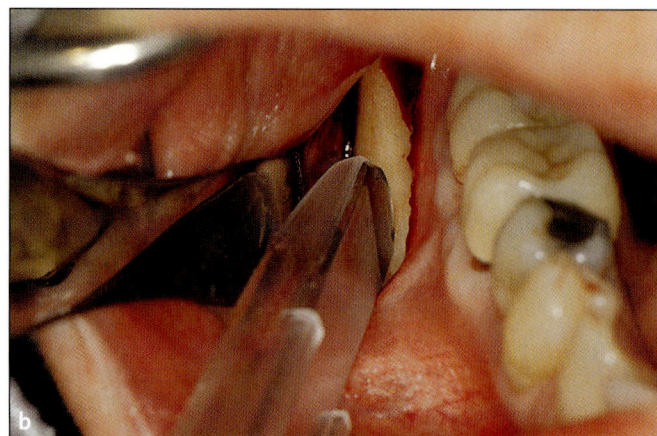
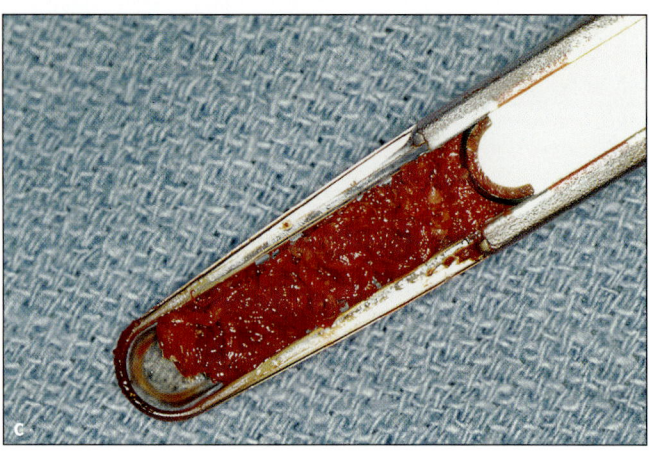

Fig 11-7a Posterior mandible donor site access.

Fig 11-7b Harvesting of bone from the posterior mandible using a scraper device (MX-Grafter).

Fig 11-7c Bone shavings collected within the scraper device.

longer strokes with the scraper blade and expedites graft harvesting. The dense cortical bone should be repeatedly lubricated with sterile saline during bone harvesting.

Potential damage to the inferior alveolar nerve, like that to the peripheral mental branches when harvesting from the chin, is a matter of concern with the ramus graft technique. For this reason, it is important to plan osteotomies in the posterior mandible to avoid the mandibular canal. In contrast to the common complaint of altered sensation of the incisors with chin bone harvest, no ramus graft patients have noted numbness of their molar teeth.[34,43] Although the posterior incision along the external oblique ridge could possibly damage the long buccal nerve, sensory loss in the buccal mucosa is rare and most likely goes unnoticed.[52] Ramus graft patients appear to have fewer problems in managing postoperative edema and pain compared with chin graft patients.[34,43] Those who experience trismus following surgery should be placed on postoperative glucocorticoids and nonsteroidal anti-inflammatory medications to reduce dysfunction. The mandibular ramus is now the preferred donor site for most clinicians.[28,34,42,43]

Biology of Autologous Bone

The embryologic origin of autologous bone grafts and its significance in graft incorporation and resorption has received much attention. Membranous bone grafts from the mandible or calvarium resorb far less than do grafts from endochondral sites such as the iliac crest.[53–56] Most studies on the influence of graft origin on resorption refer to onlay augmentation with block bone grafts. The morphology of the graft (ie, particulate or block) and whether it is used for onlay or interpositional placement are important factors to consider. Interpositional bone grafts typically resorb less

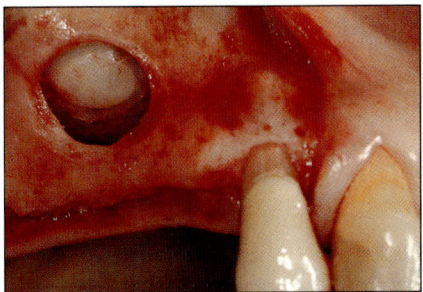 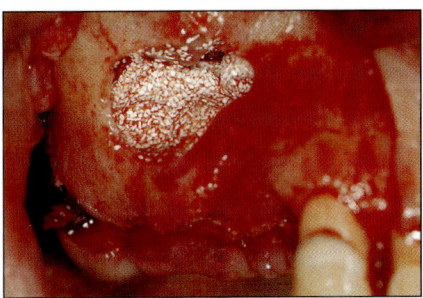 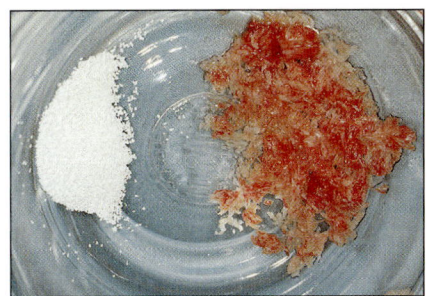

Fig 11-8a Window prepared in the lateral maxilla for sinus access.

Fig 11-8b Bovine hydroxyapatite (Bio-Oss) placed into the sinus, which has been elevated superiorly.

Fig 11-8c Bovine hydroxyapatite and rinsed bone shavings.

than bone used for onlay augmentation. The maxillary sinus is an enclosed environment well-protected by bony walls with a rich vascular supply. For these reasons, sinus floor augmentation is more comparable to an interpositional than an onlay bone graft and therefore undergoes less resorption. Block and Kent[4] found no qualitative clinical differences with regard to implant integration or maintenance of bone when comparing the use of iliac crest bone with bone from the chin, ramus, and tuberosity for sinus grafting. Recent studies challenge the hypothesis of embryologic origin and graft resorption, emphasizing the importance of the microarchitecture of the bone.[57,58] Ozaki and Buchman[58] found that cortical bone grafts lose less volume than cancellous grafts, regardless of embryologic origin. Cortical bone grafts from the mandible exhibit minimal resorption and maintain their dense quality, making them ideal for onlay augmentation.[31]

Immediately after it is harvested, the bone graft should be placed in sterile saline to maintain its cellular vitality, and minimal time should elapse between graft procurement and placement.[59] However, the number of viable cells contained in a mandibular cortical graft is probably not a significant factor in new bone formation. Some studies have found bacterial contamination of orally harvested bone grafts, especially when suction traps are used to collect drill-bone debris.[60] Preoperative antisialologue agents such as glycopyrrolate are useful to decrease salivary flow, and chlorhexidine rinsing prior to surgery has been shown to significantly reduce this problem. Particulate bone grafts may be rinsed with sterile saline. If block grafts or trephine cores are milled into particulate bone, the particle size should not be too fine. Some burs or mills pulverize the bone graft into a powder or paste, a form in which it will quickly resorb. Larger particles are less likely to resorb and are more osteoconductive.[61–63] Bone powder collected by a suction is acellular, desiccated, and relatively deproteinized, whereas bone scrapers produce ribbon-like shavings favorable for revascularization and graft incorporation.[28]

Clinical Use of Autologous Bone

Particulate autologous bone may be mixed with bone substitutes such as allografts, alloplasts, and xenografts.[3] The microarchitecture of bovine tissue has a naturally porous morphology mimicking that of human inorganic structure. Moreover, bovine bone is highly osteoconductive and undergoes physiologic remodeling when incorporated into surrounding bone. Bovine-derived resorbable hydroxyapatite (Bio-Oss, Osteohealth) combined with autologous bone provides very favorable results.[7,19,43,64,65]

A layered approach combining different types of graft materials according to their biologic properties has been advocated by Misch[5] (Figs 11-8a to 11-8l). With this approach, autologous bone is used alone or in combination with substitutes (50:50 ratio) as the bottommost layer along the sinus floor, closest to the dental implants. Platelet-rich plasma (PRP) also may be added to the particulate autograft (see chapter 25), which provides growth

chapter 11 Maxillofacial Donor Sites for Sinus Floor and Alveolar Reconstruction

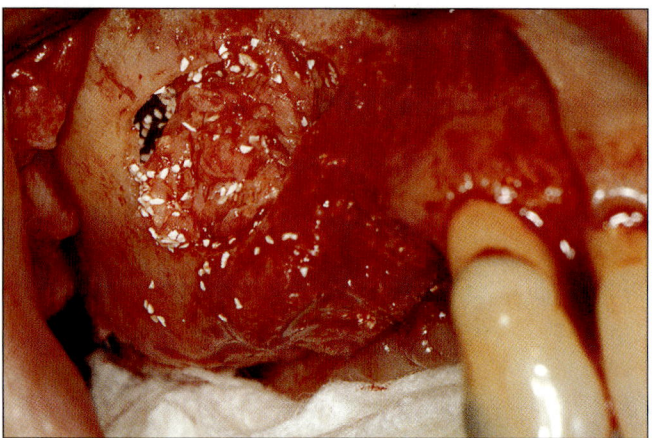

Fig 11-8d Composite graft of bovine hydroxyapatite, particulate autologous bone, and PRP.

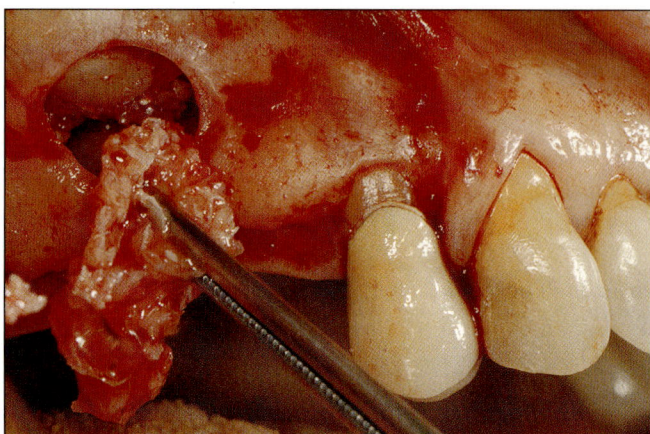

Fig 11-8e Placement of particulate autologous bone mixed with PRP and placed along the sinus floor. Note improved handling properties provided by PRP.

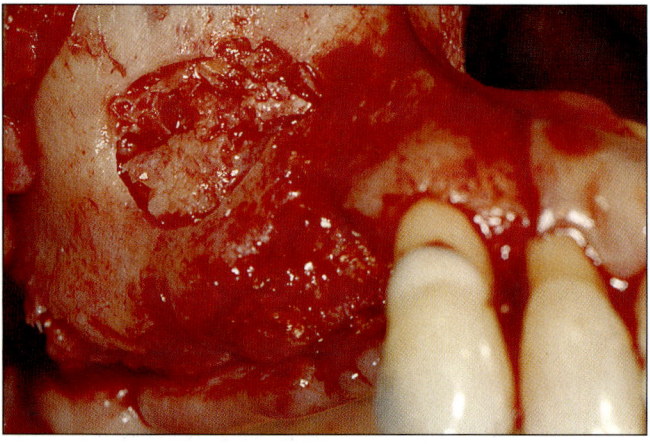

Fig 11-8f Sinus access window covered with bone harvested from the tuberosity.

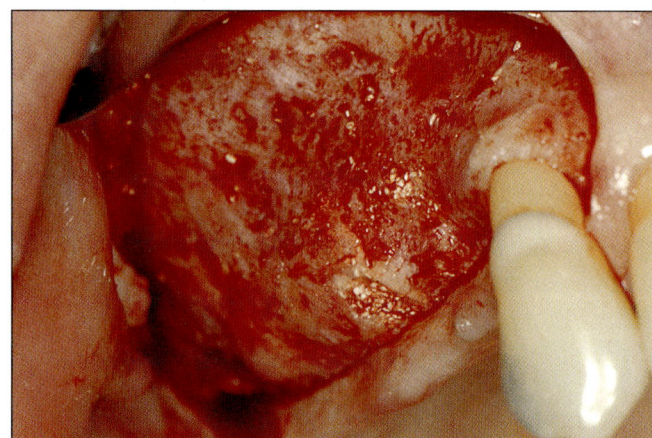

Fig 11-8g Exposure of the lateral maxilla 4 months after grafting.

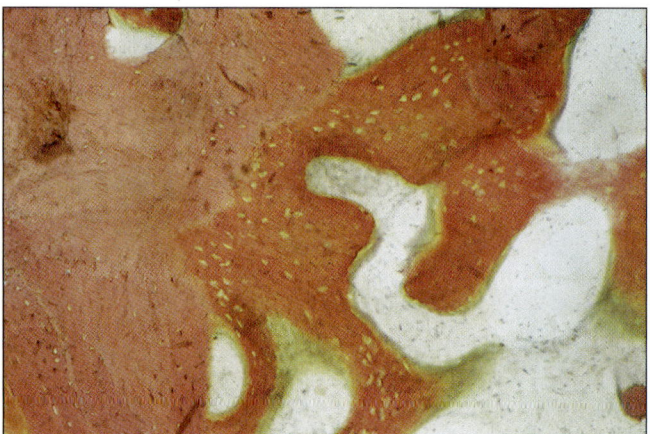

Fig 11-8h Histologic sample of the grafted sinus. New bone growth along the surface of the bone shaving is exhibited with osteoid formation *(green)* at the periphery. (Stevenel blue–van Gieson picro fuchsin stain; magnification ×20.)

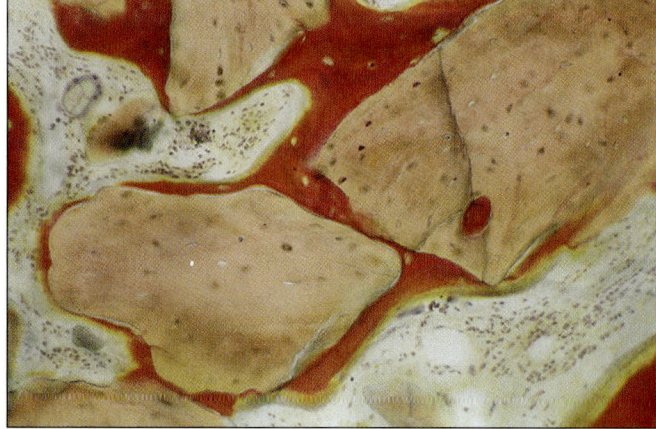

Fig 11-8i Bio-Oss particles surrounded by new bone formation. (Stevenel blue–van Gieson picro fuchsin stain; magnification ×20.)

Fig 11-8j Placement of dental implants (Replace Select, Nobel Biocare) into the grafted sinus.

Fig 11-8k Occlusal view of the implants placed into the grafted sinus.

Fig 11-8l Panoramic radiograph of the implants and grafted sinus.

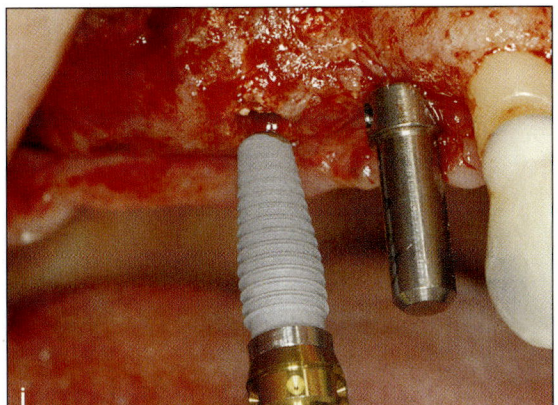
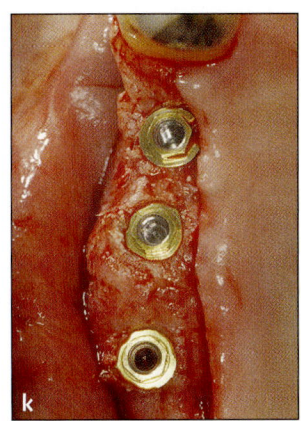
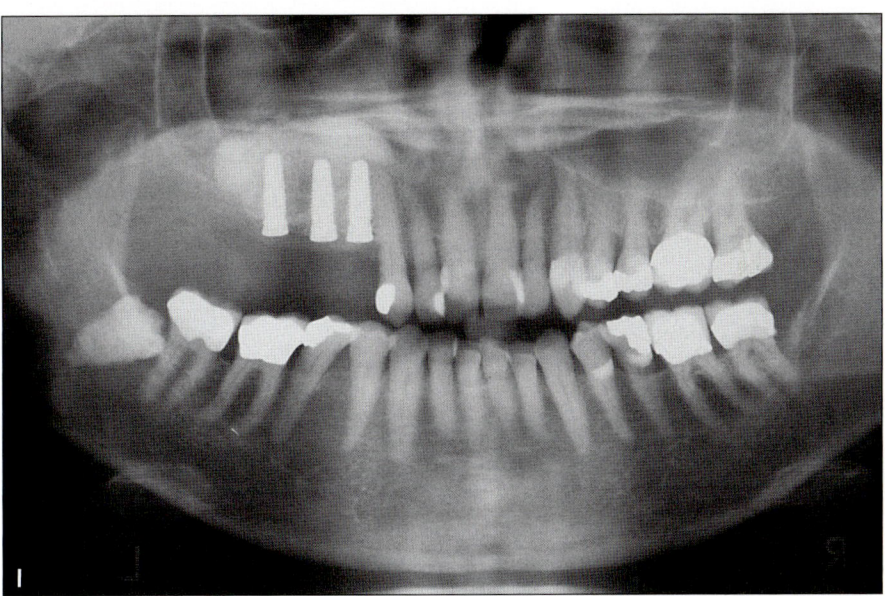

factors such as platelet-derived growth factor (PDGF) and transforming growth factor beta (TGF-β).[21] While these growth factors are not specifically osteoinductive, they are osteopromotive.[21,66] In addition to these biologic advantages, PRP improves the handling characteristics of the graft by promoting particle adherence.[67] As an alternative to a commercially prepared membrane, a thin layer of cortical bone removed from the posterior maxilla with a chisel may be used as a barrier over the window.

Alternatively, block bone grafts may be placed along the sinus floor and fixated with the dental implant(s) through the ridge.[32,35] This is difficult to accomplish with small grafts. Ramus bone, placed horizontally through the lateral maxilla, acts to contain block sinus augmentation.[68] Although some reports discuss the use of block bone in the sinus, most clinicians favor the use of particulate bone grafts for sinus floor augmentation.[32,35,38]

Block bone grafts can also be used to correct posterior maxillary ridge deficiencies at the same time as the sinus-grafting procedure (Fig 11-9) (see chapter 21). The block graft is secured to the maxilla with screws that perforate the grafted antrum. Alternatively, lateral augmentation can be accomplished with particulate bone in a titanium mesh or using a split-bone grafting technique.[69,70] Atrophic edentulous maxillae usually have adequate ridge width posteriorly for dental implants but often require bone

chapter 11 Maxillofacial Donor Sites for Sinus Floor and Alveolar Reconstruction

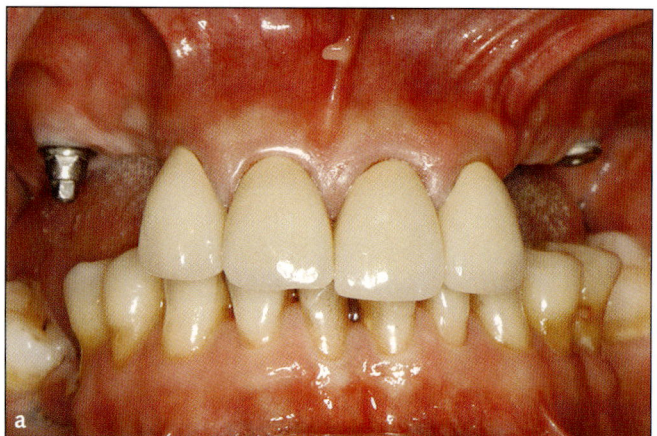

Fig 11-9a Preoperative facial view of the maxilla.

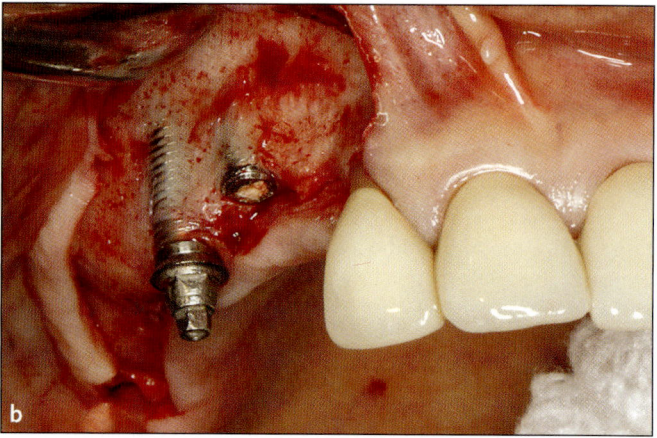

Fig 11-9b Evident bone loss around the posterior implant and fractured fixture in the premolar site.

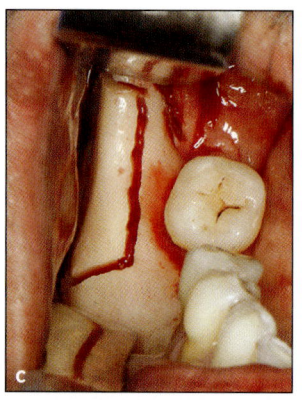
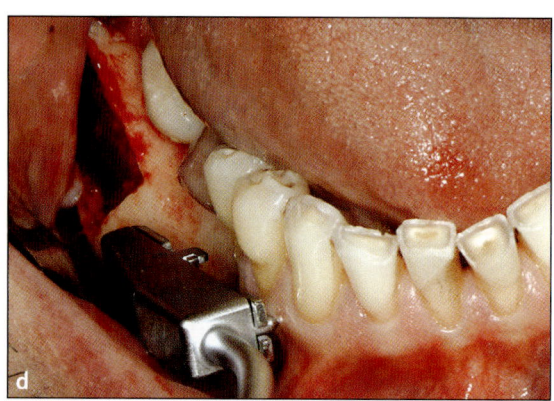

Fig 11-9c Osteotomies for harvesting of a block bone graft from the ramus.

Fig 11-9d Harvesting of particulate bone from the body of the mandible using a bone scraper (Ebner Grafter).

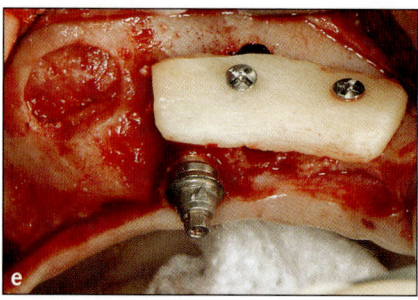
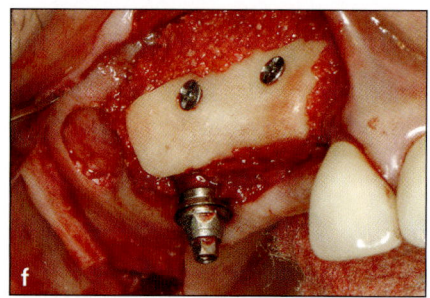

Fig 11-9e Block cortical bone graft placed over the lateral maxilla. The sinus window has been covered with tuberosity bone following sinus grafting.

Fig 11-9f Bone shavings mixed with PRP packed around the block bone graft.

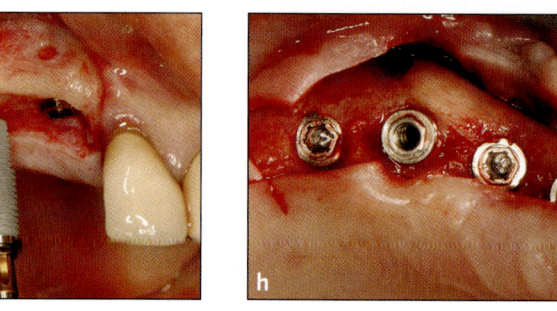

Fig 11-9g Placement of implants (Brånemark MK III, Nobel Biocare) into the grafted maxilla 4 months after grafting.

Fig 11-9h Occlusal view of the implants placed into the grafted maxilla.

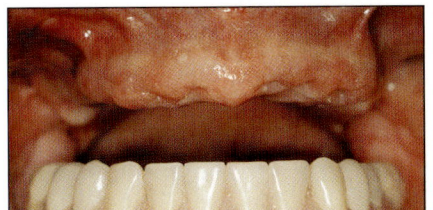

Fig 11-10a Preoperative facial view of edentulous maxilla. The mandible was restored with an immediate load prosthesis.

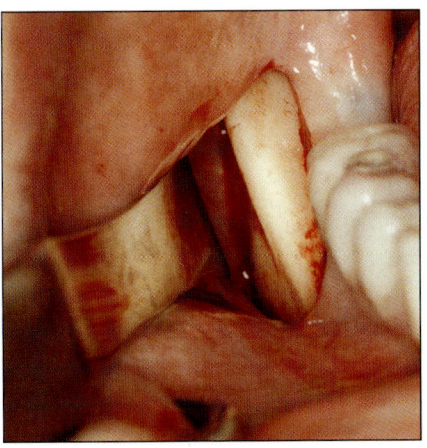

Fig 11-10b Mandibular ramus donor site.

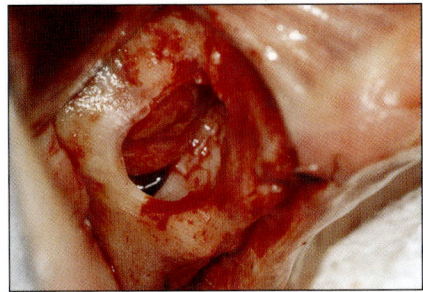

Fig 11-10c The prepared sinus window.

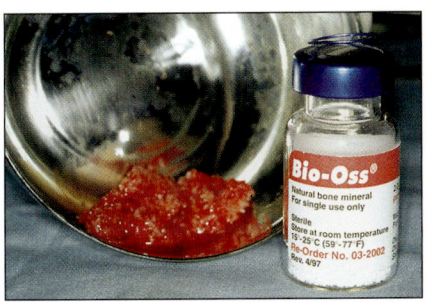

Fig 11-10d Particulate bone shavings mixed with Bio-Oss and PRP.

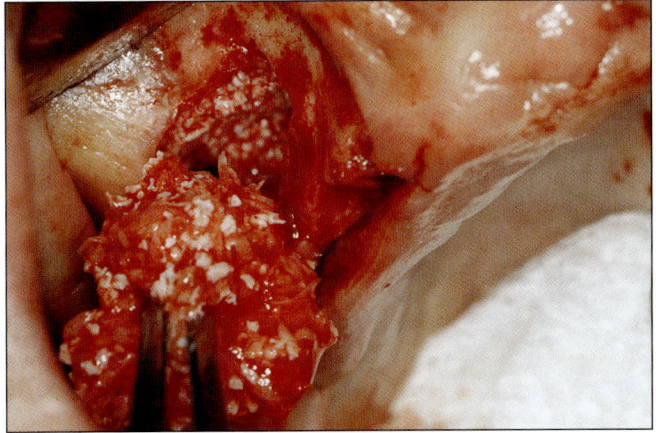

Fig 11-10e Placement of composite bone graft into the prepared sinus.

augmentation in the premolar area and/or anterior maxilla. Intraoral donor sites provide donor bone for treatment of these conditions. Reconstruction of severe atrophy in the maxilla should be resolved with bone harvested from the ilium.[32,71,72] The iliac crest would then provide sufficient bone volume for both sinus grafting and reconstruction of the anterior maxilla (see chapter 13).

The use of autologous bone, especially from the vital iliac crest, can significantly shorten the healing period following staged reconstruction of pneumatized sinuses. A general goal is to harvest sufficient autologous bone to provide at least 50% of graft volume. For unilateral sinus grafting, this can be readily obtained from one mandibular donor site such as the ramus area. Bilateral sinus grafts require two donor sites, especially if onlay bone grafting also is required. If extensive sinus grafting is needed, extraoral sources should be considered. A 4-month healing period before implant placement is generally adequate in most patients when autogenous bone is used.[31,73] Implants with textured surfaces are recommended for sinus grafts.[74] The quality of the regenerated bone in the sinus is often favorable when autograft is used. Implant healing times can be decreased and immediate implant loading may be considered when nongrafted bone is sufficiently load bearing (Figs 11-10a to 11-10l).

chapter 11 Maxillofacial Donor Sites for Sinus Floor and Alveolar Reconstruction

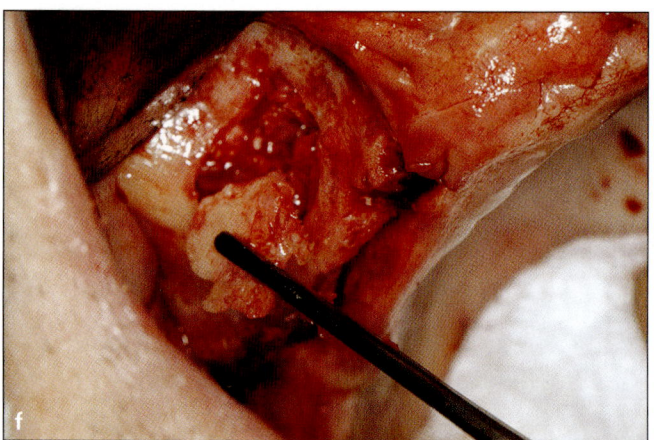

Fig 11-10f Harvesting of bone from the tuberosity region.

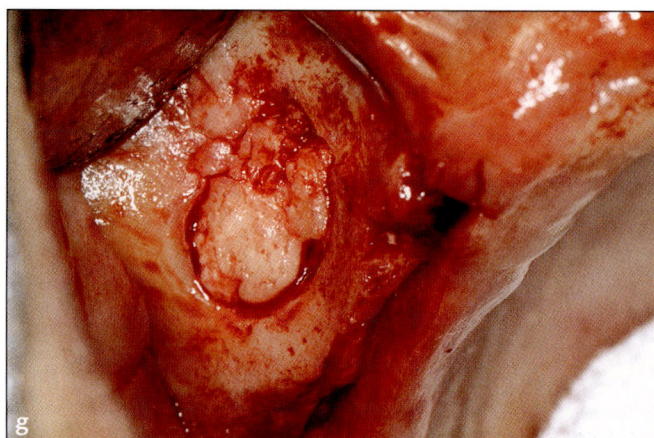

Fig 11-10g Sinus access window covered with the thin cortical graft from the tuberosity.

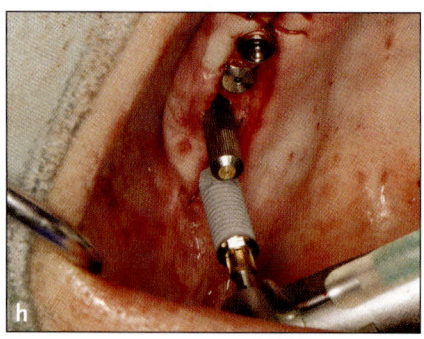
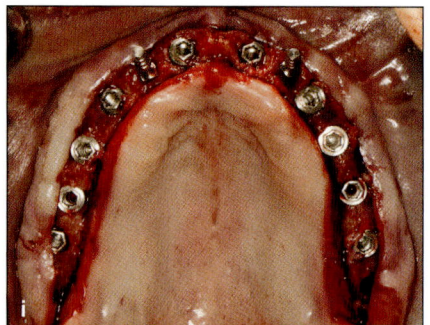

Fig 11-10h Placement of implants (Brånemark MK IV) into the grafted sinus after 4 months of healing.

Fig 11-10i Occlusal view of 12 implants placed into the grafted maxilla.

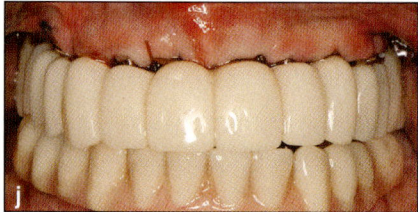
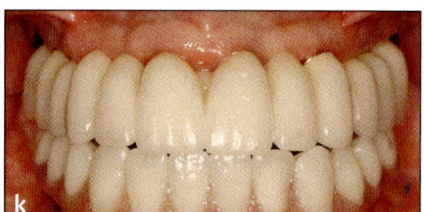

Fig 11-10j Immediate loading of implants with a metal-reinforced provisional prosthesis.

Fig 11-10k Final restoration of the maxillary implants with a porcelain-to-metal prosthesis.

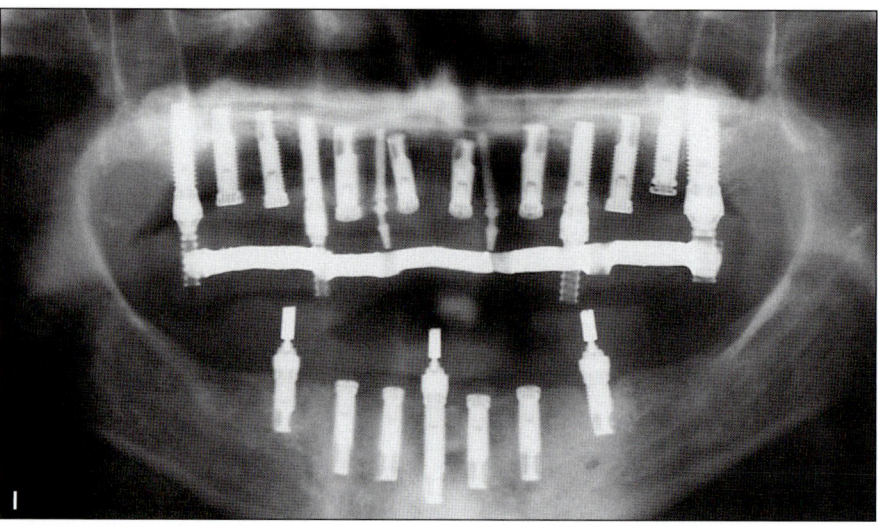

Fig 11-10l Panoramic radiograph of the implants and grafted sinuses.

Conclusion

Autologous bone grafts procured from the maxillofacial region offer several advantages in sinus bone grafting and reconstruction of the maxilla for implant placement. These include increased bone formation, shorter healing time requirements, low operator costs, no risk of disease transmission, and the ability to simultaneously perform onlay augmentation. The surgical procedures may be performed in an office setting and do not require general anesthesia. Intraoral donor bone is readily available, and several techniques are available for harvesting particulate or block bone grafts. The tuberosity and zygomatic buttress are routinely accessible during sinus graft surgery through a lateral window approach. The posterior mandible has some advantages over the mandibular symphysis as a remote donor site. Nonetheless, most intraoral donor sites are associated with minimal morbidity and offer significant benefits for sinus grafting.

References

1. Boyne PJ, James R. Grafting of the maxillary sinus floor with autogenous marrow and bone. J Oral Surg 1980;38:613–618.
2. Tatum H. Maxillary and sinus implant reconstructions. Dent Clin North Am 1986;30:207–229.
3. Jensen OT, Shulman LB, Block MS, Iacono VJ. Report of the Sinus Consensus Conference of 1996. Int J Oral Maxillofac Implants 1998;13(suppl):11–45.
4. Block MS, Kent JN. Sinus augmentation for dental implants: The use of autogenous bone. J Oral Maxillofac Surg 1997;55:1281–1286.
5. Misch CE. The maxillary sinus lift and sinus graft surgery. In: Misch CE (ed). Contemporary Implant Dentistry. St Louis: Mosby, 2002:484–487.
6. Burchardt H. The biology of bone graft repair. Clin Orthopaed Rel Res 1983;174:28–42.
7. Froum SJ, Tarnow DP, Wallace SS, Rohrer MD, Cho SC. Sinus floor elevation using anorganic bovine bone matrix (Osteo-Graf/N) with and without autogenous bone: A clinical, histologic, radiographic and histomorphometric analysis—Part 2 of an ongoing study. Int J Periodontics Restorative Dent 1998;18:529–543.
8. Moy PK, Lundgren S, Holmes RE. Maxillary sinus augmentation: Histomorphometric analysis of graft materials for maxillary sinus floor augmentation. J Oral Maxillofac Surg 1993;51:857–862.
9. Wheeler SL, Holmes RE, Calhoun CJ. Six-year clinical and histologic study of sinus-lift grafts. Int J Oral Maxillofac Implants 1996:11;26–34.
10. Lorenzetti M, Mozzati M, Campanino PP, Valente G. Bone augmentation of the inferior floor of the maxillary sinus with autogenous bone or composite bone grafts: A histologic-histomorphometric preliminary report. Int J Oral Maxillofac Implants 1998;13:69–76.
11. Jensen OT, Sennerby L. Histological analysis of clinically retrieved titanium microimplants placed in conjunction with maxillary sinus floor augmentation. Int J Oral Maxillofac Implants 1998;13:513–521.
12. Tarnow DP, Wallace SS, Froum SJ, et al. Histologic and clinical comparison of bilateral sinus floor elevations with and without barrier membrane placement in 12 patients: Part 3 of an ongoing prospective study. Int J Periodontics Restorative Dent 2000;20:116–125.
13. Wood RM, Moore DL. Grafting of the maxillary sinus with intraorally harvested autogenous bone prior to implant placement. Int J Oral Maxillofac Implants 1988;3:209–214.
14. Kent JN, Block MS. Simultaneous maxillary sinus floor bone grafting and placement of hydroxylapatite coated implants. J Oral Maxillofac Surg 1989;47:238–242.
15. Tidwell JK, Blijdorp PA, Stoelinga PJ, Brouns JB, Hinderks F. Composite grafting of the maxillary sinus for placement of endosteal implants. A preliminary report of 48 patients. Int J Oral Maxillofac Surg 1992;21:204–209.
16. Raghoebar GM, Brouwer TJ, Reintsema H, Van Ooort RP. Augmentation of the maxillary sinus floor with autogenous bone for the placement of endosseous implants: A preliminary report. J Oral Maxillofac Surg 1993;51:1198–1203.
17. Misch CE. Maxillary sinus augmentation for endosteal implants: Organized alternative treatment plans. Int J Oral Implantol 1987;4:49–58.
18. Pikos M. Block autografts for localized ridge augmentation: Part I. The posterior maxilla. Implant Dent 1999;8:279–285.
19. Hallman M, Sennerby L, Lundgren S. A clinical and histologic evaluation of implant integration in the posterior maxilla after sinus floor augmentation with autogenous bone, bovine hydroxylapatite, or a 20:80 mixture. Int J Oral Maxillofac Implants 2002;17:635–643.
20. Misch CM, Krauser J. The use of platelet-rich plasma in maxillofacial reconstruction with dental implants. Presentation at the Second Annual Platelet-Rich Plasma Symposium, San Francisco, CA, April 25–27, 2003.
21. Marx RE, Carlson ER, Eichstaedt RM, Schimmele SR, Strauss JE, Georgeff KR. Platelet-rich plasma: Growth factor enhancement for bone grafts. Oral Surg Oral Med Oral Pathol 1998;85:638–646.
22. Fennis JP, Stoelinga PJ, Jansen JA. Mandibular reconstruction: A clinical and radiographic animal study on the use of autogenous scaffolds and platelet-rich plasma. Int J Oral Maxillofac Surg 2002;31:281–286.
23. Boyne PJ, Herford AS. Distraction osteogenesis of the nasal and antral osseous floor to enhance alveolar height. J Oral Maxillofac Surg 2004;62(suppl 2):123–130.

24. Jensen OT, Leopardi A, Gallegos L. The case for bone graft reconstruction including sinus grafting and distraction osteogenesis for the atrophic edentulous maxilla. J Oral Maxillofac Surg 2004;62:1423–1428.
25. Misch CM. The pharmacologic management of maxillary sinus elevation surgery. J Oral Implantol 1992;18:15–23.
26. Ten Bruggenkate CM, Kraaijenhagen HA, van der Kwast WAM, Krekeler G, Oostenbeck HS. Autogenous maxillary bone grafts in conjunction with placement of ITI endosseous implants. Int J Oral Maxillofac Surg 1992;21:81–84.
27. Misch CM, Misch CE. Intraoral autogenous donor bone grafts for implant dentistry. In: Misch CE (ed). Contemporary Implant Dentistry. St Louis: Mosby, 2002:503–504.
28. Peleg M, Garg A, Misch CM, Mazor Z. Maxillary sinus and ridge augmentations using a surface-derived autogenous bone graft. J Oral Maxillofac Surg 2004;62:1535–1544.
29. Kainulainen VT, Sandor GK, Oikarinen KS, Clokie CM. Zygomatic bone: An additional donor site for alveolar bone reconstruction. Technical note. Int J Oral Maxillofac Implants 2002;17:723–728.
30. Sindet-Pedersen S, Enemark H. Reconstruction of alveolar clefts with mandibular or iliac crest bone grafts: A comparative study. J Oral Maxillofac Surg 1990;48:554–558.
31. Misch CM, Misch CE, Resnik R, Ismail Y. Reconstruction of maxillary alveolar defects with mandibular symphysis grafts for dental implants: A preliminary procedural report. Int J Oral Maxillofac Implants 1992;7:360–366.
32. Jensen J, Sindet-Pedersen S, Oliver AJ. Varying treatment strategies for reconstruction of maxillary atrophy with implants: Results in 98 patients. J Oral Maxillofac Surg 1994;52:210–216.
33. Lundgren S, Moy P, Johansson C, Nilsson H. Augmentation of the maxillary sinus floor with particulated mandible: A histologic and histomorphometric study. Int J Oral Maxillofac Implants 1996;11:760–766.
34. Misch CM. Comparison of intraoral donor sites for onlay grafting prior to implant placement. Int J Oral Maxillofac Implants 1997;12:767–776.
35. Khoury F. Augmentation of the sinus floor with mandibular bone block and simultaneous implantation: A 6-year clinical investigation. Int J Oral Maxillofac Implants 1999;14:557–601.
36. Buhr W, Coulon JP. Limits of the mandibular symphysis as a donor site for bone grafts in early secondary cleft palate osteoplasty. Int J Oral Maxillofac Surg 1996;25:389–393.
37. Borstlap WA, Heidbuchel KLWM, Freihofer HPM, Kuijpers-Jagman AM. Early secondary bone grafting of alveolar cleft defects: A comparison between chin and rib grafts. J Craniomaxillofac Surg 1990;18:201–205.
38. Hoppenreijs TJM, Nijdam ES, Freihofer HPM. The chin as a donor site in early secondary osteoplasty: A retrospective clinical and radiographic evaluation. J Cranio-Max-Fac Surg 1992;20:199–224.
39. Hunt DR, Jovanovic SA. Autogenous bone harvesting: A chin graft technique for particulate and monocortical bone blocks. Int J Periodontics Restorative Dent 1999;19:165–173.
40. Zide MF. Autogenous bone harvest and bone compacting for dental implants. Compend Contin Educ Dent 2000;21:585–590.
41. Raghoebar GM, Louwerse C, Kalk WW, Vissink A. Morbidity of chin bone harvesting. Clin Oral Implants Res 2001;12:503–507.
42. Nkenke E, Schultze-Mosgau S, Radespiel-Troger M, Kloss F, Neukam FW. Morbidity of harvesting of chin grafts: A prospective study. Clin Oral Implant Res 2001;12:495–502.
43. Hallman M, Hedin M, Sennerby L, Lundgren S. A prospective 1-year clinical and radiographic study of implants placed after maxillary sinus floor augmentation with bovine hydroxyapatite and autogenous bone. J Oral Maxillofac Surg 2002;60:277–284.
44. Misch CM, Misch CE. The repair of localized severe ridge defects for implant placement using mandibular bone grafts. Implant Dent 1995;4:261–267.
45. Jensen J, Sindet-Pedersen S. Autogenous mandibular bone grafts and osseointegrated implants for reconstruction of severely atrophied maxilla: A preliminary report. J Oral Maxillofac Surg 1991;49:1277–1287.
46. Rubens BC, West RA. Ptosis of the chin and lip incompetence: Consequences of lost mentalis support. J Oral Maxillofac Surg 1989;4:359–366.
47. Misch CM. Ridge augmentation using mandibular ramus bone grafts for the placement of dental implants: Presentation of a technique. Pract Periodont Aesthet Dent 1996;8:127–135.
48. Misch CM. Use of the mandibular ramus as a donor site for onlay bone grafting. J Oral Implantol 2000;26:42–49.
49. Smith BR, Rajchel JL, Waite DE, Read L. Mandibular anatomy as it relates to rigid fixation of the sagittal ramus split osteotomy. J Oral Maxillofac Surg 1991;49:222–226.
50. Rachel J, Ellis E, Fonseca RJ. The anatomic location of the mandibular canal: Its relationship to the sagittal ramus osteotomy. Int J Adult Orthod Orthognathic Surg 1986;1:37–42.
51. Crawford EA. The use of ramus bone cores for maxillary sinus bone grafting: A surgical technique. J Oral Implantol 2001;27:82–88.
52. Hendy CW, Smith KG, Robinson PP. Surgical anatomy of the buccal nerve. Br J Oral Maxillofac Surg 1996;34:457–460.
53. Smith JD, Abramson M. Membranous vs. endochondral bone autografts. Arch Otolaryngol 1974;99:203–205.
54. Zins JE, Whitaker LA. Membranous vs. endochondral bone autografts: Implications for craniofacial reconstruction. Plast Reconstr Surg 1983;72:778–785.
55. Lin KY, Bartlett SP, Yaremchuk MJ, Fallon M, Grossman RF, Whitaker LA. The effect of rigid fixation on the survival of onlay bone grafts: An experimental study. Plast Reconstr Surg 1990;86:449–456.
56. Hardesty RA, Marsh JL. Craniofacial onlay bone grafting: A prospective evaluation of graft morphology, orientation and embryologic origin. Plast Reconstr Surg 1990;85:5–14.
57. Manson PN. Facial bone healing and bone grafts. A review of clinical physiology. Clin Plast Surg 1994;21:331–348.
58. Ozaki W, Buchman SR. Volume maintenance of onlay bone grafts in the craniofacial skeleton: Micro-architecture versus embryologic origin. Plast Reconstr Surg 1998;102:291–299.

59. Steiner M, Ramp WK. Short-term storage of freshly harvested bone. J Oral Maxillofac Surg 1988;46:868–871.
60. Young MP, Korachi M, Carter DH, Worthington HV, McCord JF, Drucker DB. The effects of an immediately presurgical chlorhexidine oral rinse on the bacterial contaminants of bone debris collected during dental implant surgery. Clin Oral Implants Res 2002;13:20–29.
61. Fonseca RJ, Clark Pj, Burkes EJ Jr, Baker RD. Revascularization and healing of onlay particulate autologous bone grafts in primates. J Oral Surg 1980;38:572–577.
62. Dado DV, Izquierdo R. Absorption of onlay bone grafts in immature rabbits: Membranous versus endochondral bone and bone struts versus paste. Ann Plast Surg 1989;23:39–48.
63. Pallesen I, Schou S, Aaboe M, Hjorting-Hansen E, Nattestad A, Melsen F. Influence of particle size of autogenous bone grafts on the early stages of bone regeneration. A histologic and stereologic study in rabbit calvarium. Int J Oral Maxillofac Implants 2002;17:498–506.
64. Yildirim M, Spiekermann H, Biesterfeld S, Edelhoff D. Maxillary sinus augmentation using xenogenic bone substitute material Bio-Oss in combination with venous blood. A histologic and hiostomorphometric study in humans. Clin Oral Implants Res 2000;11:217–229.
65. Misch CM. Discussion. A prospective 1 year clinical and radiographic study of implants placed after maxillary sinus floor augmentation with bovine hydroxylapatite and autogenous bone. J Oral Maxillofac Surg 2002;60:285.
66. Hollinger J, Wong ME. The integrated processes of hard tissue regeneration with special emphasis on fracture healing. Oral Surg Oral Med Oral Pathol 1996;82:594–606.
67. Sullivan SM, Bulard RA, Meaders R, Patterson MK. The use of fibrin adhesive in sinus lift procedures. Oral Surg Oral Med Oral Pathol Oral Radiol Endod 1997;84:616–619.
68. Krekmanov L, Heimdahl A. Bone grafting to the maxillary sinus from the lateral side of the mandible. Br J Oral Maxillofac Surg 2000;38:617–619.
69. Boyne PJ, Cole MD, Stolinger D, Shafquat JP. A technique for osseous reconstruction of deficient edentulous maxillary ridges. J Oral Maxillofac Surg 1985;43:87–91.
70. Malchiodi L, Scarano A, Quaranta M, Piatelli A. Rigid fixation by means of titanium mesh in edentulous ridge expansion for horizontal ridge augmentation in the maxilla. Int J Oral Maxillofac Implants 1998;13:701–705.
71. Adell R, Lekholm U, Grondahl K, Brånemark PI, Lindstrom J, Jacobsson M. Reconstruction of severely resorbed edentulous maxillae using osseointegrated fixtures in immediate autogenous bone grafts. Int J Oral Maxillofac Implants 1990;5:233–246.
72. Keller EE, Van Roeckel NB, Desjardins RP, Tolman DE. Prosthetic-surgical reconstruction of the severely resorbed maxilla with iliac bone grafting and tissue-integrated prostheses. Int J Oral Maxillofac Implants 1987;2:155–165.
73. Matsumoto MA, Filho HN, Francischone E, Consolaro A. Microscopic analysis of reconstructed maxillary alveolar ridges using autogenous bone grafts from the chin and iliac crest. Int J Oral Maxillofac Implants 2002;17:507–516.
74. Wallace SS, Froum SJ. Effect of maxillary sinus augmentation on the survival of endosseous dental implants. A systematic review. Ann Periodontol 2003;8:328–343.

chapter 12
Tibia Bone Grafting for Sinus Augmentation

Robert E. Marx, DDS

The average volume of the maxillary sinus in a dentate individual is 15 mL. In the fully edentulous individual, however, the maxillary sinus volume increases to 21 mL due to resorption of alveolar bone at the sinus floor. The standard sinus bone graft is about 7 mL in volume, sufficient to fill about one third of the maxillary sinus (Fig 12-1). For a graft composed of 100% autogenous cancellous marrow, 10 mL of uncompressed cancellous marrow is recommended for each sinus. Proportional amounts of autogenous cancellous marrow are required for composites of autogenous cancellous marrow and nonautogenous graft materials. Obviously, oral bone sites such as the chin, ramus, and tuberosity are inadequate for harvesting the quantity of graft material necessary for this procedure.[1] Moreover, the quality of the bone in these areas may be deficient as well. The chin bone yields a maximum of about 5 mL of cancellous marrow, the ramus yields 3 mL of cortical bone, and the tuberosity yields only 2 mL of fibrofatty trabecular marrow. For office-based sinus graft surgeries, only the tibia provides the quality and quantity of cancellous bone required in an area that can be harvested with convenient access, minimal complexity, and minimal complications.[2]

Cancellous marrow obtained from the tibial plateau contains the same quantity of endosteal osteoblasts and marrow stem cells as grafts harvested from the anterior or posterior ilium (Fig 12-2). Furthermore, the harvesting technique lends itself to a one- or two-person surgical approach that can be performed with the patient seated in a dental chair. Although the surgery can be performed with the patient under local anesthesia, local anesthesia supplemented with intravenous sedation is usually recommended. Patients are able to walk out of the office without the need of a cane or walker, and they experience minimal postoperative discomfort or other harvest site morbidities.[4] Accessibility of high-quality autogenous bone in sufficient quantities for bilateral sinus grafting allows the surgeon to avoid non-osteogenic allogeneic bone sources and bone substitutes.[1,5]

Surgical Anatomy of the Tibia

Because the tibia provides the major bony support of the leg below the knee, it is important to emphasize that the approach described in this chapter for harvesting cancellous marrow does not weaken this bone substantially or place it at risk for fracture.

The entry site for marrow harvest is at Gerdy's tubercle, an easily palpable ridge located on the lateral surface of the tibia, about 1.5 cm below the articulating surface (Fig 12-3a).[1,6,7] This ridge courses obliquely for 3 cm from a superior lateral position to a more inferior medial position. The tensor fascia lata muscle and tensor fascia lata

chapter 12 Tibia Bone Grafting for Sinus Augmentation

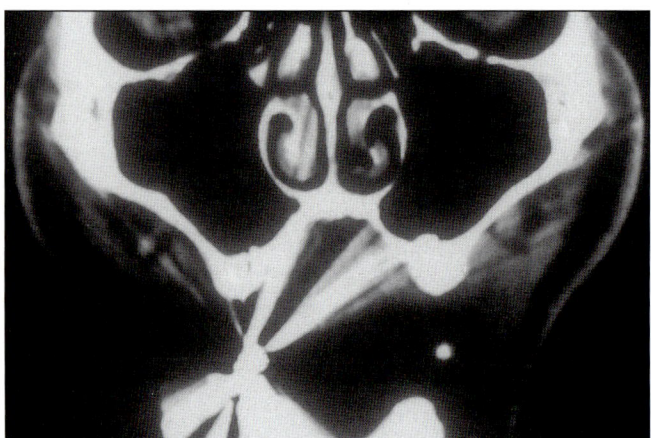

Fig 12-1 Resorption of the sinus floor toward the alveolar crest increases the volume of the edentulous maxillary sinus to 21 mL.

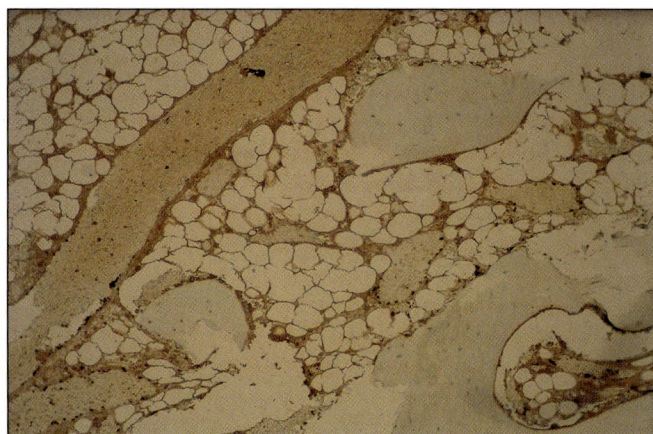

Fig 12-2 Brown-stained osteoprogenitor cells clustered around a small venule and upon the surface of trabecular bone. Osteoprogenitor cells with membrane receptors for TGF-β1 are found in equal quantities in donor bone harvested from the tibia, the anterior ilium, and the posterior ilium. (Immunoperoxidase stain). (Reprinted with permission from Marx and Garg.[3])

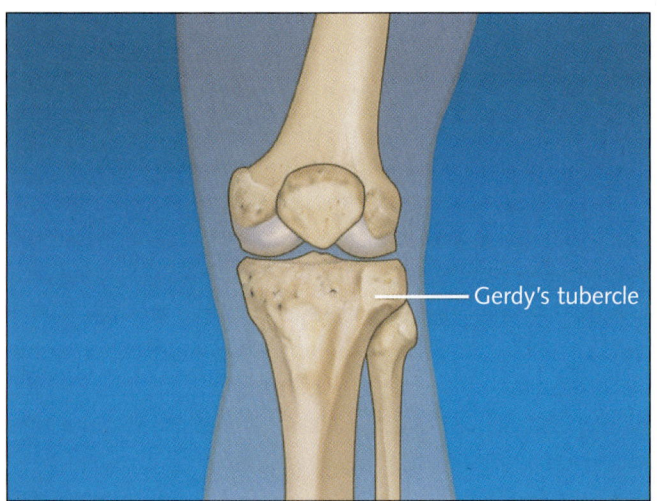

Fig 12-3a Gerdy's tubercle is located about 1.5 cm inferior to the tibial articulating surface on the lateral aspect. (Reprinted with permission from Garg.[1])

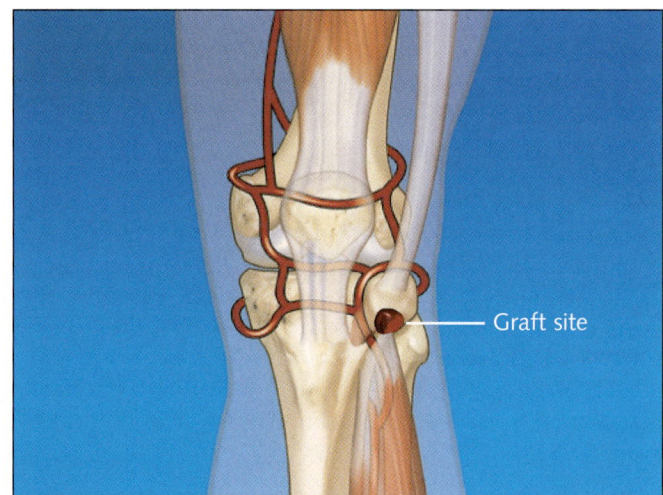

Fig 12-3b The entry point to harvest cancellous marrow from the lateral proximal tibia is just below the ridge of Gerdy's tubercle, where the uppermost fibers of the anterior tibialis attach. (Reprinted with permission from Garg.[1])

proper insert into this ridge area, which includes the tubercle immediately superior to the ridge. Since the insertion is via Sharpey's fibers, which are very tenacious, the preferred entry point into the tibia is through the fossa just inferior to the ridge, where a small portion of the anterior tibialis muscle is easily reflected (Fig 12-3b).

The bony cortex in the area of Gerdy's tubercle is only 0.6 to 1.5 cm deep to the skin surface, and there are no major sensory or motor nerves and no major blood vessels in the surgical field to pose a bleeding potential. The nerve nearest to this surgical site is the common peroneal nerve, which is located 2 cm posterior and lateral to it. The nearest blood vessel is the anterior tibial artery, which is 3 cm inferior and lateral to the surgical site and protected by the overlying anterior tibialis muscle. The soft tissue dissection is thus straightforward, progressing through the skin, the subcutaneous layer, and the periosteum.

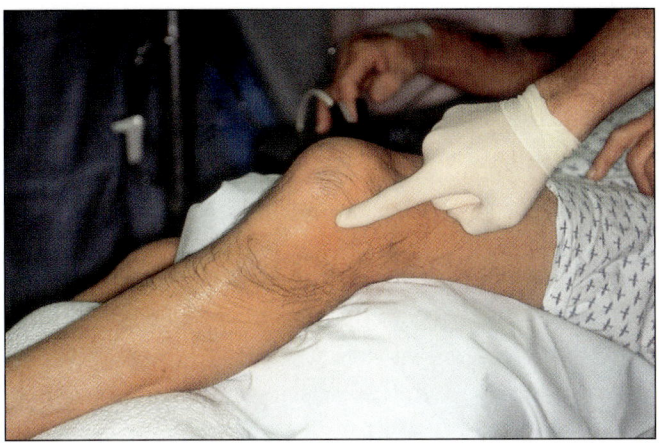

Fig 12-3c Flexion of the knee, supported by a pillow, brings Gerdy's tubercle (indicated by surgeon) into prominence and enhances the patient's comfort.

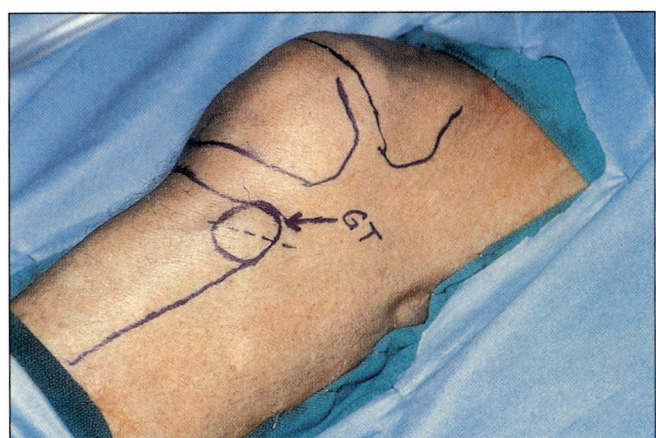

Fig 12-3d Bone harvest site draped to expose the entire knee joint, the distal third of the femur, and the proximal half of the tibia. Draping helps the surgeon to maintain orientation.

Surgical Approach

Patient positioning and preparation

Once intravenous access has been established for a blood draw, platelet-rich plasma (PRP) preparation, and intravenous sedation, the dental chair is configured for slight flexion at the knees and hips. Flexion of the knee on the operative side is reinforced by placing a pillow under the knee joint in the popliteal fossa (Fig 12-3c). This positioning also brings the surgical area to the eye level of a seated surgeon and assistant and improves the visibility and palpability of the ridge at Gerdy's tubercle. The right-handed surgeon is strongly advised to harvest cancellous marrow from the left leg and the left-handed surgeon to harvest cancellous marrow from the right leg. This will minimize the risk of knee joint entry by directing the bone-harvesting curette in a natural trajectory medially and inferiorly away from the knee joint and into the large reservoir of cancellous marrow in the tibial plateau.

The bone harvest site requires preparation with sterile Betadine (Purdue Frederick) or 4% chlorhexidine (Purdue Frederick), sterile drapes, and full sterile gowns and gloves for the surgical team. The sterile preparation and draping should encompass the entire knee joint as well as the areas 10 cm above and below the knee joint, which allows the surgeon to visualize the relationships of the femur, tibia, fibula, and patella. Use of a sterile marking pen is recommended to draw the regional anatomy on the skin so as to reinforce visual perspective throughout the procedure (Fig 12-3d). The pertinent anatomy includes the outline of the tibia and its articulating surface; Gerdy's tubercle; the patella, lower femur, and fibula; and the insertion of the tensor fascia lata and anterior tibialis muscle. The 2.5-cm incision is marked directly over the ridge at Gerdy's tubercle (see Fig 12-3d).

Anesthesia and sedation

Since the sinus bone graft site and the tibia harvest site undergo surgery simultaneously, intravenous sedation of the surgeon's preference is recommended. One suggestion is to use midazolam (Versed, Roche), fentanyl (Sublimaze, Baxter Healthcare), and propofol (Diprivan, Astra Tech Pharmaceuticals) in age- and weight-appropriate doses. Local anesthesia, such as 4% septocaine (Articaine, Septodent) with 1:100,000 epinephrine, is also recommended.

The local anesthesia is injected at the subcutaneous level in a tract along the incision line (Fig 12-3e). A second carpule is then injected deep, onto the periosteum, by inserting the needle at a right angle to the skin surface. Once the needle tip touches bone, the entire carpule (1.8 mL) is deposited on its surface (Fig 12-3f). A waiting period of 3 minutes is recommended to allow a profound nerve blockade to develop.

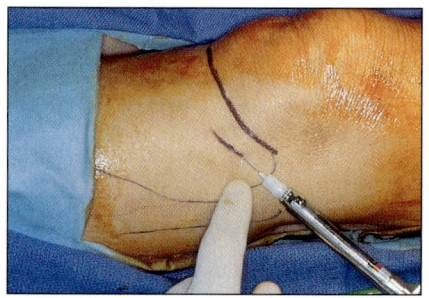

Fig 12-3e Local anesthesia injected along the incision outline.

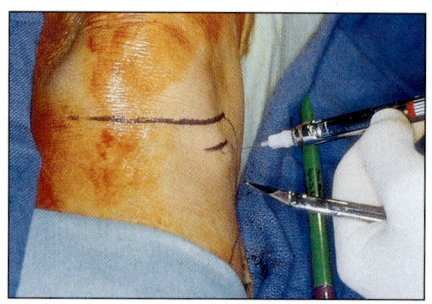

Fig 12-3f Following anesthetizing of the skin, an injection of 1 to 2 mL of local anesthesia is deposited on the periosteum-bone surface.

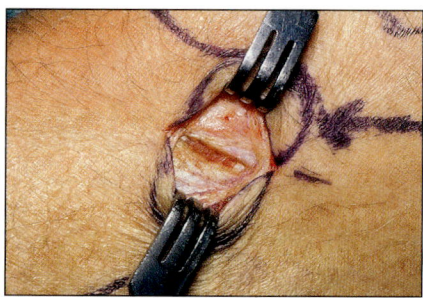

Fig 12-3g The initial incision exposes the thick white fascia extending over the ridge of Gerdy's tubercle. The upper fibers of the anterior tibialis muscle are visible below the incision, and the tensor fascia lata is visible above the incision.

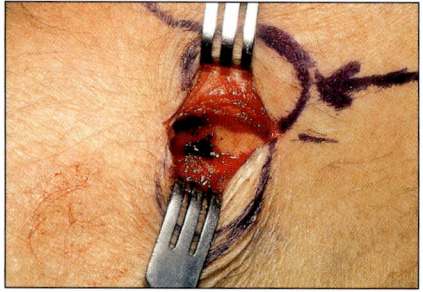

Fig 12-3h The ideal entry point is at the fossa just below the ridge of Gerdy's tubercle. The site is exposed by reflecting the uppermost fibers of the anterior tibialis muscle. The use of Senn retractors (shown here) requires the help of an assistant.

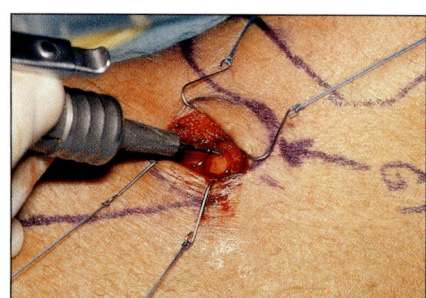

Fig 12-3i A no. 702 bur is used to make a circular 1.0- to 1.5-cm-diameter cortical opening. Here, Dura Hooks are used as self-retaining retractors.

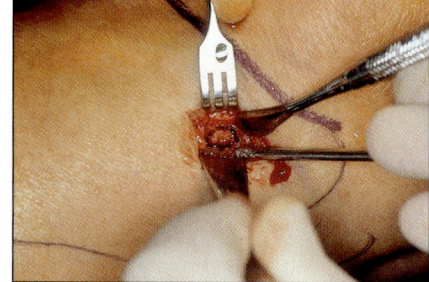

Fig 12-3j The circular piece of cortical bone is wedged out and added to the graft.

Surgical Technique

The incision is initiated through the full thickness of the skin and the subcutaneous layer. Small rake retractors such as a Senn retractor (Walter Lorenz), or self-retaining retractors such as Dura Hooks (Walter Lorenz), are inserted (Fig 12-3g). The incision will expose a glistening white layer deep to the subcutaneous fat. This represents the tensor fascia lata and its extension over the ridge at Gerdy's tubercle and the anterior tibialis muscle (see Fig 12-3g). A dry sponge or Kitner's wipe (Johnson & Johnson) is useful for wiping away subcutaneous fat lobules that might obscure the surgeon's vision.

The ridge at Gerdy's tubercle should be readily palpable, and a 2-cm incision is made through the fascia and periosteum down to bone. Releasing incisions in an inferior direction at each edge of the incision are recommended to permit maximum reflection and exposure of the tibial cortex inferior to the ridge at Gerdy's tubercle (Fig 12-3h). A Seldon or Austin retractor can be used to retract the small reflected portion of the anterior tibialis muscle and attached periosteum inferiorly, allowing a 1.5-cm-diameter cortical opening to be made. Using a no. 702 tapered fissure bur, the cortex is perforated in a 1.5-cm-diameter circle (Fig 12-3i). In this area, the cortex is only about 1.0 to 1.5 mm thick, so the bur is not buried into the marrow space. The author prefers to make individual bur hole perforations in a 1.5-cm-diameter circular pattern, which are then connected. The resulting piece of cortical bone is then wedged out (Figs 12-3j and 12-3k). No additional cortical bone is obtained from this site.

Cancellous cellular marrow is harvested through the 1.5-cm-diameter opening using a Molt curette (Walter

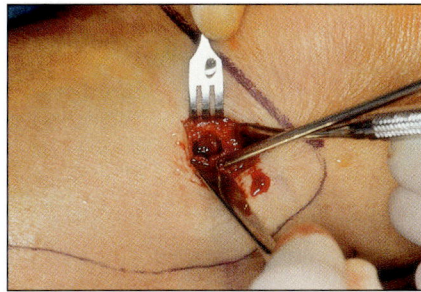

Fig 12-3k The cortical opening allows access to the large reservoir of cancellous bone located in the proximal area of the tibia.

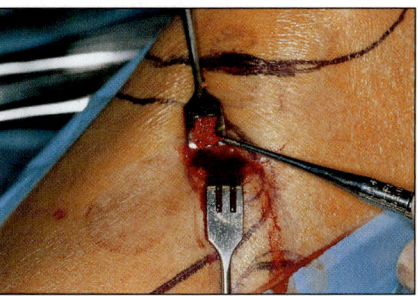

Fig 12-3l Curetted bone from the proximal area of the tibia. (Reprinted with permission from Garg.[1])

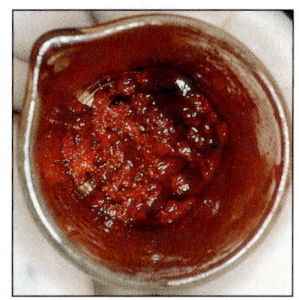

Fig 12-3m Taking this approach, an abundant amount of autogenous cancellous marrow can be curetted from the tibia.

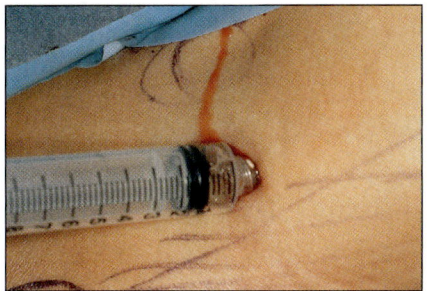

Fig 12-3n Injection of activated PPP into the hollowed cavity to assist in clot development and hemostasis. (Reprinted with permission from Garg.[1])

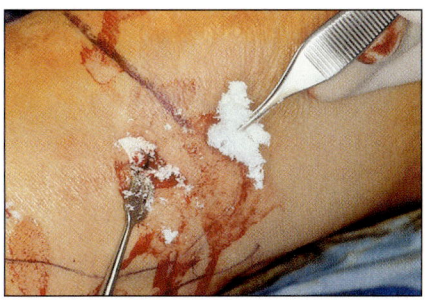

Fig 12-3o Placement of microfibrillar bovine collagen (Avitene) into the hollowed cavity to assist in clot development and hemostasis.

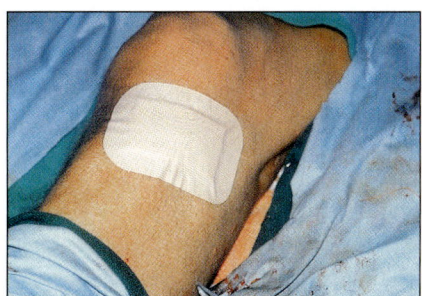

Fig 12-3p Usually, only a simple Band-Aid–type of dressing is required to cover the closed wound.

Lorenz). This proximal area of the tibia represents an abundant source of cancellous bone and cellular marrow, ranging from 75 to 100 mL in volume. Since each sinus graft requires only about 10 mL of uncompressed cancellous marrow, tibial grafts harvested for this purpose require only about 20 mL, an amount that is readily available via this approach.

Although some surgeons use orthopedic bone curettes to harvest the cancellous marrow, the no. 4 Molt curette is recommended. A curette of any type is best used with a rotational wrist motion that separates cancellous marrow from the site as it completes a 360-degree arc. The loose cancellous bone particles are worked to the cortical opening and removed either to be placed directly into the prepared sinus cavity or temporarily stored in PRP or sterile saline (Figs 12-3l and 12-3m). As noted earlier, the direction of entry is inferior and medial, which is away from the knee joint. When the quantity of harvested bone exceeds 10 to 15 mL, the hollowed cavity in the tibia makes it difficult to maneuver separated cancellous marrow to the cortical opening. This can be overcome by pinning the separated cancellous marrow against the inner lateral cortex with the curette and then withdrawing the curette through the opening.

Once the required quantity of cancellous marrow is obtained, a slow marrow ooze is likely to develop. This should be controlled with topical hemostatic agents. If available, activated platelet-poor plasma (PPP) can be placed into the bony cavity (Fig 12-3n). Otherwise, 1 g of microfibrillar bovine collagen (Avitene, Med Chem) also achieves good hemostasis (Fig 12-3o). This is followed by a layered closure where the fascia is closed first using a 3-0 resorbable suture. The subcutaneous/dermal level is closed next with the same 3-0 resorbable suture, followed by a skin surface closure using a horizontal mattress technique with 4-0 nylon or 4-0 prolene suture. The closure is then coated with an antibiotic ointment and a light cover dressing or large Band-Aid–type of dressing (Fig 12-3p). Leg wraps or pressure dressings are not necessary.

chapter 12 — Tibia Bone Grafting for Sinus Augmentation

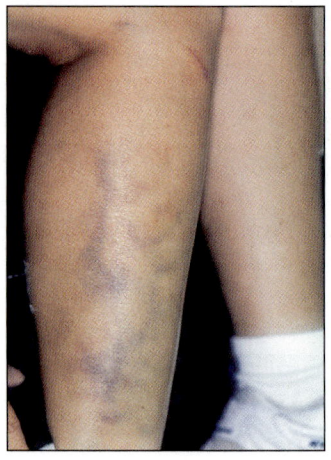

Fig 12-3q Development of ecchymosis (bruising), the most common postoperative sequela, distal to the incision and extending to about the ankle.

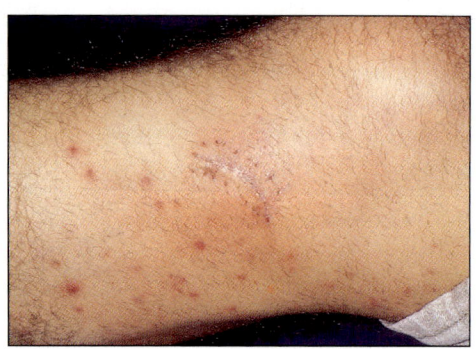

Fig 12-3r Bone harvest site 7 days after surgery. The skin sutures have been removed.

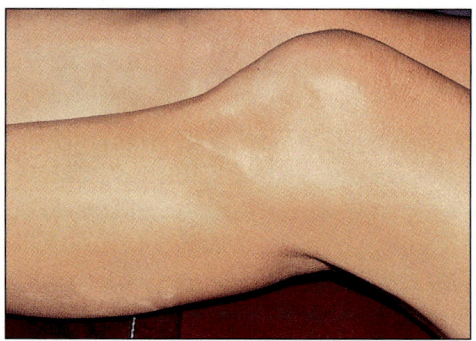

Fig 12-3s The small scar of a tibia bone harvest is acceptable to most patients.

Intraoperative Medications

The surgeon should select an antibiotic and a steroid regimen based on experience and patient history. If the patient is not allergic to penicillin, ampicillin 1 g with sulbactam 500 mg (Unasyn 1.5 g, Roerig-Pfizer) is the preferred antibiotic. This antibiotic preparation is bactericidal; well tolerated; covers the appropriate spectrum for the sinus area, oral cavity, and skin of the lower extremities; and has an extended spectrum (due to the sulbactam) to include penicillinase-producing bacteria. For the penicillin-allergic patient, cefoxitin 1 g (Mefoxin, Merck) may be prescribed. Because cefoxitin is not a true cephalosporin, but rather a cephamycin, it does not have cross allergenicity to penicillin, yet it covers nearly all of the oral anaerobes. If the penicillin allergy is an anaphylaxis, it is prudent not to challenge the patient even with cefoxitin. In such cases, second-line alternatives such as erythromycin 1 g or levofloxacin 500 mg (Levaquin, Ortho-McNeil) are reasonable choices.

A single dose of intravenous dexamethasone 8 mg (Decadron, American Pharmaceutical) given intraoperatively will suppress most of the postoperative edema. Methylprednisolone (Solu-Medrol, Pharmacia & Upjohn) 125 mg intravenously can be used as an alternative.

Postoperative Recovery and Instructions

No specific extension of the recovery time is required for a tibia bone harvest procedure. Once recovery from the intravenous sedation is sufficient, the patient can walk with an escort to an automobile or other form of transportation. Nonambulation is recommended thereafter until the next morning for full recovery from the intravenous sedation as well as the tibia harvest. Elevation of the leg with an ice pack is recommended for the first postoperative night. Ice is not needed after the first night, and cooling of the skin may even be counterproductive. The patient is instructed to engage in normal activities but to limit walking to no more than one eighth of a mile per day. For the next 6 weeks, the patient should not engage in sports, strenuous exercise, walking up more than one flight of stairs, running, or bicycle riding. This will allow time for the tensor fascia lata and anterior tibialis muscles to re-attach to the bone. A specific warning to expect ecchymosis (bruising) is given to the patient prior to the surgery and reiterated to the escort as part of the postoperative instructions. Due to gravity and the natural flow of fluids in the leg (ie, the lymphatic network), bruising and swelling are to be expected, most frequently below the

TABLE 12-1 Mean bone height of sinus grafts (n = 571) using autogenous marrow from the tibial plateau		
Starting bone height (mm)	Bone height 1 year later (mm)	Permanent gain in height (mm)
2.3	14.8	12.5

TABLE 12-2 Success rate of sinus grafts using 100% autogenous marrow from the tibial plateau			
Tibia grafts	Grafts lost due to infection	Sufficient regenerated bone	Functioning implants at 1 year
618 (100%)	26 (4.2%)	564 (91.3%)	550 (89.0%)

surgical site and extending to the ankle (Fig 12-3q). Since the ankle area is at a distance from the surgical site, swelling and ecchymosis in this area may prompt significant unnecessary concern in the patient and/or the patient's family, and such forewarning alleviates these anxieties. Postoperative analgesics and antibiotics are prescribed as necessary following the sinus graft surgery. There is no advantage in prescribing a different antibiotic for the tibia harvest site. Amoxicillin 875 mg with clavulanate 125 mg (Augmentin 875 mg, GlaxoSmith-Kline) is prescribed to be taken twice daily. In the penicillin-allergic patient, erythromycin ethylsuccinate 400 mg (EES, Abbott Laboratories) three times daily, levofloxacin 500 mg (Levaquin) once daily, or azithromycin 500 mg (Zithromax, Pfizer) once daily are reasonable second-line choices. Analgesics containing hydrocodone or oxycodone with acetaminophen or aspirin are also prescribed for about 7 days. Skin sutures may be removed on or near postoperative day 7 (Figs 12-3r and 12-3s).

Outcome Analysis of the Tibia Harvest

Sinus augmentation results

A review of 571 consecutive cases of bone grafts for sinus augmentation harvested from the tibia and accomplished in an office setting at the University of Miami Miller School of Medicine's Division of Oral and Maxillofacial Surgery program yielded the following graft outcome results (Tables 12-1 and 12-2). Of the 571 cases, 84 received prosthodontic care at the referring practitioner's site and thus were lost to follow-up. The remaining 487 patients involved 618 sinus augmentation procedures in 131 bilateral cases and 356 unilateral cases.

Of the 618 augmented sinuses, 26 (4.2%) developed infections, usually from sinusitis/upper respiratory infections, resulting in loss of the graft. Of the remaining sinuses, 28 (4.5%) were deemed to have insufficient regenerated bone into which dental implants could be placed and therefore required further augmentation. The remaining 564 sinuses (91.3%) were deemed successful. The mean initial natural bone height in these sinuses was 2.3 mm. The 1-year mean measured bone height after grafting was 14.8 mm, resulting in a mean gain in alveolar bone height of 12.5 mm. Implants placed in 14 of the sinus grafts failed to osseointegrate. The remaining 550 sinus grafts (89.0%) underwent placement of 1,388 implants, which osseointegrated and withstood functional loading.

During implant placement, bone core samples were retrieved from 411 sinus grafts. The mean viable trabecular bone area measured in these grafts was 62% (Fig 12-4a) and was superior to comparable grafts using freeze-dried bone allograft (FDBA) (University of Miami Tissue Bank) (21%) (Fig 12-4b); xenogenic bone (Bio-Oss, Osteohealth) (24%) (Fig 12-4c); hydroxyapatite (C-Graft, Clinician's Preference) (22%) (Fig 12-4d); and bioglass (BioGran, Implant Innovations Inc) (15%) (Fig 12-4e).

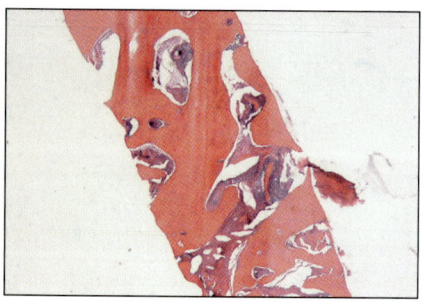

Fig 12-4a Core biopsy specimen from a sinus graft consisting of autogenous tibial cancellous marrow. The area of trabecular bone measured 62% in this specimen. (Hematoxylin-eosin; magnification ×4.)

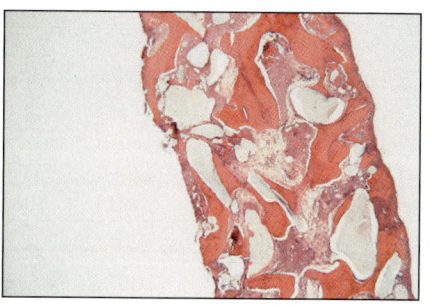

Fig 12-4b Core biopsy specimen from a sinus graft consisting of freeze-dried allogeneic bone. The area of trabecular bone measured 21% in this specimen. (Hematoxylin-eosin; magnification ×4.)

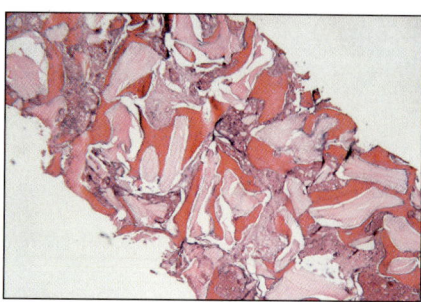

Fig 12-4c Core biopsy specimen from a sinus graft consisting of treated xenogenic bone (Bio-Oss). The area of trabecular bone measured 24% in this specimen. (Hematoxylin-eosin; magnification ×10.)

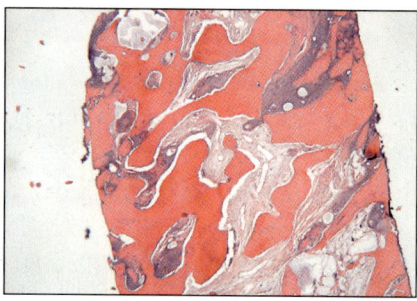

Fig 12-4d Core biopsy specimen from a sinus graft consisting of natural hydroxyapatite (C-Graft). The area of trabecular bone measured 22% in this specimen. (Hematoxylin-eosin; magnification ×10.)

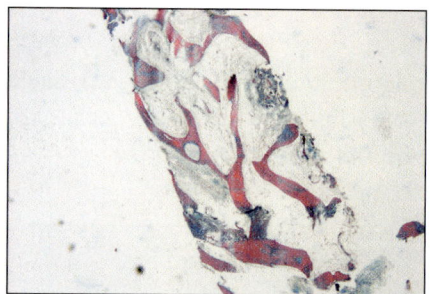

Fig 12-4e Core biopsy specimen from a sinus graft consisting of bioglass (BioGran). The area of trabecular bone measured 15% in this specimen. (Hematoxylin-eosin; magnification ×4.)

Harvest site morbidity

A review of 571 consecutive cases of tibia bone harvesting accomplished specifically for sinus graft procedures in an office setting at the University of Miami Miller School of Medicine's Division of Oral and Maxillofacial Surgery program yielded the following donor site morbidity results (Tables 12-3 and 12-4). The average volume of bone graft harvested for a unilateral sinus graft was 12 mL. This produced a blood loss ranging from 10 to 65 mL (mean, 30 mL). The average bone graft volume harvested for a bilateral sinus graft was 22.5 mL. This produced a blood loss ranging from 25 to 100 mL (mean, 55 mL) (see Table 12-3). Neither of these blood-loss calculations is considered significant, nor did they affect the patient's recovery or general physiology.

Standard orthopedic surgery morbidity parameters for tibia bone harvesting were published by O'Keefe in 1991.[3] His study of 230 cases assessed the potential morbidities of gait disturbance, hematoma, fracture, and infection as accomplished in the controlled environment of the operating room setting. His overall complication rate was 1.4%. For the 571 tibia bone harvest procedures accomplished by the author and his colleagues in the office setting for sinus grafting, ecchymosis, knee joint entrance, knee joint complaints, objectionable scar, and dehiscence were also stud-

TABLE 12-3 Bone graft volumes and related blood loss from tibia bone harvest procedures performed in the office setting	
Bone graft yield	Blood loss
Unilateral sinus graft, 12 mL	10 to 65 mL (mean, 30 mL)
Bilateral sinus graft, 22.5 mL	25 to 100 mL (mean, 55 mL)

TABLE 12-4 Morbidity parameters and their rate of occurrence in 571 tibia bone harvest procedures performed in an office setting	
Morbidity parameters	No. (%)
Fracture	0
Gait disturbance	0
Knee joint entrance	0
Knee joint complaint	0
Objectionable scar	2 (0.35%)
Hematoma	2 (0.35%)
Superficial wound infection	1 (0.18%)
Dehiscence	2 (0.35%)

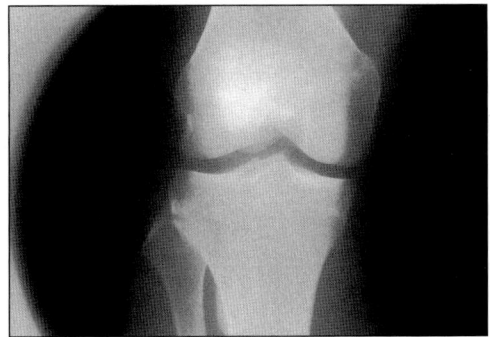

Fig 12-5a Postoperative radiograph of a tibia harvest site exhibiting minimal bone void.

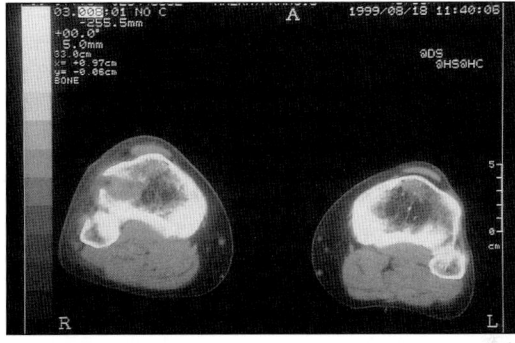

Fig 12-5b Postoperative CT scan of a tibia harvest site showing a small entry window and a small blood clot in the marrow space where bone was harvested. A large area of bone remains after the graft harvest.

ied as potential morbidities (see Table 12-4). This study documented no incidents of knee joint entrance, knee joint complaints, fractures, or permanent gait disturbance (Figs 12-5a and 12-5b). Two patients (0.35%) complained that the scar was larger than anticipated, 2 patients (0.35%) developed a hematoma, 1 patient (0.18%) developed a superficial wound infection, and 2 patients (0.35%) developed a dehiscence. Though not a true complication, 44 patients developed more significant ecchymosis than expected, which resolved without affecting healing or walking. The infection at the incision area resolved with a small secondary debridement, wound irrigations, and a 2-week extension of antibiotics. It did not progress to an osteomyelitis or an infection to the level of the bone. Of the two hematomas, one resolved without further intervention and the other required evacuation and resuturing. Of the two cases of dehiscence, both occurred in individuals who exercised in the early postoperative course. Each was treated to resolution with a revision and resuturing. The overall morbidity of 1.2% in these 571 office-based cases is lower than that published for operating room tibia harvests by O'Keefe (1.4%), which also is low. It is important to note that none of the observed morbidities required hospitalization or resulted in deformity or disability.

Conclusion

Absence of significant morbidity combined with a significant yield of high-quality cancellous cellular marrow, resulting in an average of 12.5 mm of regenerated bone, a bone graft success rate of 91.3%, and a mean trabecular bone density of 62%, makes office-based tibia bone harvesting ideally suited for the sinus graft procedure. It frees the surgeon from the limitations associated with the use of allogeneic bone, xenogenic bone, and the wide variety of bone substitutes currently in the marketplace. Moreover, it is a procedure with documented safety and a track record of predictable outcomes. The surgical technique is straightforward, and the regional anatomy is not complex. Residents and practicing oral and maxillofacial surgeons can learn and apply this procedure with available coursework, mentoring, and supervised practice.

References

1. Garg AK. Bone Biology, Harvesting, and Grafting For Dental Implants: Rationale and Clinical Applications. Chicago: Quintessence, 2004:121–170.
2. Catone GA, Reimer BL, McNeir D, Ray R. Tibial autogenous cancellous bone as an alternative donor site in maxillofacial surgery: A preliminary report. J Oral Maxillofac Surg 1992;50:1258–1263.
3. Marx RE, Garg AK. Dental and Craniofacial Applications of Platelet-Rich Plasma. Chicago: Quintessence, 2004.
4. O'Keeffe RM Jr, Riemer BL, Butterfield SL. Harvesting of autogenous cancellous bone graft from the proximal tibial metaphysic. A review of 230 cases. J Orthop Trauma 1991;5:469–474.
5. Jakse N, Seibert FJ, Lorenzoni M, Eskici A, Pertl C. A modified technique of harvesting tibial cancellous bone and its use for sinus grafting. Clin Oral Implants Res 2001;12:488–499.
6. Van Damme PA, Merkx MA. A modification of the tibial bone-graft-harvesting technique. Int J Oral Maxillofac Surg 1996;25:346–348.
7. Clemente CD. Anatomy: A Regional Atlas of the Human Body, ed 4. Philadelphia: Lippincott Williams & Wilkins, 1997:plates 541–547.

chapter 13 Sinus Augmentation with Bone Harvested from the Ilium

R. Gilbert Triplett, DDS, PhD
Sterling R. Schow, DMD

The availability of a sufficient amount of residual bone in the posterior maxilla is critical for successful endosseous implant support. When the bone between the sinus floor and the alveolar crest is less than 10 mm thick, it is necessary to graft the alveolar sinus floor to provide adequate osseous support for an implant-borne prosthesis.[1] Bone graft augmentation in the maxilla has advanced significantly over the past 20 years. Autologous, allogeneic, alloplastic, and combinations of these materials have all been advocated for use in augmenting the maxillary sinus floor and alveolus. Despite efforts to find an alternative, the patient's own bone is still the ideal graft material. The ilium is a highly desirable donor site because of the excellent quality and quantity of bone it can provide.

Iliac bone, which can be particulated, richly cellular cancellous marrow, or corticocancellous blocks, provides viable osteoblasts, osteocytes, and osteoprogenitor cells capable of osteoinduction (see chapter 28). It is also capable of osteoconduction and remodeling into mature lamellar bone. It has the ability to be shaped to reconstruct lost architecture and it is rapidly revascularized. It has low antigenicity and low risk of infection and provides predictable bone regeneration. Other donor sites for autologous bone, such as the calvarium, the mandible, and the tibia, all have their place in augmentation of the alveolar processes. However, the ilium provides access to large quantities of bone with flexibility for either particulate or corticocancellous blocks. Therefore, the iliac crest is still considered the gold standard in augmentation procedures.

The disadvantages of iliac bone grafts include increased surgical time for harvesting the graft, increased expense because the procedure must be performed in a surgical setting, and morbidity associated with donor site harvest.

Both the anterior and the posterior iliac crest are suitable for harvesting iliac bone, although the anterior crest offers some advantages. It is more accessible, allows simultaneous surgery of the hip and oral cavity, and does not require repositioning of the patient prior to exposure of the recipient site and transplantation of the bone.[2] The posterior iliac crest donor site is indicated when a large quantity of bone is needed for an onlay graft or a combination of sinus floor and onlay grafting. Approximately 2 to 2.5 times more bone can be obtained from the posterior than from the anterior iliac crest.[3] Potential contraindications for harvesting bone from this site concern the patient's physical condition, cost, and individual preference.

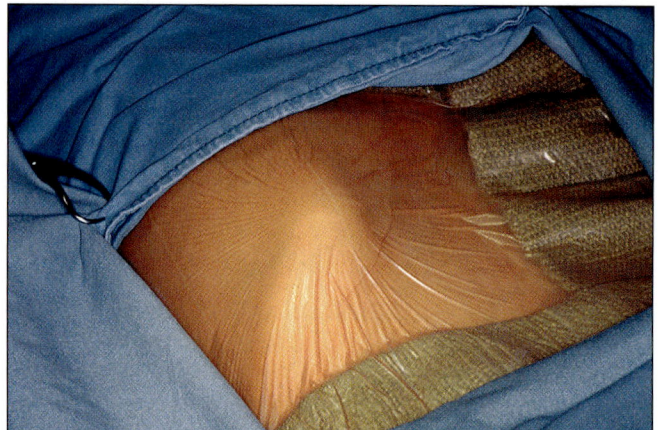

Fig 13-1a Anterior hip donor site prepared for harvesting procedure. Note the prominence of the anterior iliac spine.

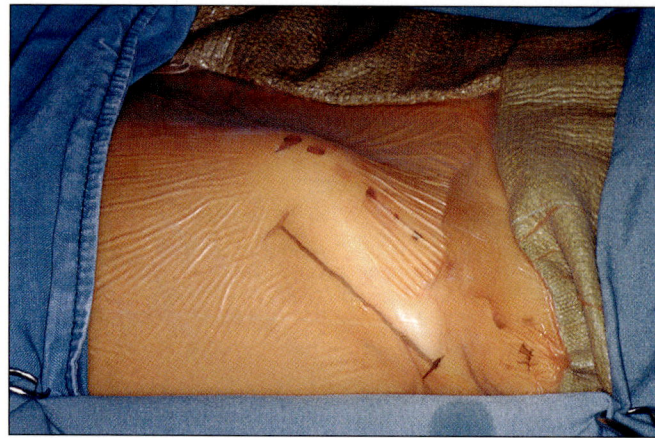

Fig 13-1b Superficial marking of the iliac crest and incision site lateral and inferior to the crest. Prior to incising, the incision line is moved over the crest by depressing the abdomen.

Harvesting Bone from the Anterior Ilium

As already noted, one of the primary advantages of the anterior over the posterior iliac crest is that surgery in the oral cavity and the iliac crest can be performed simultaneously. With the patient in a supine position, surgical rolls or sandbags are placed beneath the ilium to elevate the hip, raise the underlying bone to a more superficial level, and shift abdominal contents away from the donor site (Fig 13-1a). The anatomy is marked so that the surgical team can identify the iliac crest and tubercle, located approximately 6 cm posterior to the anterior iliac spine.[3] The incision site is marked 2 to 3 cm inferior to the iliac crest (Fig 13-1b). The skin incision (5 to 6 cm in length) begins 2 cm posterior to the anterior iliac spine.[2] This incision placement minimizes the risk of injury to the lateral femoral cutaneous and iliohypogastric nerves (Fig 13-1c). It is slightly inferior to the actual crest to avoid mechanical irritation of the scar postoperatively by tight clothing. The skin is tensed medially above the iliac crest by manually depressing the abdominal wall. An incision is made through skin, and the dissection is carried through subcutaneous tissue until Scarpa's fascia and the periosteum overlying the iliac crest are exposed (Fig 13-1d). At the iliac crest, the external abdominal oblique muscle and the tensor fascia lata muscle are attached; the incision to bone should not transsect these muscle fibers. The tensor fascia lata muscle originates from the external lip of the anterior iliac crest between the anterior superior spine and the tubercle.[3] It extends inferiorly as part of the lateral thigh and spans the hip and knee joints to insert on the lateral tibia and contracts in most walking movements. Improperly placed incisions that transsect muscle fibers and increase blood loss during the harvesting procedure cause inflammation and swelling that may be prolonged and affect the gait postoperatively.

Below the anterior iliac crest, the gluteal medius and gluteal minimus muscles originate on the lateral cortex, while the iliacus muscle originates on the medial cortex. The inguinal ligament attaches to the anterior-superior spine and the sartorius muscle and to the anterior-inferior spine (Fig 13-1e). The iliohypogastric nerve, which is a sensory nerve, passes over the area of the tubercle and is often affected during harvesting of bone from the anterior ilium. The lateral femoral cutaneous nerve (also sensory) is not close to the ilium proper but courses medially between the psoas muscle and the medial edge of the iliacus muscle.[2,3] It then courses deep to the inguinal ligament to pierce the tensor fascia lata muscle at the level of the lesser trochanter, innervating the skin in the lateral thigh. The surgeon should avoid dissection over the anterior iliac spine to minimize risk of injury to the lateral femoral cutaneous nerve. Maintaining a distance of 2 to 3 cm posterior to the anterior spine while harvesting also prevents potential fracture of the anterior iliac spine.

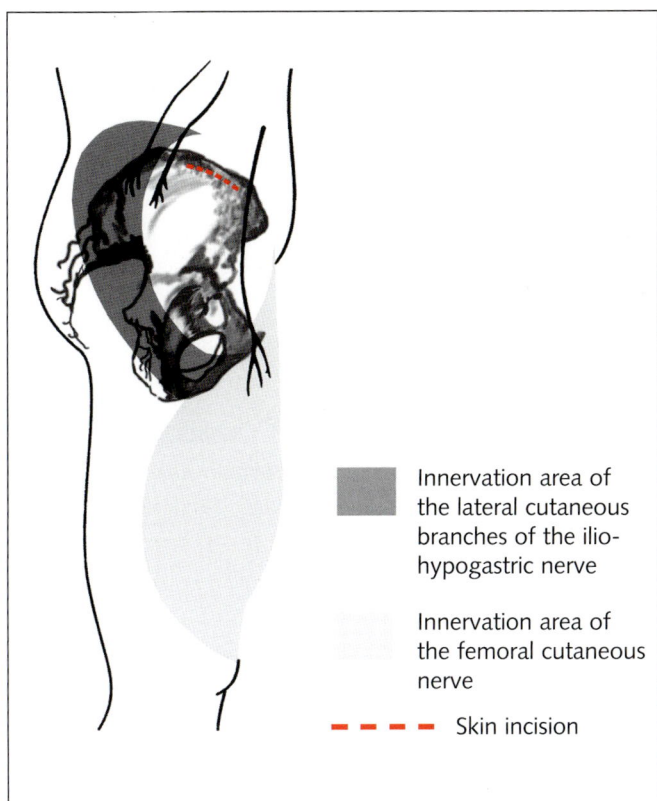

Fig 13-1c Placement of the incision line is designed to avoid injury to the sensory nerve distribution in the area.

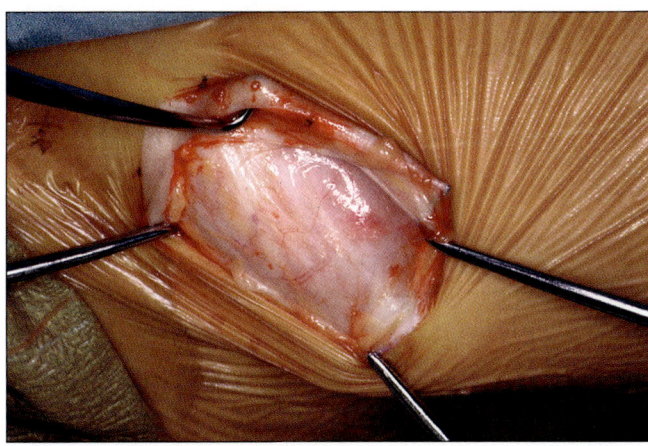

Fig 13-1d Dissection completed through skin and subcutaneous tissue, exposing Scarpa's fascia.

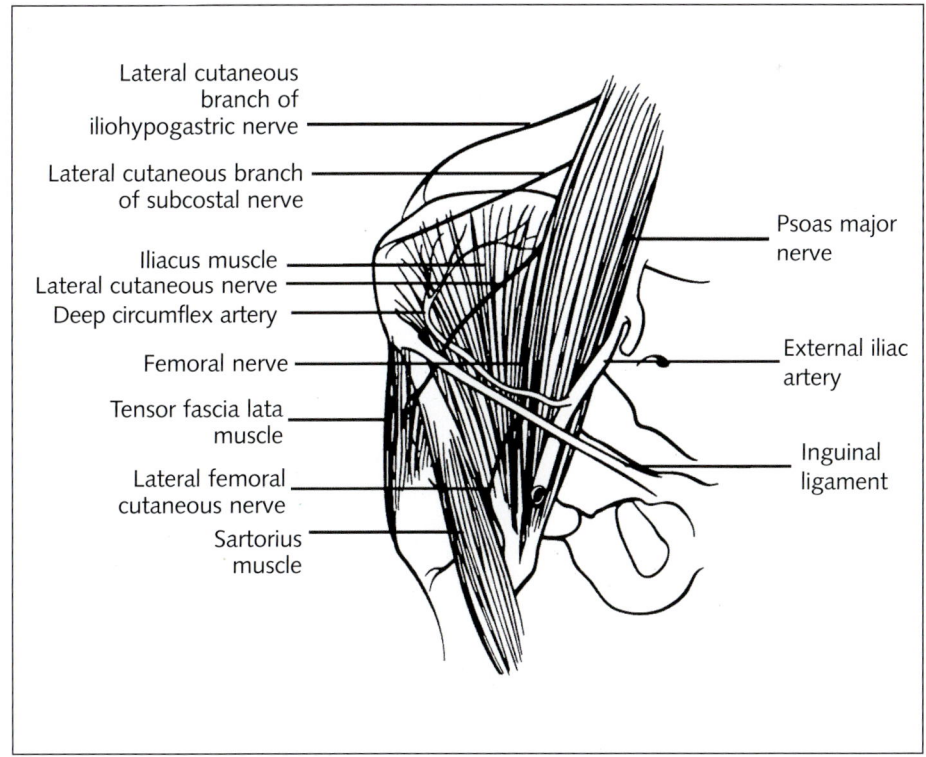

Fig 13-1e The iliohypogastric and lateral femoral cutaneous nerves are avoided during bone harvesting from the anterior ilium. To avoid fracturing the anterior iliac spine, harvesting should be limited to the area posterior to the anterior spine.[3]

chapter 13 Sinus Augmentation with Bone Harvested from the Ilium

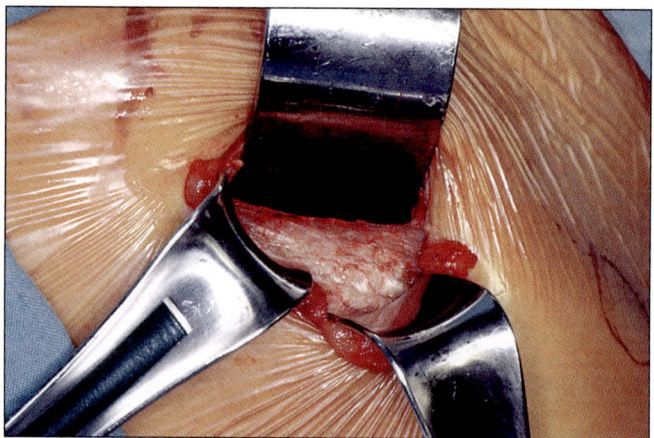

Fig 13-1f Exposure of the anterior iliac crest after dissection through Scarpa's fascia and the periosteum. The broad retractor is placed on the medial surface of the ilium subperiosteally.

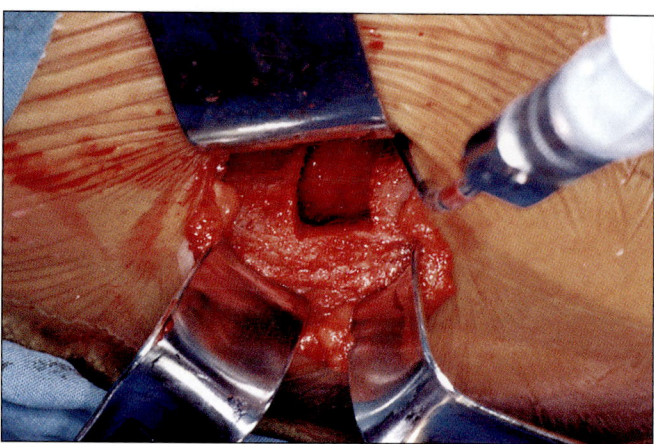

Fig 13-1g Anterior iliac crest donor site following removal of a 1 × 5 cm–block of corticocancellous bone. The lateral portion of the iliac crest is not violated.

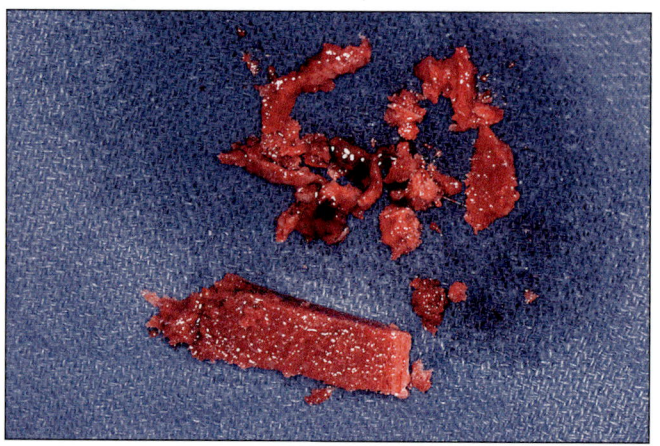

Fig 13-1h The anterior ilium will provide corticocancellous blocks of bone as well as a large volume of cancellous bone, depending on the needs at the recipient site.

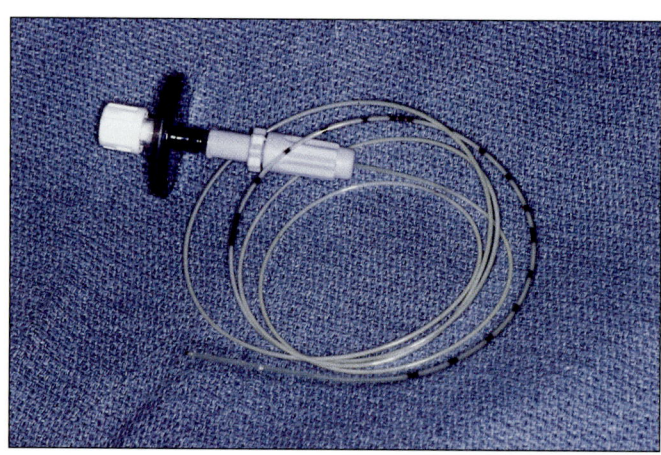

Fig 13-1i Epidural catheter with microporous filter and injection port. The catheter is placed in the iliac donor site for injection of local anesthetic at 4- to 6-hour intervals for a period of 48 to 72 hours after bone-harvesting surgery.

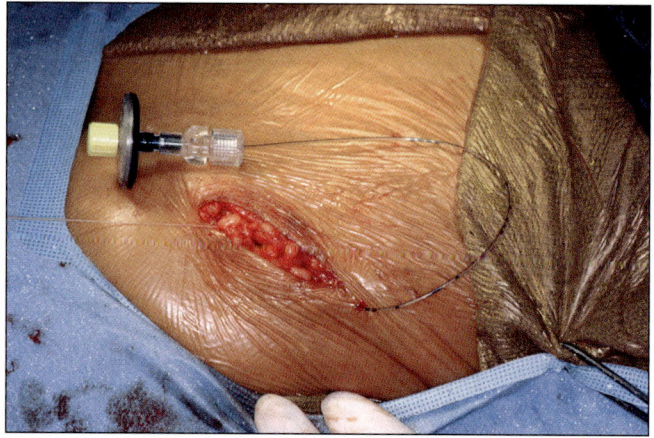

Fig 13-1j Closure of the anterior iliac crest donor site in layers after placement of the anesthetic catheter. Patients and their caregivers are trained to use the catheter during the early postoperative period.

Once the periosteum is exposed, the incision is made through the raphae between the iliacus and the tensor fascia lata muscles at the iliac crest. The incision through the periosteum allows exposure of the crest of the ilium (Fig 13-1f). For a medial approach, the iliacus muscle is reflected; for a lateral approach, a subperiosteal dissection is carried out beneath the tensor fascia lata. The surgeon must make every effort to stay within the periosteal envelope of the ilium to minimize bleeding and injury to the abdominal structures (should a medial approach be chosen). Although the lateral reflection of the anterior ilium is used by many surgeons, a medial dissection is preferred by others because it avoids reflection of the tensor fascia lata muscle and, therefore, causes the patient less difficulty in ambulation.[3]

The bony ostectomies depend on the surgeon's preference and the type of graft that is desired. For small quantities of bone, a so-called trap door or *Tschopp approach* to the anterior ilium allows cancellous bone to be harvested and minimizes the postoperative defect in the crest by repositioning the cortical crest.[3] After harvesting of particulate cancellous marrow, the elevated crest can be secured in place with either wire or sutures. Alternatively, corticocancellous blocks can be harvested from the medial table, leaving the lateral cortical table intact to maintain crestal contour and minimize bleeding and muscle injury. Several strips of corticocancellous blocks of varying width also can be harvested to a depth of 4 to 5 cm (Fig 13-1g). Particulate marrow can be harvested from the remaining exposed portions of the ilium by undermining the crest and anterior and posterior osteotomy sites that are exposed after removal of the corticocancellous blocks (Fig 13-1h).

Following the harvesting of bone, the wound should be inspected for bleeding and sharp bony edges. Particles or sheets of bovine collagen may be placed in the donor site to help control postoperative bleeding. Alternatively, if platelet-rich plasma has been used, the residual platelet-poor plasma can be placed in the wound as a hemostatic agent. Bone wax, another alternative hemostatic agent, is not preferred because of slower healing and occasional foreign body giant cell reactions. When large segments of bone are harvested, placement of allogeneic human cancellous chips of bone in the wound is recommended to aid iliac bone regeneration. These materials can be stabilized with platelet-poor plasma or a mixture of bovine collagen and blood. This is an excellent way to minimize dead space and avoid postoperative hematoma and seroma formation. When good hemostasis is achieved, a drain is not needed.

When closing the donor site, the surgeon should reapproximate the periosteum and muscle attachments and close the wound in layers. An analgesic catheter is frequently used, particularly with large harvests, to allow periodic administration of a long-acting local anesthetic in the postoperative period. For this technique, an epidural catheter is passed through the adjacent skin superior and slightly lateral to the skin incision. The catheter is attached to a bacteriostatic filter with an injection port so that local anesthetic can be administered (Figs 13-1i and 13-1j). After wound closure, a clear occlusive dressing is placed over the incision to allow the patient to shower or bathe in the postoperative period. Pressure dressings are placed over the site for the first 24 hours. The patient and escort should be provided with specific postoperative instructions. A walker is usually provided for the patient's use for the first few postoperative days. This provides safety against falling and/or injury to the opposite leg/hip.

Harvesting Bone from the Posterior Ilium

Bone harvested from the posterior iliac crest requires that the patient be placed in a prone position. Careful positioning of the patient is critical to avoid injuries to the genital area and the abdomen. Bolsters or sandbags are placed beneath the anterior ilium to position the posterior ilium superiorly for improved access. The area of harvest contains several sensory cutaneous nerves: the superior cluneal nerves originating from L1, L2, L3 and the middle cluneal nerves (S1, S2, S3). The superior cluneal nerves pierce the lumbodorsal fascia superior to the posterior crest and innervate the skin over the posterior middle buttocks (Fig 13-2a). The middle cluneal nerves emerge from foramina of the sacrum and course laterally to innervate the skin over the medial buttocks. An incision 5 to 8 cm long can be made over the posterior ilium depending on the quantity of bone needed. The incision follows a diagonal line from a cranial and medial position below, laterally crosses the posterior iliac crest, and avoids the gluteal branches of the middle and superior cluneal nerves (Figs 13-2b and 13-2c).[4] After the incision is made through skin, a blunt dissection is made to the posterior crest. An incision

chapter 13 Sinus Augmentation with Bone Harvested from the Ilium

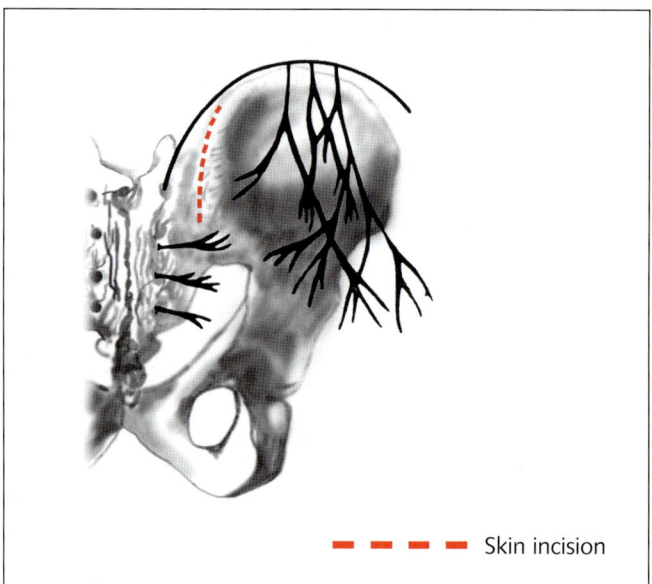

Fig 13-2a Posterior iliac incision site and the location of relevant sensory nerves.

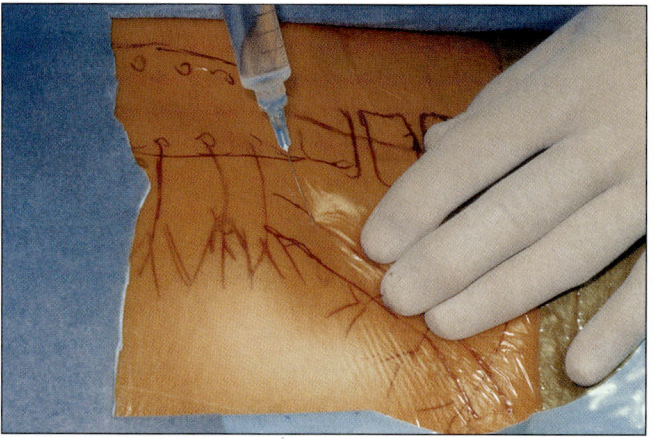

Fig 13-2b Crest, vertebrae, and ilium outlined on the skin and approximate location of superior and middle cluneal nerve branches. Local anesthesia is administered.

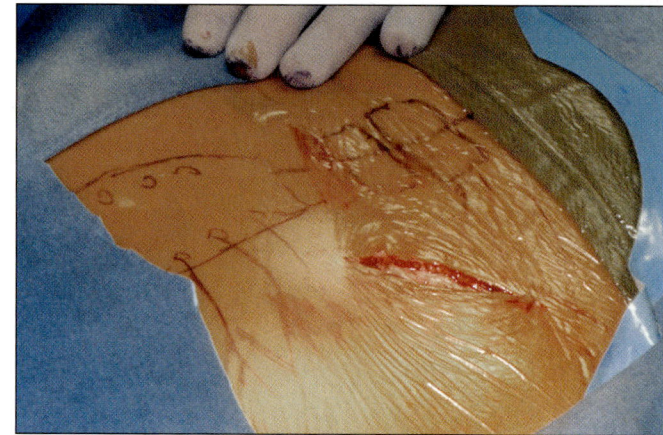

Fig 13-2c Curvilinear incision overlaying the posterior iliac crest minimizes damage to sensory nerves.

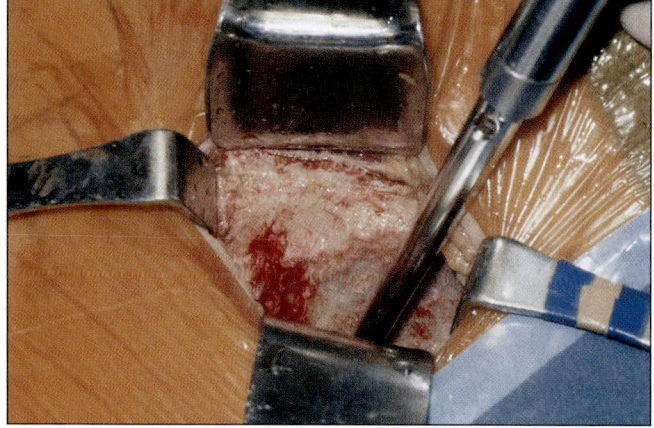

Fig 13-2d Lateral reflection of muscle to expose posterior iliac crest and lateral table.

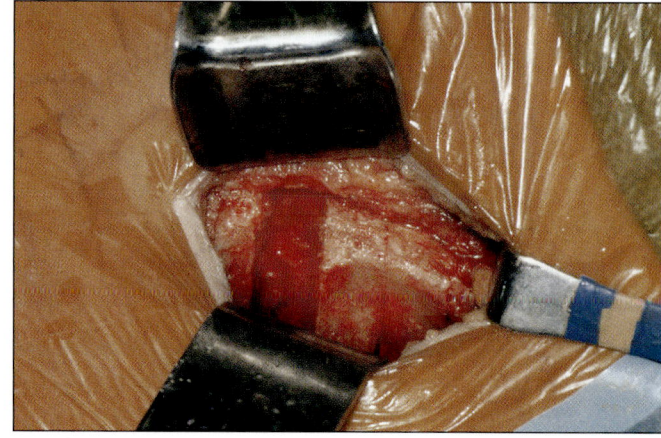

Fig 13-2e Harvesting of bone strips from the posterior lateral iliac crest.

directly over the crest, to bone, does not transsect gluteal muscle fibers. The gluteal muscles are dissected subperiosteally from their crestal attachments to expose the outer table of the posterior ilium. The lateral dissection should be continued, remaining within the periosteal envelope, reflecting periosteum both medially and laterally to expose the crest and lateral cortex for harvest (Figs 13-2d and 13-2e). The medial dissection is carried over the crest only far enough to identify the entire crest and to free periosteum for closure after harvesting of the lateral cortex.

The largest reservoir of cancellous bone is found beneath the insertion of the gluteus maximus muscle adjacent to the sacroiliac articulation. In the area of bone harvest, the posterior iliac crest beneath the gluteus maximus muscle has a well-defined, palpable bony prominence and a triangular area of insertion on the lateral aspect of the iliac wing.[3] The sacroiliac articulation lies medially and is not approached by the dissection because violation of this area may cause sacroiliac joint instability. The sciatic notch, and hence the sciatic nerve containing most of the motor innervation to the lower extremities, is located 6 to 8 cm inferior to the posterior crest. The surgeon should make every effort not to dissect inferiorly more than 5 cm to avoid injury to the sciatic nerve (ie, do not expose the sciatic notch). A posterior iliac approach allows harvesting of large segments of corticocancellous blocks as well as a large volume of particulate marrow. Blood loss is usually minimal, postoperative ambulation is improved, and pain is less than with the anterior approach.[4] The disadvantage of the posterior iliac approach is that it adds significantly to the duration of the procedure (1.5 to 2 hours) because surgery at the donor and oral recipient sites cannot be performed simultaneously. The patient must be repositioned on the operating table prior to the recipient site surgery.

Because the period between graft procurement and placement is prolonged, the graft should be kept moist in a cool environment until it is transplanted to the donor site.

Trephine Bone Grafts from the Ilium

For small grafts such as those needed for a single maxillary sinus or a smaller alveolar defect, often a series of trephines can be used to obtain adequate material from the iliac crest.[5,6] These commercially available instruments harvest an excellent quality and quantity of bone for such indications in cores ranging from 5 to 8 mm in diameter and up to 5 cm in length.[3,5,6]

Trephine bone harvesting can be carried out under local anesthesia with or without sedation. Local anesthesia is administered to the skin, subcutaneous tissue, and periosteum in the area of the ilium to be harvested. An incision is made down to the periosteum overlying the iliac crest (Fig 13-3a). A small portion of the periosteum is reflected to expose the underlying bone. The trephine is placed over the widest portion of the iliac crest and tapped approximately 6 mm into the crest. A 6-mm disc of cortical bone is harvested as part of the graft. The cylindrical osteotome is advanced into the cancellous bone by gentle tapping with a mallet to a depth of 4 to 5 cm to harvest a core of cancellous bone (Figs 13-3b and 13-3c). As many as three cancellous bone plugs can be harvested through a single cortical perforation by varying the angulation of the trephine (Fig 13-3d).

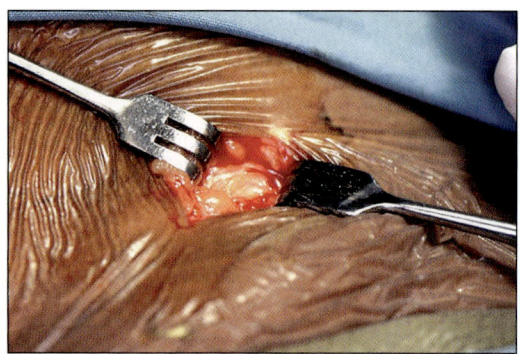

Fig 13-3a Limited incision to the anterior iliac crest for harvesting of trephine cores.

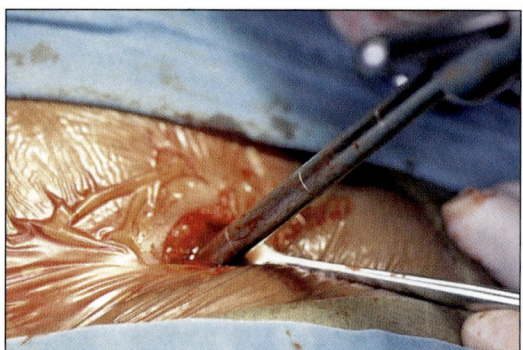

Fig 13-3b Exposure of the iliac crest allows easy access for obtaining trephine cores. Marks on the trephine allow the surgeon to gauge depth.

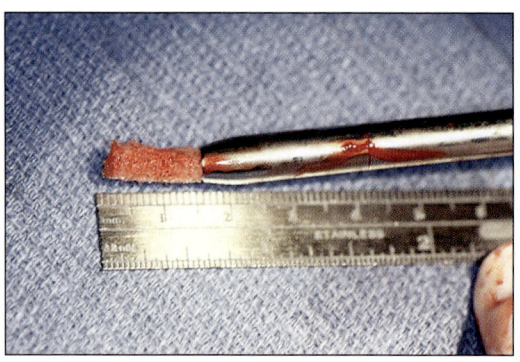

Fig 13-3c Trephine core harvested from the anterior iliac crest.

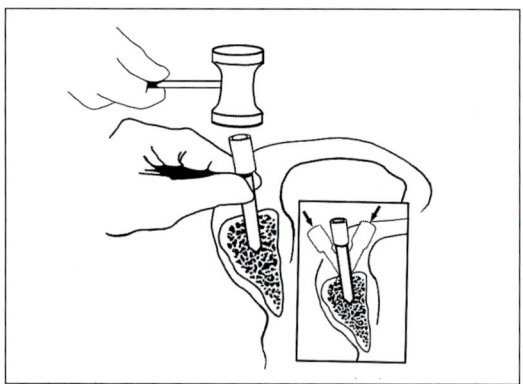

Fig 13-3d The trephine is redirected in several areas to obtain additional cores through a single entry site.

Maxillary Sinus Floor Grafting

Once autologous bone has been harvested from the ilium, it should be placed into the recipient site as soon as possible to maintain viability of the osteogenic cells. Clinical evaluation and imaging will guide the surgeon in choosing the mucosal and bony flap design for the recipient site. It is often advisable to elevate the sinus membrane before making the decision to use a particulate or corticocancellous block. In most cases, the membrane will be elevated intact or with minor tears that can be repaired; however, if the membrane is torn beyond repair, a corticocancellous block supplemented with particulate cancellous marrow should be used. The block graft can be stabilized with titanium bone screws if adequate alveolar bone for dental implants is not available. This decision should be based on the surgical anatomy, the status of the membrane, and the surgeon's preference. Delayed implant placement is preferred in most circumstances because the restorative requirements are more apparent after the graft has consolidated. Figures 13-4a and 13-4b present examples of a bone window and graft placement for stabilization of a corticocancellous block with dental implants. The implants effectively stabilize the block graft, and voids are filled with particulate cancellous marrow. The technical challenge of stabilizing the graft and simultaneously placing the implants should not be underestimated by those embarking on this technique. Consideration of the position and angulation of the implants required for prosthetic restoration must be balanced with the need for adequate residual alveolar bone to achieve initial implant stability.

In most circumstances, clinical and surgical findings allow for access to the sinus and elevation of the membrane to accommodate a particulate cancellous marrow graft (Figs 13-5a and 13-5b). It is important to protect the membrane

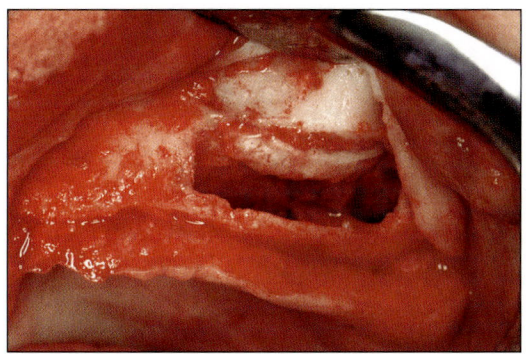

Fig 13-4a Elevation and infracture of the left maxillary sinus wall with sinus membrane for sinus floor grafting. The recipient area is ready for placement of the graft.

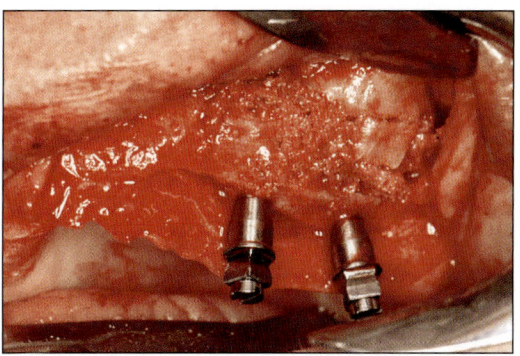

Fig 13-4b Placement of an autologous iliac corticocancellous graft and stabilization with two dental implants.

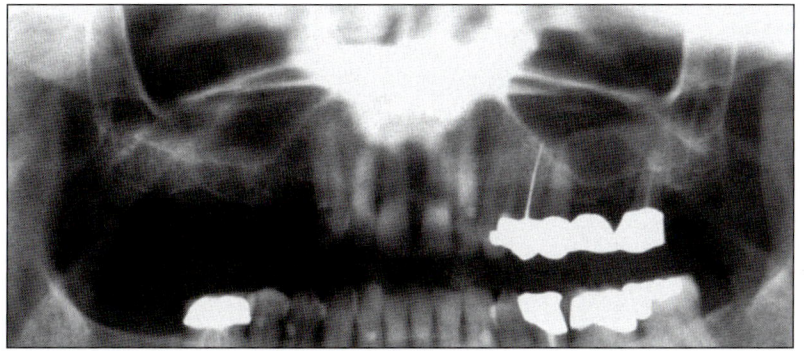

Fig 13-5a Preoperative panoramic radiograph showing edentulous space and pneumatized sinus in the right maxillary area.

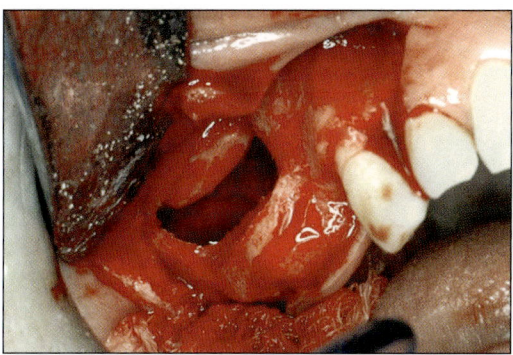

Fig 13-5b Infracture of sinus window in preparation for bone graft.

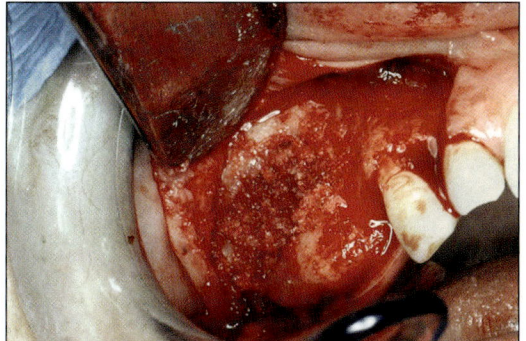

Fig 13-5c Placement of bone graft from anterior iliac crest into maxillary sinus floor.

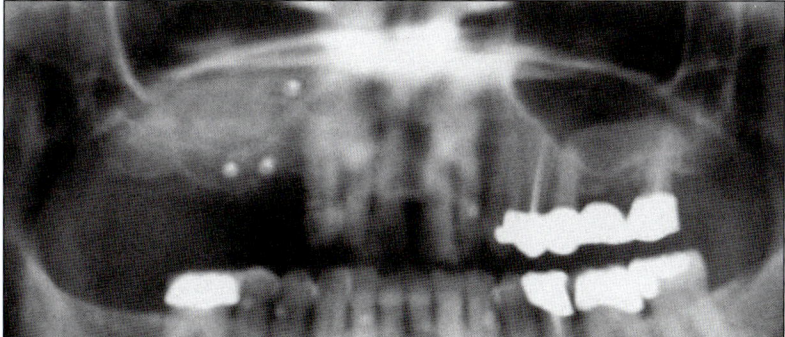

Fig 13-5d Postoperative panoramic radiograph showing the three miniature screws used to stabilize the barrier membrane.

during graft placement; the temptation to overpack the sinus, which could result in a loss of membrane integrity or obstruction of the sinus ostium, must be resisted (Fig 13-5c). Following graft placement, a barrier membrane can be placed over the access window to promote repair of the lateral maxillary wall. If there is sufficient graft to reconstruct the entire lateral maxillary wall, a membrane is not needed. However, if there are large voids surrounding the graft, then membrane placement will allow for an intact repair following consolidation of the graft (Fig 13-5d). Subsequently, implant placement and routine restorative procedures will complete the case (Figs 13-5e to 13-5h).

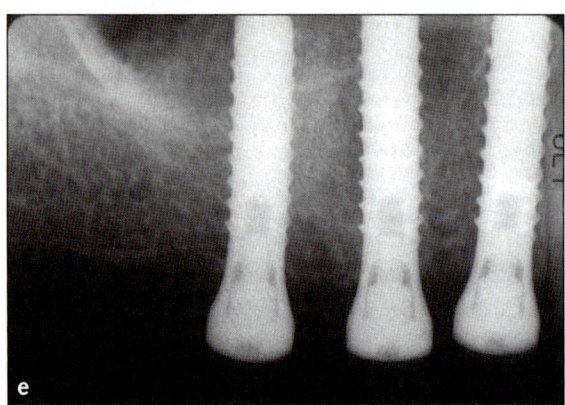

Fig 13-5e Implants placed in the grafted sinus floor.

Fig 13-5f Four months after grafting, a bone core specimen removed at the time of implant site preparation shows excellent bone growth.

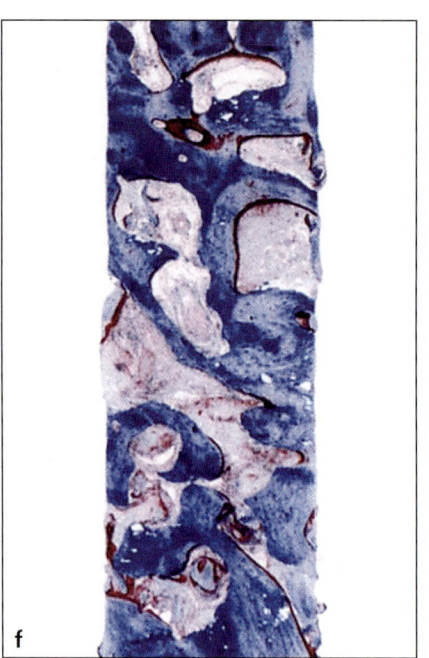

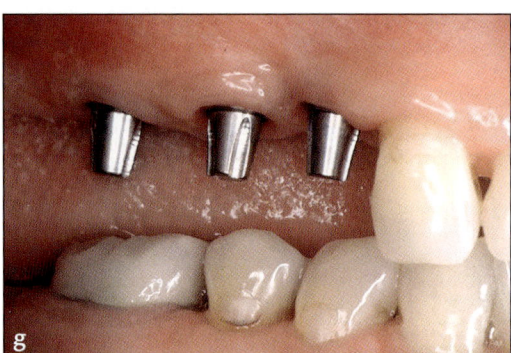

Fig 13-5g Abutments in place prior to final restoration.

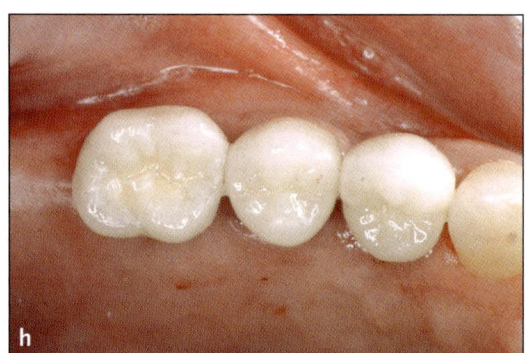

Fig 13-5h Occlusal view of the final restoration of three implants supported by a maxillary sinus floor bone graft harvested from the anterior iliac crest.

Clinical Experience

Ninety-two patients (30 men and 62 women; age range, 29 to 76 years) who received augmentation of the maxillary sinus floor with autologous bone from the iliac crest were included in this study. The criterion for inclusion was a subantral bone height less than or equal to 8 mm from the alveolar crest to the sinus floor in the area of the proposed implant site. In most instances, the subantral height was 5 mm or less. Altogether, they received 145 bone grafts to the maxillary sinus floor (Table 13-1). Patients who required additional augmentation of the subantral sites were counted as failures. An infracture technique (n = 31) and a modified Caldwell-Luc technique (n = 114) were used for access to the maxillary sinus floor. Data collection extended over a period of 12 years (1990–2002).

Early in the series, implants were used to stabilize block grafts; however, the procedure was technically difficult and often did not result in ideal implant positioning. Subsequently, implants were placed simultaneously with the graft if there was sufficient subantral bone to achieve pri-

TABLE 13-1 Classification of grafts by harvest site and type

Harvest type	Corticocancellous bone	
	Block (n = 33)	Particulate (n = 112)
Anterior iliac crest	25	79
Posterior iliac crest	8	24
Trephine	0	9

TABLE 13-2 Success rates for maxillary sinus floor augmentation with autologous iliac bone grafts

	No. placed	No. of failures	Success (%)
Autologous corticocancellous block and particulate grafts*	145	11	92.4

*38 bilateral, 107 unilateral

mary stability of the implants as well as adequate positioning for prosthetic construction. In these cases, at least 6 mm of residual subantral bone was required at the implant sites. A total of 122 implants were placed into the subantral sites simultaneously with autologous grafting. The augmentation was completed with particulate cancellous marrow condensed around the apical portion of the implant to ensure complete implant coverage.

The criteria for bone graft success were twofold: *(1)* radiographic evidence of bone augmentation compared with pregrafting images, and *(2)* stability of the new bone under functional loading. Criteria for implant success included *(1)* implant stability (nonmobility), *(2)* freedom from pain (in and out of function), *(3)* freedom from persistent peri-implant inflammation and infection, and *(4)* functional loading for more than 1 year. If the implant survived for more than 1 year yet the patient experienced pain and/or inflammation and infection, it was considered a failure. Data were evaluated statistically using Fisher's exact test for 95% confidence limits.

Results

Of the 145 autologous iliac grafts placed in 92 patients to augment the maxillary sinus floor, 92.4% were deemed successful (Table 13-2).

Implant success was evaluated for 370 implants placed in the grafted sites and followed over the period of observation. Of these, 122 implants were placed simultaneously at the time of bone grafting, and 19 failed for an 84.4% success rate. Of the 248 delayed implants placed, 18 failed for a 92.7% success rate. The pooled data for implant placement in the sinus floor grafts revealed a 10% failure rate (Table 13-3). These data were further evaluated for implant survival according to their surface characteristics (rough or smooth) (all implants were threaded) (Table 13-4). The surviving implants have been under functional load for a minimum of 2 years. Statistical analysis revealed that there was a difference in implant survival between those implants placed simultaneously with the autologous iliac bone graft in the maxillary sinus floor and those implants placed in a delayed fashion ($P < .05$). The implants placed in a delayed fashion were more successful than those place simultaneously with the graft (pooled data). A statistical difference also was found between the smooth-surfaced implants that were placed simultaneously with bone grafting and those that had delayed placement ($P < .05$). The smooth-surfaced delayed implants were more successful than the smooth-surfaced immediately placed implants. However, there was no significant difference between the rough-surfaced implants placed simultaneously and those placed after graft consolidation ($P > .41$) (see Table 13-4).

TABLE 13-3 Survival rate for implants placed in autologous (iliac) bone grafts to maxillary sinus floor (n = 370)

	No. placed	No. of failures	Success (%)
Simultaneous graft implant	122	19	84.4
Delayed implant	248	18	92.7
Total	370	37	90.0

TABLE 13-4 Survival rate of implants by surface characteristics

	No. placed	No. of failures	Success (%)
SMOOTH-SURFACED IMPLANTS			
Simultaneous graft implant	98	16	83.7
Delayed implant	188	14	92.6
Subtotal	286	30	89.5
ROUGH-SURFACED IMPLANTS			
Simultaneous graft implant	24	3	87.5
Delayed implant	60	4	93.3
Subtotal	84	7	91.7
TOTAL	370	37	90.0

Complications

Minor complications of iliac bone harvesting include superficial infection, seroma or hematoma formation, (transient) hyperaesthesia, and (short-term) irregularities of gait. Major complications include donor defect hernias, vascular injuries, nerve injuries, deep infections, deep hematomas, iliac wing fractures, permanent gait disturbances, and deep vein thrombosis.[3,4,7] These risks are minimized by a thorough understanding of the anatomy, meticulous surgery, good hemostasis, and careful reapproximation of the soft tissues in layers. Prophylactic antibiotics are indicated for the bone harvest to oral cavity graft procedure, but not necessarily when grafting to other extraoral sites. Postoperative analgesic requirements are minimized by the use of the anesthetic catheters previously described. The catheter is retained for 4 to 7 days. The patient and a family member are instructed in its use and supplied with syringes and a long-acting local anesthetic solution to inject into the catheter every 6 to 8 hours as needed. Ambulation within 24 hours is encouraged; the use of a walker is recommended until the patient is comfortable and stable.

Using techniques similar to those described in this chapter, Kessler et al harvested bone from both the anterior and posterior iliac crest.[4] They measured the quantity of bone harvested, the operating time (including trephine harvesting), and the donor site morbidity, comparing the anterior approach (n = 81) with the posterior approach (n = 46). The study included 65 males and 53 females ranging in age from 8 to 90 years. The mean operating time for the anterior approach was 35 minutes (range, 22 to 48 minutes). The mean operating time for the posterior approach was 40 minutes (range, 32 to 55 minutes). (In the authors' experience, these operating times are significantly shorter than expected for the techniques described in this chapter.) The mean volume of bone harvested from the anterior ilium was 9 cm^3 (mean, 5 to 25 cm^3) and from the posterior iliac crest 25.5 cm^3 (mean, 17 to 29 cm^3), which was less than the volumes harvested in the authors' series. Larger amounts of bone harvested from both sites may account for longer surgical times.

TABLE 13-5 Complications associated with harvesting of bone from the anterior (n = 81) and posterior (n = 46) iliac crest (Kessler et al[4])

Complication	Anterior (%)	Posterior (%)	Total (%)	p value
Seroma	1 (1.2)	3 (6.5)	4 (3.1)	
Hematoma	7 (8.6)	2 (4.3)	9 (7.1)	
Infection	1 (1.2)	0	1 (0.8)	
Hyperaesthesia	1 (1.2)	0	1 (0.8)	
Total	**10 (12.3)**	**5 (10.9)**	**15 (11.8)**	
Pain	57 (70.4)	15 (32.6)	72 (56.7)	< .001
Gait irregularities				
After 2 weeks	26 (32.1)	3 (6.5)	29 (22.8)	< .002
After 4 weeks	8 (9.9)	1 (2.1)	9 (7.1)	

TABLE 13-6 Complications associated with harvesting of bone from the anterior (n = 186) and posterior (n = 18) iliac crest (Triplett and Schow)

Complication	Anterior (%) Standard (n = 180)	Anterior (%) Trephine (n = 6)	Posterior (%)	Total (%)	p value
Seroma	10 (5.6)	0	1 (5.6)	11 (5.4)	
Hematoma	7 (3.9)	0	1 (5.6)	8 (3.9)	
Infection	1 (0.6)	0	1 (5.6)	2 (1.0)	
Neurosensory disturbance	4 (2.2)	0	0	4 (2.0)	
Deep vein thrombosis	2 (1.1)	0	0	2 (1.1)	
Total	**24 (13.3)**	**0**	**3 (16.7)**	**27 (13.2)**	
Pain					
w/o catheter (n = 61)	45 (25.0)	2 (33.3)	3 (16.7)	50 (24.5)	< .01
w/ catheter (n = 125)	28 (15.6)	0	1 (5.6)	29 (14.2)	
Gait irregularities					
After 2 weeks	21 (11.7)	0	2 (11.1)	23 (11.3)	< .001
After 4 weeks	5 (2.8)	0	0	5 (2.8)	

Kessler et al reported 15 complications (Table 13-5) for a complication rate of 11.8% (15/127). Complications were limited to those patients from whom the volume of bone harvested exceeded 17 cm³. A significant difference was noted between the anterior and posterior donor sites in the amount of postoperative pain and irregularities of gait experienced after 2 weeks. The bone harvested from the anterior site had a 70.4% incidence of pain compared to a 32.1% incidence of pain in the posterior site. Irregularities of gait after 2 weeks occurred in 32.1% of the patients who had surgery in the anterior and in only 6.5% of the patients who had posterior surgery. Marx[3] and others have reported similar complication rates associated with posterior versus anterior iliac bone harvesting.

The present authors observed a complication rate of 13.2% (27/204) (Table 13-6), excluding pain or gait disturbances. An 11.3% incidence of gait irregularity at 2 weeks and a 2.8% incidence at 4 weeks were found in our patients. There were no irregularities of gait in the trephine harvests. These results compare favorably with reports in the literature.[3,4]

Conclusions

The harvesting of autologous bone from the iliac crest for augmentation in the maxillofacial region is a well-established procedure. Complications at the donor site must be anticipated, however, and when they occur they must be recognized and resolved. The ilium offers cortical, cancellous, and corticocancellous bone in volumes sufficient for most indications in the maxillofacial area. The overall complication rate of iliac bone harvest, as reported by numerous authors, is approximately 12%. The use of an anesthetic catheter port to improve patient comfort during the postoperative period has been an outstanding addition to our techniques. Both the anterior and posterior approaches to the ilium are appropriate harvest sites that should be selected based on the quantity of bone that is needed. When a relatively small volume is required, the trephine technique is a rapid, easy, and efficient method for harvesting good-quality bone with excellent osteogenic potential. Both smooth-surfaced threaded and rough-surfaced threaded implants were successful in augmented sinuses when placement was delayed to allow graft consolidation. However, when placed simultaneously with the bone grafts, the smooth-surfaced threaded implants had a higher failure rate than when placement was delayed. No differences in success were found between simultaneous and delayed implant success with rough-surfaced implants. Our recommendation has generally been that a more predictable prosthetic placement can be achieved when the implants are placed secondarily after bone grafts have consolidated.

Acknowledgment

Statistics provided by Larry Bellinger, PhD.

References

1. Block MS, Kent JN. Simultaneous placement of hydroxyapatite-coated implants and autogenous bone grafts. In: Jensen OT (ed). The Sinus Bone Graft. Chicao, IL: Quintessence, 1999:129–143.
2. Nkenke E, Weisbach V, Winckler E, et al. Morbidity of harvesting of bone grafts from the iliac crest for preprosthetic augmentation procedures: A prospective study. Int J Oral Maxillofac Surg 2004;33:157–163.
3. Marx RE. Philosophy and particulars of autogenous bone grafting. Oral Maxillofac Surg Clinics North Am 1993;5:599–612.
4. Kessler P, Thorwarth M, Bloch-Birkholz A, Nkenke E, Neukam FW. Harvesting of bone from the iliac crest—Comparison of the anterior and posterior sites. Br J Oral Maxillofac Surg 2005;43:51–56.
5. Kinsel RP, Turbow MM. The use of a trephine biopsy needle to obtain autogenous corticocancellous bone from the iliac crest: Technical note. Int J Oral Maxillofac Implants 2004;19:438–442.
6. Shepard GH, Dierberg WJ. Use of cylinder osteotome for cancellous bone grafting. Plast Reconstr Surg 1987;80:129–132.
7. Kalk WW, Raghoebar GM, Jansma J, Boering G. Morbidity from iliac crest bone harvesting. J Oral Maxillofac Surg 1996;54:1424–1429.

chapter 14
Sinus Augmentation with Bone Harvested from the Calvarium

Jean F. Tulasne, MD

The cranial vault has always been a valuable site for the harvesting of bone grafts. Ease of harvesting, low morbidity, and a high success rate make calvarial bone grafts ideal material for the sinus floor.

Bone from the cranial vault was used as early as 1890 as part of an osteocutaneous flap by Konig[1] and Muller,[2] and the first autogenous cranial bone graft was performed by Dandy[3] in 1929. Tessier,[4] however, was the first to popularize the calvarium as a donor site for grafts used in cranial and facial reconstruction. Results of maxillary sinus grafting using cranial bone were first published in 1993.[5]

This chapter describes the outcome to date of the use of more than 1,000 bone grafts harvested from the calvarium to augment the sinus floor and alveolar process in a staged approach.

Criteria for sinus grafting included an alveolar bone height of 7 mm or less, inadequate bone density, and/or deficient alveolar width. Implant loading for each patient also was taken into account. In some cases, a bridge supported by three well-stabilized implants[6,7] (including a pterygomaxillary implant[6–8]) was considered as an alternative.

First-Stage Surgery: Reconstruction of the Maxilla

Alveolar-sinus reconstruction proceeded in four steps: *(1)* elevation of the sinus membrane, *(2)* harvesting of the cranial bone grafts, *(3)* grafting of the sinus floor, and *(4)* reconstruction of the alveolar ridge.

Patients received general anesthesia administered via orotracheal intubation. Before the grafting procedure, any dental or sinus pathosis was treated and resolved. A panoramic radiograph and a computerized tomography (CT) scan (coronal and axial views) (Dentascan, General Electric) were obtained preoperatively to ascertain the precise state of the sinuses, their walls, and, of particular interest, the floor.

The presence and localization of septa were noted. The patient was prepared, and a limited zone of the scalp (approximately 1.0 to 1.5 cm wide × 20 cm long) in the temporoparietal region was shaved.

chapter 14 Sinus Augmentation with Bone Harvested from the Calvarium

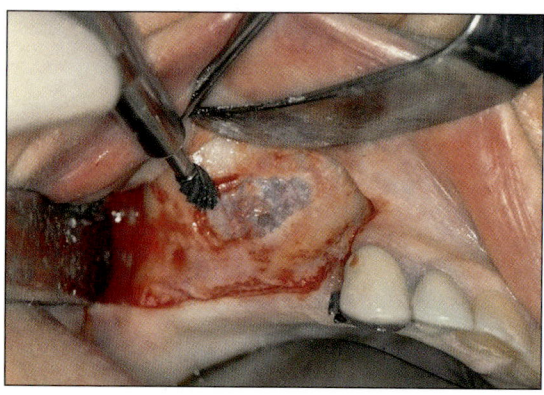

Fig 14-1a Exposure of the sinus mucosa through an anterolateral window.

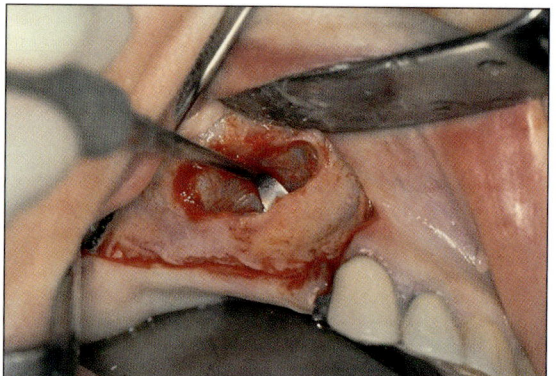

Fig 14-1b Elevation of the mucosa from the floor of the sinus cavity.

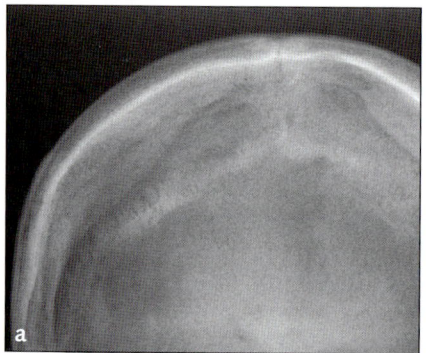
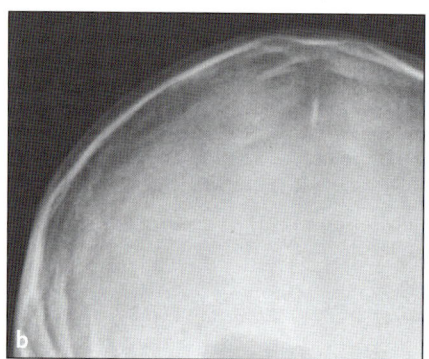
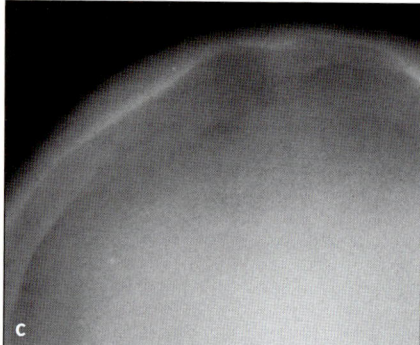

Figs 14-2a to 14-2c The thickness and density of the cranial vault varies considerably: (a) thick vault; (b) thin vault; (c) vault of variable thickness.

Dissection of the sinus floor

The anterolateral area of the maxilla is exposed, either by a vestibular incision or, preferably, by an incision on the alveolar crest that continues in the vestibule via one or two vertical releasing incisions, thus creating a pedicled mucoperiosteal flap. The latter approach allows for a more precise and direct reconstruction of the alveolar region. The flap is raised by sharp dissection close to the bone surface.

A wide window is subsequently made with a large bur in the anterior wall of the sinus until the sinus mucosa is exposed over a surface of approximately 2 cm^2 (Fig 14-1a). The mucosa is elevated by careful dissection, first from the lateral wall of the sinus cavity, then progressing to the entire floor, and finally by the medial and posterior walls (Fig 14-1b). If the sinus mucosa tears, the defect is gently contoured with the dissector to prevent further tearing.

The floor and lateral walls of the sinus are completely cleared of all epithelial and fibrous debris with a rasp.

Harvesting of the cranial bone grafts

The bone is harvested in the parietal region, in the nondominant hemisphere (generally the right side) behind the coronal suture and approximately 3 cm lateral to the sagittal suture or midline of the skull. (The sagittal suture is where the sagittal sinus is located, constituting a significant risk.) Preoperative skull radiographs are essential for determining the thickness and density of the vault, which varies greatly from one individual to the next (Fig 14-2). Generally, parietal bone is thin immediately behind the coronal suture but becomes progressively thicker as you move posteriorly.

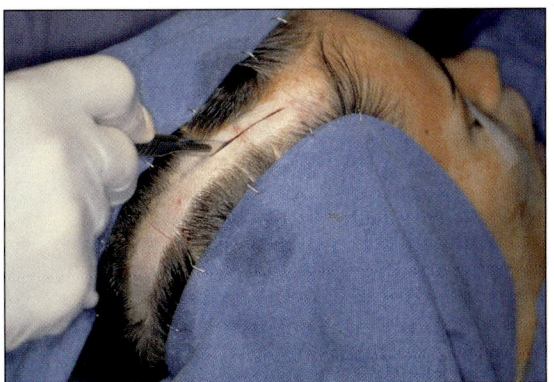

Fig 14-3a Incision of the scalp in the right parietal area.

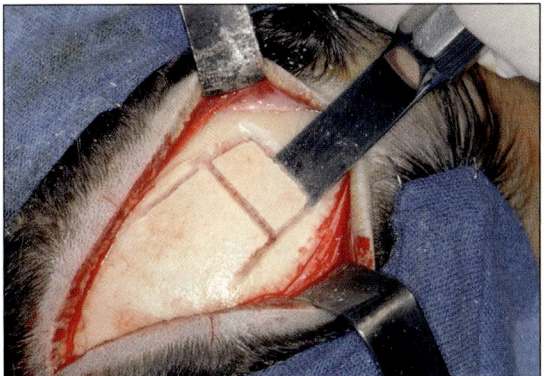

Fig 14-3b Splitting and elevation of rectangular (outer cortex) corticocancellous grafts.

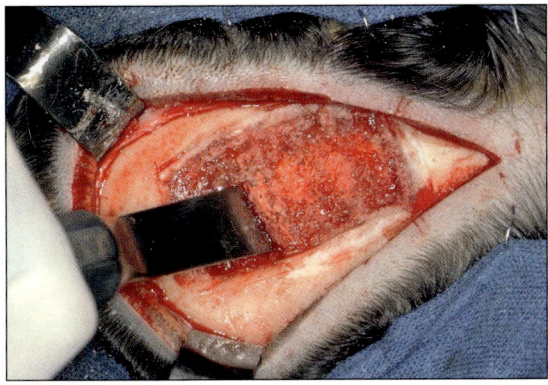

Fig 14-3c Harvesting of shavings of diploic bone with an osteotome.

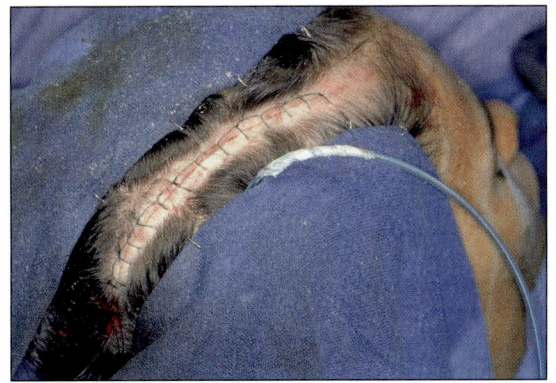

Fig 14-3d Scalp closure with suction drain.

The scalp incision is made along a parasagittal axis midway between the midline and the temporal crest, and it extends about 20 cm (depending on the quantity of bone needed) (Fig 14-3a). The incision should be full-thickness to the bone, which is subsequently exposed by raising the pericranium.

Outer table grafts are harvested as follows: The outline of the proposed donor site is traced with an oscillating saw held perpendicular to the skull, giving special attention to the internal (medial) limit of this zone. Each graft is then contoured, usually in the form of rectangular strips, each measuring approximately 45 × 15 mm. The groove created with the oscillating saw is deepened down to the diploë with a bur.

The outer edge of the groove is feathered to facilitate the introduction of an osteotome between the inner and outer cortices, within the diploic space and tangential to the surface of the vault. The splitting and elevation are done progressively, graft by graft, with a 10 or 15 mm straight osteotome. A narrower osteotome is used in the presence of brittle bone. When the splitting progresses toward the internal table, a slightly curved osteotome is used (Fig 14-3b). A minimum of three corticocancellous grafts and as many fragments or shavings of diploë as possible are harvested for one sinus (Fig 14-3c).

The peripheral edges of the donor site are beveled and smoothed, first with the osteotome and then with a large oval bur so that sharp bone edges will be less palpable through the scalp. The donor site is well irrigated, and hemostasis is usually unnecessary, although bone wax may be conservatively applied to areas of brisk bleeding (emissary veins). Any full-thickness defects are covered with the remaining bone chips, which are held in place with a single sheet of absorbable hemostatic gauze. Dural tears should be repaired and managed appropriately and require neurosurgical consultation. Scalp closure is accomplished in two layers after placement of a suction drain, and the area is then covered by a sterile drape that slightly compresses the region (Fig 14-3d).

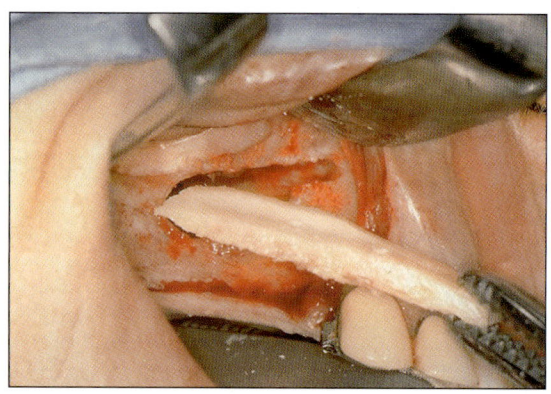

Fig 14-3e Insertion of the transmaxillary graft into the sinus.

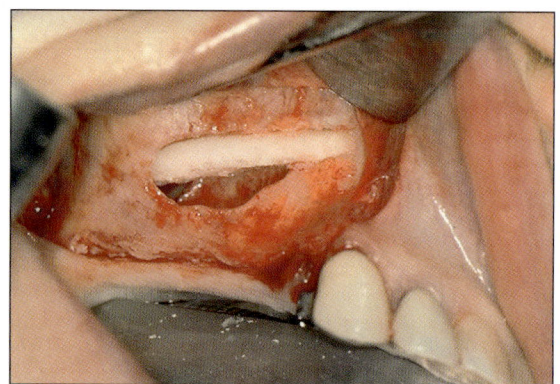

Fig 14-3f Stabilization of graft embedded in an anterior cutout notch.

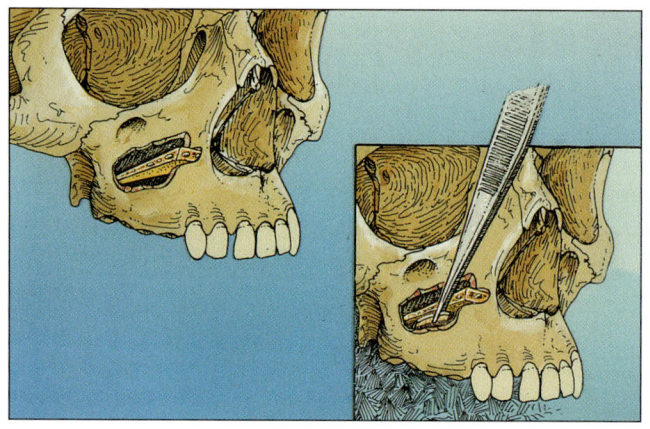

Fig 14-3g Transmaxillary graft in place. (*Inset*) Packing of the sinus with compressed bone fragments.

Grafting of the sinus floor

The sinus graft starts with the positioning of a large rectangular strut that is placed 10 to 15 mm above the sinus floor and is also used to aid in restructuring the alveolar process. Before its insertion, the cortical side of the graft is thinned with a bur, and several holes are made to facilitate revascularization. One end is shaped to a triangular point so that it can be lodged in an osseous trench that is chiseled into the posterior wall and extends to the pterygomaxillary suture. The strut is placed into the sinus (Fig 14-3e), the triangular end is gently forced into the posterior groove with a mallet, and the other end is embedded anteriorly into a notch made in the canine pillar (Fig 14-3f). In this manner, a perfectly stable foundation is established.

The unused portions of the grafts are milled into tiny fragments using the Tessier osseomicrotome or prepared for use in alveolar reconstruction. Corticocancellous bone fragments are placed beneath the inserted rectangular strut to fill the prepared cavity (Fig 14-3g). The volume of the cavity is generally between 10 and 15 cm^3. Bone fragments are tightly compressed into the space contained by the floor of the sinus below and by the transmaxillary graft above until it is completely filled and no dead space remains.

Reconstruction of the alveolar ridge

When alveolar reconstruction is required, a presurgical guide is made from the patient's denture to evaluate the degree of atrophy in both the vertical and horizontal planes. An antrostomy onlay alveolar graft is then placed *over* the antrostomy window and rests beneath the foundation of the transmaxillary graft. The "overgraft" is secured by one or two screws and is then perforated in several places to promote vascular invasion (Fig 14-3h).

For advanced atrophy of the alveolar ridge, a second graft is placed palatally. The cancellous sides of the two grafts are oriented toward each other and then affixed with screws and/or wires (Figs 14-3i and 14-4a to 14-4m).

First-Stage Surgery: Reconstruction of the Maxilla

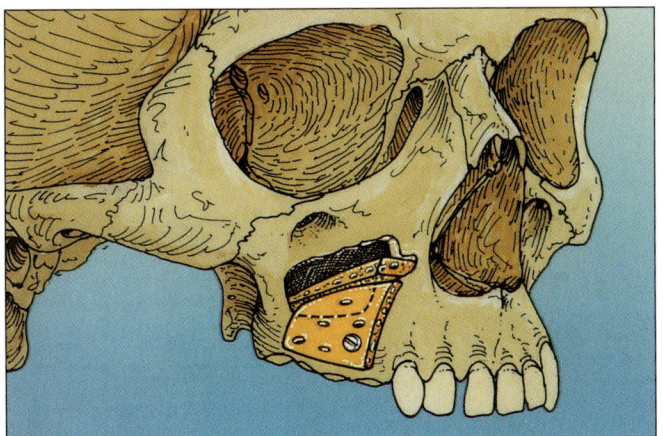

Fig 14-3h Onlay vestibular graft secured by one screw.

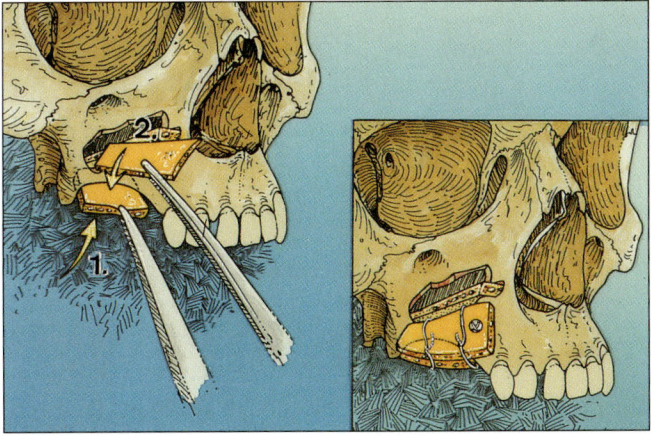

Fig 14-3i Ridge augmentation with fixation of two onlay grafts, one palatal and one vestibular. *(Inset)* Immobilization at the base of the maxilla by circumferential double metal wiring and one screw.

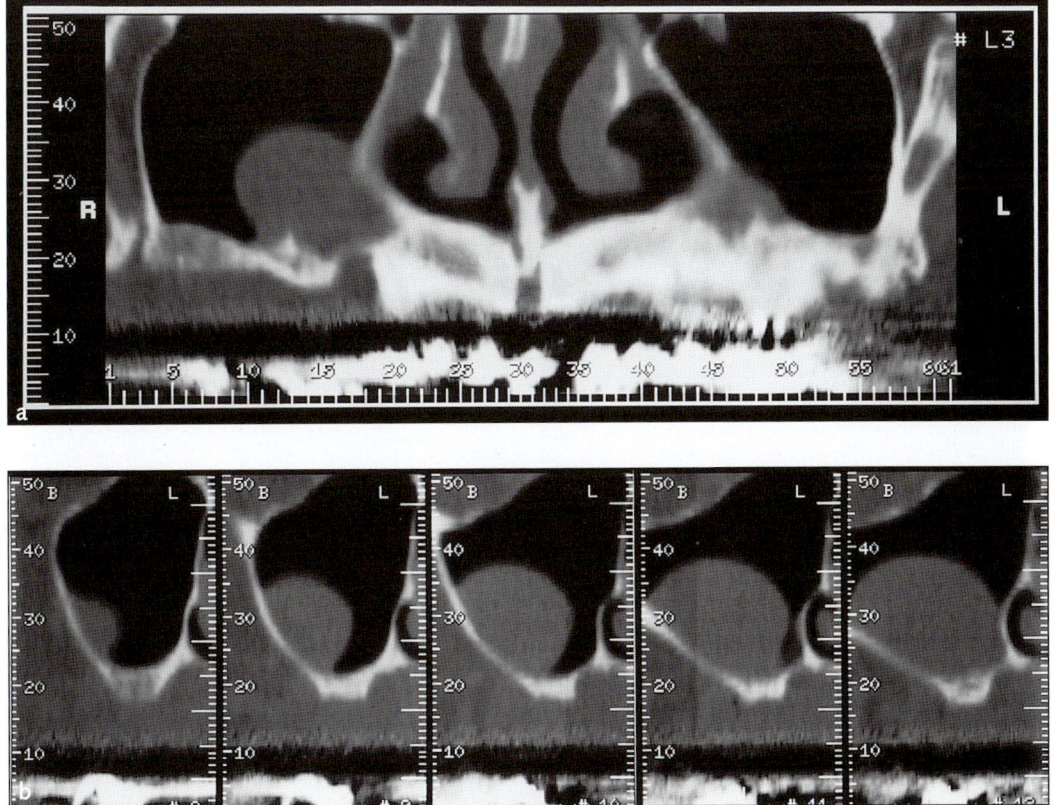

Figs 14-4a and 14-4b CT scans of patient missing the right second premolar and molars with atrophy of the alveolar ridge.

175

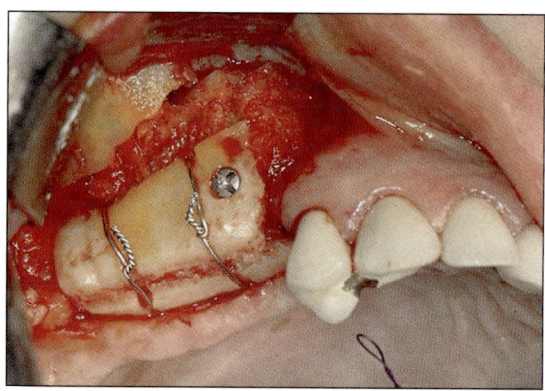

Fig 14-4c Sinus graft and augmentation of the alveolar ridge with two affixed onlay grafts, one palatal and one vestibular (see Fig 14-3i).

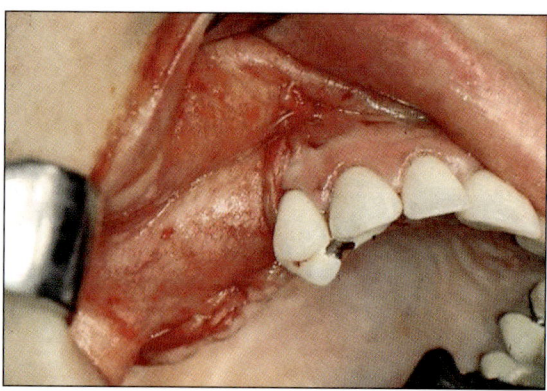

Fig 14-4d Appearance after closure of the vestibular flap. An abscess diagnosed 4 weeks later was treated by drainage under local anesthesia and antibiotic. Resolution of the infectious event was rapid. (The abscess was related to absorbable sutures.)

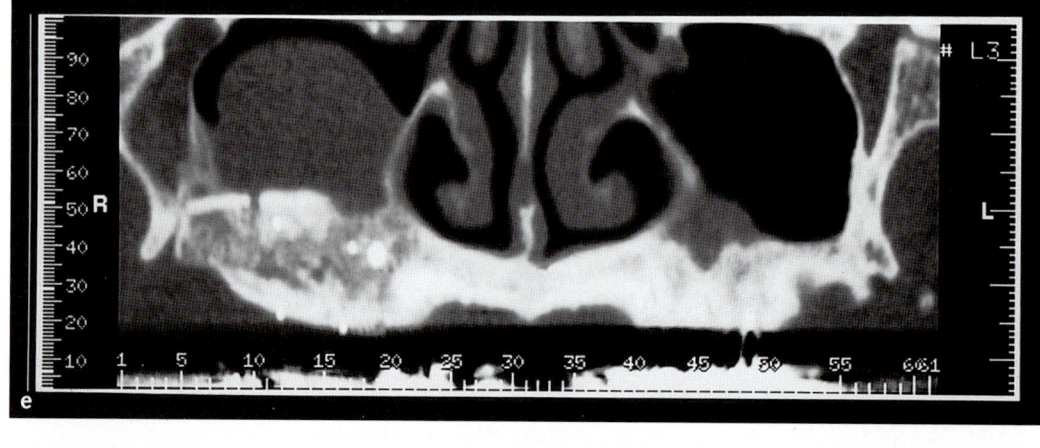

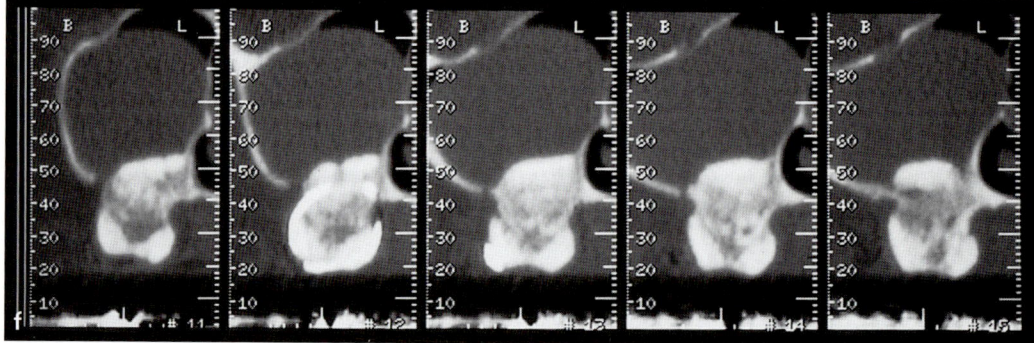

Figs 14-4e and 14-4f Appearance 7 months after surgery. The endosinusal cyst has progressed, but there are no signs of sinusitis either clinically or endoscopically.

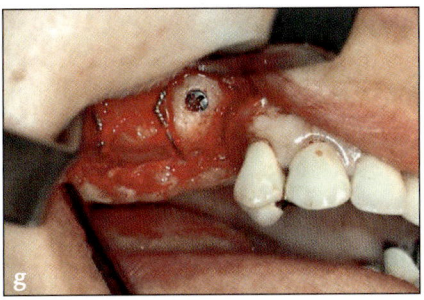

Fig 14-4g Exposure of the reconstructed area shows no resorption of the grafts at 7 months.

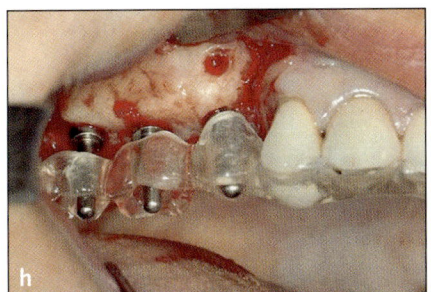

Figs 14-4h and 14-4i Placement of three Brånemark implants, all 10 mm in length.

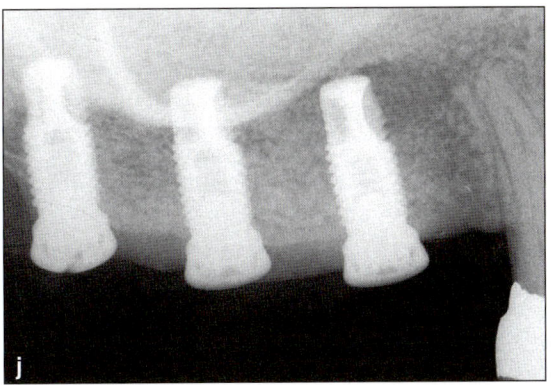

Fig 14-4j Osseointegration of implants at 6 months.

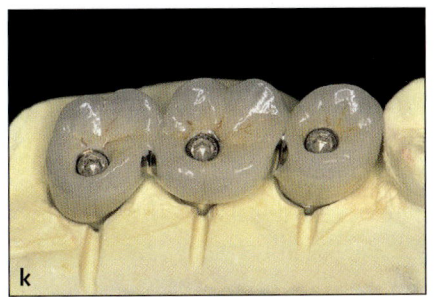

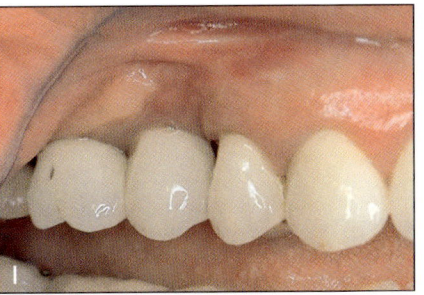

Figs 14-4k and 14-4l Prosthetic reconstruction (Dr Simonet, Paris, France).

Fig 14-4m A new prosthesis was constructed in 2004 (7 years after the sinus graft surgery).

The protruding edges of the bone graft are smoothed, and dead space is filled with fragments of diploë. The periosteum of the mucoperiosteal flap is then mobilized for coverage and suturing without tension. Finally, a pressure dressing is used to compress the area.

This alveolar reconstruction approach highlights the advantage of calvarial bone grafting: it provides bone mass equivalent to that of iliac block bone grafting, but without the microarchitectural tendency for substractive remodeling.

Postoperative period

The postoperative period generally passes with little or no morbidity, and the patient usually experiences minimal discomfort. The dressing and suction drain are removed the day after surgery, and at that time the patient's hair can be washed. The patient is released 1 day postsurgery with a 15-day antibiotic regimen. Edema of the scalp is virtually nonexistent, but there may be significant edema at the maxillary site. Sutures of the scalp are removed 10 days postsurgery. The partial denture is generally relined after 2 to 3 weeks.

Second-Stage Surgery: Placement of Implants

The second stage of treatment consists of the placement of implants. Implants are placed after a *minimum period of 3 months* following the calvarial grafting procedure, but only after the quality of the maxillary reconstruction has been verified by means of a CT scan.

Results

Implant survival

From 1990 to 1997, 249 implants were examined after at least 6 months of loading, and the overall retention rate was 94.8%. Five implants failed to osseointegrate. One had been placed in a very heterogenous zone of the sinus that probably consisted more of fibrous than osseous tissue. An infection developed 6 weeks after placement of an implant in another patient, but the implant was not removed because it was clinically stable at the time of drainage of the abscess. The implant later became mobile and was removed. Eight implants were lost after loading, six in patients presenting with severe bruxism (see chapter 7). In spite of these complications, prosthetic rehabilitation was accomplished in all patients according to the treatment plan. Since 1997, placement of the implants has generally been performed by other practitioners and has therefore not been followed.

Marginal bone loss

Radiographic evaluations every 12 months have shown no peri-implant bone loss.

Stability of the sinus bone graft

Density of the sinus bone graft is best evaluated with CT scan cross sections. CT scans of seven patients who received calvarial bone grafts revealed excellent stability of the reconstructed zones more than 5 years postsurgery (mean follow-up, 4 to 6 years).

Complications

Thirty-two patients presented with sinus infections that developed early (less than 2 months postoperative) in the healing period. One patient had a sinusitis that evolved subclinically. It was eventually diagnosed by CT scan 6 months postsurgery, necessitating removal of the cranial bone graft. The patient later underwent regrafting with cancellous bone from the iliac crest.

Two patients had vestibular abscesses at 4 and 6 weeks postoperative that were treated by incision and drainage. Healing was uneventful.

Another vestibular abscess developed 6 weeks after implant placement in a patient with a previously grafted sinus. Complete healing was obtained after drainage and sequestrectomy. One of three implants was lost.

Another patient presenting with a vestibular abscess underwent drainage under local anesthesia 4 weeks after the graft placement (see Fig 14-4d). Healing afterward was successful even in the presence of osteosynthesis hardware. A control CT scan obtained at 6 months showed a well-healed reconstruction (see Figs 14-4e and 14-4f).

During the past 3 years, 438 sinuses (269 patients) were grafted. Only one vestibular abscess (in a heavy smoker who resumed smoking on the seventh postoperative day) and necrosis of a very small part of the graft in another patient were observed, without serious damage to the sinus graft.

There was no relationship found between tearing of the sinus mucosa and a postsurgical sinus infection. There was one cranial complication: An epidural hematoma developed following a 1-cm^2 defect of the cranial vault, from bleeding in the immediate postoperative period. Immediate reoperation resulted in complete recovery after a few hours. No other complications (seroma, infection, or dural tears) were encountered at the donor site, although a few patients complained of scalp depression or skull irregularity.

Discussion

Rationale for using calvarial grafts

Autogenous bone is a safe and reliable graft material for reconstructive skeletal surgery. Among the donor sites currently used in facial surgery, the cranial vault has been preferred by many surgeons, including Tessier (who popularized the procedure),[4] since the early 1980s. Among its advantages are the simplicity of harvesting the graft, the near absence of patient discomfort during the postoperative period, and most importantly, the high density and low resorption of the reconstruction, resulting in long-term stability (see Figs 14-4a to 14-4m).

Experimental studies confirm that calvarial bone grafts have a better retention of the graft[9] and more than twofold the radiographic density compared with iliac crest bone grafts.[10] Moreover, membranous bone has been shown to resorb less readily than endochondral bone.[11,12]

Although these differences correlate with the embryonic origin of the bone, the reason for increased retention of calvarial graft remains unclear. It has been suggested that because of early revascularization of the membranous bone (calvarial graft), as demonstrated by Zins and Whitaker[12] and then by Kusiak et al,[13] a greater percentage of the graft is preserved as living bone. However, experimental studies[14] have conversely demonstrated that revascularization of cancellous bone, particularly that taken from the iliac crest,[15] is greater and more rapid than that taken from the cranium.

Hardesty and Marsh[9] hypothesized that the differences observed in graft resorption and incorporation were directly related to the three-dimensional osseous architecture of the graft. With earlier vascular penetration made possible in the rather loose, abundant cancellous portion of iliac bone, as compared to the dense and relatively thin diploic space of calvarium, osteoclastic resorption may be more pronounced, thereby allowing inward collapse of the iliac cortical plate. This architectural explanation was reinforced by the experimental studies of Sullivan and Szwajkun,[15] which showed that cortical bone does appear to be a barrier to vessel ingrowth. Moreover, the relatively thin cortical plate of the iliac graft is probably more susceptible to resorption prior to appositional bone formation than the more robust calvarial graft.[9]

To summarize, calvarial bone is considered better able to retain its volume because it is predominantly cortical. Nevertheless, as suggested by Hardesty and Marsh,[9] it must be remembered that "current concepts of bone graft survival are largely based on clinical observations and extrapolations from non-primate animal experimentation."

Osseointegration in calvarial grafts

There are only a few reports in the literature of dental implants inserted into cranial grafts. Donovan et al[16] report on 93 Brånemark implants placed in 24 patients reconstructed with calvarial bone grafts. Reconstruction was limited to the alveolar ridge and the nasal floor, without opening the sinus. They achieved various success rates (86% to 98%), depending on the type of reconstruction. A vertical grafting technique with delayed implant placement had an 86% success rate in 13 patients who had 50 implants placed. A horizontal grafting technique with immediate implant placement (43 implants in 13 patients) had a success rate of 98%. Two patients had a combination of grafting techniques.[16]

Jensen and Sindet-Pedersen[17] report a 94.5% success rate in severely atrophied maxillary alveolar ridges reconstructed with bone grafts from the mandibular symphysis. These cortical grafts respond in a manner comparable to calvarial bone when placed on the sinus floor. Zerbib[18] has reported a failure rate of 22 of 530 implants placed in sinus grafts of iliac or cranial origin.

Similarly, Daelemans (personal communication, 1997) and Malevez (personal communication, 1997) have observed excellent integration of implants placed into sinuses grafted with calvarial or iliac bone. Comparable results have been obtained with both iliac and cranial bone grafts, with no significant late-term resorption found on the CT scan at 5 years.

Lenzen et al[19] reported on augmentation of the maxilla and mandible with calvarial bone grafts in 63 patients. After 1 year, the resorption rate was approximately 10%, with no resorption occurring between 6 and 12 months after augmentation. The resorption rate was low and constant around the 32 implants placed in 12 patients.

Orsini et al[20] took biopsies 4 months after maxillary augmentation with calvarial onlay grafts in two patients, at the time of implant placement. Histologic and histomorphometric studies demonstrated living bone well-incorporated into the pre-existing bone. Implants were loaded at 5 months and well-integrated after 15 months of function.

Le Lorc'h-Bukiet et al[21] examined 24 bone specimens of the sinus 10 months after grafting with cranial bone. The boundary between new bone and the recipient bed was indiscernible. The grafted particles were incorporated in new bone and almost completely resorbed.

Iizuka et al[22] observed minimal bone resorption after alveolar ridge reconstruction with calvarial split bone in 13 patients. The mean follow-up time was 19.6 months. None of the 42 dental implants placed into the bone grafts was lost.

Advantages of calvarial bone grafts

The greatest surgical advantage of cranial bone is its high rate of success in the reconstruction of the alveolar ridge. This is where the cranial bone harvest is justified (see Fig 14-4i). Although intrasinus iliac bone also retains mass (the essential difference being in the density), it does not respond as well as cranial bone when placed on the alveolar crest. A significant degree of resorption of onlay iliac grafts is a common finding. On the other hand, resorption of cranial bone grafts is usually minimal, comparable to that of cortical bone harvested from the chin.

Cranial bone grafts offer distinct advantages for combined alveolar and sinus reconstruction (see chapter 21). A high-quality reconstruction as well as a relatively low incidence of postsurgical morbidity is promoted by calvarial bone. Indeed, the donor site is relatively pain-free and exhibits minimal local reaction, which is not the case with oral or iliac crest harvest sites.

All patients treated by Donovan et al[16] who answered a questionnaire reported experiencing no pain from the cranial harvest site.

Disadvantages of calvarial bone grafts

Cranial bone harvesting requires the use of general anesthesia and somewhat weakens the cranial vault. If the amount of bone needed is limited, an alternative is to harvest from the chin, which can be accomplished under local anesthesia. Patients presenting with advanced baldness will benefit from filling the donor site with acrylic implant to avoid visible deformation of the parietal region. This type of implant is perfectly tolerated, and the scar is not visible.

Although harvesting of bone from the calvarium is not difficult, it requires special training to avoid major complications such as those described by Cannella and Hopkins[23] and Frodel et al.[24] From a multicenter study in which more than 13,000 cranial bone grafts were harvested, Kline and Wolfe[25] identified seven temporary and four permanent neurologic complications, all of which (except for three temporary deficits) took place in patients treated by surgeons who had little or no experience in this field.

To avoid exposing or tearing the dura, it is important to evaluate the thickness of the cranial vault before proceeding. Pensler and McCarthy[26] measured skull thickness on 200 fresh adult cadavers. The mean value was a little more than 7 mm, with maximum thickness found in the posterior parietal region. Two or three frontal teleradiographs with different views allow a direct measurement of the thickness and the localization of irregularities. If the cranial vault is too thin or made purely of cortical bone (no diploic space), which is rare, another harvest site (eg, the iliac crest) should be chosen.

Finally, the extreme cortical nature of calvarial bone can compromise healing of the graft, especially if the volume of the graft exceeds the body's capacity to revascularize it. Tessier[4] observed cases of sequestration of the central portion of otherwise well-vascularized bone grafts. He hypothesized that no part of a graft should be located more than 10 mm from recipient bone (see chapter 24). It is likely that the complications observed in two of the patients in the present study were related to excessively large bone grafts. In addition to a prosthetic work-up, the specific amount of bone augmentation required should be based on local and anatomic conditions of the patient, the experience of the surgeon, and the physiologic distance to the recipient bed.

Two-stage approach

The risk of losing not only dental implants but also the bone graft in the event of infection is sufficient reason to delay implant placement. A two-stage approach enables the surgeon to assess the quality of the reconstruction clinically and radiographically prior to placement of implants. This is a safe and conservative course and more likely to achieve orthoalveolar form. Moreover, it is technically and physiologically dangerous to consider simultaneous placement in complex cases. When there is primary stabilization of the implants, a combined approach is justified. But even in this situation, implants cannot occupy an ideal axial position because of alveolar atrophy. For this reason, it is often preferable to reconstruct first, then place implants in the most favorable alveolar position, waiting only *3 months* between the two surgeries, as implants seem to stabilize the bone and thus prevent additional resorption.

Conclusion

Reconstruction of the sinus floor and resorbed alveolar ridge with calvarial bone has proven to be a safe and reliable procedure. The major advantages of harvesting bone from the calvarium is the lack of donor site morbidity, the large quantity of available bone, the high density (quality) of the healed graft, the relatively low incidence of resorption when bone is placed on the alveolar crest, and the short hospitalization required compared to harvesting from the iliac crest. However, calvarial harvesting must be reserved for those with surgical experience who have received appropriate training and work in consultation with a neurosurgeon.

Acknowledgments

I am greatly indebted to Dr Jose Mario Camelo Nunes for collecting the data and to Dr Caroline Plamondon for reviewing the French manuscript and translating it into English. I also express gratitude to my medical artist, Mrs Merri Scheitlin, for her excellent drawings, and to Dr Alain Lacan for the follow-up CT scans of my patients.

References

1. Konig F. Der knocherne Ersatz grosser Schadeldefekte. Zentralbl Chir 1890;17:497.
2. Muller W. Zur Frage der temporanen Schadelresektion an Stelle der Trepanation. Zentralbl Chir 1890;17:65.
3. Dandy WE. An operative treatment for certain cases of meningocele (or encephalocele) into the orbit. Arch Ophthalmol 1929;2:123.
4. Tessier P. Autogenous bone grafts taken from the calvarium for facial and cranial applications. Clin Plast Surg 1982;9:531.
5. Tulasne J-F, Saade J, Riachi A. Greffe osseuse du sinus maxillaire et implants de Brånemark. Implant 1993;May:101–114.
6. Tulasne J-F. Osseointegrated fixtures in the pterygoid region. In: Worthington P, Brånemark P-I (eds). Advanced Osseointegration Surgery: Applications in the Maxillofacial Region. Chicago: Quintessence, 1992:182–188.
7. Tulasne J-F. Implant treatment of missing posterior dentition. In: Albrektsson T, Zarb G (eds). The Brånemark Osseointegrated Implant. Chicago: Quintessence, 1989:103–115.
8. Tulasne J-F. Implants pterygo-maxillaires. Experience sur 7 ans. Implant 1992;Oct:39.
9. Hardesty RA, Marsh JL. Craniofacial onlay bone grafting: A prospective evaluation of graft morphology, orientation, and embryonic origin. Plast Reconstr Surg 1990;85:5.
10. Donovan MG, Dickerson NC, Hellstein JW, Hanson LJ. Autologous calvarial and iliac onlay bone grafts in miniature swine. J Oral Maxillofac Surg 1993;51:898.
11. Smith JD, Abramson M. Membranous vs. endochondral bone autografts. Arch Otolaryngol 1974;99:203.
12. Zins JE, Whitaker LA. Membranous versus endochondral bone: Implications for craniofacial reconstruction. Plast Reconstr Surg 1983;72:778.
13. Kusiak JF, Zins JE, Whitaker LA. The early revascularization of membranous bone. Plast Reconstr Surg 1985;76:510.
14. Albrektsson T. Repair of bone grafts. A vital microscopic and histological investigation in the rabbit. Scand J Plast Reconstr Surg 1980;14:1.
15. Sullivan WG, Szwajkun PR. Revascularization of cranial versus iliac crest bone grafts in the rat. Plast Reconstr Surg 1991;87:1105.
16. Donovan MG, Dickerson NC, Hanson LJ, Gustafson RB. Maxillary and mandibular reconstruction using calvarial bone grafts and Brånemark implants: A preliminary report. J Oral Maxillofac Surg 1994;52:588.
17. Jensen J, Sindet-Pedersen S. Autogenous mandibular bone grafts and osseointegrated implants for reconstruction of the severely atrophied maxilla: A preliminary report. J Oral Maxillofac Surg 1991;49:1277.
18. Zerbib R. Greffes osseuses autogenes en chirurgie pre-implantaire. Rev Odontol Stomatol 1996;25:437.
19. Lenzen C, Meiss A, Bull HG. Augmentation of the extremely atrophied maxilla and mandible by autologous calvarial bone transplantation [in German]. Mund Kiefer Gesichtschir 1999;3(Suppl 1):S40–S42.
20. Orsini G, Bianchi AE, Vinci R, Piattelli A. Histologic evaluation of autogenous calvarial bone in maxillary onlay bone grafts: A report of 2 cases. Int J Oral Maxillofac Implants 2003;18:594–598.
21. Le Lorc'h-Bukiet I, Tulasne J-F, Llorens A, Lesclous P. Parietal bone as graft material for maxillary sinus floor elevation: Structure and remodelling of the donor and recipient sites. Clin Oral Implants Res 2005;16:244–249.
22. Iizuka T, Smolka W, Hallermann W, Mericske-Stern R. Extensive augmentation of the alveolar ridge using autogenous calvarial split bone grafts for dental rehabilitation. Clin Oral Implants Res 2004;15:607–615.

23. Cannella DM, Hopkins LN. Superior sagittal sinus laceration complicating an autogenous calvarial bone graft harvest: Report of a case. J Oral Maxillofac Surg 1990;48:741.
24. Frodel JL, Marentette LJ, Quatela VC, Weinstein GS. Calvarial bone graft harvest. Techniques, considerations, and morbidity. Arch Otolaryngol Head Neck Surg 1993;119:17.
25. Kline RM, Wolfe SA. Complications associated with the harvesting of cranial bone grafts [discussion by Paul Tessier]. Plast Reconstr Surg 1995;95:5.
26. Pensler J, McCarthy JG. The calvarial donor site: An anatomic study in cadavers. Plast Reconstr Surg 1985;75:648.

chapter 15
Safety and Efficacy of Bone Allograft for Sinus Grafting

Laureen Langer, DDS
Burton Langer, DMD, MSD
James T. Mellonig, DDS, MS

Since the introduction of the sinus elevation technique, autogenous bone has been the grafting material of choice for clinicians worldwide. However, allograft also has been used successfully for many years by many clinicians for a wide variety of situations. Allograft offers the means to repair and augment lost bone in many applications without the need to harvest autogenous bone from a secondary site. Approximately 350,000 to 400,000 bone allograft procedures are performed annually in the United States. Of these, about 100,000 are dental-related and involve the use of allograft in freeze-dried or mineralized form. The use of cadaver bone for bone grafting is avoided in much of the world despite the fact that in the 25 years that this material has been in use in its freeze-dried form, there have been no incidents of disease transfer reported to date.

The use of allogenic bone for the sinus floor graft is now in its third decade and is the subject of this chapter, but first a thorough discussion of safety is warranted, because safety trumps efficacy.

Safety of Freeze-Dried Bone Allograft

The possible transmission of infectious diseases by the transplantation of contaminated tissue is an overriding concern of clinicians and patients alike. Viral, bacterial, and fungal infections have been transmitted via a variety of tissue allografts, such as bone, skin, cornea, heart valves, whole organs, blood, and semen.[1,2] The most widely discussed infectious diseases are HIV, hepatitis B virus (HBV), hepatitis C virus (HCV), bacterial infection, and the agent or "prion" responsible for Creutzfeldt-Jakob disease (CJD); these diseases form the basis for concern in the dental and medical communities, as well as in the media.[3] Over the past decade, improvements in donor screening criteria—such as excluding potential donors who either have an infection or engage in behaviors that place them at risk for HIV-1 and hepatitis infection—and the introduction of new donor blood tests have significantly reduced the risk of transmitting HIV or hepatitis and have nearly eliminated the risk of transmitting CJD.

The transfer of disease from bone allograft is of particular concern. However, it is extremely important to recognize that there are several different types of allograft and that the risks associated with their use vary. Bone allograft is available fresh frozen and in mineralized and demineralized freeze-dried forms. In terms of safety, the greatest differences are found between frozen and freeze-dried bone allografts.

Procurement of bone allograft for dental procedures

More than 85% of all bone allografts are processed by one of six US tissue banks,[4] which in itself provides some measure of safety. The first step in procurement involves the selection of an acceptable donor. The development of

> **BOX 15-1 Exclusionary criteria for bone allograft donors**
>
> 1. Omission of donors from high-risk groups by medical and social screening. Unless reliable information regarding previous hospitalizations, blood transfusions, serious illnesses, and lifestyle can be ascertained, the donor must be regarded as unacceptable.
> 2. HIV antibody and antigen testing
> 3. Autopsy or biopsy to rule out occult disease, such as carcinoma
> 4. Special lymph node studies beyond those usually performed at autopsy. Such studies are performed to recognize changes characteristic of early HIV infection and provide another opportunity to exclude individuals with morphologic nodal changes typical of nonspecific infection (eg, bacterial, viral, parasitic, or fungal, and chronic infection or drug abuse).
> 5. Blood cultures for bacterial contamination
> 6. Serologic tests for syphilis and all types of hepatitis
> 7. Follow-up studies of grafts from the same donor. One third of the donors are concomitant donors of vital organs, such as heart, kidneys, and liver. With the exception of fresh bone allografts, frozen and processed bone allografts are not ready for clinical use until several months after procurement. If the recipient of a vital organ were to be identified as having HIV or another related illness, the bone from the donor would not be released for clinical use.

exclusionary criteria for donor procurement significantly improved the safety of allografts of all types. The chance of obtaining a fresh bone allograft from an HIV-infected donor who failed to be excluded by one of the screening techniques described in Box 15-1 is calculated to be 1 in 1.67 million.[5]

To ensure that they are sterile, bone allografts are procured in a sterile fashion, usually within 12 hours of death of the donor (after which time the incidence of bacterial contamination significantly increases). If it is found to be bacterially contaminated, the bone is subjected to secondary methods of sterilization. Irradiation and ethylene oxide are currently used as end-stage sterilizing agents. The use of irradiation is controversial[6-9]; however, it is generally acknowledged that doses above 2.0 to 2.5 megarads of gamma irradiation are destructive to new bone formation.[10]

Ethylene oxide, a powerful alkylating agent, has significant deleterious effects on bone induction.[11,12] An ethylene-oxide sterilization procedure of sufficient dosage to kill spores will render a bone allograft incapable of inducing new bone formation. Furthermore, residual levels of ethylene oxide will cause morphologic changes in fibroblasts cocultured with the allograft.[12]

Although processing of a freeze-dried bone allograft varies to some degree among tissue banks, it generally includes the following steps:

1. Cortical bone is harvested under sterile procedure. Long bones are the source of mineralized freeze-dried bone allograft (FDBA) and demineralized or decalcified freeze-dried bone allograft (DFDBA). The cortical bone is harvested because it has been found to be less antigenic than cancellous bone.[13,14] Bone-inductive proteins are located in the bone matrix,[15,16] and since cortical bone has more bone matrix than cancellous bone, cortical bone is the material of choice.
2. All soft tissue is removed from the bones. The cortical bone is rough cut to a particle size ranging from 500 μm to 5 mm and subjected to repeated washings to remove the bone marrow. This fragmentation increases the efficiency of defatting the cortical bone and subsequent decalcification, if the allograft is to be demineralized.
3. The graft is immersed in 100% ethanol for 1 hour to remove fat that may inhibit osteogenesis[17] and to inactivate virus. Viral infectivity is undetectable within 1 minute of treatment with 70% ethyl alcohol.[18] This process is usually repeated at various stages during processing.
4. The bone is frozen in liquid nitrogen for 1 to 2 weeks to interrupt the degradation process. During this time, the results of bacterial cultures, serologic tests, and antibody and antigen tests are analyzed. If contamination is found, the bones are most likely sterilized by irradiation or ethylene oxide.
5. The sterile, infection-free graft material is freeze-dried. Freeze-drying is a process by which dehydration is achieved by removing water directly from a frozen state to a vapor state, thus bypassing the liquid state. The process takes place in a vacuum and is termed *sublimation*.[19] Freeze-drying removes more than 95%

of the bone's moisture content. Although freeze-drying kills all cells (rendering the bone lacunae empty spaces), it offers the advantage of facilitating long-term storage and markedly reducing antigenicity. In one study, patients who received multiple periodontal grafts did not develop anti–human lymphocyte antigen (HLA) antibodies when evaluated by sensitive microcytotoxicity assays.[14]

6. The cortical bone is ground and sieved to a particle size of approximately 250 to 750 μm. Particle sizes within this range have been shown to promote osteogenesis,[20,21] whereas particles smaller than 125 μm are quickly engulfed by multinucleated foreign body giant cells.[21]

7. If the bone allograft is to be decalcified, it is immersed in 0.6 N of hydrochloric acid. Demineralization removes the calcium and exposes the bone-inductive proteins collectively known as *bone morphogenetic protein* (BMP).[22] This step is unnecessary in the processing of FDBA, which is used in orthopedic and oral surgical procedures where structural stability is more important than bone induction. Cortical FDBA has the same amount of BMP as DFDBA, but the calcium must be biologically removed over a long period of time before induction can take place. DFDBA forms new bone by *osteoinduction*, which is the differentiation of host mesenchymal or stem cells into bone-forming cells. FDBA forms bone by *osteoconduction*, a process by which the graft acts as a lattice network or matrix and passively assists the host in forming new bone.

8. The bone is washed in a sodium phosphate buffer to remove residual acid. Repeated washing with various solutions is frequently done throughout the processing.

9. If the bone is demineralized, it is re–freeze-dried. Some banks arrange the processing steps so that only a single freeze-drying cycle is necessary.

10. Vacuum sealing in glass containers protects the material against contamination and degradation while permitting storage at room temperature for an indefinite period of time.

Preventing transmission of infectious disease

HIV

Laboratory tests for detection of the AIDS virus are mandatory for the screening of bone allograft donors. An enzyme-linked immunosorbent assay (ELISA) is the standard test used to detect the presence of HIV antibody.[23] Its major disadvantage is the possibility that a prolonged period of time may pass between infection with the virus and seroconversion with subsequent development of antibodies to HIV. Antibody to HIV usually forms in HIV-infected persons within 6 months,[24] whereas most individuals seroconvert within 6 weeks of inoculation.[25] Based on blood bank data, the chance of a patient who has a negative ELISA antibody test to be an HIV viral carrier is estimated as 1:40,000 to 1:153,000.[26,27] The HIV antigen (p24) test is another blood test that screens for the AIDS virus and is sometimes used as an adjunct to the ELISA antibody test.[23] A third test used for AIDS screening is based on polymerase chain reaction (PCR) technology and provides the most reliable screening possible. It is extremely accurate in the diagnosis of patients who are HIV carriers and decreases the window of vulnerability to 1 week or less.[28] PCR tests amplify portions of genetic makeup of HIV, thereby making the virus more easily detectable.[29] There are four known cases of HIV transmission from a bone allograft donor, all of them involving *unprocessed fresh frozen bone*.[30] There has never been a reported case of disease transfer from FDBA or DFDBA.[31]

Both FDBA and DFDBA are perceived to pose a lower risk for viral transmission than large, unprocessed fresh frozen osteochondral allografts. This perception is attributed to an expectation that the chemical agents used in the processing, such as ethanol and hydrochloric acid, produce a virucidal effect on tissue-borne HIV.

The ability of chemical agents to inactivate HIV under clinical and laboratory conditions is well known.[18,32] Exposure of 7 to 10 logs of infectious dose of virus to alcohol at 70% concentration inactivated HIV below detectable levels within 1 minute.[18] During processing, allograft bone is defatted by soaking in a bath containing 100% ethanol for 1 hour. It has been demonstrated that ethanol will completely penetrate cortical bone (5.5 × 2.5 cm) within 15 minutes following introduction of this virucidal agent.[33] Further evidence of the effectiveness of chemical decontamination was provided by the implantation of the simian immunodeficiency virus (SIV). Bone procured from an SIV-infected monkey was processed several ways. The contaminated bone was either treated with ethanol or frozen. Monkeys receiving non–ethanol-treated frozen bone allograft all tested positive for SIV within 2 weeks. No animal receiving ethanol-treated bone became infected with SIV.

Furthermore, exposure of HIV to a low pH such as that obtained with hydrochloric acid also will inactivate the virus.[32,34] Strongly acidic solutions have been shown to disrupt the phosphodiester bonds of nucleic acids.[35] It has been demonstrated that HIV, HBV, HCV, cytomegalovirus, and poliovirus can all be inactivated by the demineralization process used in the preparation of DFDBA. Reports indicated that freezing[36] and freeze-drying[37] also may result in a reduction of HIV infectivity.

To determine if processing could inactivate HIV in a bone allograft, bone that was free of HIV infection was spiked both with HIV and with bone obtained from a donor who died of AIDS.[38] The spiked and the infected bone were treated with a virucidal agent and demineralization. Replication of viable HIV could not be demonstrated after treatment. This study and other evidence indicates that even if an HIV-infected donor somehow was able to escape detection by the various exclusionary techniques now in force, processing a bone allograft with a virucidal agent such as ethanol, hydrochloric acid, or another suitable chemical agent will render the processed bone allograft safe for human implantation. The probability that any particular brand of DFDBA contains HIV has been calculated to be 1 in 2.8 billion.[39]

Hepatitis

Hepatitis A is spread by person-to-person contact and is highly unlikely to be transmitted via tissues.[23,40] In addition, hepatitis A is usually a mild subclinical illness and is unlikely to result in a chronic carrier state. Patients who have a history of hepatitis A are eliminated as allograft donors.

Hepatitis B is almost always transmitted via blood and blood products. Screening for hepatitis B is mandatory. The standard test for hepatitis B is hepatitis B surface antigen (HBsAg).[41] As with HIV infection, hepatitis B has a window of approximately 6 weeks between infection and antibody development. However, acute hepatitis B infection is easily recognizable, and donor screening via blood testing history and physical examination are very sensitive. Antibody to hepatitis B surface antigen (anti-HBsAg) also is performed because its level begins to peak approximately 6 months after infection.[42] Antibody to hepatitis B core antigen (anti-HBc) is another test that detects all but the earliest phases of HBV infection. This antibody is detectable in more than 95% of HBsAg-positive donors and may be the only marker for hepatitis B infection.[43] Ethanol soaks will effectively inactivate HBV.[44,45] Since 1954, there have been no reported cases of hepatitis transmission by a bone allograft.[46]

Hepatitis C (or hepatitis non-A, non-B) is the chief cause of post-transfusion hepatitis.[23] Screening for hepatitis C is mandatory. The standard test is antibody to hepatitis C virus (anti-HCV). The introduction of PCR in testing for HCV has improved screening methods.[47] Because HCV is a lipid-containing virus, alcohol may inactivate it.[3] No cases of any type of hepatitis transmission with either FDBA or DFDBA have been reported.

Other transmissible diseases

Syphilis, caused by the organism *Treponema pallidum*, is not known to be transmissible via bone or soft tissue; moreover, the causative agent is sensitive to antibiotics, heat, and drying. Tissue banks test for syphilis primarily because blood banks do so,[40] generally using the rapid plasma reagin (RPR) test, the Venereal Disease Research Laboratories (VDRL) test, or the fluorescent treponemal antibody absorption (FTA-ABS) test. There has been no report of any sexually transmitted disease associated with FDBAs.

Bacterial infection was reported in 7% of a series of 303 applications of small FDBAs.[48] Of the 21 infections, 12 were minor, characterized by local wound erythema; therefore, the overall incidence was 3.6%. The organism most commonly isolated was *Staphylococcus epidermidis*. Only 1 of 11 patients who had positive wound cultures showed the same organism that had been cultured postoperatively from the allograft.[48] The infection rate of 3.6% compares favorably with the 3.9% infection rate reported for autogenous bone grafts.[49]

CJD disease is a slow progressive encephalopathy. It is caused by a prion, a novel self-replication protein and the smallest known infectious particle.[50] In the US and Europe, the estimated crude annual incidence is 1 case in 1 million.[51] The principle routes of disease transmission are through infected neurologic tissue such as dura mater, pituitary growth hormone, and cornea.[1] Bone has never been known to have transmitted CJD. Excluding donors with a past medical history of neurologic disease has nearly eliminated the risk of CJD from all allografts. Transmission of CJD has never been reported with any type of bone allograft.

In summary, the safety of freeze-dried allogeneic bone is excellent due to rigorous hard tissue bank standards and protocols that should make both clinicians and patients feel safe and secure.

Sinus Allograft Procedures

For the sinus graft procedure, allogeneic bone is placed using any of three generally accepted techniques: *(1)* the osteotome technique, *(2)* the simultaneous sinus elevation and implant placement technique, or *(3)* a two-stage lateral approach to sinus elevation and implant placement for more challenging cases. Access to the sinus is usually made via a paracrestal incison, in which the wound margin is removed from the osseous site of surgery.[52]

For all three techniques, the authors use a variation of the crestal approach to flap elevation, known as the *overlapped flap*. A split-thickness flap is reflected from the palatal side of the edentulous ridge. The flap widens apically until it reaches the alveolar bone to minimize vascular embarrassment to the coronal edge of the flap. Next, two beveled vertical incisions are made on the outer portion of the flap to facilitate mucoperiosteal elevation. If the tuberosity is included in the flap, the distal releasing incision is omitted. This "double" flap is raised buccally to reveal the bone overlying the sinus cavity. Vertical incisions may be extended to ease reflection without significant compromise to the blood supply (Fig 15-1).

When a lateral approach with infracture and sinus membrane elevation is used, the allograft is packed onto the sinus floor using direct vision. The buccal flap, including the epithelium and connective tissue extension, is then coapted over the graft site. If implants or membranes are employed, they will lie under the flap. Should the crest height or a lateral deficiency require augmentation, it may be necessary to lengthen the vertical incisions facially for flap mobility. Additional tissue length can be obtained by incising the undersurface of the flap. The palatal flap is then coapted over the connective tissue extension of the buccal flap to close the surgical site by primary intention.

If vertical augmentation is not required, a crestal incision with one or two vertical incisions is a satisfactory approach to the sinus. Both methods provide adequate periosteal covering for the graft.

While some clinicians report that the window is incompletely healed upon re-entry unless an occlusive membrane is used, this has not been our experience.[53,54] A membrane was rarely used in the series of patients reported here, and yet complete closure of the lateral sinus wall is routine.

Lateral approach for sinus elevation

The lateral window approach is used for both delayed and simultaneous implant placement. Once the tissue covering the lateral wall of the maxillary sinus has been elevated, the contour and anatomy of the antrum can usually be identified by its convex appearance. Variations in the thickness of the bone on the lateral wall mask its perimeter, which can sometimes be revealed by transillumination. Autogenous bone is harvested from the lateral wall of the antrum for use in conjunction with allograft. In addition, by thinning out the lateral wall, the full extent of the sinus cavity is made visible. The osteotomy is then performed using a multifluted finishing bur. The finishing bur is particularly suitable because it reduces the incidence of membrane tears. When the osteotomy is completed, infracture and membrane elevation are accomplished and the graft procedure is performed.

If bony septa are encountered, they should not be removed; instead, the sinus can be grafted into two compartments and the septum can be used as an interior border.[55] Special effort should be made to retain as much original bone as possible to take full advantage of its endosseous capacity for bone repair.

Whenever possible, at least 3 mm of bone should be left between the inferior border of the window and the crest of the ridge to preserve the shape of the original outer wall and to prevent flap collapse into the graft site.

The question as to the amount of sinus membrane elevation necessary for implant placement remains controversial. The average height of an adult sinus is approximately 18 to 30 mm, allowing adequate room to graft for a standard-sized implant. Allograft is densely packed onto the sinus floor beneath the elevated membrane (Fig 15-2). The volume of the graft affects the potential for new bone formation. Therefore, the parts of the graft positioned furthest from host bone have a much lower potential for ossification. Grafted bone ultimately relies on proximate vasculature that perfuses host bone for revascularization. In most cases, membrane elevation should not exceed 15 mm, and some height should be expected to be lost through remodeling.

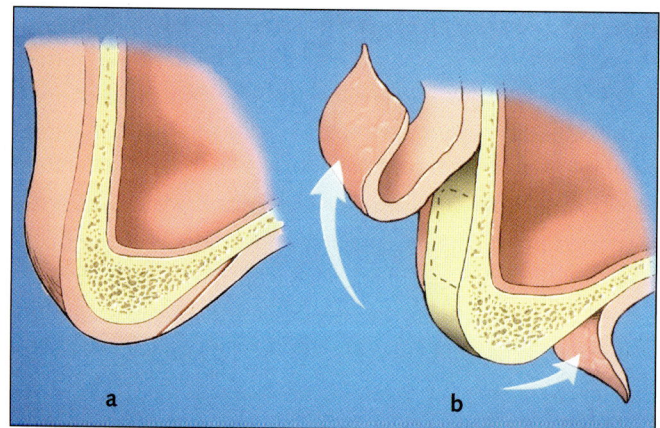

Fig 15-1 (a) Delayed sinus elevation with 1 to 4 mm of residual bone. A partial-thickness flap is beveled to the palate. (b) Elevation of split-thickness buccal and palatal flaps exposes the underlying bone. The osteotomy is made in the lateral wall of the sinus.

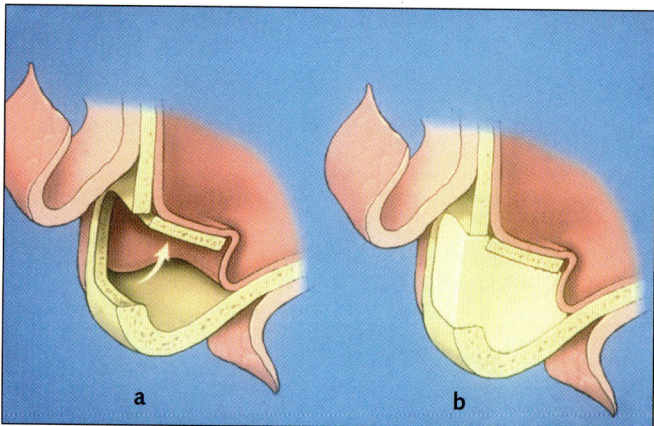

Fig 15-2 (a) Infracturing of the external wall of the sinus and elevation of the membrane. (b) Dense packing of bone allograft into the cavity created by the membrane elevation.

Success of allograft versus other graft materials

There are very few long-term studies on loaded osseointegrated implants in grafted sinuses. Autogenous hematopoietic marrow grafts were considered the gold standard because of their osteoinductive properties.[56–63] Subsequently, allografts, xenografts, and alloplasts were tested. Non-autogenous materials are osteoconductive rather than osteoinductive.[64–70]

Long-term studies on loaded osseointegrated implants in grafted sinuses followed for significant periods of time are now being published. Most reviews, however, include data pooled from many studies of implants with at least 1 year of loading in grafted sinuses.[59,71–74] Based on analysis, the survival rate of implants placed in sinuses variously augmented using the lateral approach ranged from 61.7% to 100%, with an average survival rate of 91.8%.[75] Grafts consisting of 100% autogenous bone or including autogenous bone as a component of a composite graft did not affect implant survival.[71]

Thus, it seems that the use of autogenous bone was not required for sinus graft success at all. In fact, the area inferior to the maxillary sinus is so conducive to new bone formation that a number of different augmentation materials permitted adequate bone growth for implant loading. Allograft is one such material.

Two-stage delayed approach

In the most challenging cases where there is less than 3 or 4 mm of residual bone, a two-stage protocol using a lateral approach is preferred. Treatment time is increased by 6 to 9 months to allow for graft maturation. Another 6 months may be required for osseointegration in large graft-reliant implant sites.

Clinical performance

The following case reports exemplify the successful use of allograft, specifically demineralized freeze-dried bone, in the sinus floor. The choice of demineralized (instead of mineralized) allograft is based on medical safety. The demineralization process reportedly adds an extra margin of safety that prevents viral pathogens from being transmitted to the patient.[37,75–78] Demineralized allograft has some osteoinductive capacity, perhaps more than that found in mineralized allograft, and it has been reported that BMP is released from the demineralized bone.[79,80] While mineralized allograft adds mineral content to the graft about 3 months sooner than demineralized allograft, this benefit is probably not clinically significant after 9 months of healing.

Case 1

A 58-year-old female patient presented for treatment wearing a well-made complete denture with porcelain teeth. She had well-controlled diabetes but was otherwise healthy.

Sinus Allograft Procedures

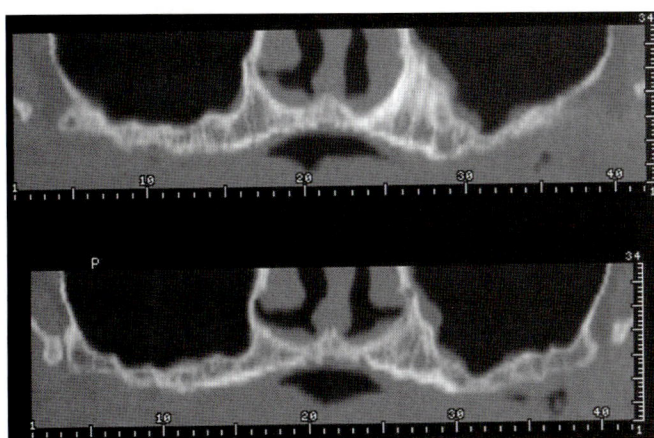

Fig 15-3a Preoperative CT scan reveals 1 to 3 mm of bone bilaterally.

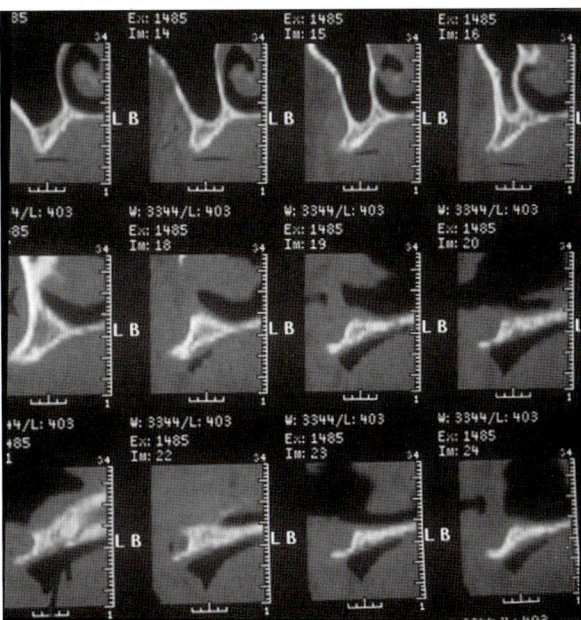

Fig 15-3b Axial CT scans reveal a very thin and severely resorbed premaxilla.

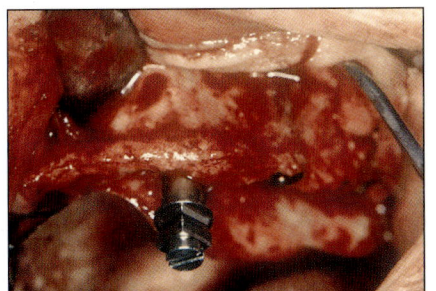

Fig 15-3c Implant placement 9 months after bilateral sinus elevations. The severe undercut of the premaxilla necessitated a more palatal placement of the implant in the canine position.

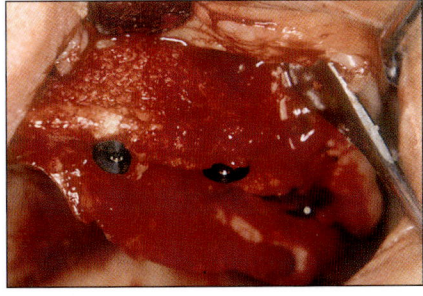

Fig 15-3d Placement of DFDBA on the buccal surface of the ridge.

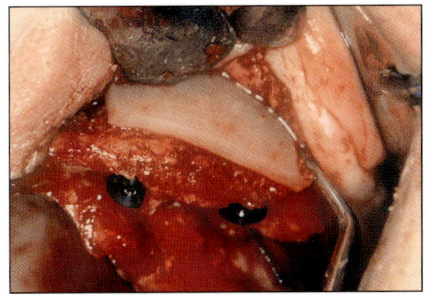

Fig 15-3e Placement of a thick piece of laminar bone over the DFDBA to cushion the graft site from denture pressure.

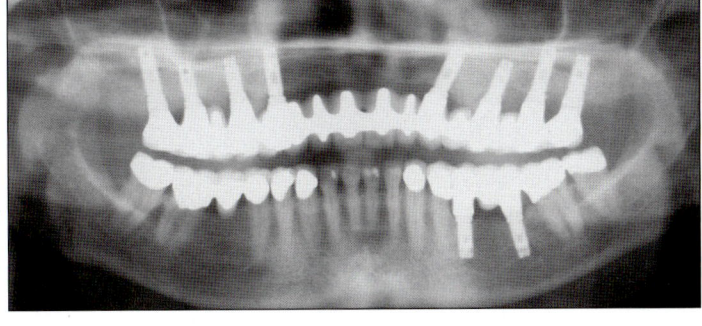

Fig 15-3f Twelve-year postoperative radiograph of the eight machined screw-type implants supporting a porcelain-fused-to-metal fixed partial denture. The implants are 10 and 13 mm in length. The bone profile demonstrates a long-term steady state.

A computerized tomography (CT) examination revealed less than 1 mm of bone bilaterally beneath the sinuses as well as a severely resorbed anterior maxilla (Figs 15-3a and 15-3b). The patient wished to become denture free. Bilateral sinus elevations using freeze-dried allografts were accomplished. In addition, the concave anterior ridge was augmented with freeze-dried bone overlayed with laminar bone (Figs 15-3c to 15-3e). Healing was uneventful. *Nine months later*, a total of eight machined-surface screw-type implants ranging in height from 10 to 13 mm were placed. A 12-year postoperative panoramic radiograph reveals a steady level of crestal bone (Fig 15-3f).[81]

chapter 15 — Safety and Efficacy of Bone Allograft for Sinus Grafting

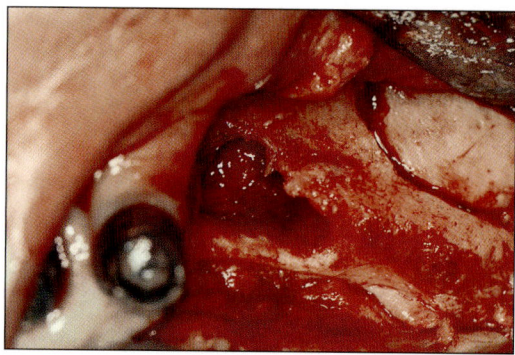

Fig 15-4a Maxillary left posterior bone defect in the area of the first premolar and deficiency of bone in the first molar region. This patient, who has implants in the anterior maxilla, lost the posterior teeth due to recurrent caries and root fractures.

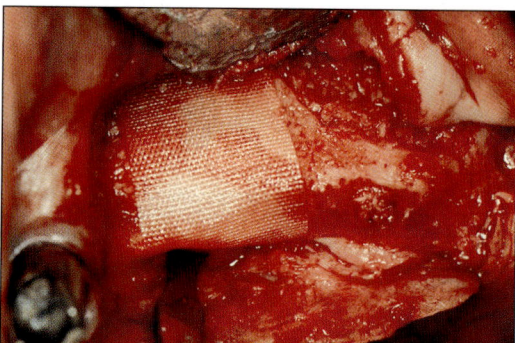

Fig 15-4b Elevation of the sinus and grafting of the sinus as well as the defect in the premolar region with demineralized allograft. Note that the premolar is the only area to receive a membrane.

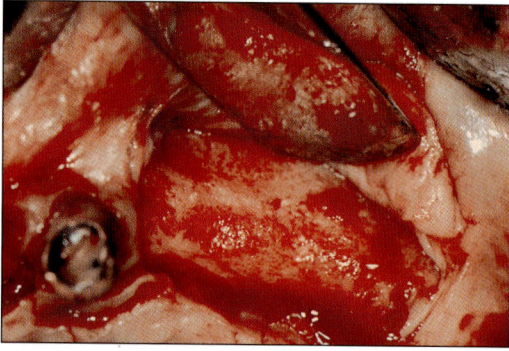

Fig 15-4c Re-entered 6 months later, the area shows well-mineralized bone on the lateral window and vertical bone growth in the premolar area.

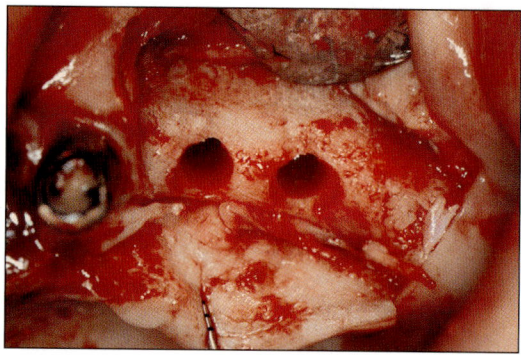

Fig 15-4d Two osteotomy sites prepared to receive implants.

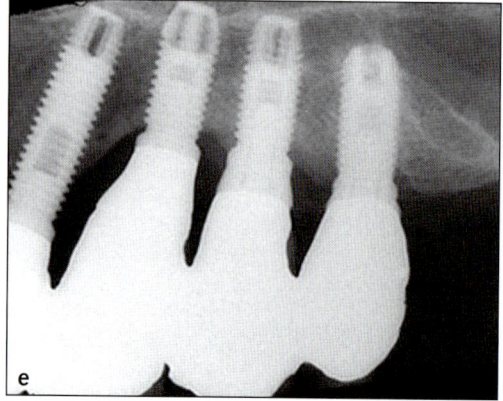

Fig 15-4e Restoration of the areas with two 10-mm machined-surface titanium implants in demineralized allograft.

Fig 15-4f Ten years after loading, the area shows no visible change in the bone height around the implants.

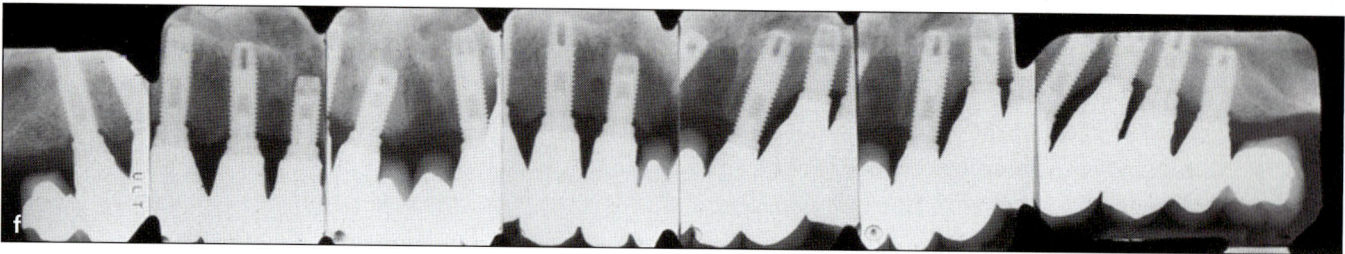

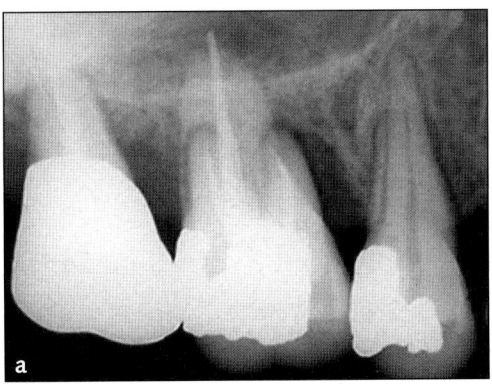 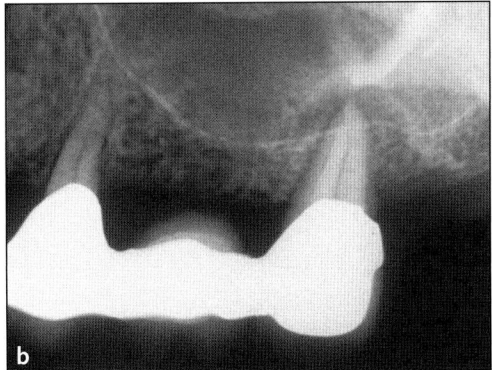

Figs 15-5a and 15-5b Bilateral advanced bone loss and pneumatized sinus in a 38-year-old patient with aggressive periodontal breakdown despite continued professional care.

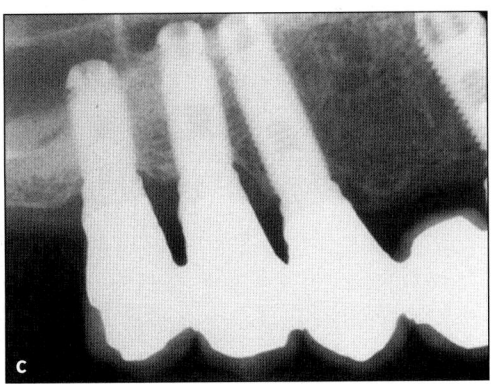 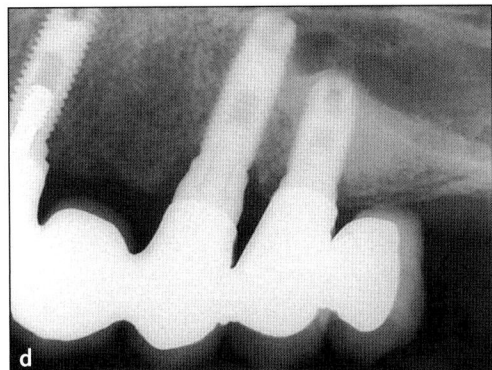

Figs 15-5c and 15-5d Definitive prosthesis 10 years after loading.

Case 2

A 42-year-old female patient had been under periodontal care for 10 years. As a result of tooth loss and mobility, her maxillary teeth were splinted with a full-coverage prosthesis. Endodontic abscess, recurrent caries, and vertical tooth fractures developed (Fig 15-4a). The patient was advised to have implants placed to restore her dentition. She was skeptical because her natural teeth failed despite extensive efforts to save them. She consented to have implants placed in the anterior region. After these proved successful, bone augmentation and sinus grafting were performed (Figs 15-4b to 15-4f). All implants were successful. The steady state of bone was maintained in the same manner as those placed in nongrafted bone.

Case 3

A 38-year-old female patient had been treated for recalcitrant periodontitis since age 20. Recurrent abscesses and loose prostheses led the patient to seek alternative treatment. Radiographs revealed inadequate bone to restore the posterior dentition (Figs 15-5a and 15-5b). Tooth removal and bilateral sinus elevation were performed; the canines were retained to anchor a fixed provisional splint. Machined-surface titanium implants were placed 6 months after the sinus elevation procedure and uncovered 6 months later. The 10-year posterior radiograph shows no apparent changes in the bone levels around the implants placed in augmented bone (Figs 15-5c and 15-5d).

chapter 15 Safety and Efficacy of Bone Allograft for Sinus Grafting

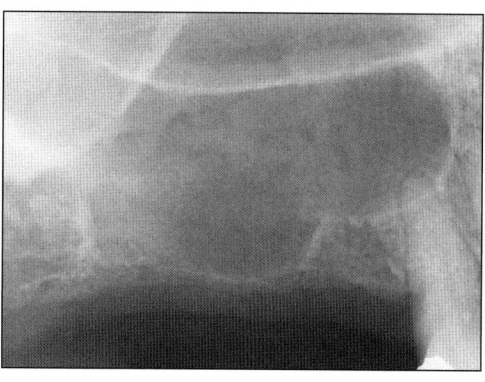

Fig 15-6a Preoperative radiograph showing 1 to 2 mm of residual bone.

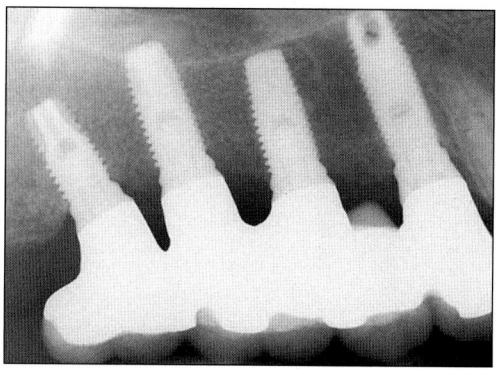

Fig 15-6b Ten-year postoperative radiograph of four machined-surface implants, 8.5 to 13 mm in length, supporting a freestanding partial denture.

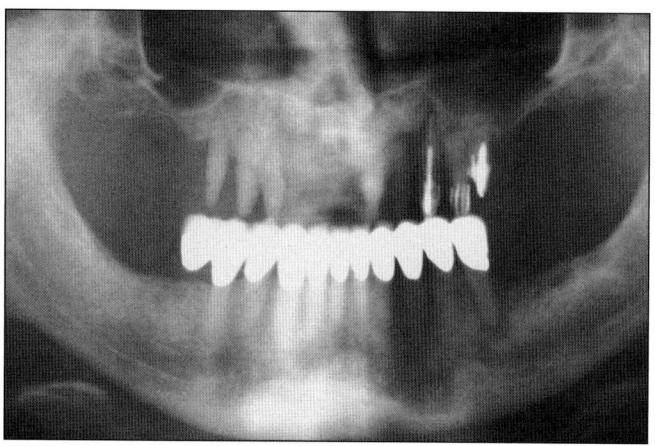

Fig 15-7a Preoperative view of severe bone loss around premolars and residual periapical radiolucency around the canine.

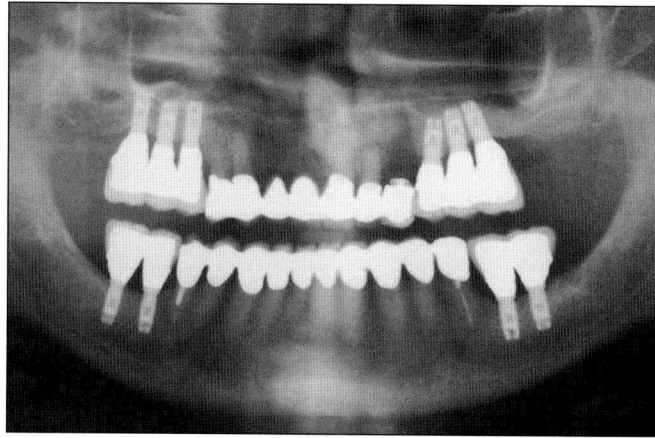

Fig 15-7b Postoperative view of two freestanding posterior implant-supported fixed partial dentures and an anterior splint on natural teeth.

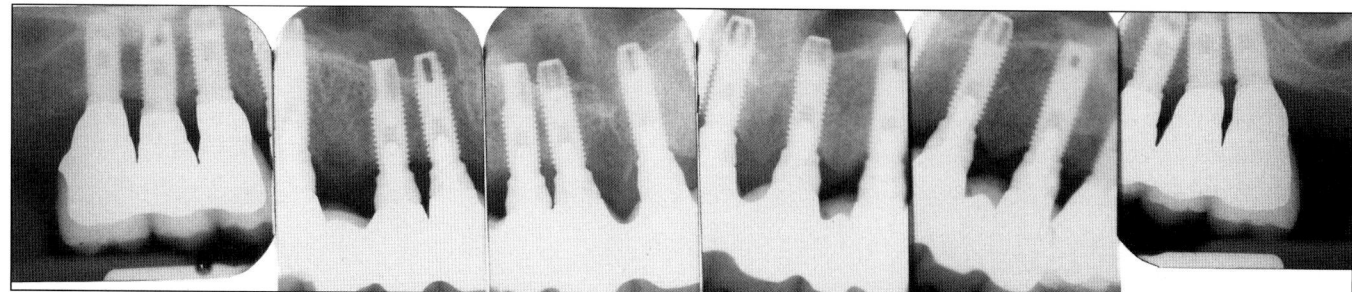

Fig 15-7c Replacement of the anterior teeth and splint with a third freestanding implant-supported fixed partial denture. Ten-year follow-up of the posterior implants.

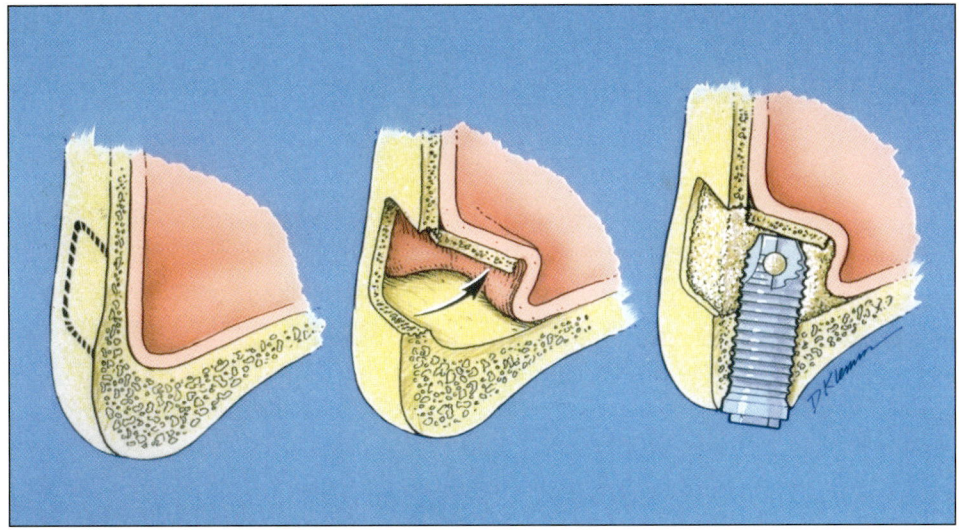

Fig 15-8 Simultaneous lateral window sinus elevation and implant placement. Demineralized allograft is densely packed into the sinus cavity and around the implant.

Case 4

A 56-year-old female patient, who was told that she lacked the amount of bone needed to hold implants, remained edentulous in the maxillary right posterior area for 15 years. She also had bone loss and tooth mobility on the left side, and large pneumatized sinuses encompassed the entire posterior alveolar crest (Fig 15-6a). At 68 years of age, feeling that her appearance and chewing ability were severely compromised, she agreed to undergo sinus elevation. The radiograph shows a 10-year follow-up of four implants placed to support a freestanding fixed partial denture (Fig 15-6b).

Case 5

A 78-year-old man presented with advanced bone loss around his remaining maxillary premolars. The left canine and first premolar showed periapical radiolucencies. Bilaterally, all the molars were absent, and the amount of bone below the maxillary sinus ranged from 1 to 5 mm (Fig 15-7a).

Since the patient did not wish to wear a removable prosthesis, bilateral sinus grafts consisting of DFDBA were placed above the premolars and in the edentulous molar region. Six months postoperatively, the premolars were removed, and three 10-mm machined-surface implants were placed bilaterally. The left canine underwent an apicoectomy.

The implants were uncovered 6 months later, and the definitive prosthesis, consisting of two freestanding posterior implant-supported partial dentures, was inserted in conjunction with an anterior fixed splint (Fig 15-7b).

Additional implants were later placed anteriorly to support a fixed partial denture. At the 10-year follow-up, there was no perceptible change in the bone level of the posterior implants (Fig 15-7c).

Simultaneous sinus elevation and implant placement

When the amount of residual bone is 5 to 6 mm, sinus grafting with allograft and simultaneous placement of implants may be performed (Fig 15-8). Instead of the osteotome procedure, the surgeon may wish to have direct view of the sinus cavity and to maintain control of the graft site. The success of this procedure depends on the surgeon's ability to adequately stabilize the implant in the residual native bone.

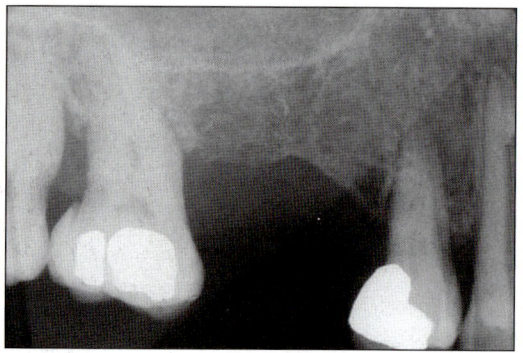

Fig 15-9a Preoperative radiograph of a 37-year-old female patient with advanced periodontitis. There were 5 mm of bone available beneath the sinus.

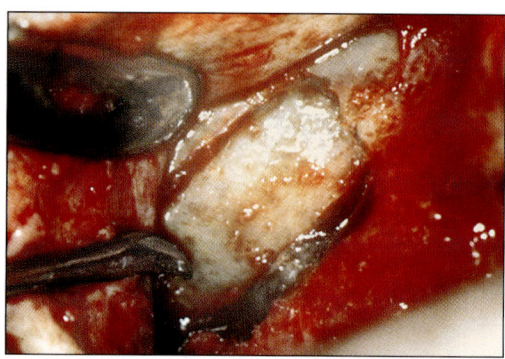

Fig 15-9b Infracture of the lateral wall and elevation of the membrane as the wall moves superiorly.

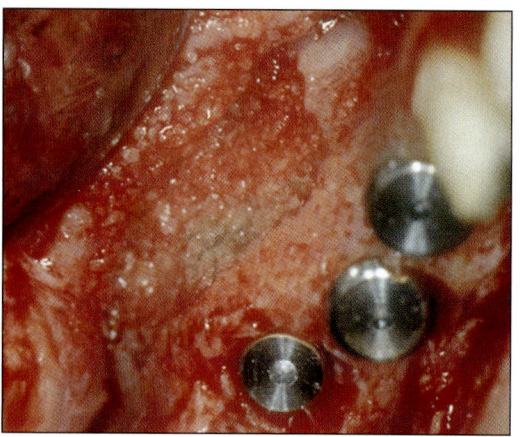

Fig 15-9c Demineralized graft. Two of the implants are faintly visible beneath the graft.

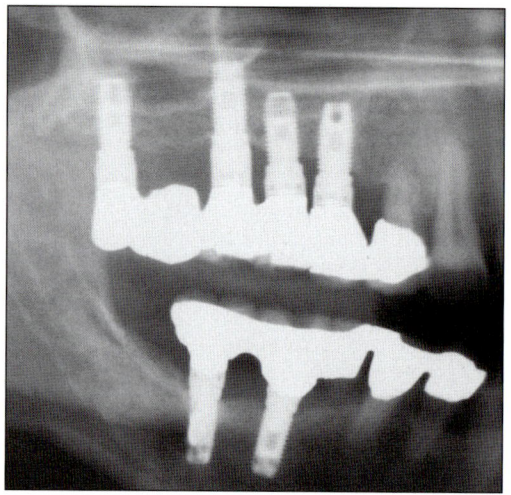

Fig 15-9d Freestanding porcelain-fused-to-metal fixed partial denture 13 years postsurgery.

Case 6

A 37-year-old female patient presented with several missing teeth, advanced periodontal disease, and second- and third-degree mobility throughout her dentition. The exam revealed that there was 5 mm of available bone below the sinus. The treatment plan therefore consisted of sinus elevation combined with simultaneous implant placement (Fig 15-9a).

The osteotomy was made with a round bur, and the access window was tapped in with light pressure (Fig 15-9b). Freeze-dried allograft was packed into the sinus cavity and around the implants (Fig 15-9c). No membrane was placed over the site, and healing was allowed to progress for 8 months. The postoperative radiograph demonstrates the 13-year survival of the freestanding fixed partial denture (Fig 15-9d).

Case 7

A 34-year-old female patient presented with approximately 5 mm of maxillary bone immediately distal to the maxillary canine (Fig 15-10a). In the molar area, the bone height was only 2 mm. Because the patient was anxious to eliminate the removable prosthesis, the treatment plan called for combined simultaneous and delayed implant placement.

Two 10-mm implants were placed in 1991 and uncovered in 1992 (Figs 15-10b and 15-10c). At the uncovering appointment, two additional implants were placed and allowed to heal for 6 months (Fig 15-10d). The original implants were loaded with an acrylic resin provisional prosthesis. At the designated time, the remaining implants were uncovered and loaded with a definitive prosthesis (Fig 15-10e). By 2005, radiographs reveal that all of the implants continue in an osseous steady state of health (Fig 15-10f).

Fig 15-10a Left maxilla. There was 5 mm of bone in the premolar area and 2 mm of bone height in the molar area.

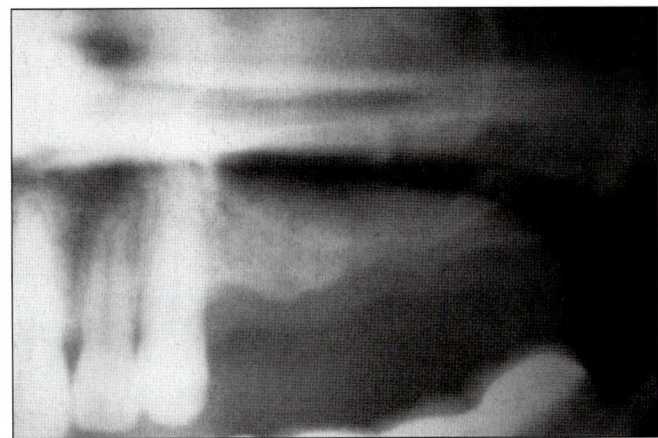

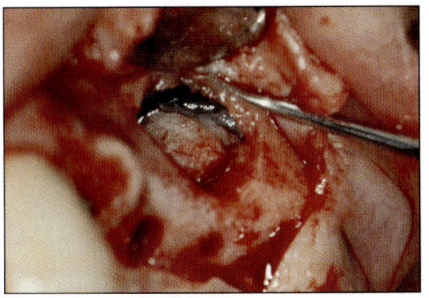

Fig 15-10b Combined simultaneous and delayed implant placement procedure. Two implants were placed in the premolar area, and 6 months later, two additional implants were placed in the molar area.

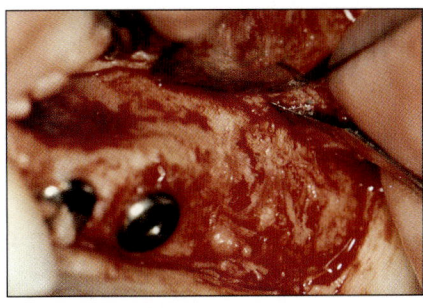

Fig 15-10c Complete reconstitution of the buccal wall shown at uncovering of the simultaneously placed implants.

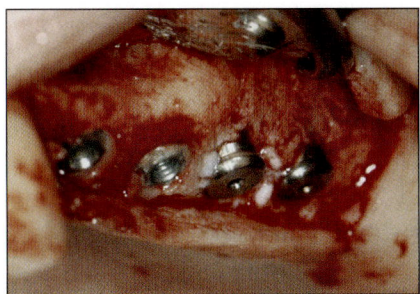

Fig 15-10d Placement of two additional implants.

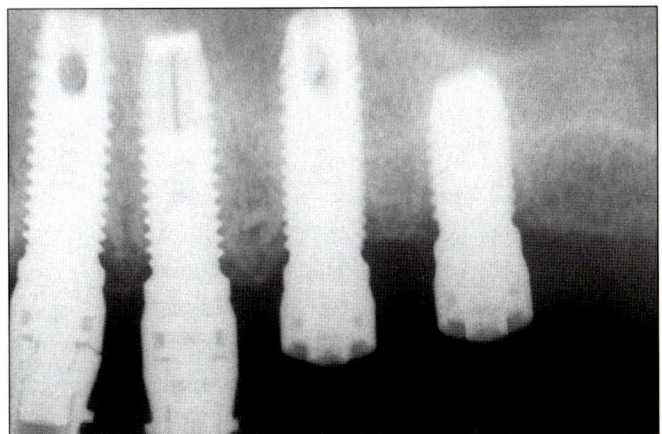

Fig 15-10e Uncovering and provisional restoration of the two premolar implants 6 months after placement. Two additional implants were then placed in the previously grafted sinus.

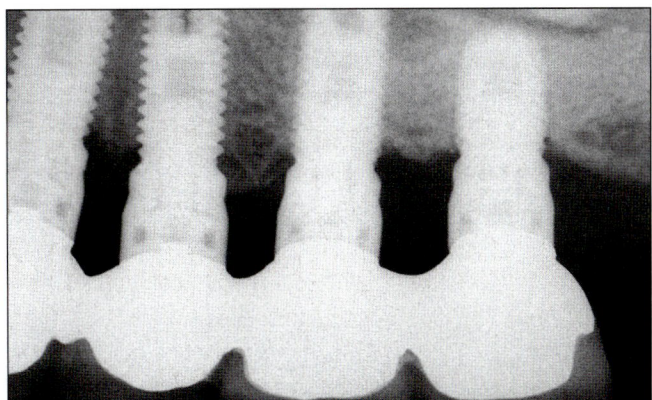

Fig 15-10f Thirteen- and twelve-year follow-up views of the premolar and molar implants, respectively.

TABLE 15-1 Implant distribution by group and type of sinus elevation procedure

	Simultaneous		Delayed		
	Placed/failed	Survival (%)	Placed/failed	Survival (%)	Period of follow-up
Group I (1/94–12/99)	390/32	91.8	663/55	91.7	Up to 11 yrs
Group II (1/00–8/03)	112/5	95.5	609/24	96.1	Up to 4.5 yrs

Results

Over a 15-year period (1989–2004), 2,402 implants were placed in consecutive patients in conjunction with sinus elevation procedures. All patients were treated with either the osteotome, simultaneous lateral window, or delayed lateral window sinus elevation technique previously described. Implants were loaded and followed for periods ranging from 1 to 15 years. Patients were treated in one of two private practice locations by two surgeons (Langer and Langer). The only exclusion criterion was active sinus infection.

The follow-up consisted of periodontal maintenance visits and periodic radiographs. Not all implant-retained fixed partial dentures were removed on an annual basis. The collected data were divided into three groups: The early developmental group, from 1989–1993, has previously been reported.[82] Group I, consisting of 507 patients, included implants placed between January 1994 and December 1999. Group II included 307 patients who underwent treatment between January 2000 and August 2003. The implants in the developmental group patients have been loaded for up to 15 years, those in Group I for up to 11 years, and those in Group II for up to 4.5 years.

There are few studies that have reported long-term results for sinus elevation with a minimum number of variables.[71] Most prospective studies have an observation period of 1 to 3 years, and medium-term retrospective studies typically observe implants for up to 5 years. To limit the number of variables in the present studies, the subgroup of 1,774 implants (Groups I and II) were all placed in DFDBA using the lateral window approach (Table 15-1).

The remaining 630 implants are not included in this review for one of the following reasons: (a) placed with the osteotome sinus elevation technique, (b) utilized xenograft or autogenous hip or chin graft, (c) included the use of a variety of implant surfaces, or (d) have not been loaded for more than 1 year. The survival rate for Group I (92%) is consistent with reports using a variety of bone graft material, implant types, and surfaces from smooth to rough, albeit for a longer time period than most other reports.[71] The survival rate is higher for Group II (96%). The implants in Group II have been followed for up to 4.5 years compared to up to 11 years of follow-up for the implants in Group I; however, it is well established that the vast majority of failed implants are lost either before or at the time of abutment connection or within the first year of loading. Interestingly, the survival rate appears not to be dependent on the surgical technique used, since the implants placed with either the simultaneous lateral window technique or the delayed lateral window technique have comparable survival rates within their respective groups. However, the implants placed simultaneously with the sinus augmentation technique have more residual bone from the outset.

Albrektsson and Wennerberg[83] analyzed a continuum of implant surface topography, including those with minimal surface roughness (defined as between 0.5 and 1.0 µm in Sa value), moderate surface roughness (those 1 to 2 µm in Sa value), and high surface roughness (those > 2 µm in Sa value). They report that implants with moderate surface roughness show a stronger bone response than either the turned (smoother) or plasma-sprayed (rougher) implants. Potential drawbacks of rough surfaces are a greater incidence of peri-implantitis and a risk of ion leakage. They conclude that while moderately roughened surfaces have some advantages over smoother or rougher surfaces, the differences are small and often not statistically significant. Since the implants in Group I are machined commercially pure titanium, the improved survival rate between Group I and Group II appears to be due solely to the increased use of a moderately rough (anodized) implant surface (Table 15-2 and Fig 15-11).

TABLE 15-2 Implants with varying surface roughness placed between January 2000 and August 2003

Implant type	No. placed/no. lost	Survival rate (%)
Machined (minimally rough)	279/21	92.5
Acid-etched (minimally rough)	114/5	95.6
Anodized (moderately rough)	326/3	99.1

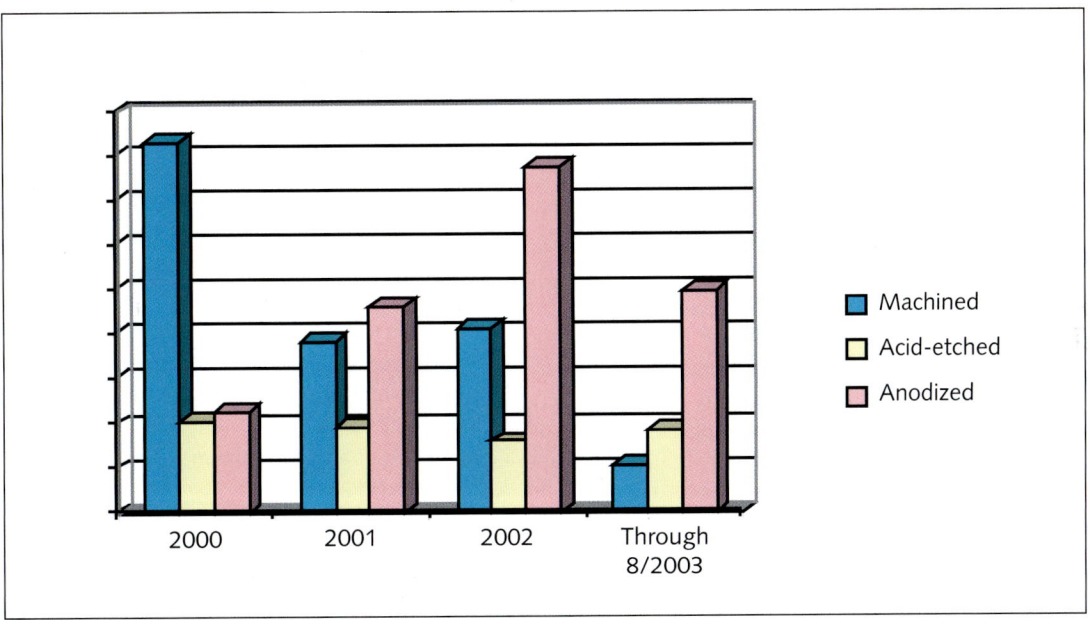

Fig 15-11 Relative proportions of implants placed according to surface topography, 2000–2003. Only implants placed up to August 2003 are included in order to have a follow-up of at least 1 year after loading.

Conclusions

Allogeneic bone grafting onto the sinus floor for implant anchorage is highly successful. Additionally, the results reported here indicate that a small difference in implant surface topography had a significant impact on osseointegration success in allograft bone graft sites. There was no apparent difference, however, between simultaneous and delayed implant placement when selective about the amount of native bone necessary to place implants simultaneous to bone grafting.

The use of allograft for augmentation of the maxillary sinus is a highly viable option. Implant survival, as assessed over an 11-year period, is well within acceptable standards compared to other grafting modalities. The widely held belief that autogenous bone grafting is the true gold standard is not valid when measured by implant survival, functionality of the bone graft, or sustained long-term peri-implant or sinus bone levels. Thus, bone substitutes appear to be equal to or better than autogenous bone for the sinus graft procedure provided there is an extended healing period.

While we have not seen any reason to change grafting material, we have added anodized titanium screw-type implants to our implant armamentaria with shorter-term (up to 4.6 years) but more positive results.

The majority of those working in the field of osseointegration have made changes in the surface roughness of the implants they use. Those who were using rough-surfaced implants have gravitated to a moderately rough implant, and many of those using a minimally rough implant surface are also using a moderately rough variety. The ultimate goal is to improve osseointegration while preserving the long-term success and steady state of bone that we have been accustomed to achieving with machined-surfaced titanium implants.

Acknowledgment

Special thanks to Ulrika Peterson, DDS, PhD, Clinical Researcher, Nobel Biocare AB, Gothenburg, Sweden, for her assistance in statistical analysis.

References

1. Gottesdiener KM. Transplanted infections: Donor-to-host transmission with the allograft. Ann Intern Med 1989;110:1001–1010.
2. Kayaiga R, Miller WV, Gudino MDL. Tissue transplant transmitted infections. Transfusion 1991;31:277–284.
3. Eastiund T. Infectious disease transmission through tissue transplantation: Reducing the risk through donor selection. J Transplant Coordination 1991;1:23–30.
4. Buck BE, Malinin TL. Human bone and tissue allografts. Clin Orthop 1994;303:8–17.
5. Buck BE, Malinin T, Brown MD. Bone transplantation and human immunodeficiency virus. Clin Orthop 1989;240:129–136.
6. Wientroub S, Reddi AH. Influence of irradiation on the osteoinductive potential of demineralized bone matrix. Calif Tissue Int 1988;42:255–260.
7. Munting E, Wilmart J, Wijne A, Hennebert P, Delloye C. Effect of sterilization on osteoinduction. Comparison of five methods in demineralized bone matrix gelatin. Acta Odontol Scand 1988;59:34–38.
8. Schwarz N, Redl H, Schiesser A, et al. Irradiation-sterilization of rat bone matrix gelatin. Acta Orthop Scand 1988;59:165–167.
9. Conway B, Tomford WW, Mankin HJ, Hirsch MS, Schooley RT. Radiosensitivity of HIV-1 potential application to sterilization of bone allografts. AIDS 1991;5:608–609.
10. Forsell JH. Irradiation of musculoskeletal tissues. In: Tomford WW (ed). Musculoskeletal Tissue Banking. New York, NY: Raven, 1993:149–180.
11. Aspenberg P, Johnsson E, Thorngren K. Dose-dependent reduction of bone-inductive properties by ethylene oxide. J Bone Joint Surg [B] 1992;72:1036–1037.
12. Zislis T, Martin SA, Cerbas E, Heath JR, Mansfield JL, Hollinger JO. A scanning electron microscopic study of in vivo toxicity of ethylene oxide sterilized bone repair materials. J Oral Implantol 1989;1:41–46.
13. Friedlaender G, Strong M, Sell K. Studies on the antigenicity of bone. I. Freeze-dried and deep frozen bone allografts in rabbits. J Bone Joint Surg [A] 1976;58:854–858.
14. Quattlebaum J, Mellonig JT, Hansel N. Antigenicity of freeze-dried cortical bone allograft in human periodontal osseous defects. J Periodontol 1988;59:394–397.
15. Urist M, Iwata H. Preservation and biodegradation of bone morphogenetic property of bone matrix. J Theoret Biol 1973;38:155–167.
16. Urist M, Jurist J, Dubuc D, Strates B. Quantitation of new bone formation in intramuscular implants of bone matrix in rabbits. Clin Orthop 1970;68:279–293.
17. Aspenberg P, Thoren K. Lipid extraction enhances bank bone incorporation. Acta Orthop Scand 1990;61:546–548.
18. Resnick L, Veren K, Salahuddin S, Tondreau S, Markhan P. Stability and inactivation of HTLV-111/LAV under clinical and laboratory environments. JAMA 1986;255:1887–1891.
19. Flosdorf EW, Hyatt GW. The preservation of bone grafts by freeze-drying. Surgery 1952;31:716–719.
20. Mellonig JT, Levey R. The effect of different particle sizes of freezedried bone allograft on bone growth. J Dent Res 1984;63:222.
21. Fucini SE, Quintero G, Gher ME, Black BS, Richardson RC. Small versus large particles of demineralized freeze-dried bone allograft in human intrabony periodontal defects. J Periodontol 1993;64:844–847.
22. Urist MR, Strates BS. Bone morphogenetic protein. J Dent Res 1971;50:1392–1406.
23. Tomford WW. Surgical bone banking. In: Tomford WW (ed). Musculoskeletal Tissue Banking. New York: Raven, 1993:19–60.
24. Sandler SG, Chyang F, Williams A. Retroviral infections transmitted by blood transfusion. Yale J Bio Med 1990;63:353–360.
25. Ward JW, Schable C, Dickinson GM, et al. Acute human immunodeficiency virus infection. Antigen detection and seroconversion in immunosuppressed patients. Transplantation 1989;47:722–724.
26. Cumming PD, Wallace EL, Schorr JB, Dodd RY. Exposure of patients to human immunodeficiency virus through the transfusion of blood components that test antibody-negative. N Engl J Med 1989;321:941–946.
27. Ward JW, Holmberg SD, Allen JR, et al. Transmission of human immunodeficiency virus (HIV) by blood transfusions screened as negative for HIV antibody. N Engl J Med 1988;318:473–478.
28. Wolinsky SM, Rinaldo CR, Kwok S, et al. Human immunodeficiency virus type 1 (HIV-1) infection a median of 18 months before a diagnostic western blot. Evidence from a cohort of homosexual men. Ann Intern Med 1989;111:961–972.
29. Eisenstein BI. The polymerase chain reaction: A new method of using molecular genetics for medical diagnosis. N Engl J Med 1990;322:178–183.
30. Simonds RJ, Holmberg SD, Hurwitz RL, et al. Transmission of human immunodeficiency virus type 1 from a seronegative organ and tissue donor. N Engl J Med 1992;326:726–732.
31. Centers for Disease Control. Transmission of HIV through bone transplantation: Case report and public health recommendation. MMWR 1988;37:587–599.

32. Martin LS, McDougal JS, Loskoski SL. Disinfection and inactivation of the human T lymphotropic virus type III/lymphadenopathy associated virus. J Infec Dis 1985;152:400–403.
33. Prewett AB, O'Leary R, Harrell J. Kinetic evaluation of the penetration of ethanol solutions containing virucidal agents through mid-diaphyseal cortical bone. Osteotech Tech Report. Shrewsberry, NJ: Osteotech, 1991.
34. Ongradi A, Ceccheini-Neilli L, Pistello M, Specter S, Bendinelli M. Acid sensitivity of cell-free associated HIV-1: Clinical implications. AIDS Res Human Retrovirus 1990;12:1433–1436.
35. Vodicka P, Hemminki K. Phosphodiester cleavage in apurinic dinucleotides. Chem Biol Interactions 1988;68:153–164.
36. Buch BE, Resnick L, Shah SM, Malinin T. Human immunodeficiency virus cultured from bone. Implications for transplantation. Clin Orthop 1990;251:249–253.
37. Quinnan GV Jr, Wells MA, Wittek AE, et al. Inactivation of human-cell lymphotropic virus, type III by heat, chemicals, and irradiation. Transfusion 1986;26:481–483.
38. Mellonig JT, Prewett AB, Moyer MP. HIV inactivation in a bone allograft. J Periodontol 1992;63:979–983.
39. Russo R, Scarborough N. Inactivation of viruses in demineralized bone matrix. FDA Workshop on Tissue for Transplantation and Reproductive Tissue. June 20–21, 1995, Bethesda, MD.
40. Tomford WW. Cadaver donor musculoskeletal tissue banking. In: Tomford WW (ed). Musculoskeletal Tissue Banking. New York, NY: Raven, 1993:61–148.
41. Centers for Disease Control. Public health service interagency guidelines for screening donors of blood, plasma, organs, tissue, and semen for evidence of hepatitis B and hepatitis C. MMWR 1991;40:1–17.
42. Hollinger FB. Specific and surrogate screening tests for hepatitis. In: Menitov HE (ed). Arlington, VA: American Association of Blood Banks, 1987:69–86.
43. Dodd RY, Popovsky MA. Members of the scientific sections coordinating committee: Antibodies to hepatitis B core antigen and the infectivity of the blood supply. Transfusion 1991;31:433–449.
44. Kobayashi H, Tsuzuki M, Koshimizu K, et al. Susceptability of hepatitis B virus to disinfectants or heat. J Clin Microbiol 1984;20:214–216.
45. Bond WW, Favero MS, Peterson NJ, Ebert JW. Inactivation of hepatitis B virus by intermediate to high level disinfectant chemicals. J Clin Micro 1983;18:535–538.
46. Shutkin NM. Homologous serum hepatitis following the use of refrigerated bone-banked bone. J Bone Joint Surg [A] 1954;36:160–162.
47. Cha TA, Kolberg J, Irvine B, et al. Use of a signature nucleotide sequence of hepatitis C virus for detection of viral RNA in human serum and plasma. J Clin Microbiol 1991;29:2528–2534.
48. Tomford WW, Starkweather RJ, Goldman MH. A study of the clinical incidence of infection in the use of banked allograft bone. J Bone Joint Surg [A] 1981;63:244–248.
49. Cruse PJE. Incidence of wound infection on the surgical services. Surg Clin North Am 1975;55:1269–1275.
50. Prusiner SB, Scott M, Foster D, et al. Transgenetic studies implicate interactions between homologous PrP isoforms in scrapie prion replication. Cell 1990;63:673–686.
51. Brown P, Preece MA, Will RG. "Friendly fire" in medicine: Hormones, homografts, and Creutzfeldt-Jacob disease. Lancet 1992;340:24–27.
52. Langer B, Langer L. The overlapped flap: A surgical modification for implant fixture installation. Int J Periodontics Restorative Dent 1990;10:209.
53. Wallace S, Froum S, Tarnow D. Histologic evaluation of sinus graft materials. In: Proceedings of American Academy of Periodontology Regenerative Conference. Chicago: American Academy of Periodontology, 1997.
54. Tarnow DP, Wallace SS, Froum SJ, Rohrer MD, Cho S-C. Histologic and clinical comparison of bilateral sinus floor elevations with and without barrier membrane placement in 12 patients: Part 3 of an ongoing prospective study. Int J Periodontics Restorative Dent 2000;20:116–125.
55. Watzek G, Ulm CW, Haas R. Anatomic and physiologic fundamentals of sinus floor augmentation. In: Jensen OT (ed). The Sinus Bone Graft. Chicago: Quintesssence, 1999:31–47.
56. Jensen J, Sindet-Pederson S. Autogenous mandibular bone grafts and osseointegrated implants for reconstruction of the severely atrophied maxilla: A preliminary report. J Oral Maxillofac Surg 1991;49:1277–1287.
57. Wood RM, Moore DL. Grafting of the maxillary sinus with intraorally harvested autogenous bone prior to implant placement. Int J Oral Maxillofac Implants 1988;3:209–214.
58. Block MS, Kent JM. Sinus augmentation for dental implants: The use of autogenous bone. Int J Oral Maxillofac Surg 1997;55:1281–1286.
59. Tolman DE. Reconstructive procedures with endosseous implants in grafted bone: A review of the literature. Int J Oral Maxillofac Implants 1995;10:275–294.
60. Hirsch JM, Ericsson I. Maxillary sinus augmentation using mandibular bone grafts and simultaneous installation of implants: A surgical technique. Clin Oral Implants Res 1991;2:91–96.
61. Johansson B, Wannfors K, Ekenbéck J, Smedberg J-l, Hirsch J. Implants and sinus inlay bone grafts in a one-stage procedure on severely atrophied maxillae: Surgical aspects of a 3-year follow-up study. Int J Oral Maxillofac Implants 1999;14:811–818.
62. Keller EE, Tolman DE, Eckert SE. Maxillary antral-nasal autogenous bone graft reconstruction of the compromised maxilla: A 12-year retrospective study. Int J Oral Maxillofac Implants 1999;14:707–721.
63. Khoury F. Augmentation of the sinus floor with mandibular bone block and simultaneous implantation: A 6-year clinical investigation. Int J Oral Maxillofac Implants 1999;14:557–564.
64. Tawil G, Mawla M. Sinus floor elevation using a bovine bone mineral (Bio-Oss) with or without the concomitant use of a bilayered collagen barrier (Bio-Gide): A clinical report of immediate and delayed implant placement. Int J Oral Maxillofac Implants 2001;16:713–721.

65. Froum SJ, Tarnow DP, Wallace SS, Rohrer MD, Cho S-C. Sinus floor elevation using anorganic bovine bone matrix (Osteo-Graf/N) with and without autogenous bone: A clinical, histologic, radiographic, and histomorphometric analysis—Part 2 of an ongoing prospective study. Int J Periodontics Restorative Dent 1998;18:529–543.
66. Valentini P, Abensur D. Maxillary sinus floor elevation for implant placement with demineralized freeze-dried bone and bovine bone (Bio-Oss): A clinical study of 20 patients. Int J Periodontics Restorative Dent 1997;17:233–241.
67. Haliman M, Hedin M, Sennerby L, Lundgren S. A prospective 1-year clinical and radiographic study of implants placed after maxillary sinus floor augmentation with bovine hydroxyapatite and autogenous bone. J Oral Maxillofac Surg 2002;60:277–284.
68. Hallman M, Sennerby L, Lundgren S. A clinical and histologic evaluation of implant integration in the posterior maxilla after sinus floor augmentation with autogenous bone, bovine hydroxyapatite, or a 20:80 mixture. Int J Oral Maxillofac Implants 2002;17:635–643.
69. Valentini P, Abensur D, Wenz B, Peetz M, Schenk R. Sinus grafting with porous bone mineral (Bio-Oss) for implant placement: A 5-year study on 15 patients. Int J Periodontics Restorative Dent 2000;20:245–253.
70. van den Bergh JP, ten Bruggenkate CM, Krekeler G, Tuinzing DB. Maxillary sinus floor elevation and grafting with human demineralized freeze dried bone. Clin Oral Implants Res 2000;11:487–493.
71. Wallace SS, Froum SJ. Effect of maxillary sinus augmentation on the survival of endosseous dental implants. A systematic review. Ann Periodontol 2003;8:328–343.
72. Del Fabbro M, Testori T, Francetti L, Weinstein R. Meta-analysis of survival rates for implants placed in the grafted maxillary sinus. Int J Periodontics Restorative Dent 2004;24:565–577.
73. Jensen OT, Shulman LB, Block MS, Iacono VJ. Report of the Sinus Consensus Conference of 1996. Int J Oral Maxillofac Implants 1998;13(suppl):11–32.
74. Tong DC, Rioux K, Drangsholt M, Beime OR. A review of the survival rates for implants placed in grafted maxillary sinuses using meta-analysis. Int J Oral Maxillofac Implants 1998;13:175–182.
75. Buck B, Malinin T, Brown M. Bone transplantation and human immunodeficiency virus. Clin Orthop 1988;240:129.
76. Martin LS, McDougal JS, Loskoski SL. Disinfection and inactivation of the human T lymphotropic virus type III/lymphadenopathy-associated virus. J Infect Dis 1985;152:400–403.
77. Resnick L, Veren K, Salahuddin SZ, Tondreau S, Markham PD. Stability and inactivation of HTL-III/LAV under clinical and laboratory environments. JAMA 1986;255:1887–1891.
78. Mellonig J, Prewett A, Moyer M. HIV inactivation in a bone allograft. J Periodontol 1992;63:979–983.
79. Urist M, Iwata R. Preservation and biodegradation of the morphogenetic property of bone matrix. J Theor Biol 1973;38:155.
80. Urist M, Jurist J, Dubuc F, Strates B. Quantitation of new bone formation in intramuscular implants of bone matrix in rabbits. Clin Orthop 1970;68:279.
81. Albrektsson T, Zarb G, Worthington P, Eriksson AR. The long-term efficacy of currently used dental implants: A review and proposed criteria of success. Int J Oral Maxillofac Implants 1986;1:11–25.
82. Langer B, Langer L. Use of allografts for sinus grafting. In: Jensen O (ed). The Sinus Bone Graft. Chicago: Quintessence, 1999:69–72.
83. Albrektsson T, Wennerberg A. Oral implant surfaces: Part I—Review focusing on topographic and chemical properties of different surfaces and in vivo responses to them. Int J Prosthodont 2004;17:536–543.

chapter 16
Use of Alloplasts for Sinus Floor Grafting

Ole T. Jensen, DDS, MS
Giuliano Garlini, DDS
Dieter Bilk, DDS
Fabian Peters, PhD, MS

Hydroxyapatite (HA), beta-tricalcium phosphate (β-TCP), bioactive glass, and xenograft have demonstrated almost equal efficacy both clinically and scientifically for use in sinus floor grafting procedures.[1–4] Resorbable and nonresorbable alloplasts are more or less indistinguishable in terms of their capacity for space maintenance, osteoconduction, and facilitation of bone migration from the sinus floor. From a biologic perspective, then, the question we must ask is not which material to use, but how to achieve the most favorable bone-healing capacity. Endosteal proliferation in the sinus floor does not depend on the type of graft material used,[5] and sinus bone graft "success" is generally measured by dental implant restorability, a highly indirect method of measuring bone graft integrity.[6]

The question has been raised as to whether sinus elevation and implant placement *without* a bone graft is sufficient for sinus floor augmentation. Figure 16-1 documents a case study performed at the University of Colorado School of Dentistry in 1995 to test this theory.[7] Sinus elevation and implant placement were accomplished without bone grafting, and an expanded polytetrafluoroethylene (e-PTFE) (ie, Teflon) membrane was used to cover the osteotomy site (see Figs 16-1a to 16-1d). The 4-year progression of sinus floor bone "growth" was measured using subtraction radiography. By year 4, the sinus floor bone had migrated up and over the apex of the distal implant, which initially had five screw threads exposed to the sinus cavity. This 5-mm migration suggests the *intrinsic* capacity of the sinus floor to proliferate without graft placement. Some of the height gain was passive migration (Fig 16-1e) that occurred prior to loading, and some was active "growth" stimulated by biomechanical bone strain from occlusal function over time (Fig 16-1f). These few millimeters of additional sinus floor bone may provide sufficient clinically significant osseointegration to sustain occlusal forces (see chapter 9). Based on this finding, large sinus bone grafts may be superfluous or even contraindicated since most implant load is confined to the crestal 5 mm of the implant.[8–11]

This raises another question: Whether it is xenograft, allograft, or autograft, why use biologically derived graft material at all? While autograft is the so-called gold standard for reconstruction of discontinuity defects, what about the sinus floor? If alloplasts provide the necessary few millimeters of bone augmentation in the majority of cases, why subject patients to the added risk—be it ever so small—of implanting *materia biomedica*?

chapter 16 Use of Alloplasts for Sinus Floor Grafting

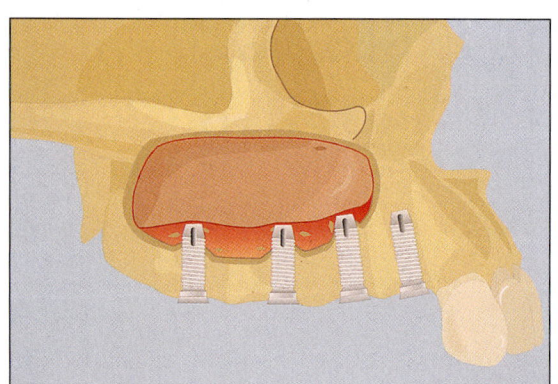

Fig 16-1a Minor elevation of the sinus may be accomplished through a small lateral antrostomy, and then implants can be placed to "tent up" the sinus membrane. Bone will fill some of the space by passive migration from the sinus floor. Following biomechanical loading, bone strain–mediated active migration will occur over time.

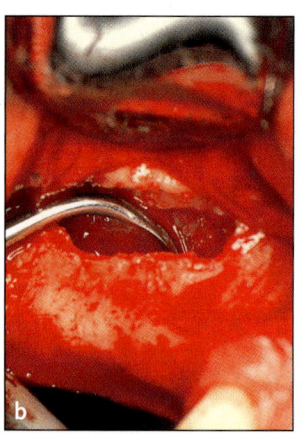 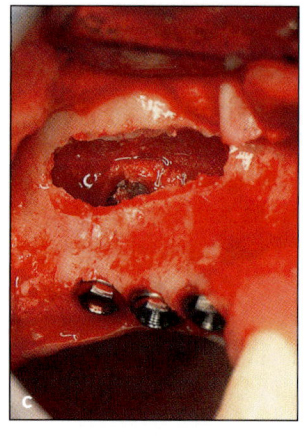

Figs 16-1b and 16-1c *(b)* The sinus membrane is elevated through a narrow antrostomy window. *(c)* Placement of three smooth-surfaced screw-form implants in the sinus cavity with five, six, and eight screw threads exposed *(front to back). No bone graft is placed.* Primary implant stability is obtained.

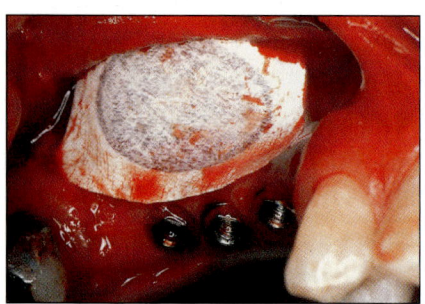 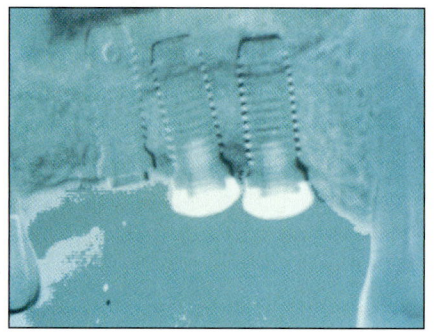 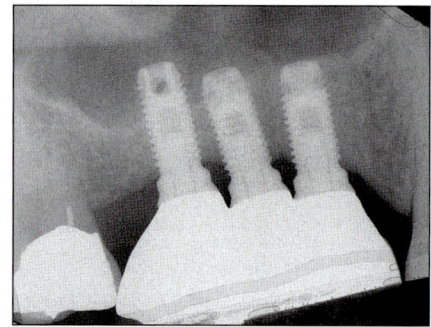

Fig 16-1d Lateral placement of Teflon membrane. The wound is closed primarily. (Figs 16-1b to 16-1d courtesy of Dr Brian Brada, Lakewood, Colorado.)

Fig 16-1e Four-month postsurgical radiograph shows screw thread exposures of two, three, and seven *(front to back)*.

Fig 16-1f Four-year postsurgical radiograph shows screw thread exposures of five, two, and zero *(front to back)*. Overall bone augmentation over the 4-year period is 5 mm.

Comparison of Alloplast Materials

Hydroxyapatite

HA in its various permutations has demonstrated excellent osteoconductive capacity (Fig 16-2).[12–15] A recent study compared the degree of marginal bone resorption and implant longevity when HA or xenograft was used in sinus augmentation and found no significant difference in terms of bone resorption around implants or osseointegration success rates in a 4-year follow-up study.[16] In this study, a 97% success rate was reported for treatment of 34 patients with 26 sinus grafts and 37 implants placed, with 1 implant lost. Marginal bone loss was 1 mm for both HA and xenograft. This and other similar studies throw into doubt the microarchitectural advantage long associated with the use of deproteinized bovine bone.[16]

In another study, HA in the form of solid bioceramic discs was used to treat critical-sized defects in rat craniums that were allowed to heal primarily. The ceramic achieved

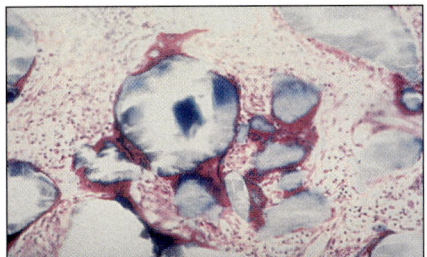

Fig 16-2a Early woven bone (red) growing on the osteoconductive surface of HA (Biostite) (magnification ×25).

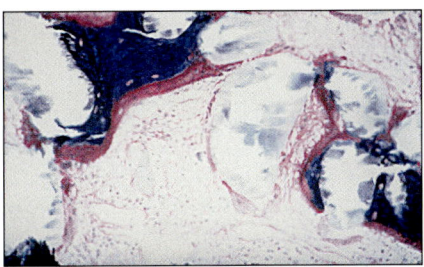

Fig 16-2b Lamellar bone formation (blue) and continued expansion of osseous density by woven bone (red) in intermediate healing phase of HA (magnification ×160).

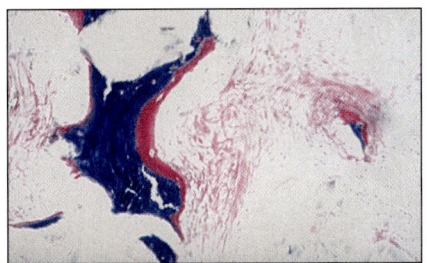

Fig 16-2c Newly forming bone encircles the HA particles (magnification ×160).

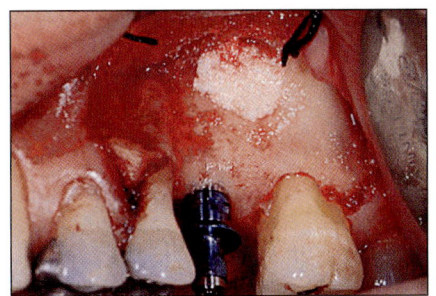

Fig 16-2d Simultaneous implant placement with HA sinus graft from a lateral antrostomy approach.

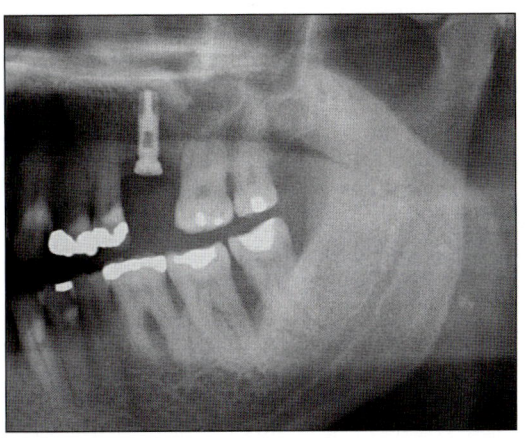

Fig 16-2e Radiopaque shadow evident of HA-grafted sinus.

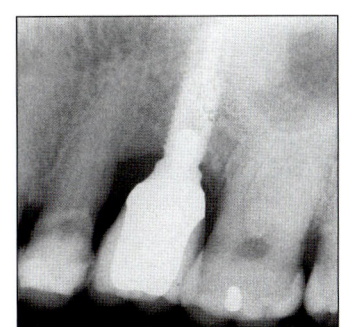

Fig 16-2f Stable osseous graft and osseointegration 3 years postrestoration.

better results than autogenous graft alone. Such findings indicate that when ceramic is placed in close approximation with native bone, as it is in the sinus floor, excellent results can be obtained if the microarchitecture is favorable. Porous ceramic in pore sizes ranging from 50 to 300 μm is most optimal for bone growth.[17]

Ewers used Algipore (Friadent), an unusual HA-like product made of porous calcified plant matrix, for sinus grafting. Over a period of 15 years, more than 1,000 sinus-directed implants were placed and overall retention was greater than 90%.[18,19] These results coincide with the findings of Hurzeler et al,[20] who used porous corraline for sinus floor grafts followed by dental implant placement and reported greater than 90% retention after 12 years of follow-up.

Bioactive glass

Bioglass (BioGran, Implant Innovations Inc) is a silicon dioxide material that contains calcium, phosphate, and sodium ions (45% SiO_2, 24.5% CaO, 24.5% Na_2O and 6% P_2O_5) in particle sizes ranging from 90 to 710 μm.[21]

When bioglass particles come into contact with tissue fluid, hydroxycarbonate apatite (HCA) forms on their surface, making them highly conducive to osteoblast attachment via chondroitin sulfate and glycosamine protein bonds. Mineralization progresses rapidly under these conditions, resulting in dense bone formation. Bioactive glass bonds directly to bone, but because of the amorphous nature of its structure, it is not a true ceramic. Through osteoconduction, glass becomes wholly incorporated and

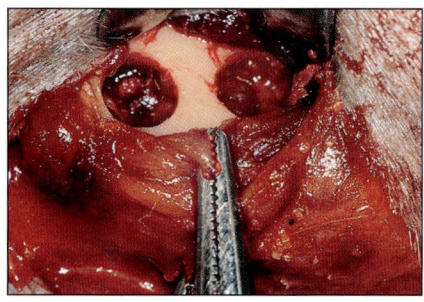 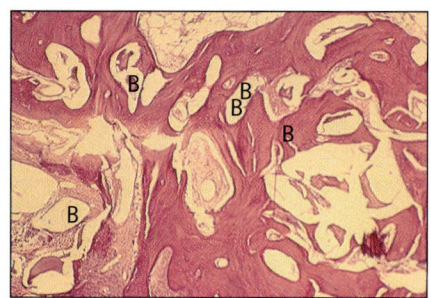 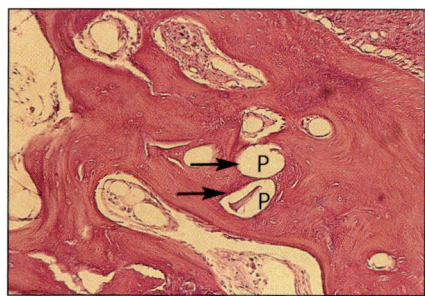

Fig 16-3a Brown capuchin *(Cebus apella)* monkey mandible prepared with 5-mm critical-sized defects for comparison of the use of alloplasts in bone grafting. (Figs 16-3a to 16-3c reprinted from Cancian et al[26] with permission.)

Fig 16-3b Placement of granules of bioglass with irregular shapes and sizes demonstrates osteoconductivity and bone formation. Many residual glass particles are completely enclosed in bone. At 26 weeks, there is no evidence of an inflammatory process. (B = bioglass.)

Fig 16-3c Placement of small, regular, particle-sized granules of bioglass (PerioGlas, US Biomaterials) completely fills the defect with bone. Smaller amounts of regular-shaped particles remain. At 12 weeks, an absence of inflammation is noted. (P = PerioGlas.)

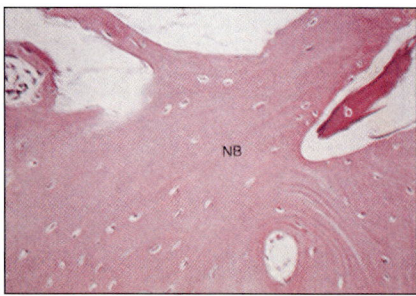 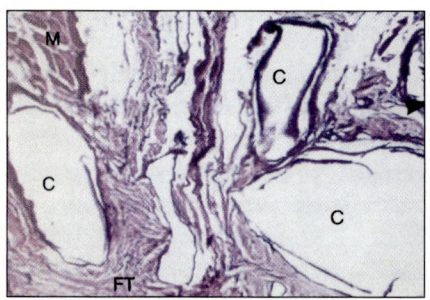

Fig 16-3d Placement of bioglass (BioGran, Orthovita) resulted in complete bone replacement in 180 days. (NB = new bone.) (Figs 16-3d and 16-3e reprinted from Cancian et al[25] with permission.)

Fig 16-3e Placement of nonporous HA (Calcitite) resulted in a predominance of scar formation at 180 days. (C = *Calcitite*; FT = *fibrous tissue*.)

is then resorbed and replaced by bone.[22–24] In one study, the dissolution of glass particles resulted in bone formation centrally within the glass granule, but most reports describe a simple peripheral dissolution of glass and its replacement with bone in a noninflammatory process. Cancian et al compared the use of HA (Calcitite, Zimmer Dental) with bioglass in monkey mandibular defects and observed replacement of bioglass with new bone after 180 days, whereas scar tissue and a foreign body reaction developed around the HA over the same period (Fig 16-3).[25,26]

Furusawa and Mizunuma used bioglass in 25 grafted sinuses and reported that 7 months later, trephine biopsies demonstrated bone formation in all cases.[27]

Beta-tricalcium phosphate

β-TCP is a highly biocompatible, resorbable, osteoconductive grafting material that has been tested in many animal studies and used extensively for repair of bone defects and to expand autograft for sinus grafting. This material has performed extremely well in space maintenance and as a graft replacement and has been successfully used in the sinus.[6,28]

Following tooth extraction in a beagle dog, Suba et al used β-TCP (Cerasorb, Curasan) to fill the sockets and showed that lamellar bone formed without an inflammatory process even as the β-TCP resorbed (Fig 16-4).[29]

Artzi et al placed β-TCP (Cerasorb) or bovine bone in critical-sized defects in mongrel dog mandibles. Both showed excellent bone bridging, but the β-TCP had entirely resorbed by 24 months and was completely replaced by lamellar bone (Fig 16-5).[30]

Engelke et al used β-TCP to place sinus-directed implants and reported that 200 implants osseointegrated for a 95% success rate.[31]

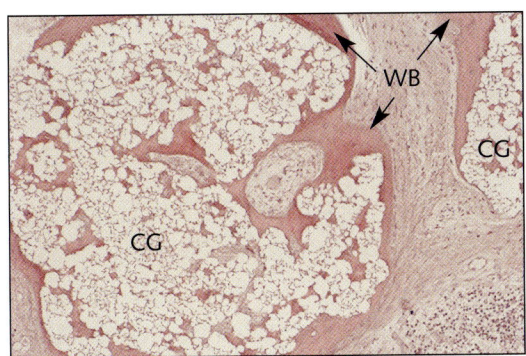 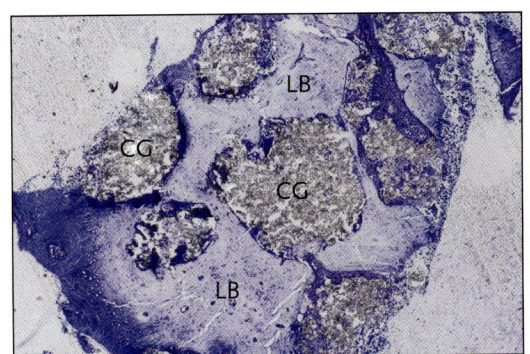

Fig 16-4a Beagle dog extraction sockets treated with resorbable β-TCP (Cerasorb) at 12 weeks, showing osteogenic mesenchyma and woven bone while osteoclastic action is observed; it is not on the graft material itself. Channels within the porous β-TCP are partially filled with osteoid (CG = β-TCP; WB = woven bone) (hematoxylin-eosin; magnification ×10).

Fig 16-4b Beagle dog extraction sockets treated with β-TCP at 24 weeks, showing newly formed lamellar bone with embedded but resorbing β-TCP. No inflammatory reaction is noted (CG = β-TCP; LB = lamellar bone) (toluidine blue; magnification ×2). (Figs 16-4a and 16-4b reprinted from Suba et al[29] with permission.)

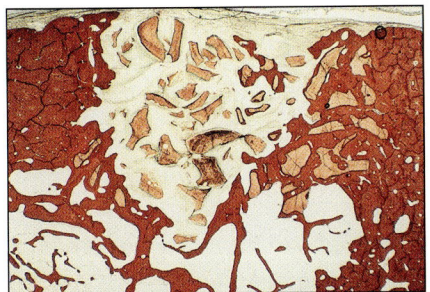 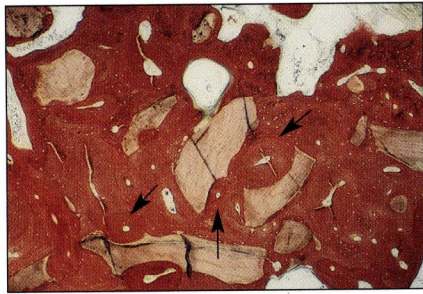 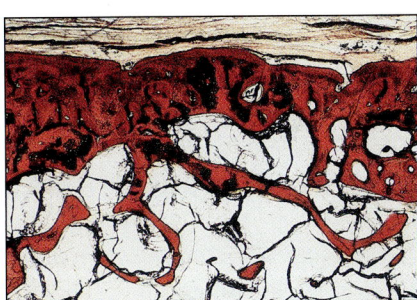

Fig 16-5a Critical-sized defects in mongrel dog mandible implanted with inorganic bovine bone matrix. Healing from the periphery of the defect via osteoconductive bone formation is observed by 3 months (Stevenel blue and Van Gieson picro fuchsia; magnification ×20).

Fig 16-5b Haversian systems *(arrows)* in close approximation to xenograft particles at 24 months.

Fig 16-5c Incorporation of β-TCP (Cerasorb) and bone bridging across the defect at 6 months (magnification ×20).

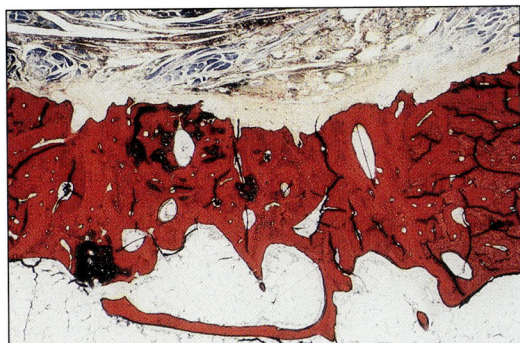 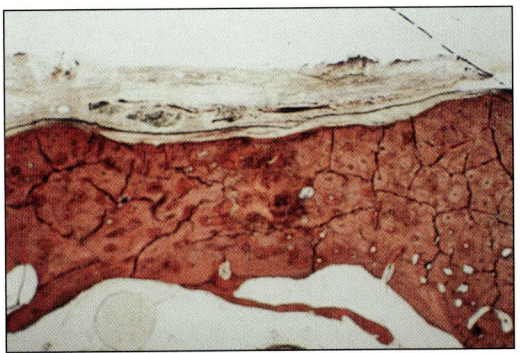

Fig 16-5d Substantial replacement of the β-TCP with bone at 12 months.

Fig 16-5e Complete resorption of the β-TCP particles and replacement by lamellar bone at 24 months. (Figs 16-5a to 16-5e reprinted from Artzi et al[30] with permission.)

The success of bone regeneration using different β-TCP products varies because of differences in phase purity, porosity, and particle size. During biodegradation of β-TCP, two processes can affect graft performance: hydrolytic *degradation* and osteoclastic *resorption*. These are the processes that are determined by phase purity, porosity, and particle size and stability.

Phase purity
TCP can be divided into two phases based on atom position in the crystal lattice. The chemical formula $Ca_3(PO_4)_2$ is transformed by heat from the beta (β) phase to the alpha (α) phase, which leads to changes of material characteristics. The α phase is much more soluble than the β phase.[32] When α-TCP is used in bone grafting, it dissolves and then recrystallizes as a thermodynamically stable calcium, and the result is a nonresorbable HA ($Ca_{10}(PO_4)_6(OH)_2$). By modifying the phases of the material and increasing its porosity, the rate at which it undergoes degradation and resorption can be adapted somewhat to accommodate the rate of bone regeneration.[33,34]

HA remains after resorption of β-TCP if two phases are present. If HA particles are finely dispersed within the β-TCP biomaterial, they provoke an inflammatory reaction. More soluble calcium phosphate phases, such as calcium pyrophosphate or α-TCP, will disintegrate before bone is replaced and scar tissue forms. Therefore, phase purity should be at least 99% in order to avoid an unfavorable biologic response.[35]

Porosity
The dissolution speed of a resorbable biomaterial is controlled by porosity. Higher porosity leads to more rapid resorption. Pores and cavities are important for perfusion. Blood vessels and newly formed bone grow through porous biomaterial, provided it has a minimum pore size of 60 μm.[36] Bone ingrowth is also supported by interconnections of 20 μm to augment cell nutrition of pores optimally sized from 50 to 100 μm.[31] Long-winding pores do not fill with bone. A basic biologic principle formulated by De Groot is that the maximum length of an open pore should not exceed 10 times its width.[37]

Modulation of resorption/degradation rates may be required to treat different types of defects.[38] Mandibular defects associated with dental implant preparation demand rapid resorption and therefore a high porosity, while periodontal defects require treatment with a low porosity for optimal bone healing.

Particle size and stability
In 1985, De Groot observed that implants made of macro- and microporous β-TCP disintegrated rapidly into particles that could be found in neighboring lymph nodes.[37] Particulate disintegration was the result of mechanical instability of the material. The relationship between particle size and foreign body reactions shows that small particles of a few micrometers undergo giant cell reaction.[35,36] Phagocytosed particles are transported to the lymph nodes. To minimize the risk of this inflammatory reaction, the average particle size should be larger than 7 to 10 μm. A β-TCP made up of small-sized particles must have mechanically stable interconnection to prevent phagocytic disintegration. Formation of new bone requires material degradation, not fragmentation, which provokes an inflammatory response.[38] Over the past 30 years, different temperatures and pressures have been used to modify β-TCP (Fig 16-6).[39] Granular and block forms are now available for regeneration of bone throughout the endoskeleton, but only β-TCP with a validated phase purity of at least 99%[39] is recommended for use in the sinus graft. Round granules with a porosity of 30 ± 5% (pore size 0.1 to 50 μm), or with a porosity of 60 ± 5% (maxipore size 0.1 to 500 μm) can be used alone or mixed with autograft. In the future, patient-specific resorbable block-form implants made from pure-phase β-TCP will be available. Data derived through computerized tomography will be sent for shaping using computer-aided design/computer-assisted manufacturing technology to fit specific surgical defects, such as those made for the interpositional bone graft[40] or advance Le Fort osteotomy in conjunction with sinus grafting (Fig 16-7) (see chapter 20).[41–45]

Particulate porous β-TCP is well suited for osteotome sinus floor intrusion with simultaneous implant placement (Fig 16-8). It can also be used in conjunction with a lateral approach (Fig 16-9) as an adjunct expander with autograft (Fig 16-10).

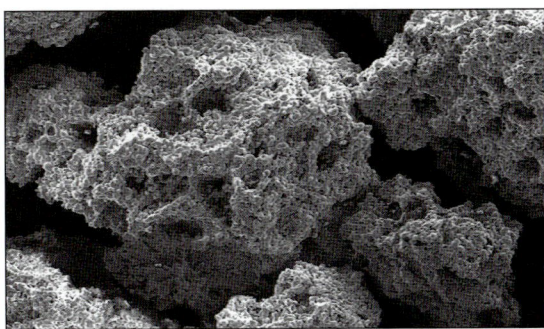

Fig 16-6 Scanning electron micrograph (SEM) of β-TCP granules (Cerasorb M) of 1,000 to 2,000 μm (magnification ×70.5).

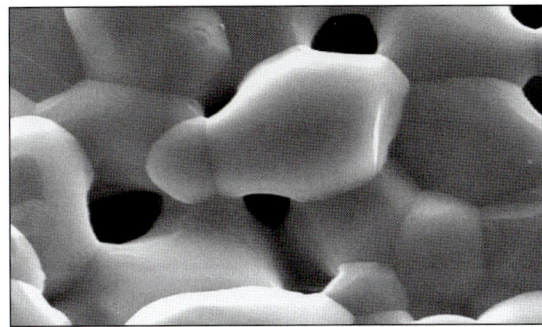

Fig 16-7 Primary particles of Cerasorb β-TCP have an average size of at least 10 μm with interconnecting porous scaffold formed via sinternecks. The material is both porous and mechanically stable (SEM; magnification ×3,000).

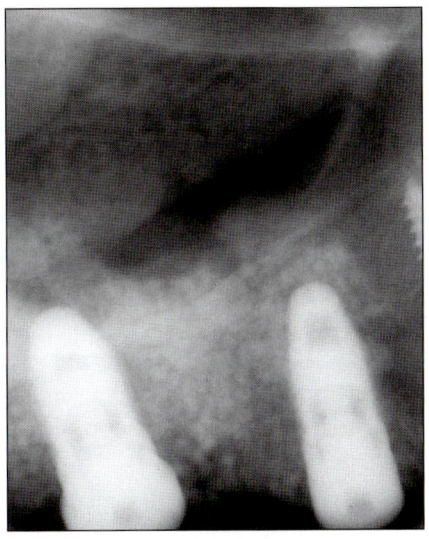

Fig 16-8 β-TCP used as an extender of the sinus floor in the osteotome technique. This may be useful in highly trabecular bone.

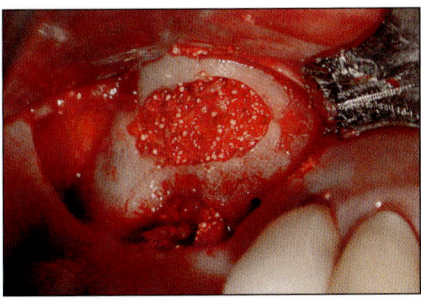

Fig 16-9 Sinus graft site packed with β-TCP and autograft in a 50:50 ratio.

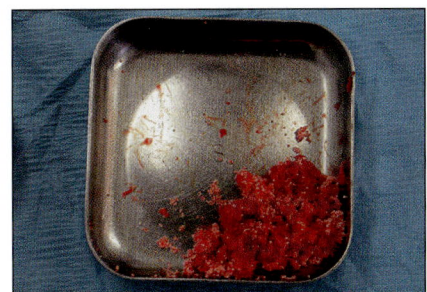

Fig 16-10 Autograft mixed with β-TCP in a 50:50 ratio. This is an effective strategy for sinus augmentation.

Summary

Calcium phosphates, bioactive glasses, and hydroxyapatites have now been used successfully for sinus graft augmentation in the vast majority of situations, either alone or as an expander.

Pure-phase β-TCP offers ready availability in unlimited supply of a material that is free of allergens and foreign proteins and avoids second-site surgery for bone harvest. The material is resorbable, easy to handle, predictable, and compatible with the barrier membrane. It also reduces surgical treatment time. Bioglass, too, is a highly osteoconductive material that resorbs over time with a high ratio of bone replacement. HA, when porous, is a favorable bone conductor as well. All of these alloplasts are excellent at forming bone sufficient for osseointegration, mostly due to the favorable bone-growing capacity of the sinus floor.

References

1. Wheeler SL. Sinus augmentation for dental implants: The use of alloplastic materials. J Oral Maxillofac Surg 1997;55:1287–1293.
2. Scher EL, Day RB, Speight PM. New bone formation after a sinus lift procedure using demineralized freeze-dried bone and tricalcium phosphate. Implant Dent 1999;8:49–53.
3. Chanavaz M. Sinus graft procedures and implant dentistry: A review of 21 years of surgical experience (1979–2000). Implant Dent 2000;9:197–206.
4. Block MS, Kent JN. Sinus augmentation for dental implants: The use of autogenous bone. J Oral Maxillofac Surg 1997;55:1281–1286.
5. Jensen OT, Sennerby L. Histologic analysis of clinically retrieved titanium microimplants placed in conjunction with maxillary sinus floor augmentation. Int J Oral Maxillofac Implants 1998;13(4):513–521.
6. Jensen OT, Shulman L, Block M, Iacono VJ. Report of the Sinus Consensus Conference of 1996. Int J Oral Maxillofac Implants 1998;13(suppl):11–45.
7. Jensen OT. Treatment planning for sinus grafts. In: Jensen OT (ed). The Sinus Bone Graft. Chicago: Quintessence, 1999:49–68.
8. Akca K, Cehreli MC, Iplikcioglu H. A comparison of three-dimensional finite element stress analysis with in vitro strain gauge measurements on dental implants. Int J Prosthodont 2002;15:115–121.
9. Pierrisnard L, Renouard F, Renault P, Barquins M. Influence of implant length and bicortical anchorage on implant stress distribution. Clin Implant Dent Relat Res 2003;4:254–262.
10. Renouard F, Nisand D. Short implants in the severely resorbed maxilla—A 2-year retrospective clinical study. Clin Implant Dent Relat Res 2005;7(suppl 1):S104–S110.
11. Tawil G, Younan R. Clinical evaluation of short, machined-surface implants followed for 12 to 92 months. Int J Oral Maxillofac Implants. 2003;18:894–901.
12. Kokubun S, Kashimoto O, Tanaka Y. Histological verification of bone bonding and ingrowth into porous hydroxyapatite spinous process spacer for cervical laminoplasty. Tohoku J Exp Med 1994;173:337–344.
13. Martin RB, Chapman MW, Sharkey NA, Zissimos SL, Bay B, Shores EC. Bone ingrowth and mechanical properties of coralline hydroxyapatite 1 yr after implantation. Biomaterials 1993;14:341–348.
14. Ono I, Ohura T, Murata M, Yamaguchi H, Ohnuma Y, Kuboki Y. A study on bone induction in hydroxyapatite combined with bone morphogenetic protein. Plast Reconstr Surg 1992;90:870–879.
15. Ono I, Tateshita T, Nakajima T. Evaluation of a high density polyethylene fixing system for hydroxyapatite ceramic implants. Biomaterials 2000;21:143–151.
16. Marorana C, Sigurta D, Mirandola A, Garlini G, Santoro F. Bone resorption around dental implants placed in grafted sinuses: Clinical and radiologic follow-up after up to 4 years. Int J Oral Maxillofac Implants 2005;20:261–266.
17. Silva RV, Camilli JA, Bertran CA, Moreira NH. The use of hydroxyapatite and autogenous cancellous bone grafts to repair bone defects in rats. Int J Oral Maxillofac Surg 2005;34:178–184.
18. Schopper C, Moser D, Sabbas A, et al. The fluorohydroxyapatite (FHA) FRIOS Algipore is a suitable biomaterial for the reconstruction of severely atrophic human maxillae. Clin Oral Implants Res 2003;14:743–749.
19. Schopper C, Moser D, Wanschitz F, et al. Histomorphologic findings on human bone samples six months after bone augmentation of the maxillary sinus with Algipore. J Long Term Eff Med Implants 1999;9:203–213.
20. Hurzeler MB, Kirsch A, Ackermann KL, Quinones CR. Reconstruction of the severely resorbed maxilla with dental implants in the augmented maxillary sinus: A 5-year clinical investigation. Int J Oral Maxillofac Implants 1996;11:466–475.
21. Wilson J, Pigott GH, Schoen FJ, Hench LL. Taxicology and biocompatibility of bioglasses. J Biomed Mater Res 1981;15:805–817.
22. Anderegg CR, Alexander DC, Freidman MA. A bioactive glass particulate in the treatment of molar furcation invasion. J Periodontol 1999;70:384–387.
23. Schepers E, Ducheyne P. Bioactive glass particles of narrow size range for the treatment of oral bone effects: A 1–24 month experiment with several materials and particle sizes and size ranges. J Oral Rehabil 1997;3:171–181.
24. Shimizu Y, Sugawara H, Furusawa T, Mizunuma K, Inada K, Yamashita S. Bone remodeling with resorbable bioactive glass and hydroxyapatite. Implant Dent 1997;6:269–274.
25. Cancian DC, Hochuli-Vieira E, Marcantonio RA, Marcantonio E. Use of BioGran and Calcitite in bone defects: Histologic study in monkeys (Cebus apella). Int J Oral Maxillofac Implants 1999;14:859–864.
26. Cancian DCJ, Hochuli-Vieira E, Mercantonio RAC, Garcia, Jr IR. Utilization of autogenous bone, bioactive glasses, and calcium phosphate cement in surgical mandibular bone defects in Cebus apella monkeys. Int J Oral Maxillofac Implants 2004;19:73–79.
27. Furusawa T, Mizunuma K. Osteoconductive properties and efficacy of resorbable bioactive glass as a bone-grafting material. Implant Dent 1997;6(2):93–101.
28. Williams DF. The biocompatibility and clinical uses of calcium phosphate ceramics. In: Williams DF (ed). Biocompatibility of Tissue Analogs, vol 2. Boca Raton, FL: CRC Press, 1985:44–65.
29. Suba Z, Takacs D, Gyulai-Gaal S, Kovacs K. Facilitation of β-tricalcium phosphate–induced alveolar bone regeneration by platelet-rich plasma in beagle dogs: A histologic and histomorphometric study. Int J Oral Maxillofac Implants 2004;19:832–838.
30. Artzi Z, Weinreb M, Givol N, et al. Biomaterial resorption rate and healing site morphology of inorganic bovine bone and β-tricalcium phosphate in the canine: A 24-month longitudinal histologic study and morphometric analysis. Int J Oral Maxillofac Implants 2004;19:357–368.
31. Engelke W, Schwarzwaller W, Behnsen A, Jacobs HG. Subantroscopic laterobasal sinus floor augmentation (SALSA): An up-to-5-year clinical study. Int J Oral Maxillofac Implants 2003;18:135–143.

32. Elliott JC. Structure and Chemistry of the Apatities and Other Calcium Orthophosphates, Studies in Inorganic Chemistry, 18. New York: Elsevier, 1994.
33. Wiltfang J, Merten HA, Schlegel KA, et al. Degradation characteristics of α and β tri-calcium-phosphate (TCP) in minipigs. J Biomed Mater Res 2002;63:115–121.
34. ASTM F 1088-04. Standard Specification for Beta Tricalcium Phosphate for Surgical Implantation. ASTM International.
35. Peters F, Reif D. Functional materials for bone regeneration from beta-tricalcium phosphate. Mat Wiss U Werkstofftech 2004;35:203–207.
36. Eggli PS, Mueller W, Schenk RK. The role of pore size on bone ingrowth and implant substitution in hydroxyapatite and tricalcium phosphate ceramics: A histologic and morphometric study in rabbits. In: Pizzoferrato A, Marchetti PG, Ravigiolo A, Lee AJC (eds). Biomaterials and Clinical Applications. Amsterdam: Elsevier Science, 1987:53–56.
37. De Groot K. Effect of porosity and physicochemical properties on the stability, resorption, and strength of calcium phosphate ceramics. Ann N Y Acad Sci 1988;523:227–233.
38. Klawitter JJ, Hulbert SF. Application of porous ceramics for the attachment of load bearing internal orthopedic applications. J Biomed Mater Res Symposium 1971;2:161–229.
39. Lu J, Descamps M, Dejou J, et al. The biodegradation mechanism of calcium phosphate biomaterials in bone. J Biomed Mater Res 2002;63:408–412.
40. Shimizu S. Subcutaneous tissue responses in rats to injection of fine particles of synthetic hydroxyapatite ceramic. Biomed Res 1988;9:95–111.
41. Heide H, Koster K, Lukas H. Neuere Werstoffe in der medizinischen Technik. Chemie-Ing Techn 1975;47:327–333.
42. Tadic D, Epple M. A thorough physicochemical characterization of 14 calcium phosphate-based bone substitution materials in comparison to natural bone. Biomaterials 2004;25:987–994.
43. Jensen OT. Combined sinus grafting and Le Fort I procedures. In: Jensen OT (ed). The Sinus Bone Graft. Chicago: Quintessence, 1999:191–200.
44. Jensen OT, Kuhlke L, Bedard JF, White D. Alveolar segmental sandwich osteotomies for vertical maxillary augmentation prior to implant placement. J Oral Maxillofac Surg 2006 (in press).
45. Jensen OT. Posterior alveolar segmental "sandwich" osteotomies of edentulous sites for dental implants. J Oral Maxillofac Surg 2006 (in press).

chapter 17
Use of Xenografts for Sinus Augmentation

Stuart J. Froum, DDS
Stephen S. Wallace, DDS
Sang-Choon Cho, DDS, BDS, MS
Dennis P. Tarnow, DDS

The use of xenografts has been demonstrated to be effective for increasing bone height and bone volume in the deficient posterior maxilla.[1] Anorganic bovine bone matrix alone and in combination with autogenous bone is the graft material of choice for many practitioners who perform sinus augmentation procedures. In fact, a survey of the literature on bone replacement grafts (BRGs) showed that studies of the use of xenografts are the most complete and well documented.[2,3] This chapter presents the clinical and scientific reasons for the gradual shift from using autogenous bone alone to substituting xenografts for part or all of the graft, as shown in two recently published evidence-based reviews[2,3] and other recent literature.

Criteria for Evaluation and Comparison

The success of the sinus elevation procedure is best evaluated by considering therapeutic goals and patient outcomes. The goals of sinus augmentation include formation of vital bone where no bone existed and the long-term survival and success of functionally loaded implants placed in graft bone. From a clinical perspective, the latter is determined by prospective long-term studies of implant survival. The problem with this approach is that while the comparison of efficacy of different graft materials is multifactorial, it is most often measured indirectly by a single variable: implant longevity.

Variations in technique and materials combined with timing of implant placement, differences in sinus anatomy, residual alveolar height, and host factors such as smoking and compliance make it impossible to compare disparate results from the myriad array of bone graft regimens.[3]

This is why no definitive data have established the minimal amount of vital bone that is necessary for implant integration (see chapter 5). Addressing this question, histologic measurements of vital bone formation in sinuses filled with either a xenograft (BRG) or a composite graft were compared to define the grafts' capacity for healing as well as osseointegration.

Data from evidence-based reviews correlated with histologic studies formed the basis of this review, focusing on the percentage of vital bone formed after grafting with xenograft alone, with xenograft combined with autogenous bone, and with autogenous bone alone.

Implant survival rates in sinuses grafted with these different materials were also compared. Given the paucity of randomized controlled clinical trials, the review also considered noncontrolled human trials, case series, retrospective studies, and selected case reports that included human histologic data. However, this review relies most heavily on evidence-based reviews.[2,3]

Evolution of Graft Material

In 1996, the Sinus Consensus Conference evaluated 2,997 implants placed in 1,007 augmented sinuses. Five-year data revealed that 229 implants failed, resulting in a 92.4% implant survival rate.[1]

A consensus statement from the conference concluded that "autogenous bone is appropriate for sinus grafting." The majority opinion concerning allografts, alloplasts, and xenografts, alone or in combination with each other, stated that "these materials may be effective as a graft material in selected clinical situations" but that "there are limited published data to make a statement about their use in severely atrophic situations."[1]

A literature review by Tolman[4] covered 58 articles, 591 patients, 733 grafts, and 2,315 implants. Another review by Tong et al[5] analyzed 10 articles (those that met their inclusion criteria), including 484 implants in 130 patients followed for 6 to 60 months. Implant survival was reported as follows: 90% for autogenous bone, 94% for hydroxyapatite (HA) combined with autogenous bone, 98% for demineralized freeze-dried bone combined with HA, and 87% for HA alone.[5] Neither of these review articles included xenograft as a grafting material, instead focusing primarily on success rates with autogenous bone.

Since these reviews were published, a large body of research on xenografts as bone replacement material for sinus augmentation has been documented and analyzed.

The use of 100% autogenous bone harvested extraorally from the ilium, tibia, and cranium or intraorally from the ramus, symphysis, or maxillary tuberosity has been deemed the gold standard of sinus grafting materials, for good reason. Autogenous bone contains all of the elements necessary to promote vital bone formation, including mineral, collagen matrix, growth factors, and, depending on the source and time of delivery, vital cells. Moreover, autograft is osteoinductive as well as osteoconductive. However, the use of 100% autogenous bone as a graft has certain disadvantages. For example, the need for a second surgical site increases postsurgical morbidity and surgical risks. Further, depending on the size of the sinus and the selected donor site, the postsurgical pain from the donor site may be significant. Use of autogenous bone also increases the surgical time, costs, and logistics of the surgical intervention.

A recent evidence-based review of the sinus augmentation by Wallace and Froum[2] included a total of 5,267 implants followed for a minimum period of 1 year after loading. The studies included 34 lateral window approaches of which 11 used xenograft alone or in combination with autogenous bone (composite) or mixed with platelet-rich plasma (PRP). The survival rate of the implants placed in xenografts was statistically the same as for implants placed in particulate autogenous bone grafts. This comparison is significant because implants placed into sinuses augmented with particulate grafts show a higher rate of survival than those placed in sinuses augmented with block grafts.[2] Del Fabbro et al[3] conducted a systematic review of survival rates in 39 articles that met their inclusion criteria, which consisted of 6,913 implants in 2,046 subjects with follow-up times ranging from 12 to 75 months. They reported an average survival rate of 87.7% for implants placed in 100% autogenous grafts of all categories, including block grafts, block plus particulate grafts, and particulate grafts alone. This was significantly lower than the 94.9% survival rate of implants placed in composite grafts of xenograft and autogenous bone and the 96% survival rate of implants placed in 100% xenograft.

Comparative studies by Hising et al,[6] Hallman et al,[7] and Valentini and Abensur[8] report higher survival rates for implants placed in sinuses augmented with 100% xenograft than for those augmented with 100% autogenous bone or composite grafts of xenograft and autogenous bone.

Hising et al[6] studied 231 implants placed in 92 augmented sinuses. The implant survival rate in sinuses grafted with 100% xenograft (Bio-Oss, Osteohealth) was 92.2% compared to a 77.2% survival rate of implants placed in sinuses augmented with a composite of Bio-Oss and autogenous bone.

Hallman et al[7] reported an overall survival rate of 91.0% for 111 implants placed in 36 sinuses and loaded for at least 1 year. The survival rate in sinuses augmented with 100% autogenous bone in this limited study was 82.4%. With a 20:80 composite of autogenous bone and bovine bone, the survival rate was 94.4%, and in sinuses grafted with 100% xenograft (Bio-Oss), the survival rate was 96.0%.

A recent retrospective study by Valentini and Abensur[8] evaluated the survival rate of titanium plasma spray-coated cylindrical and machined screw-type implants placed in sinus grafts in 59 consecutively treated patients. A total of 187 implants were placed in 78 grafted sinuses. The overall implant survival rate was 94.5% after a mean period of 6.5 ± 1.9 years of function. The implant survival

> **BOX 17-1** Technical considerations for the use of xenografts in sinus augmentation
>
> 1. Elevate the sinus membrane from the floor and medial sinus walls to the height of the lateral window osteotomy.
> 2. Use a 1:1 mixture of small (0.25–1.00 mg) and large (1.00–2.00 mg) particles. This results in optimal interparticle spacing. Using only small particles under compression may impede vascular ingrowth, while using only large particles may delay resorption and new bone formation.
> 3. Hydrate the xenograft particles with sterile saline.
> 4. After hydration, remove any excess saline. Placing the xenograft material in a relatively dry state makes it easier to control the placement and allows the material to hydrate with blood.
> 5. Fill the anterior compartment first to reduce the possibility of leaving empty voids.
> 6. Visualizing the medial wall, compress the xenograft particles against the floor and medial wall but not superiorly against the sinus membrane.
> 7. Place the membrane barrier over the window and extend approximately 3 mm over remaining bone.
> 8. Achieve tension-free suturing of the flap, including vertical and periosteal releasing incisions where necessary.

rate was 96.8% in sinuses grafted with xenograft alone versus 90% in sinuses grafted with a composite of xenograft and demineralized freeze-dried bone allograft.

A histologic report by Froum et al[9] showed that the addition of PRP resulted in only a 2% increase in vital bone formation when the same graft material was used in bilateral sinuses. A recent animal study by Roldan et al[10] similarly showed that the addition of PRP to xenograft was less effective in improving bone-implant contact in sinus graft procedures than was recombinant human bone morphogenetic protein-7 (rhBMP-7) and xenograft. Based on all of the data analyzed, a recent evidence-based review concludes that insufficient evidence exists to recommend the use of PRP in sinus graft surgery.[2]

When sinus grafting is followed by bone augmentation using autografts or demineralized allografts, a tendency for volumetric resorption on the order of 25% has been noted, along with a change in the density of the grafted sinus similar to that found in native bone. The result is an implant site that features type 3 or 4 bone. Histologic studies by Ulm et al,[11] Moy et al,[12] and Hanisch et al[13] report average posterior maxillary bone density of 17.1% to 23.4%, 45%, and 32.6%, respectively. Ulm et al reported that the mean trabecular bone counts may be as low as 6.73% in the maxillary molar area.[11] In addition, significant graft resorption has been reported with iliac autografts.[12,14] Recent studies in animals[15] and humans[16] showed significant reduction in bone height when either autogenous bone alone or a 2:1 mixture of autogenous bone and xenograft was used. In contrast, the cases submitted to the 1996 Sinus Consensus Conference showed minimal evidence of re-pneumatization in 3-year postoperative panoramic radiographs when sinuses were augmented with xenograft compared to allograft.[1]

Unpublished data from sinus studies conducted at New York University also show no significant change in the height of sinuses grafted with xenograft over a 3-year period. Such stability may perhaps be explained by the fact that the grafts do not completely resorb, but persist even as new vital bone is forming.

To study the performance of a material in human histomorphometric studies, bilateral sinuses of similar size should be used, and only one variable (graft type) should be altered. This is the principle applied in ongoing sinus augmentation studies at the New York University Department of Implant Dentistry. The sinus augmentation procedure utilizes a lateral window technique with adherence to certain clinical considerations (Box 17-1; Figs 17-1a to 17-1h). At the time of implant placement, new bone formation in the sinus is evaluated based on cores taken with a trephine from the healed lateral window (to avoid the possibility of including native bone) (Figs 17-1i to 17-1k). The cores are sent to an independent laboratory for nondecalcified sectioning, and the percentages of vital bone, connective tissue, and residual xenograft are reported for each specimen.[17–19]

The osteoconductive properties of xenograft in human sinus grafts[17,19,20] derive from its chemical composition as

chapter 17
Use of Xenografts for Sinus Augmentation

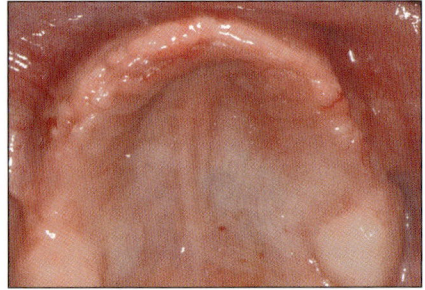

Fig 17-1a Presurgical site.

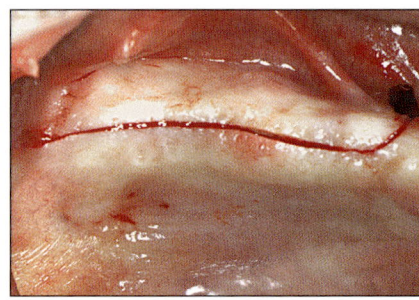

Fig 17-1b Crestal incision.

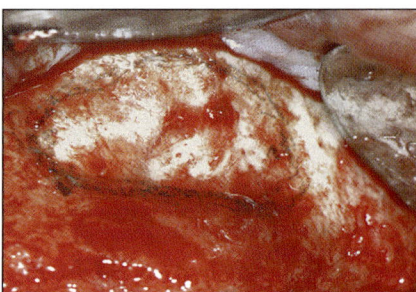

Fig 17-1c Presurgical outline of osteotomy in lateral sinus wall.

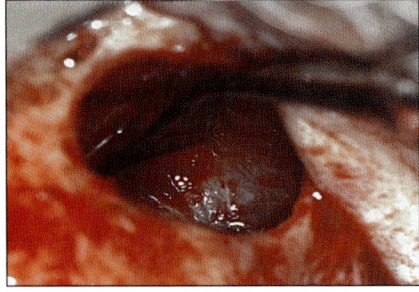

Fig 17-1d Sinus membrane elevated prior to graft placement.

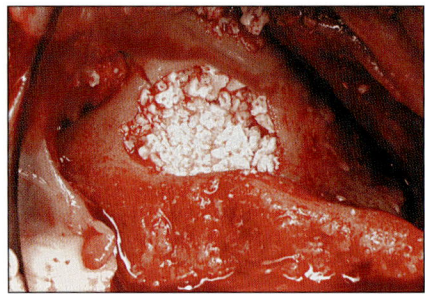

Fig 17-1e Sinus filled with xenograft.

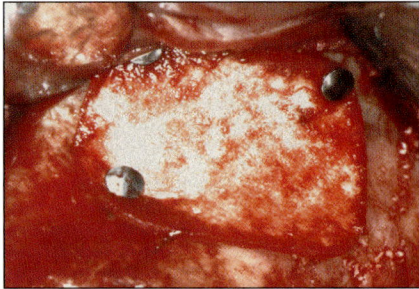

Fig 17-1f Barrier membrane placed over the lateral window.

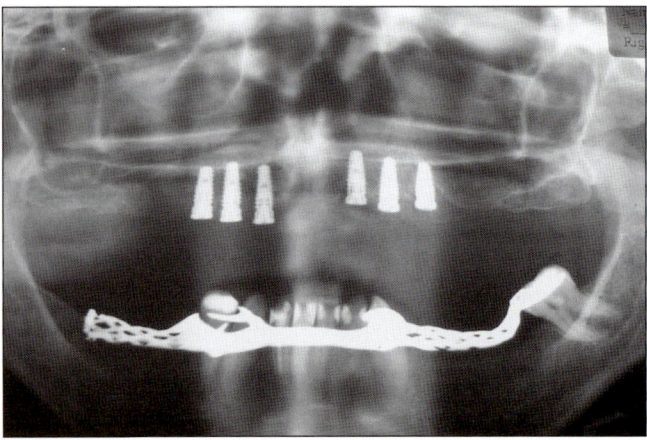

Fig 17-1g Panoramic radiograph prior to bilateral sinus graft surgery.

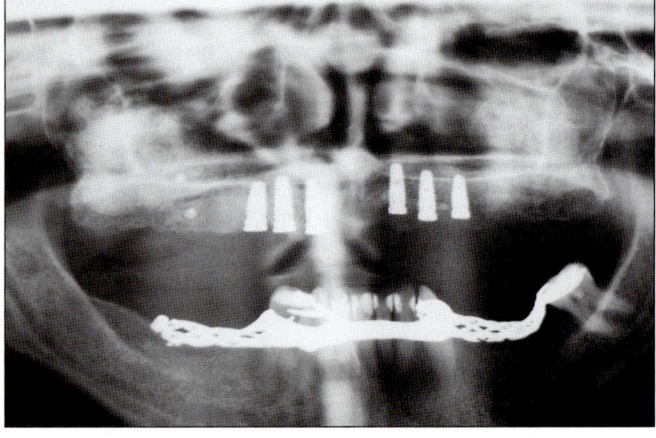

Fig 17-1h Panoramic radiograph following bilateral sinus graft surgery, demonstrating the fill of the sinus cavities with xenograft particles on one side and xenograft with autogenous bone on the other side.

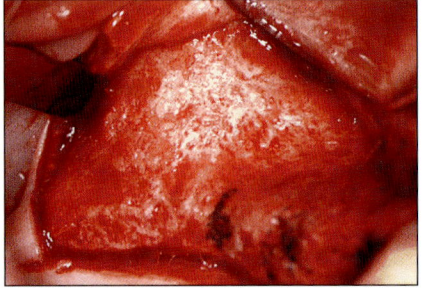

Fig 17-1i Re-entry at 12 months to harvest bone core for histologic study.

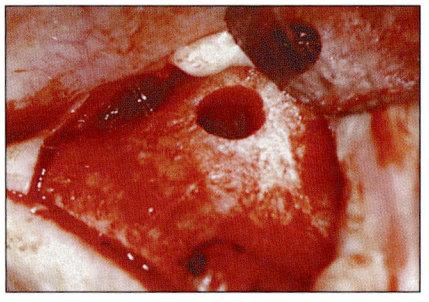

Fig 17-1j Donor site following core harvesting.

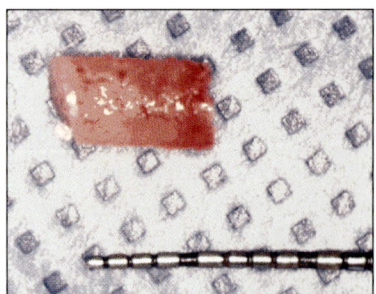

Fig 17-1k Core prior to histologic processing.

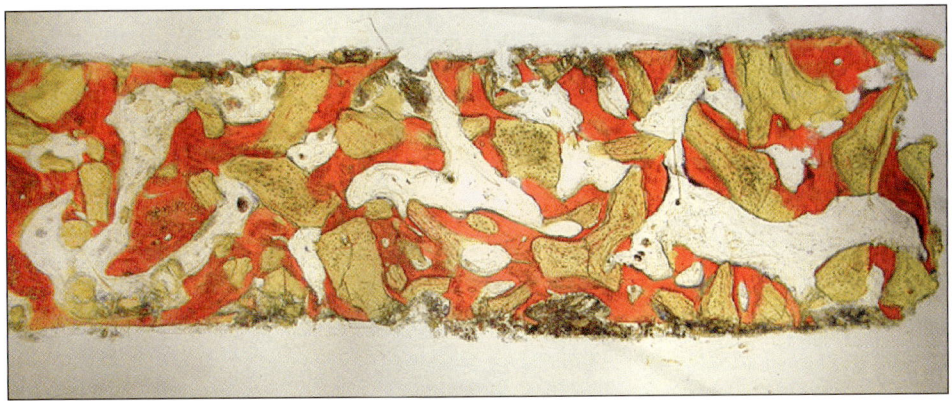

Fig 17-2a Low-power histologic view of sinus core specimen demonstrating bone growth *(red)* surrounding xenograft particles *(yellow)* at 6 months. (Stevenel blue and picric acid fuchsin; original magnification ×4.)

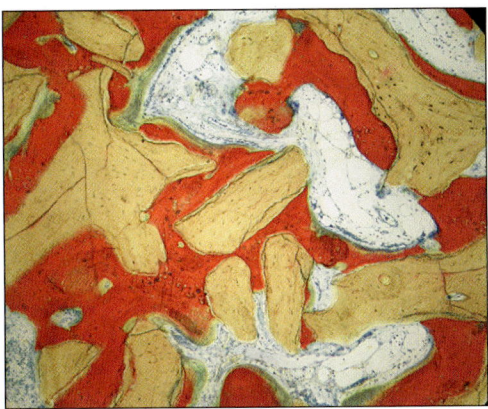

Fig 17-2b High-power histologic view of sinus core specimen demonstrating bone deposition *(red)* directly on Bio-Oss particles *(yellow)*. Note that "bridging" bone growth connects the particles (green = osteoid). (Stevenel blue and picric acid fuchsin; original magnification ×20.)

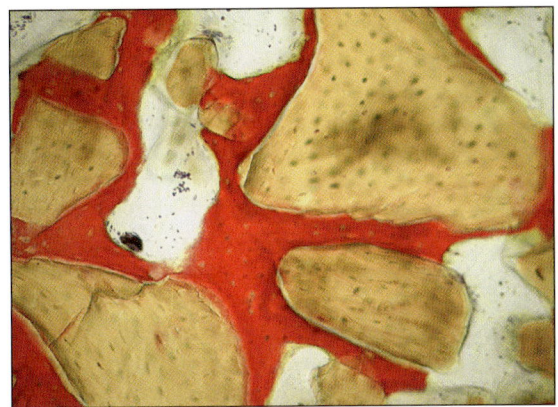

Fig 17-2c Higher-power view (original magnification ×40) of the histology shown in Fig 17-2b.

well as its macro- and micromorphology. Histologic sections of sinus cores (Fig 17-2) in studies by Froum et al[17] and Wallace et al[19] reveal the presence of osteoblasts and osteoid, as well as bone apposition directly on the surface of the xenograft particles. Vital bone is observed to "bridge" the gaps between xenograft particles and has been shown histologically to increase over time.[21] Moreover, while the formation of vital bone occurs more rapidly in sinuses grafted with 100% autogenous bone[22,23] and to a greater extent[17] initially than it does when bone replacement grafts are used, these studies also show that bone formation with xenografts equalize over time. As previously noted, xenografts have been shown to resorb slowly and incompletely (Table 17-1). For example, Piatelli et al[24] retrieved 20 biopsy specimens at time intervals ranging from 6 months to 4 years from sinuses augmented with 100% Bio-Oss. Findings at 6 to 9 months showed them to be composed of about 40% marrow space, about 30% newly formed bone, and about 30% residual Bio-Oss particles. Four-year specimens showed that Bio-Oss particles were still easily recognizable. Also present were osteoclasts in the process of resorbing Bio-Oss particles adjacent to newly formed bone[24] (Fig 17-3). In no way does this inhibit osseointegration of the implant[28–30]; in fact, the resorption of xenograft is accompanied by an increase in vital bone. Valentini et al,[20] for example, published a 6-month histology showing that proportions of bone and Bio-Oss were 21% and 39%, respectively; at 12 months, the proportion of bone had increased to 28% while the relative proportion of Bio-Oss decreased to 27%.

TABLE 17-1 Histologic composition of sinuses grafted with anorganic bovine bone (Bio-Oss) alone and with autogenous bone

Author	Graft material	Time (mos)	Bone (%)	Residual Bio-Oss (%)	Connective tissue (%)
Piatelli et al, 1999[24]	Bio-Oss alone	6–12	30	30	40
Valentini et al, 2000[20]	Bio-Oss alone	6	21	39	40
Valentini et al, 2000[20]	Bio-Oss alone	12	28	27	45
Yilderman et al, 2001[25]	Bio-Oss + autog	7.1	18.9	29.6	51.5
Yilderman et al, 2000[26]	Bio-Oss + blood	6.8	14.7	29.7	55.6
John and Wenz, 2004[27]	Bio-Oss alone	3–8	29.5	14.9	55.6
John and Wenz, 2004[27]	Bio-Oss + autog	3–8	32.2	17.8	50
NYU (unpub), 2005	Bio-Oss alone	6–12	18.5	28	53.5
NYU (unpub), 2005	Bio-Oss + autog	6–12	15.7	29.6	54.7

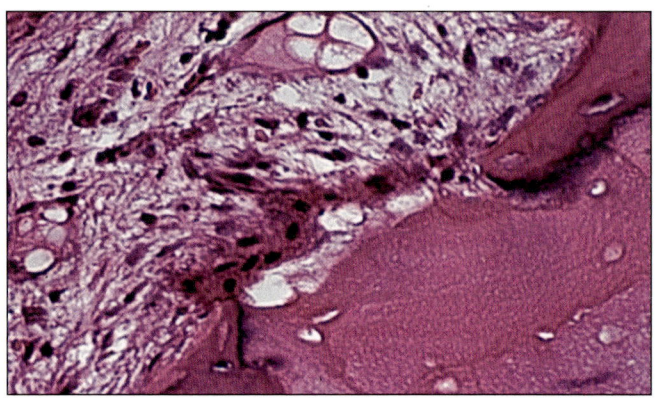

Fig 17-3a High-power histologic view of direct contact of new vital bone to xenograft (Bio-Oss) and osteoclasts adjacent to the xenograft. Bone cores harvested from augmented sinus at New York University Department of Implant Dentistry. (Hematoxylin and eosin; original magnification ×20.)

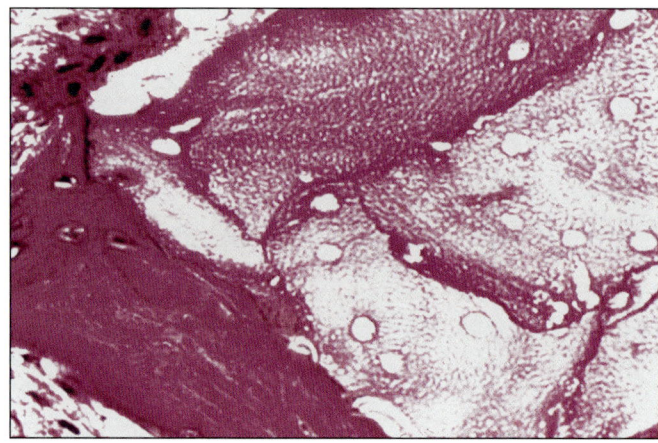

Fig 17-3b Higher-power view (original magnification ×40) of histology shown in Fig 17-3a.

Histomorphometric studies[17,19,20,25,26] at 6 to 12 months after grafting consistently report findings of relative proportions of vital bone, connective tissue, and residual xenograft to be approximately 25%, 50%, and 25%, respectively. Due to this residual volume of xenograft, the *matured graft functions as type 2 bone*. This contrasts with demineralized allograft material, which cannot mechanically support implants under function.

Disease Transmission Risk

Questions have been raised about whether xenografts increase the risk of transmitting bovine spongiform encephalopathy (BSE) to humans. While there has never been a case of disease transmission associated with the use of a xenograft, clinicians should review the processing and

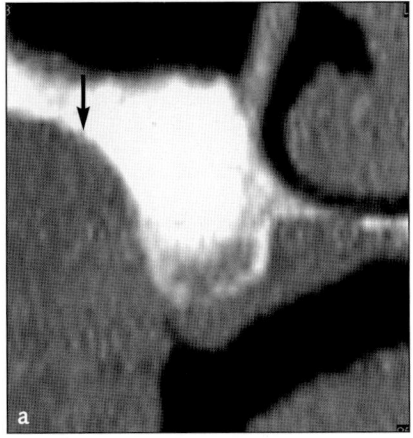 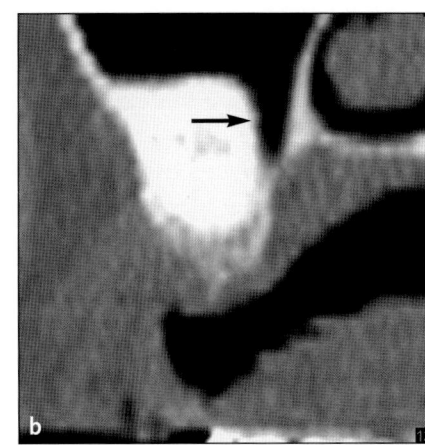

Fig 17-4a Reflection of the sinus membrane from the medial wall of the sinus, indicating complete fill of the sinus with xenograft particles *(arrow)*.

Fig 17-4b Inadequate reflection of sinus membrane, indicating the presence of a void and an unfilled area *(arrow)*.

sterilization procedures for these materials to be confident of their safety and to address any patient concerns about them. Rigorous, thorough, and extensive testing and regulation of xenograft materials are performed by the companies that manufacture them. Raw material consisting of long bones is obtained only from US cattle, and not from European sources. No case of BSE traced to long bones from bovine sources has ever been reported anywhere in the world. The material is processed either by high heat alone or by both high heat and chemicals to ensure that it is prion-free. Proof of anorganification is obtained through BioRad assay, SDS-PAGE testing, and SDS-PAGE and Western blotting.[31,32] Sogal and Tofe[33] calculated the risk of disease transmission based upon the testing model of the German Ministry of Health as 1 infection per 1.3×10^{19} 1-g doses, an infinitesimal rate.

Conductive Efficacy

Based on the preceding factors, Del Fabbro et al concluded that "Grafts utilizing bone substitute materials are as effective as autogenous bone, either when used alone or when used in combination with autogenous bone."[3] However, the clinician must remain aware that xenografts are osteoconductive, not osteoinductive, and thus the bony walls of the sinus must provide the vascularity, cells, and growth factors responsible for bone formation. To obtain the best results, the sinus membrane should be elevated medially as well as from the floor of the sinus so that the entire graft can be vascularized and a maximum number of graft particles are in contact with bony walls (Fig 17-4). Autogenous bone also provides growth factors that stimulate new bone formation during bone turnover. Because it lacks such growth factors, xenograft requires a longer period of graft healing to achieve new vital bone.[2,20,21] This essential difference was emphasized by Merkx et al,[34] who reported that autogenous grafts had produced a higher percentage of vital bone than anorganic bone replacement grafts at 4 to 6 months. However, at 3 to 8 months, John and Wenz[27] showed only a small difference in vital bone sections of sinuses grafted with Bio-Oss plus autogenous bone (vital bone = 32.2%) compared to those grafted with Bio-Oss alone (vital bone = 29.5%). A recent histomorphometric study by Degidi et al[35] compared new bone formation following sinus grafting in 7 patients at an average of 7 months. Autogenous bone (50%) harvested from intraoral sources was combined with two different xenografts (50%); new bone formation was similar in both groups. However, in a large sinus, graft maturation may be 1.5 to 2 times longer for delayed implant placement with 100% xenograft than with 100% autogenous bone (ie, 8 to 12 months compared to 4 to 6 months).

Looking toward the future, a recent study by Fuerst et al[36] in minipigs showed that cultured bone cells derived from the iliac crest, then combined with bovine bone mineral significantly increased the amount of new bone formed in sinus augmentations compared with bovine bone alone. This may have implications in humans for earlier and more rapid bone formation when cultured bone-derived cells are used with xenograft in sinus augmentation procedures.

Conclusion

Xenograft is the unheralded success story of sinus graft augmentation. When used by the prescribed methods elucidated here, xenograft is better than autograft or allograft at maintaining load-bearing bone volume, with a high percentage of vitality, safety, and lack of complication. Though xenograft is not the material of choice for bone graft reconstruction in general, for the sinus floor graft site and for the sole purpose of dental implant osseointegration, it may be the graft material of choice.

References

1. Jensen OT, Shulman LB, Block MS, Iacono VJ. Report of the Sinus Consensus Conference of 1996. Int J Oral Maxillofac Implants 1998:13(suppl)11–45.
2. Wallace SS, Froum SJ. Effect of maxillary sinus augmentation on the survival of endosseous dental implants. A systematic review. Ann Periodontol 2003;8:328–343.
3. Del Fabbro M, Testori T, Francetti L, Weinstein R. Systematic review of survival rates for implants placed in the grafted maxillary sinus. Int J Periodontics Restorative Dent 2004;24:565–578.
4. Tolman DE. Reconstructive procedures with endosseous implants in grafted bone: A review of the literature. Int J Oral Maxillofac Implants 1995;10:275–294.
5. Tong DC, Rioux K, Drangsholt M, Beirne OR. A review of the survival rates for implants placed in grafted maxillary sinuses using meta-analysis. Int J Oral Maxillofac Implants 1998;13:175–182.
6. Hising P, Bolin A, Branting C. Reconstruction of severely resorbed alveolar crests with dental implants using a bovine mineral for augmentation. Int J Oral Maxillofac Implants 2001;16:90–97.
7. Hallman M, Sennerby L, Lundgren S. A clinical and histologic evaluation of implant integration in the posterior maxilla after sinus floor augmentation with autogenous bone, bovine hydroxyapatite, or a 20:80 mixture. Int J Oral Maxillofac Implants 2002;17:635–643.
8. Valentini P, Abensur DJ. Maxillary sinus grafting with anorganic bovine bone: A clinical report of long-term results. Int J Oral Maxillofac Implants 2003;18:556–560.
9. Froum SJ, Wallace SS, Tarnow DP, Cho S-C. Effect of platelet-rich plasma on bone growth and osseointegration in human maxillary sinus grafts: Three bilateral case reports. Int J Periodontics Restorative Dent 2002;22:45–53.
10. Roldan JC, Jepsen S, Schmidt C, et al. Sinus floor augmentation with simultaneous placement of dental implants in the presence of platelet-rich plasma or recombinant human bone morphogenetic protein-7. Clin Oral Implants Res 2004;15:716–723.
11. Ulm C, Kneissel M, Schedle A, et al. Characteristic features of trabecular bone in edentulous maxillae. Clin Oral Implants Res 1999;10:459–467.
12. Moy PK, Lundgren S, Holmes RE. Maxillary sinus augmentation: Histomorphometric analysis of graft materials for sinus floor augmentation. J Oral Maxillofac Surg 1993;51:857–862.
13. Hanisch O, Lozada JL, Holmes RE, Calhoun CJ, Kan JYK, Spiekermann H. Maxillary sinus augmentation prior to placement of endosseous implants: A histomorphometric analysis. Int J Oral Maxillofac Implants 1999;14:329–336.
14. Garg AK. Current concepts in augmentation grafting of the maxillary sinus for the placement of dental implants. Dent Implantol Update 2001;12:17–22.
15. Schlegel KA, Fichtner G, Schultze-Mosgau S, Wiltfang J. Histologic findings in sinus augmentation with autogenous bone chips versus a bovine bone substitute. Int J Oral Maxillofac Implants 2003;18:53–58.
16. Hatano N, Shimizu Y, Ooya K. A clinical long-term radiographic evaluation of graft height changes after maxillary sinus floor augmentation with a 2:1 autogenous bone/xenograft mixture and simultaneous placement of dental implants. Clin Oral Implants Res 2004;15:339–345.
17. Froum SJ, Tarnow DP, Wallace SS, Rohrer MD, Cho S-C. Sinus floor elevation using anorganic bovine bone matrix (OsteoGraf/N) with and without autogenous bone: A clinical, histologic, radiographic, and histomorphometric analysis—Part 2 of an ongoing prospective study. Int J Periodontics Restorative Dent 1998;18:529–543.
18. Tarnow DP, Wallace SS, Froum SJ, Rohrer MD, Cho S-C. Histologic and clinical comparison of bilateral sinus floor elevations with and without barrier membrane placement in 12 patients: Part 3 of an ongoing prospective study. Int J Periodontics Restorative Dent 2000;20:116–125.
19. Wallace SS, Froum SJ, Tarnow DP, Cho S-C. Sinus augmentation utilizing ABBM (Bio-Oss) with and without osteotomy site coverage with various membranes. Int J Periodontics Restorative Dent 2005;25:551–559.
20. Valentini P, Abensur D, Wenz B, Peetz M, Schenk R. Sinus grafting with porous bone mineral (Bio-Oss) for implant placement: A 5-year study on 15 patients. Int J Periodontics Restorative Dent 2000;20:245–253.
21. Wallace SS, Froum SJ, Tarnow DP. Histologic evaluation of sinus elevation procedure. A clinical report. Int J Periodontics Restorative Dent 1996;16:47–51.
22. Tadjoedin ES, DeLange GL, Holzmann PJ, Kuiper L, Burger EH. Histologic observations on biopsies harvested following sinus floor elevation using a bioactive glass material of narrow size range. Clin Oral Implants Res 2000;11:334–344.
23. Tadjoedin ES, DeLange GL, Lyaruu DM, Kuiper L, Burger EH. High concentrations of bioactive glass material (BioGran) vs. autogenous bone for sinus floor elevation. Clin Oral Implants Res 2002;13:428–436.
24. Piatelli M, Favero G, Scarano A, Orsini G, Piatelli A. Bone reactions to anorganic bovine bone (Bio-Oss) used in sinus augmentation procedures: A histologic long-term report of 20 cases in humans. Int J Oral Maxillofac Implants 1999;14:835–840.

25. Yilderman M, Spiekermann H, Handt S, Edelhoff D. Maxillary sinus augmentation with the xenograft Bio-Oss and autogenous intraoral bone for qualitative improvement of the implant site: A histologic and histomorphometric clinical study in humans. Int J Oral Maxillofac Implants 2001;16:23–33.
26. Yilderman M, Spiekermann H, Biesterfeld S, Edelhof D. Maxillary sinus augmentation using xenogenic bone substitute material (Bio-Oss) in combination with venous blood: A histologic and histomorphometric study in humans. Clin Oral Implants Res 2000;11:217–229.
27. John H-D, Wenz B. Histomorphometric analysis of natural mineral for maxillary sinus augmentation. Int J Oral Maxillofac Implants 2004;19:199–207.
28. Valentini P, Abensur D, Densari D, Graziani JN, Hammerle C. Histological evaluation of Bio-Oss in a sinus floor elevation and implantation procedure: A human case report. Clin Oral Implants Res 1998;9:59–64.
29. Rosenlicht J, Tarnow DP. Human histologic evidence of functionally loaded hydroxyapatite-coated implants placed simultaneously with sinus augmentation: A case report 2½ years post-placement. Int J Oral Implantol 1999;25:7–10.
30. Scarano A, Pecora G, Piattelli M, Piattelli A. Osseointegration in a sinus augmented with bovine porous bone mineral: Histological results in an implant retrieved 4 years after insertion. A case report. J Periodontol 2004;75:1161–1166.
31. Benke D, Olah A, Möhler H. Protein-chemical analysis of Bio-Oss bone substitute and evidence on its carbonate content. Biomaterials 2001;22:1005–1012.
32. Wenz B, Oesch B, Horst M. Analysis of the risk of transmitting bovine spongiform encephalopathy through bone grafts derived from bovine bone. Biomaterials 2001;22:1599–1606.
33. Sogal A, Tofe AJ. Risk assessment of bovine spongiform encephalopathy transmission through bone graft material derived from bovine bone used for dental applications. J Periodontol 1999;70:1053–1063.
34. Merkx MAW, Maltha JC, Stoelinga PJW. Assessment of the value of anorganic bone additives in sinus floor augmentation: A review of clinical reports. Int J Oral Maxillofac Surg 2003;32:1–6.
35. Degidi M, Piatelli M, Scarano A, Iezzi G, Piattelli A. Maxillary sinus augmentation with a synthetic cell-binding peptide: Histological and histomorphometrical results in humans. J Oral Implantol 2004;30:376–383.
36. Fuerst G, Tangl S, Gruber R, Gahleitner A, Sanroman F, Watzek G. Bone formation following sinus grafting with autogenous bone-derived cells and bovine bone mineral in minipigs: Preliminary findings. Clin Oral Implants Res 2004;15;733–740.

Section 3

Technical Variations and Auxiliary Procedures

chapter 18
Effect of Surface Morphology on Implant Survival in the Grafted Maxillary Sinus

Dennis P. Tarnow, DDS
Sang-Choon Cho, DDS, BDS, MS
Stephen S. Wallace, DDS
Stuart J. Froum, DDS

The design of an implant affects its success in the grafted bone at the maxillary sinus floor. Among other design characteristics, the surface texture of implants has been shown to have a significant effect on the amount of bone-implant contact; this effect may be even more significant in the bone graft situation. Early landmark studies, such as those by Buser et al[1] and by Wennerberg et al,[2–4] and a more recent study by Lazzara et al,[5] show that rough-surfaced implants achieve greater bone-implant contact than machine-surfaced implants. This now well-established principle has led implant manufacturers away from the production of smooth, untextured surfaces toward more macroscopically and microscopically textured surfaces.

Whereas blood clot contact is maintained by a textured surface, it contracts from a machined surface during early wound healing. This phenomenon helps the endosteum maintain contact with the foreign body implant, which leads to faster bone formation directly on the surface by the process known as *osteogenesis*. Once a clot detaches from the surface of smooth or machined implants, the clot must regrow contact back to the implant surface, a process that Davies calls *distance osteogenesis*.[6] Direct apposition of the clot to the implant surface during the initial stages of healing speeds implant integration and modeling for earlier and more complete osseointegration, resulting in a higher rate of implant survival in grafted bone and allowing the adoption of earlier loading protocols.[7–10] In a study that compared machine-surfaced implants with acid-etched implants, the machined side achieved a lower-than-expected amount of implant-bone interface based on the receptor site bone quality, while the acid-etched side achieved a greater-than-expected interface.[11]

This phenomenon is extremely important clinically, particularly in softer bone such as that found in the posterior maxilla or healed sinus floor grafts. The formation of a stable bone-implant interface in type 3 or 4 bone such as that normally resulting from sinus augmentation surgery is a key factor in the success rate of implants placed in these grafts and loaded after integration. Histologic studies have confirmed the superiority of textured implants as compared to machined implants in the posterior maxillae of humans.[5]

When the floor of the sinus is grafted, the membrane is elevated from the lateral, anterior, and medial walls of the lower third of the sinus cavity. After the graft is placed, a clot forms within and around the graft particles, with vascularization from the vessels in the surrounding bony walls from which the sinus membrane has been elevated. The manner in which new bone forms in the grafted site may be compared to the manner in which bone forms in an extraction socket. The bone quality ultimately

Table 18-1 Vital bone formation in sinuses grafted with Bio-Oss alone and combined with autogenous bone (AB) or blood

Author	Graft material	Time (mos)	Bone (%)	Bio-Oss (%)	CT* (%)
Valentini, 2000[16]	Bio-Oss alone	6.0	21.0	39.0	40.0
Valentini, 2000[16]	Bio-Oss alone	12.0	28.0	27.0	45.0
Yilderim, 2001[17]	Bio-Oss + AB	7.1	18.9	29.6	51.5
Yilderim, 2000[18]	Bio-Oss + blood	6.8	14.7	29.7	55.6
John, 2004[19]	Bio-Oss alone	3.0–8.0	29.5	14.9	55.6
John, 2004[19]	Bio-Oss + AB	3.0–8.0	32.2	17.8	50.0
NYU (unpub)	Bio-Oss alone	6.0–12.0	18.5	28.0	53.5
NYU (unpub)	Bio-Oss + AB	6.0–12.0	15.7	29.6	54.7
Average			**23.0**	**27.0**	**50.0**

*CT = connective tissue.

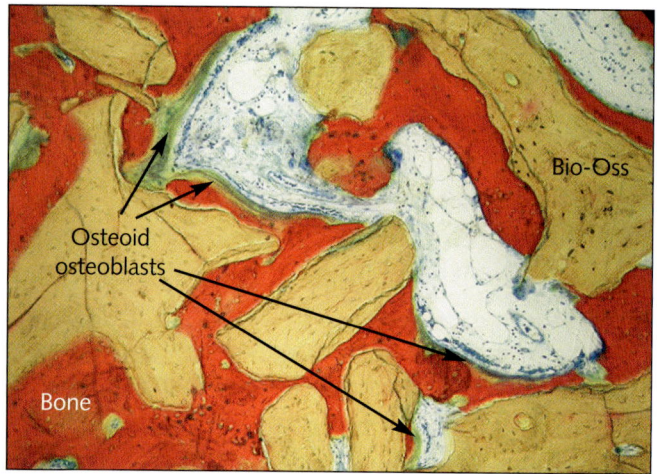

Fig 18-1 Sinus grafted with 100% Bio-Oss, 6 months after surgery, demonstrating 30% vital bone *(red)* and 24% residual Bio-Oss *(yellow)*. High-power view shows new vital bone formation directly on the residual Bio-Oss particles. (Stevenel blue and picric acid fuchsin; original magnification ×20.)

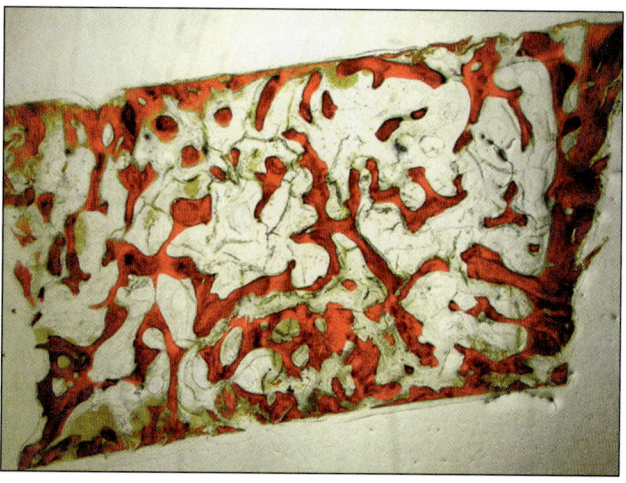

Fig 18-2 Sinus grafted with 100% Puros (Zimmer Dental) mineralized allograft at 6 months, demonstrating 25% vital bone *(red)*. Medium-power view shows vital bone formation and residual Puros particles *(brown)*. (Stevenel blue and picric acid fuchsin; original magnification ×10.)

achieved after sinus graft healing is genetically and biomechanically predetermined by the density of the natural bone in that anatomic location. In a study by Moy et al[12] in which particulated bone harvested from the chin was grafted into the sinus, the matured graft did not exhibit the same density as the grafted chin bone, but had a lower density such as that normally found in the posterior maxilla. Histologically, native bone in the posterior maxilla is composed of approximately 30% calcified bone and 70% marrow.[13] An anatomic study by Ulm et al[14] showed that bone in the maxillary molar region has an average density of 17.1% in females and 23.4% in males. The quality of the bone that migrates into and around a sinus graft appears to be determined initially by the density of the bone at the crest below the sinus.[15] Density of the bone then increases with implant function. Histologic reports in the literature show a wide range of bone graft densities; however, the prevailing average is close to 25% (Table 18-1; Figs 18-1 and 18-2).

TABLE 18-2 Implant survival classified by surface texture and type of graft (block or particulate)

Implant surface/graft type	SE	Mean (%)	Least square mean* (%)
Machined/iliac block	2.5	78.8	78.8
Machined/particulate	3.3	89.5	90.0
Rough/iliac block	6.1	90.9	89.5
Rough/particulate	1.2	94.5	94.6

*Least square mean includes adjustments for other variables.

This explanation corresponds with our knowledge of the healing of tooth extraction sites. When a mandibular canine and a maxillary second molar are extracted and all the bony walls are present, the mandibular canine socket fills with dense bone (type 1 or 2) after 6 months of healing, while the posterior maxillary socket fills with type 3 or 4 bone. This epigenetic and biomechanic phenomenon is a consistent biologic principle. Bone regeneration is consistent within each host location. The same phenomenon has been observed in the bone graft situation, where modeling and remodeling substantially replace the bone graft with nativelike bone. Thus, sinus bone grafts generally heal with type 3 or 4 bone. The significance of the choice of implant increases as bone density decreases, such as in grafted areas where primary stabilization is reduced and the capacity for osseointegration is relatively compromised.

Two systematic literature reviews on sinus grafting revealed consensus regarding the poorer rate of survival of machine-surfaced implants compared to textured implants placed in the augmented sinuses.[20–22]

Wallace and Froum[20] reported the survival of machine-surfaced implants and rough-surfaced implants as 82.4% and 95.2%, respectively. Del Fabbro et al[21] found survival rates for machine- and rough-surfaced implants of 85.6% and 95.9%, respectively. These reviews conclude that the surface texture of an implant is clinically significant.

Furthermore, rough-surfaced implants were more successful than machine-surfaced implants regardless of graft material used (Table 18-2). Del Fabbro et al[21] reported that 69.5% of all implants placed in 100% autogenous bone grafts had machined surfaces, accounting for 87.8% of the failures. The large disparity is probably owing at least in part to the fact that a majority of implants placed had machined surfaces.

Clinical Experience

At New York University, a total of 400 patients had 1,134 implants placed in grafted sinuses. Implants were classified according to their surface morphology: acid etched (724), hydroxyapatite-coated (20), machined (104), sandblasted, large grit, acid-etched (SLA [Straumann]) (105), titanium oxide–blasted (TiOblasted [Nobel Biocare]) (28), or titanium plasma-sprayed (TPS) (153) (Fig 18-3). Of the 1,134 implants placed, 1,030 had some type of roughened surface and the remaining 104 were machine turned. Minimum loading time for inclusion in this retrospective study was 6 months.

Seventy-six of the 1,134 implants placed in this study group failed, yielding an overall survival rate of 93.3%. However, a clear and significant difference was noted when the data for the rough-surfaced and machined implants were separated. A survival rate of only 70.2% was found for the machined implants versus 95.6% for all rough-surfaced implants combined. Table 18-3 presents a breakdown of implant survival by surface type.

The overall survival rate observed in this clinical investigation (93.3%) is comparable to that reported in previous studies for implants placed in grafted maxillary sinuses. The report of the Sinus Consensus Conference of 1996[23] analyzed retrospective data from 1,007 sinus floor augmentation bone grafts collected from 38 surgeons, involving the placement of 2,997 implants over a 10-year period. The complete data demonstrated a 90.0% success rate and revealed reduced success with machined implants, comparable in both regards to the NYU data.

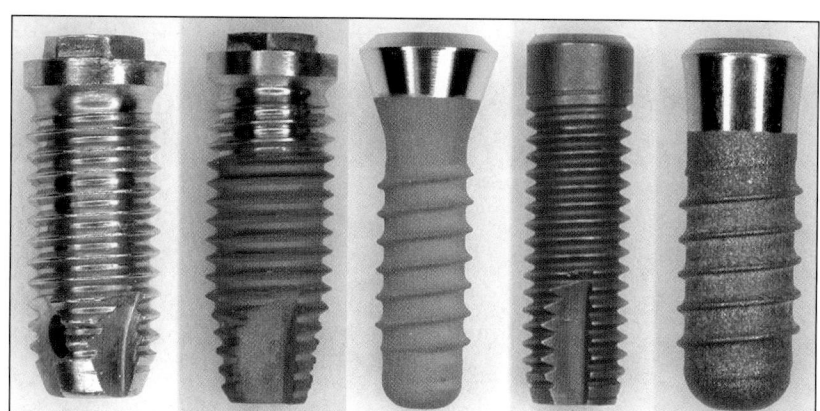

Fig 18-3 Five different implant surfaces. *From left*: machined, acid-etched, SLA, TiOblasted, TPS.

Table 18-3 Survival rates of implants classified by surface texture

Implant surface	Acid-etched	HA	SLA	TiOblasted	TPS	Machined
Survival rate	95.8% (694/724)	90.0% (18/20)	96.1% (101/105)	96.4% (27/28)	94.8% (145/153)	70.2% (73/104)

Conclusions

Implants can be placed and subsequently loaded in augmented maxillary sinuses. A high survival rate depends on the surface texture of the implant. The machined implants have a relatively poor survival rate as compared to that of rough-surfaced implants.

Future research will isolate the many confounding variables in sinus augmentation surgery for the purpose of verifying the results and conclusions reported here.

References

1. Buser D, Schenk RK, Steinemann S, Fiorellini JP, Fox CH, Stich H. Influence of surface characteristics on bone integration of titanium implants. A histomorphometric study in miniature pigs. J Biomed Mater Res 1991;25:889–902.
2. Wennerberg A, Albrektsson T, Andersson B, Kroll JJ. A histomorphometric and removal torque study of screw-shaped titanium implants with three different surface topographies. Clin Oral Implants Res 1995;6:24–30.
3. Wennerberg A, Albrektsson T, Lausmaa J. Torque and histomorphometric evaluation of commercially pure titanium screws blasted with 25- and 75-mm-sized particles of Al_2O_3. J Biomed Mater Res 1996;30:251–260.
4. Wennerberg A, Albrektsson T, Andersson B. Bone tissue response to commercially pure titanium implants blasted with fine and coarse particles of aluminum oxide. Int J Oral Maxillofac Implants 1996;11:38–45.
5. Lazzara RJ, Testori T, Trisi P, Porter S, Weinstein RL. A human histologic analysis of Osseotite and machined surfaces using implants with 2 opposing surfaces. Int J Periodontics Restorative Dent 1999;19:117–129.
6. Davies JE. Mechanisms of endosseous integration. Int J Prosthodont 1998;11:391–401.
7. Testori T, Del Fabbro M, Feldman S, et al. A multicenter prospective evaluation of 2-months loaded Osseotite implants placed in the posterior jaws: Three-year follow-up results. Clin Oral Implants Res 2002;13:154–161.
8. Cochran DL, Buser D, ten Bruggenkate CM, et al. The use of reduced healing times on ITI implants with a sandblasted and acid-etched (SLA) surface: Early results from clinical trials on ITI SLA implants. Clin Oral Implants Res 2002;13:144–153.
9. Cooper L, Felton DA, Kugelberg CF, et al. A multicenter 12-month evaluation of single-tooth implants restored 3 weeks after one-stage surgery. Int J Oral Maxillofac Implants 2001;16:182–192.

10. Roccuzzo M, Bunino M, Prioglio F, Silvio D, Bianchi F. Early loading of sandblasted and acid-etched (SLA) implants: A prospective split-mouth comparative study. Clin Oral Implants Res 2001;12:572–578.
11. Trisi P, Lazzara RJ, Rao W, Rebaudi A. Bone-implant contact and bone quality: Evaluation of expected and actual bone contact on machined and Osseotite implants. Int J Periodontics Restorative Dent 2003;23:535–546.
12. Moy PK, Lundgren S, Holmes RE. Maxillary sinus augmentation: Histomorphometric analysis of graft materials for sinus floor augmentation. J Oral Maxillofac Surg 1993;51:857–862.
13. Trisi P, Rao W. Bone classification: Clinical-histomorphometric comparison. Clin Oral Implants Res 1999;10:1–7.
14. Ulm C, Kneissel M, Schedie A, et al. Characteristic features of trabecular bone in edentulous maxillae. Clin Oral Implants Res 1999;10:459–467.
15. Valentini P, Abensur D, Densari D, Graziani JN, Hammerle C. Histological evaluation of Bio-Oss in a sinus floor elevation and implantation procedure. A human case report. Clin Oral Implants Res 1998;9:59–64.
16. Valentini P, Abensur D, Wenz B, Peetz B, Schenk R. Sinus grafting with porous bone mineral (Bio-Oss) for implant placement: A 5-year study on 15 patients. Int J Periodontics Restorative Dent 2000;20:245–253.
17. Yildirim M, Spiekermann H, Handt S, Edelhoff D. Maxillary sinus augmentation with the xenograft Bio-Oss and autogenous intraoral bone for qualitative improvement of the implant site: A histologic and histomorphometric clinical study in humans. Int J Oral Maxillofac Implants 2001;16:23–33.
18. Yildirim M, Spiekermann H, Biesterfeld S, Edelhoff D. Maxillary sinus augmentation using xenogenic bone substitute material Bio-Oss in combination with venous blood. A histologic and histomorphometric study in humans. Clin Oral Implants Res 2000;11:217–229.
19. John HD, Wenz B. Histomorphometric analysis of natural bone mineral for maxillary sinus augmentation. Int J Oral Maxillofac Implants 2004;19:199–207.
20. Wallace SS, Froum SJ. Effect of maxillary sinus augmentation on the survival of endosseous dental implants: An evidence-based literature review. Ann Periodontol 2003;8:328–343.
21. Del Fabbro M, Testori T, Francetti L, Weinstein R. Systematic review of survival rates for implants placed in the grafted maxillary sinus. Int J Periodontics Restorative Dent 2004;24:565–577.
22. Cho S-C, Yang HS, Elian N, Wallace S, Froum S, Tarnow DP. Survival rates of implants with different surface morphologies in grafted sinuses: Six-month loading data. Int J Periodontics Restorative Dent 2005;(Submitted for publication).
23. Jensen OT, Shulman LB, Block MS, Iacono VJ. Report of the Sinus Consensus Conference of 1996. Int J Oral Maxillofac Implants 1998;13:11–45.

chapter 19
Use of Barrier Membranes in Sinus Augmentation

Stephen S. Wallace, DDS
Stuart J. Froum, DDS
Dennis P. Tarnow, DDS

When a lateral window approach is used, the sinus bone graft benefits from the placement of a barrier membrane over the osteotomy site. Using a resorbable membrane to repair inadvertent perforation of the sinus membrane within the sinus also has therapeutic rationale. This chapter discusses the somewhat controversial use of barrier membranes in the course of sinus grafting.

History of Barrier Therapy

The concept of placing a barrier membrane over the lateral sinus window is a logical extension of barrier applications in orthopedics, periodontal guided tissue regeneration, and preprosthetic guided bone regeneration.

In 1959, Murray[1] described bone growth under a plastic "cage" in the spine in which bone filled a cavity where soft tissue was excluded. This finding foreshadowed what we now call *guided bone regeneration*. Murray and subsequent dental practitioners who are experienced in guided bone regeneration provided the theoretical and practical basis for membrane-protected maxillary sinus surgery.

Guided tissue regeneration is based on Melcher's[2] concept of selective cell repopulation and on later studies by Nyman et al[3] and Gottlow et al[4]. The regeneration of the attachment apparatus by selective cell repopulation evolved from these seminal studies. When applied to human periodontal defects, this technique includes the placement of a physical barrier (membrane) between the gingival flap and the root surface just coronal to the periodontal defect. The barrier retards repopulation of the root by gingival epithelium and gingival connective tissue and favors healing by cells from within the periodontal ligament. Human histology of cases treated with barrier membranes demonstrates regeneration of cementum, bone, and a functionally oriented periodontal ligament.[3-5] A requirement for the success of guided tissue regeneration includes the creation of a space apical to the membrane that isolates the treated root surface and the defect so that desired cells migrate and populate the wound. Nonabsorbable and bioabsorbable barrier membranes are effective for periodontal regeneration.[6-8] The ability to keep the membrane submerged and covered by the gingival flap influences clinical outcome.[9,10] Evidence-based reviews show that guided tissue regeneration with membranes is more effective than controls in the treatment of intrabony and furcation defects.[11,12]

The principles of guided tissue regeneration were later modified to regenerate bone for the repair of alveolar ridge defects.[13-15] This technique, known as *guided bone regeneration*, has been successfully used for site develop-

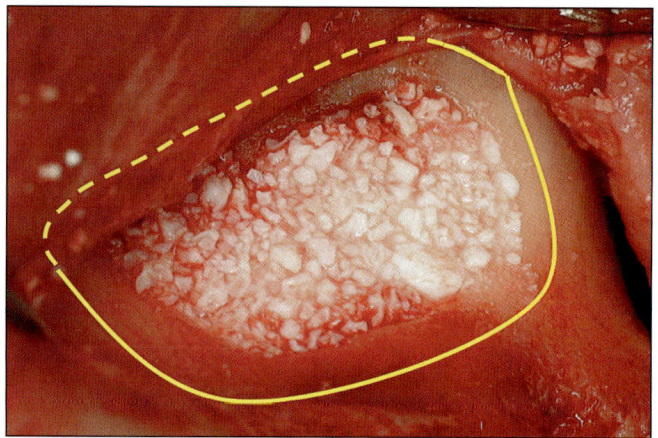

Fig 19-1 Sinus grafted with a xenograft (Bio-Oss, Osteohealth). Proposed barrier membrane placement is outlined in yellow.

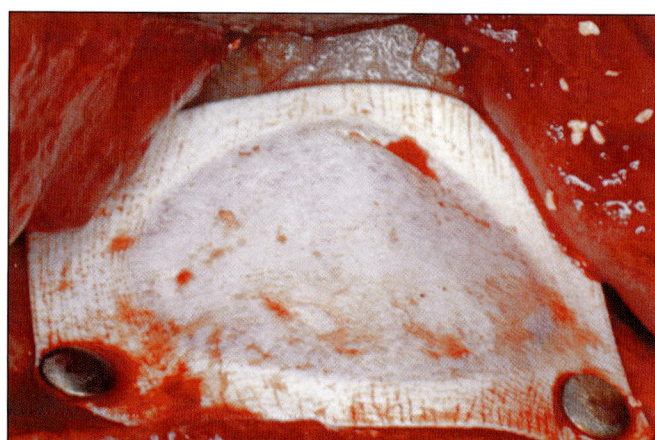

Fig 19-2 Placement and stabilization of a nonabsorbable expanded polytetrafluoroethylene (e-PTFE) barrier membrane (Gore-Tex, W. L. Gore) so as to avoid incision lines.

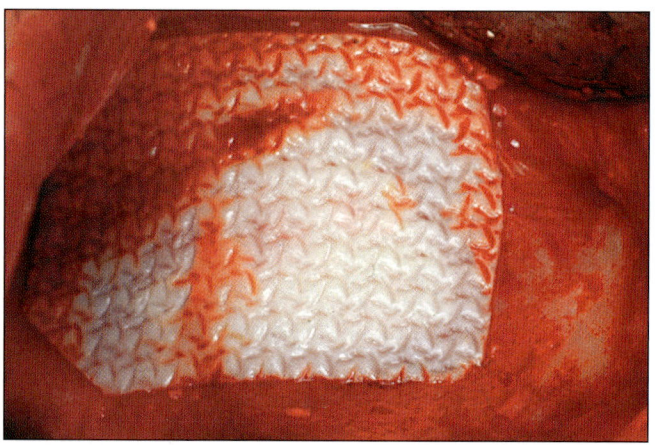

Fig 19-3 Placement of a bioabsorbable barrier membrane (Ossix, ColBar R&D) so as to avoid incision lines.

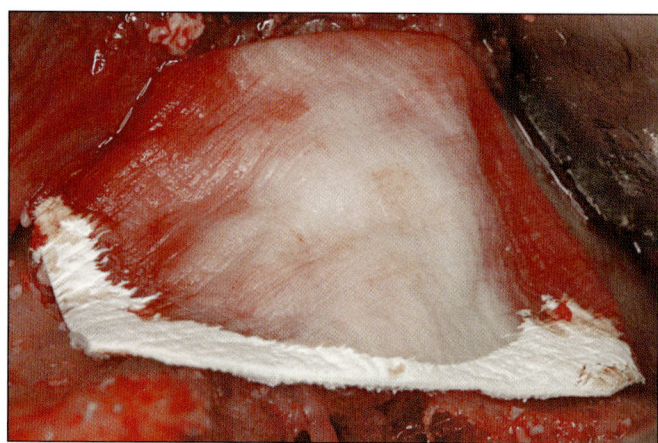

Fig 19-4 Placement of a bioabsorbable barrier membrane (Bio-Gide, Geistlich Biomaterials) so as to avoid incision lines.

ment prior to,[16,17] at the time of,[18,19] and after implant placement. The success of guided bone regeneration depends on the maintenance of space, the stability of the membrane, the duration of barrier function, and the prevention of membrane exposure. Implants placed into regenerated bone demonstrate excellent success rates.[20–26] A recent evidence-based review by Fiorellini and Nevins[27] shows an implant survival rate of 97.3% for implants placed into grafted bone.

Membrane Placement over Lateral Window

When used in sinus grafting, the surgical objective is to position an effective barrier membrane over the lateral window in such a manner as to exclude the connective tissue from the wound. Various materials have been used as barriers over the lateral window antrostomy, including nonresorbable e-PTFE membranes, long- and short-term bioabsorbable cross-linked collagen membranes, synthetic membranes, titanium mesh membranes, freeze-dried lamellar bone sheets, calcium sulfate barriers, and the repositioned original lateral bony window.

The membrane should cover the window by a minimum of 3 to 5 mm (Fig 19-1). Placing the membrane under the incision line should be avoided, as this may lead to the complication of exposure. Many membranes are packaged with templates that can be cut to the appropriate size after the window is made and the sinus membrane elevated. Using this template, the barrier membrane is then cut to size and hydrated prior to grafting the sinus. Once grafting is complete, the shaped membrane can be applied immediately.

Experience with guided bone regeneration has shown that e-PTFE membranes must be stabilized with tacks or screws (Fig 19-2) to prevent shifting, which results in loss of barrier function as well as difficulty in removal.

Depending on their stiffness, bioabsorbable barrier membranes may have the ability to remain in place without mechanical stabilization. The more adaptable (thin) membranes conform well to the surface of the lateral sinus wall (Figs 19-3 and 19-4). Most of the bioabsorbable membranes can be stabilized with tacks; however, unless the tacks are bioabsorbable, re-entry for tack removal will be required. At New York University, clinical experience has shown that these long-term, bioabsorbable membranes are still in position over the window at the time of bone core harvesting.

Studies of the effectiveness of bioabsorbable barriers have found them to be similar to e-PTFE membranes with regard to vital bone formation (see below). An advantage of the bioabsorbable membrane is elimination of the re-entry procedure required for e-PTFE.

Membranes for Perforation Repair

Perforation of the sinus membrane is a common complication of the sinus elevation procedure; reports of the incidence of membrane perforation range from 10%[28] to 44%.[29] Techniques for repairing membrane perforations include suturing, and "patching" of the perforation with biomaterials such as Gelfilm (Pfizer), CollaTape (Integra), fibrin glue, Lambone (Pacific Coast Tissue Bank), and, most commonly, bioabsorbable collagen barrier membranes. Repair techniques using collagen barriers have been reported in the literature by Vlassis and Fugazzotto,[30] Pikos,[31] and Proussaefs and Lozada.[32]

The purpose of the repair is strictly for the containment of particulate graft material. Small perforations will generally close by folding the elevated membrane back upon itself, and no further action is necessary. However, larger perforations will not close, and thus some form of corrective action must be taken. Suturing a torn membrane, while difficult, is sometimes possible, especially if the membrane is thickened. The cost of failure, however, is high. Most often, suturing merely increases the size of the perforation.

A bioabsorbable collagen membrane is an effective way to seal a perforation. The barrier acts to confine the graft material until a biologic repair can take place. It is critical that the repair effort not compromise vascularization of the sinus graft. Since the blood supply to the graft comes from the bony walls (lateral wall, crest, and medial wall), the membrane must not be placed over the endosteal blood supply.

When the sinus membrane is elevated, it forms the superior and distal walls of a regenerative space or compartment that is subsequently filled with graft material. The anterior, medial, lateral, and inferior walls of this space are the bony surfaces that contain the vascular supply. Once the membrane is elevated, the perforation usually occurs superiorly or distally (Fig 19-5a). The collagen membrane should be placed so that it rests predominantly on the elevated sinus membrane (Fig 19-5b). If the perforation is close to the area of the superior hinge, the membrane is likely to shift medially as the graft material is being added, thus leaving the perforation unrepaired. This problem can be avoided by tacking the membrane outside the sinus, superior or distal to the window as the case presents, and then folding the membrane into the sinus (Fig 19-6). The membrane can be cut so that part of it remains outside the window and the other part fits in the sinus and unfolds (Fig 19-7). In extreme cases, small holes can be drilled into the lateral wall for the placement of sutures that, along with tacks, will help stabilize the reparative membrane (Fig 19-8).

A membrane technique by Pikos[31] for the repair of larger perforations involves modifying the membrane with diagonal slits (Fig 19-9) so that it will form a tent over the graft, thus containing the particulate graft crestally. Also

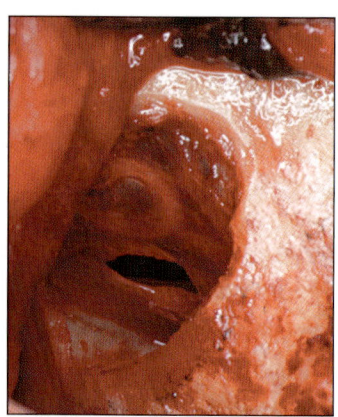

Fig 19-5a Sinus membrane perforation superiorly after elevation.

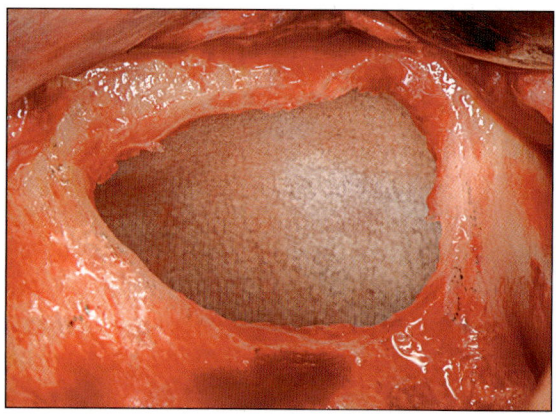

Fig 19-5b Collagen membrane positioned against elevated sinus membrane. Perforation will be stabilized against the sinus membrane by graft material.

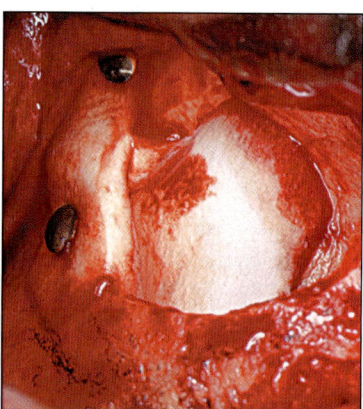

Fig 19-6 Stabilized membrane for repair of a distal perforation.

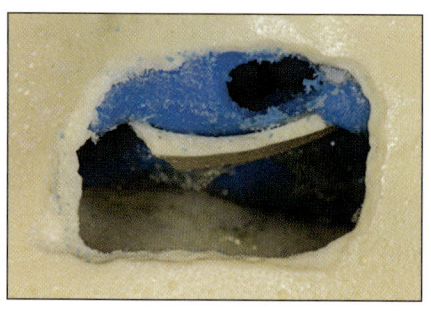

Fig 19-7a Perforation at superior osteotomy (model).

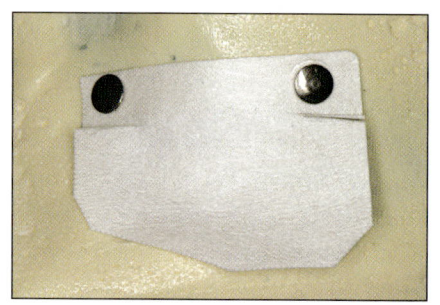

Fig 19-7b Membrane fixated external to sinus with titanium tacks and modified by lateral cuts extending to the superior corners of the window (model).

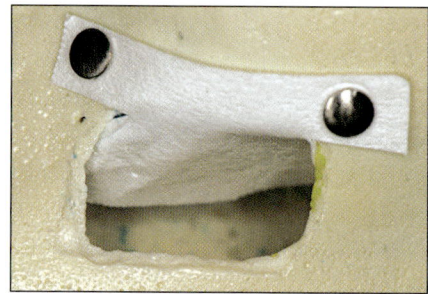

Fig 19-7c Membrane folded into position to establish a superior repair (model).

designed for large perforations is the so-called Loma Linda Pouch technique,[32] which uses a bioabsorbable membrane to completely encapsulate the graft inside the sinus. The corners of the membrane extend circumferentially to the outside of the sinus, but the graft is isolated from the endosteum.

Covering the elevated sinus membrane with a collagen barrier does not compromise the graft. A histologic animal study by Haas et al[33] has shown the sinus membrane to be an avascular tissue, and a primate study by Hürzeler et al[34] has shown it to have minimal negative effects on bone formation.

The size of the membrane used for repair should be large enough to accommodate the size of the perforation and to stabilize the membrane in place. It should be sized so that it will neither be displaced through the perforation when the graft material is being placed or forced through the perforation by changes in sinus air pressure resulting from breathing, sneezing, etc. This requires either placing the edges of the barrier membrane against areas where the sinus membrane is still intact or using additional means of stabilization.

Evidence of the efficacy of perforation repair is provided by studies showing similar outcomes for implant survival in

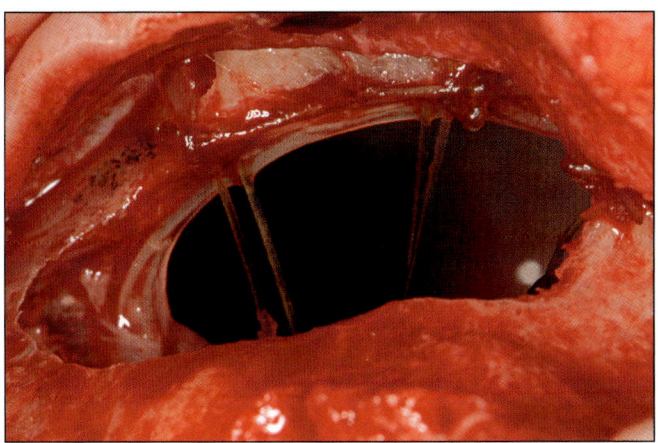

Fig 19-8a Stabilization of membrane with horizontal supporting sutures.

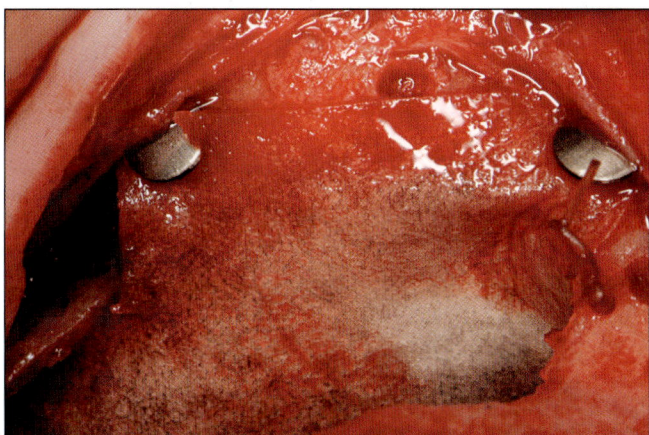

Fig 19-8b Reparative membrane positioned below suture supports and tacked externally.

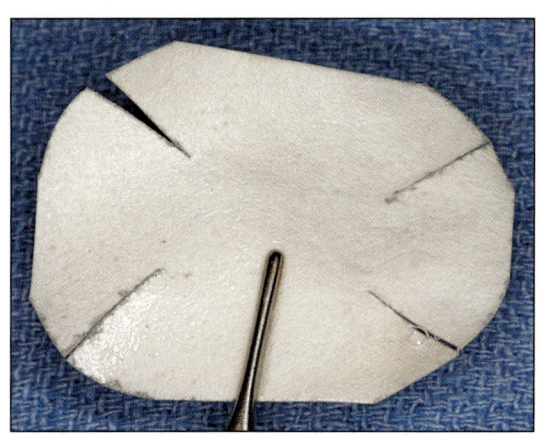

Fig 19-9 Modified membrane (Pikos technique) for use as a barrier to contain the particulate graft material.

perforated and nonperforated cases. Only 3 of 12 studies that reported perforation rates found an increased rate of implant failure associated with perforated membranes.[35–37] If a repair is successful, membrane perforation does not appear to be strongly associated with postoperative complication or reduced implant survival. Unsuccessful repairs may ultimately lead to inadequate graft density, sinusitis, and postoperative sinus infection due to loss of graft containment. Postsurgical complications result in reduced implant survival, and if the surgery is aborted an additional sinus surgery will be required.

If the repair does not work, the procedure should be aborted. In such cases, the clinician should consider placing a barrier membrane over the lateral window to prevent adhesion of the repairing sinus membrane to the periosteum, which would make re-entry more difficult.

Evidence for Using a Membrane over the Lateral Window

The efficacy of membrane placement over the lateral window is best evaluated indirectly by comparing histologic data and survival rates of implants placed in the grafted maxillary sinuses with and without the use of a membrane.

Histologic data

Bone grafts placed in the maxillary sinus are vascularized by the blood vessels and surrounding perivascular progenitors in the bony walls and within the floor of the sinus. Vascularization is not significantly affected by the periosteum that resides outside the sinus bone graft site. An

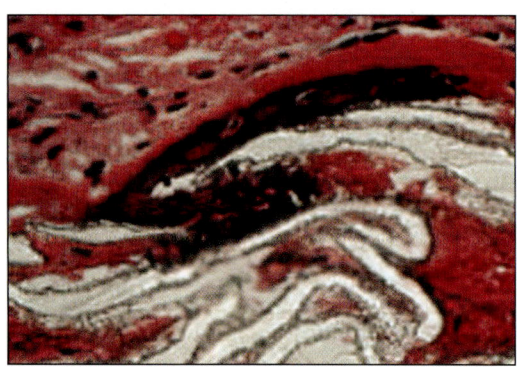

Fig 19-10a Osteoblasts and bone formation directly on (and within) the e-PTFE membrane surface (hematoxylin and eosin; original magnification ×40).

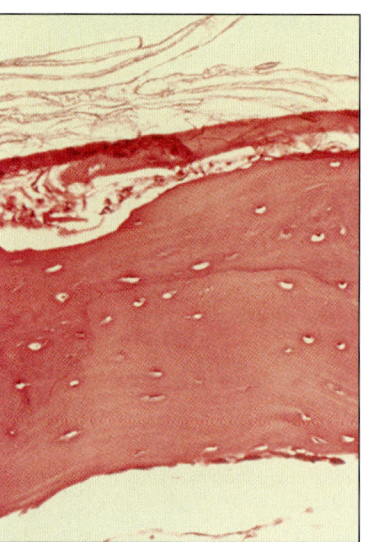

Fig 19-10b Vital bone formation in contact with e-PTFE membrane surface in area of lateral window (Stevenel blue, picric acid fuchsin; original magnification ×40).

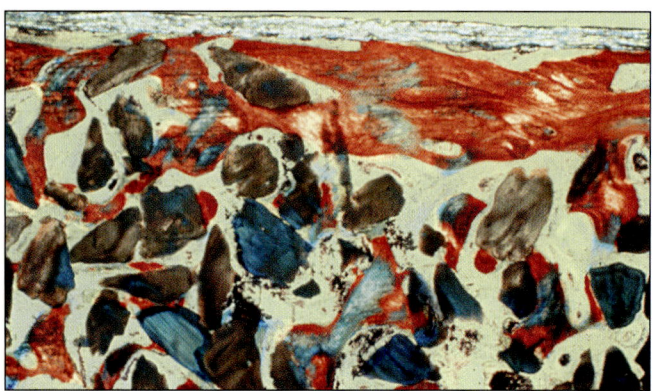

Fig 19-10c Polarized light reveals bone formation directly beneath the e-PTFE membrane. Note osteoblasts on bone surface and enclosed osteocytes (Stevenel blue, picric acid fuchsin; original magnification ×50). (Reprinted with permission from Tarnow et al[47]).

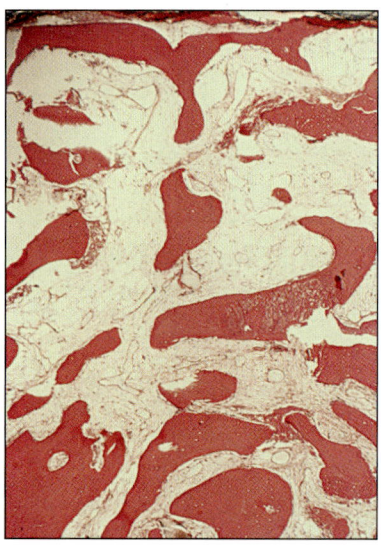

Fig 19-10d Vital bone in contact with membrane and throughout core (hematoxylin and eosin; original magnification ×31.5). (Reprinted with permission from Tarnow et al[47]).

early fluorescence microscopy study by Boyne and Kruger[38] (1962) demonstrated that the floor of the maxillary sinus responded to stimulation with reactive bone formation. Misch and Dietsch[39] and Quiñones et al[40] obtained the same response from sinus bony walls in primates after sinus membrane elevation. This pattern of bone formation was also demonstrated radiographically in a primate study by Margolin et al[41] and in humans by Boyne et al[42] and Nevins and Fiorellini.[43] Bone formation from the sinus floor occurred at a rate of about 1 mm per month in four human core samples measured by Smiler et al.[44]

TABLE 19-1 Average vital bone formed in sinuses grafted with and without a membrane

Membrane type	No. of sinuses	Average vital bone formed (%)	Marrow (%)	Residual Bio-Oss (%)
e-PTFE (Gore-Tex)	21	16.9	51.2	31.9
Collagen (Bio-Gide)	37	17.6	56.0	26.4
No membrane	6	12.1	63.6	24.3

Just as they function in guided bone regeneration, membranes prevent nonosteogenic connective tissue from developing in the grafted area and hence in the sinus, which could lead to loss of graft ossification. Soft tissue ingrowth, or encleftation, has been demonstrated in both primates and humans,[45,46] and it is similar to the problems observed in periodontal ridge defects when a membrane barrier is not used or when the barrier is prematurely lost during a regenerative procedure.

From a biologic point of view, the exclusion of connective tissue cells should favor the population of the sinus graft with perivascular osteoblasts emanating from the adjacent bony walls and the now-exposed vascular supply. Histologic sections taken through the lateral window that contain the barrier membrane reveal *bone formation in contact with the membrane* in such a manner as to restore the bony wall (Fig 19-10).

Histomorphometric evidence of enhanced bone formation following membrane placement over the lateral window is available from one random controlled trial and two controlled trials conducted at the New York University Department of Implant Dentistry. A random controlled trial by Tarnow et al[47] in which bilateral sinus grafts were accomplished with and without a membrane in each patient showed vital bone formation to be 25.5% with and 11.9% without a membrane. Six cases showed dramatic benefits, five cases were similar but favored the membrane side, and one case slightly favored the nonmembrane side. A controlled trial by Froum et al[48] measured vital bone formation in 113 sinuses grafted with either a xenograft or a combined autograft-xenograft. Average vital bone formation was 27.6% when a membrane was used and 16% when a membrane was not used.

One of the drawbacks of membrane use is the necessity to remove it after graft maturation. Nonabsorbable membranes are generally stabilized with tacks or screws, which also must be removed. Removal of membranes and tacks generally requires a surgical entry that is much more invasive than that required either for implant placement alone (delayed placement) or for stage-two surgery (simultaneous placement). If both types of membranes are equally effective, the bioabsorbable membranes would offer the clear advantage of avoiding the need for an additional surgical intervention.

A recent study by Wallace et al[49] compared vital bone formation in sinuses grafted with 100% Bio-Oss (Osteohealth) with different membranes placed over the lateral window. The nonabsorbable Gore-Tex membrane (W. L. Gore) and the bioabsorbable Bio-Gide membrane (Osteohealth) were compared to controls with no membrane coverage. No statistical differences were found between the absorbable (17.6%) and nonabsorbable (16.9%) membranes, and both were better than the no-membrane controls (12.1%) in vital bone development as well as implant survival rates (Table 19-1, Figs 19-11 to 19-13).

Clinical efficacy

Because of the relatively small number of randomized controlled human clinical trials in sinus graft surgery that have been conducted to date,[50] those that have been done do not allow for evidence-based decision making. To evaluate the efficacy of membrane placement, it would be best to have more studies that use a split-mouth design to compare the survival of implants placed in grafted sinuses with and without a membrane over the lateral window. Other relevant data may be extracted from well-conducted studies that offer lower levels of evidence (controlled trials, consecutive case series, and retrospective analyses).

Sufficient clinical evidence exists to justify the use of a barrier membrane over the lateral window in sinus graft surgery. A systematic review confirmed the importance of membrane placement in sinus augmentation surgery,[51] citing the controlled clinical trials by Tarnow et al[47] and

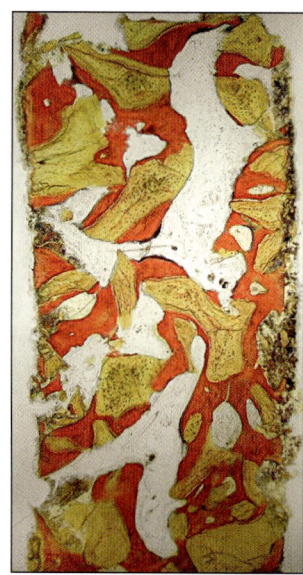 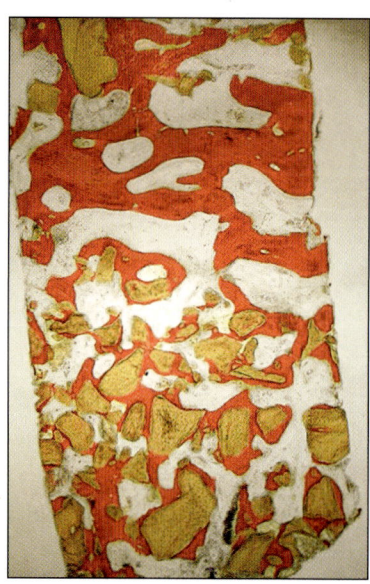 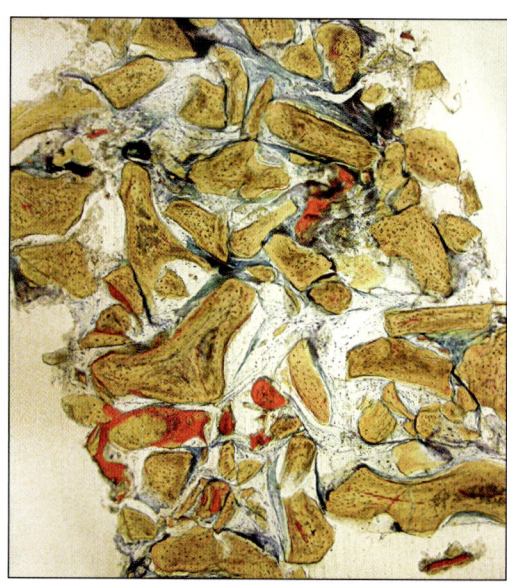

Fig 19-11 Histologic core of graft placed with a Gore-Tex e-PTFE membrane (Stevenel blue, picric acid fuchsin; original magnification ×4). (yellow, Bio-Oss; green, osteoid; red, new bone).

Fig 19-12 Histologic core of graft placed with a Bio-Gide membrane (Stevenel blue, picric acid fuchsin; original magnification ×4). (yellow, Bio-Oss; green, osteoid; red, new bone).

Fig 19-13 Histologic core of graft placed without a membrane (Stevenel blue, picric acid fuchsin; original magnification ×4). (yellow, Bio-Oss; green, osteoid; red, new bone).

Froum et al[48] in which more favorable bone formation and higher implant survival rates were obtained when a membrane was used. A controlled trial by Tawil and Mawla[52] also achieved a higher implant survival rate with membrane use. Results from these three controlled trials are provided in Table 19-2.

The aforementioned review[51] also identified 20 additional studies (15 without membrane, 5 with membrane) in which higher implant survival rates were obtained when a barrier membrane was placed over the lateral window in sinuses grafted with particulate grafts (93.6% with membrane versus 88.7% without membrane). A recent study by Wallace et al[49] has shown similar implant survival rates when e-PTFE (Gore-Tex) (97.8%) and Bio-Gide membranes (97.6%) were used in sinus grafts composed of 100% Bio-Oss xenograft (Table 19-3). Likewise, a 5-year prospective study on guided bone regeneration by Zitzmann et al[53] showed no statistical differences in implant survival rates following guided bone regeneration procedures with either Bio-Oss/Gore-Tex or Bio-Oss/Bio-Gide.

The increased vital bone formation achieved when a membrane is placed over the window can be observed clinically (Fig 19-14) and most likely accounts for the improved implant outcomes reported in the literature. When a membrane is not placed over the window, it is not uncommon to find a lack of corticalization of the graft surface. The incidence of this finding may increase with the size of the window. This phenomenon may be explained by the fibrogenic nature of the adult periosteum once it has been elevated from the bone surface, combined with the increased distance of the mid-window from the blood supply from the cut lateral wall. Tawil and Mawla have reported that in their study, implant survival was related to the quality of the reconstructed cortical plate.[52] Additionally noted in nonmembrane cases is the finding of encleftation through the sinus window.[45]

Conclusions

Systematic literature reviews have documented successful outcomes for both guided tissue regeneration around teeth[11,12] and preprosthetic guided bone regeneration prior to implant placement.[27] An evidence-based literature review by Wallace and Froum[51] on implant survival follow-

TABLE 19-2 Rates of implant survival in sinuses grafted with and without a membrane

Study	Survival rate with membrane	Survival rate without membrane
Tarnow et al (2000)[47]	100%; n = 28 implants	92.6%; n = 27 implants
Tawil and Mawla (2001)[52]	93.1%; n = 29 implants	78.1%; n = 32 implants
Froum et al (1998)[48]	99.2%; n = 133 implants	96.3%; n = 82 implants

TABLE 19-3 Rates of implant survival in sinuses grafted with absorbable and nonabsorbable membranes

Membrane	No. of implants placed	Failures	Survival (%)
e-PTFE (Gore-Tex)	46	1	97.8
Collagen (Bio-Gide)	83	2	97.6
Total	129	3	97.7

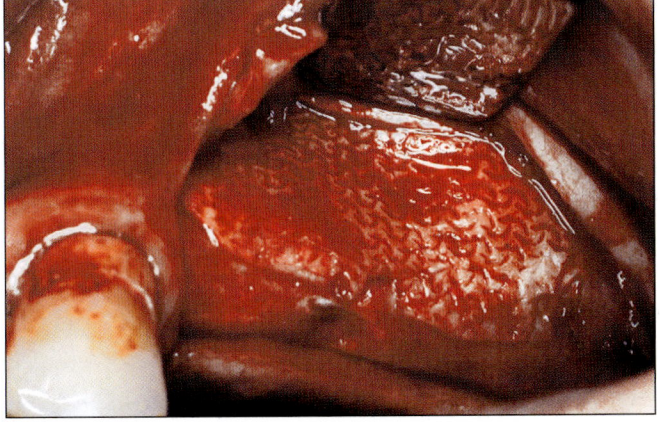

Fig 19-14a Six months after placement, the bioabsorbable Ossix membrane remains intact.

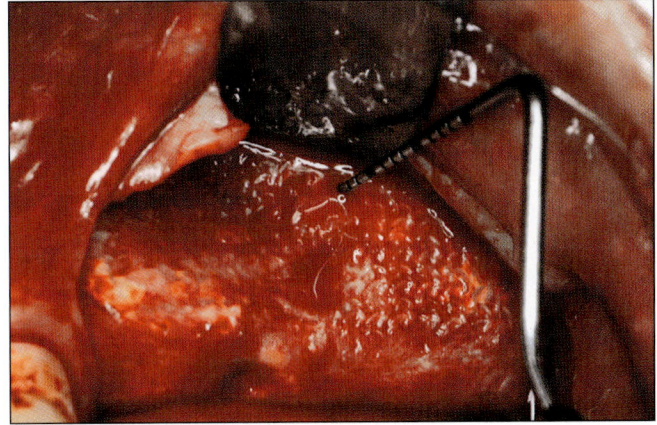

Fig 19-14b Beneath the membrane, corticalization of the graft surface can be seen.

ing sinus augmentation and histologic/histomorphometric data documents the benefits of using a membrane over the lateral window.

Following are the positive effects that have been obtained by placing a membrane over the lateral window:

1. Excludes nonosteogenic connective tissue
2. Contains particulate graft material
3. Prevents soft tissue encleftation
4. Increases vital bone formation (guided bone regeneration effect)
5. Increases implant survival rate
6. Results in positive outcomes when used for perforation repairs.

The available evidence suggests that the use of a membrane over the lateral window should be considered in all sinus graft procedures that use a lateral approach.

References

1. Murray G, Holden R, Roachlau W. Experimental and clinical study of new growth of bone in a cavity. Am J Orthop Surg 1959;93:385–387.
2. Melcher AH. On the repair potential of periodontal tissues. J Periodontol 1976;47:256–260.
3. Nyman S, Lindhe J, Karring T, Rylander H. New attachment following surgical treatment of human periodontal disease. J Clin Periodontol 1982;9:290–296.
4. Gottlow J, Nyman S, Lindhe J, Karring T, Wennstrom J. New attachment formation in the human periodontium by guided tissue regeneration. J Clin Periodontol 1986;13:604–616.
5. Stahl SS, Froum SJ, Tarnow DP. Human histologic responses to guided tissue regenerative techniques in intrabony lesions. J Clin Periodontol 1990;17:191–198.
6. Gian-Grasso J. Tooth isolation for new attachment procedures—A surgical and suturing method: Three case reports. J Periodontol 1987;58:819.
7. Shanaman R. A retrospective study of 237 sites treated consecutively with guided tissue regeneration. Int J Periodontics Restorative Dent 1994;14:293–301.
8. Laurell L, Falk H, Fornell J, Johard G, Gottlow J. Clinical use of a bioresorbable matrix barrier in guided tissue regeneration therapy. Case series. J Periodontol 1994;65:967–975.
9. Tonetti MS, Pini-Prato G, Cortellini P. Periodontal regeneration in human periodontal intrabony defects. IV. Determinants of response. J Periodontol 1993;64:934–940.
10. Murphy KG. Incidence, characterization and effect of surgical complications using Gore-Tex periodontal membranes. Effect of complications on regeneration. Int J Periodontics Restorative Dent 1995;15:549–561.
11. Reynolds MA, Aichelmann-Reidy ME, Branch-Mays GL, Gunsolley JC. The efficacy of bone replacement grafts in the treatment of periodontal osseous defects. A systematic review. Ann Periodontol 2003;8:227–265.
12. Murphy KG, Gunsolley JC. Guided tissue regeneration for the treatment of periodontal intrabony and furcation defects. A systematic review. Ann Periodontol 2003;8:266–302.
13. Dahlin C, Linde A, Gottlow J, Nyman S. Healing of bone defects by guided tissue regeneration. Plast Reconstr Surg 1988;81:672–676.
14. Dahlin C, Gottlow J, Linde A, Nyman S. Healing of maxillary and mandibular bone defects using a membrane technique [abstract 385]. J Dent Res 1989;68:918.
15. Siebert J, Nyman S. Localized ridge augmentation in dogs: A pilot study using membranes and hydroxyapatite. J Periodontol 1990;61:157–165.
16. Becker W, Becker B, Handlesman M, et al. Bone formation at dehisced dental implant sites treated with implant augmentation material: A pilot study in dogs. Int J Periodontics Restorative Dent 1990;10:93–101.
17. Buser D, Brägger U, Lang NP, Nyman S. Regeneration and enlargement of jawbone using guided tissue regeneration. Clin Oral Implants Res 1990;1:22–32.
18. Nyman S, Lang NP, Buser D, Brägger U. Bone regeneration adjacent to titanium dental implants using guided tissue regeneration: A report of cases. Int J Oral Maxillofac Implants 1990;5:9–14.
19. Lazzara RJ. Immediate implant placement into extraction sites: Surgical and restorative advantages. Int J Periodontics Restorative Dent 1989;9:333–343.
20. Buser D, Dula K, Lang NP, Nyman S. Long-term stability of osseointegrated implants in bone regenerated with the membrane technique. Five-year results of a prospective study with 12 implants. Clin Oral Implants Res 1996;7:175–183.
21. Fugazzotto PA, Shanaman R, Manos T, Shectman R. Guided bone regeneration around titanium implants: Report of the treatment of 1,503 sites with clinical re-entries. Int J Periodontics Restorative Dent 1997;17:293–299.
22. Nevins M, Mellonig JT, Clem DS, Reiser GM, Buser DA. Implants in regenerated bone: Long-term survival. Int J Periodontics Restorative Dent 1998;18:35–45.
23. Becker W, Dahlin C, Lekholm U, et al. Five-year evaluation of implants placed at extraction and with dehiscences and fenestration defects augmented with e-PTFE membranes: Results from a prospective multicenter study. Clin Implant Dent Relat Res 1999;1:27–32.
24. Simion M, Jovanovic SA, Tinti C, Parma Benfenati S. Long-term evaluation of osseointegrated implants inserted at the time of or after vertical ridge augmentation. A retrospective study of 123 implants with 1–5 year follow-up. Clin Oral Implants Res 2001;12:35–45.
25. Corrente G, Abundo R, Cardaropoli D, Cardaropoli G, Martuscelli G. Long-term evaluation of osseointegrated implants in regenerated and nonregenerated bone. Int J Periodontics Restorative Dent 2000;20:391–397.
26. Zitzmann NU, Schärer P, Marinello CP. Long-term results of implants treated with guided bone regeneration: A 5-year prospective study. Int J Oral Maxillofac Implants 2001;16:355–366.
27. Fiorellini JP, Nevins ML. Localized ridge augmentation/preservation. A systematic review. Ann Periodontol 2003;8:321–327.
28. Misch CE. The maxillary sinus lift and sinus graft surgery. In: Misch CE. Contemporary Implant Dentistry. St Louis: Mosby, 1999;469–495.
29. Schwartz-Arad D, Herzberg R, Dolev E. The prevalence of surgical complications of the sinus graft procedure and their impact on implant survival. J Periodontol 2004;75:511–516.
30. Vlassis JM, Fugazzotto PA. A classification system for sinus membrane perforations during augmentation procedures with options for repair. J Periodontol 1999;70:692–699.
31. Pikos MA. Maxillary sinus membrane repair: Report of a technique for large perforations. Implant Dent 1999;8:36–46.
32. Proussaefs P, Lozada J. The "Loma Linda Pouch": A technique for repairing the perforated sinus membrane. Int J Periodontics Restorative Dent 2003;23:593–597
33. Haas R, Baron M, Donath K, Zechner W, Watzek G. Porous hydroxyapatite for grafting the maxillary sinus: A histomorphometric study in sheep. Int J Oral Maxillofac Implants 2002;17:337–346.

34. Hürzeler MB, Quiñones CR, Kirsch A, et al. Maxillary sinus augmentation using different grafting materials and dental implants in monkeys. Part I. Evaluation of anorganic bovine-derived matrix. Clin Oral Implants Res 1997;8:476–486.
35. Jensen OT, Shulman LB, Block MS, Iacono VJ. Report of the Sinus Consensus Conference of 1996. Int J Oral Maxillofac Implants 1998;13(suppl):11–45.
36. Khoury F. Augmentation of the sinus floor with mandibular bone block and simultaneous implantation: A 6-year clinical investigation. Int J Oral Maxillofac Implants 1998;14:557–564.
37. Proussaefs P, Lozada J, Kim J, Rohrer MD. Repair of the perforated sinus membrane with a resorbable collagen membrane: A human study. Int J Oral Maxillofac Implants 2004;19:413–420.
38. Boyne PJ, Kruger GO. Fluorescence microscopy of alveolar bone repair. Oral Surg 1962;15:265–281.
39. Misch CE, Dietsch F. Subantral augmentation in *Maccaca fasicularis*: A pilot study. Int J Oral Implantol 1991;17:340.
40. Quiñones CR, Hürzeler MB, Schüpbach P, et al. Maxillary sinus augmentation using different grafting materials and osseointegrated dental implants in monkeys. Part II. Evaluation of porous hydroxyapatite as a grafting material. Clin Oral Implants Res 1997;8:487–496.
41. Margolin MD, Cogan AG, Taylor M, et al. Maxillary sinus augmentation in the non-human primate: A comparative radiographic and histologic study between recombinant human osteogenic protein-1 and natural bone mineral. J Periodontol 1998;89:911–919.
42. Boyne PJ, Lilly LC, Marx RE, et al. *De novo* bone induction by recombinant human bone morphogenetic protein-2 (rhBMP-2) in maxillary sinus floor augmentation. J Oral Maxillofac Surg 2005;63:1693–1707.
43. Nevins M, Fiorellini JP. The maxillary sinus floor augmentation procedure to support implant prostheses. In: Nevins M, Mellonig JT (eds). Implant Therapy: Clinical Approaches and Evidence of Success. Chicago: Quintessence, 1998:171–195.
44. Smiler DG, Johnson PW, Lozada JL, et al. Sinus lift grafts and endosseous implants: Treatment of the posterior atrophic maxilla. Dent Clin North Am 1992;36:151–186.
45. McAllister BS, Margolin MD, Cogan AD, Taylor M, Wollins J. Residual lateral wall defects following sinus grafting with recombinant human osteogenic protein-1 or Bio-Oss in the chimpanzee. Int J Periodontics Restorative Dent 1998;18:227–239.
46. Jensen OT, Greer RO. Immediate placement of osseointegrated implants into the maxillary sinus augmented with mineralized cancellous allograft and Gore-Tex: Second stage surgical and histological findings. In: Laney WR, Tolman DE (eds). Tissue Integration in Oral, Orthopedic, and Maxillofacial Reconstruction. Chicago: Quintessence, 1992:321–333.
47. Tarnow DP, Wallace SS, Froum SJ. Histologic and clinical comparison of bilateral sinus floor elevations with and without barrier membrane placement in 12 patients: Part 3 of an ongoing prospective study. Int J Periodontics Restorative Dent 2000;20:116–125.
48. Froum SJ, Tarnow DP, Wallace SS, Rohrer MD, Cho S-C. Sinus floor elevation using anorganic bovine bone matrix (OsteoGraf/N) with and without autogenous bone: A clinical, histologic, radiographic and histomorphometric analysis—Part 2 of an ongoing prospective study. Int J Periodontics Restorative Dent 1998;18:529–543.
49. Wallace SS, Froum SJ, Cho S-C, et al. Sinus augmentation utilizing anorganic bovine bone (Bio-Oss) with absorbable and nonabsorbable membranes placed over the lateral window: A histomorphometric and clinical analysis. Int J Periodontics Restorative Dent 2005;25:551–559.
50. Graziani F, Donos N, Needleman I, Gabriele M, Tonetti M. Comparison of implant survival following sinus floor augmentation procedures with implants placed in pristine posterior maxillary bone: A systematic review. Clin Oral Implants Res 2004;15:677–682.
51. Wallace SS, Froum SJ. Effect of maxillary sinus augmentation on the survival of endosseous dental implants. A systematic review. Ann Periodontol 2003;8:328–343.
52. Tawil G, Mawla M. Sinus floor elevation using a bovine bone mineral (Bio-Oss) with or without the concomitant use of a bilayered collagen barrier (Bio-Gide): A clinical report of immediate and delayed implant placement. Int J Oral Maxillofac Implants 2001;16:713–721.
53. Zitzmann N, Schärer P, Marinello CP. Long-term results of implants treated with guided bone regeneration: A 5-year prospective study. Int J Oral Maxillofac Implants 2001;16:355–366.

chapter 20
Le Fort I Downgraft with Sinus Elevation

Ole T. Jensen, DDS, MS
Richard Branca, DDS, MS

Reconstruction of the edentulous, highly resorbed, retrodisplaced maxilla via iliac bone graft augmentation also presents an opportunity to adjust maxillary position simultaneously using a Le Fort I osteotomy.[1] If deficiency of the maxilla is extensive (ie, Cawood and Howell Class IV, V, or VI), bone harvested from the ilium to support the interpositional osteotomy procedure is primarily used for sinus floor augmentation. The extent of Le Fort I advancement as suggested by articulator-mounted casts is usually not achievable and is usually limited to a maximum of 5 to 10 mm.

The first treatment-planning decision for the edentulous maxilla is whether to use a fixed hybrid or a removable definitive prosthesis. Since it is difficult to reconstruct a highly resorbed maxilla to accommodate a fixed prosthetic restoration, a coordinated effort between prosthodontic and surgical disciplines will be needed to establish an achievable goal.[2]

Overzealous alveolar onlay augmentation poses a long-term risk for the development of wound dehiscence and is prone to resorption[3] (see chapter 14). A Le Fort I approach reduces this risk by allowing for a more modest alveolar augmentation of about 5 mm and at the same time establishes primary implant support from bone grafted onto the sinus floor. Vertical height from the sinus floor usually increases by more than 10 mm and volumetric stability is maintained over the long term, unlike the resorption-prone alveolar onlay graft.

Modest vertical augmentation of the alveolus combined with sinus grafting *without* a Le Fort I osteotomy has demonstrated excellent vertical dimensional stability in long-term studies that now extend over a 20-year time period[4] (Fig 20-1). Given such results, it is logical to consider moving the maxilla down and forward to improve interarch jaw position and to reduce the amount of onlay grafting required.

Surgical Procedure

Modification of the surgical approach for Le Fort I osteotomy with sinus membrane preservation proceeds as follows:

1. A circumvestibular incision is accomplished, and lateral antrostomy windows are made over the sinus bilaterally. The antrostomy windows are long and narrow to provide access posteriorly and yet make bone plating possible. Sinus membrane elevation of the *entire* sinus floor is accomplished. The sinus membrane is generally elevated about 10 mm.

2. A relatively low-level Le Fort I osteotomy, protecting both sinus and nasal membranes, is completed (Fig 20-2a).

3. Osteotomes are used to free the lateral nasal walls after membrane elevation. A trans-sinal approach may be needed if the lateral nasal wall is robust.

4. The nasal septum and the pterygomaxillary sutures also are freed using osteotomes, and the maxilla is *carefully* downfractured and mobilized. (Thin maxillae will frequently fracture across the posterior palate).

chapter 20 Le Fort I Downgraft with Sinus Elevation

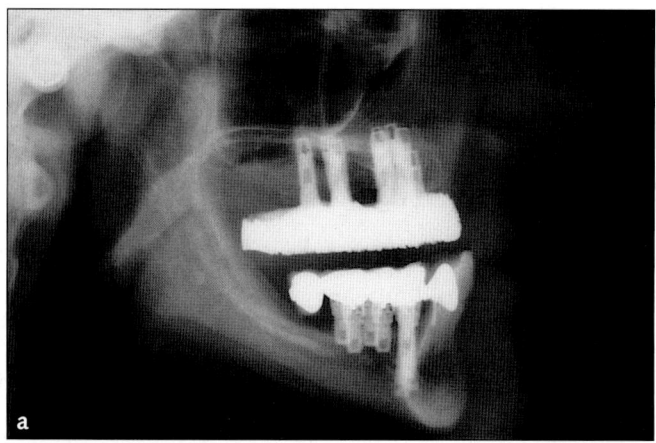

Figs 20-1a and 20-1b Radiographic views 9 years after combined vertical augmentation and sinus grafting with bone harvested from the ilium. (Figs 20-1a to 20-1g courtesy of Dr Ronald Yaros, Aurora, Colorado.)

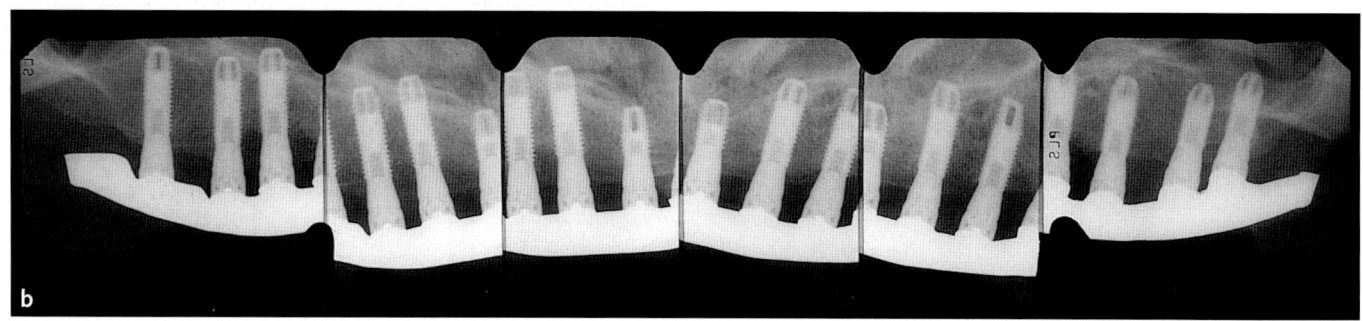

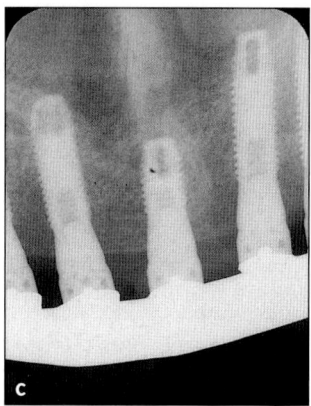

Fig 20-1c Note the stability of alveolar augmentation anteriorly, where there had been initially only a sliver of alveolar bone.

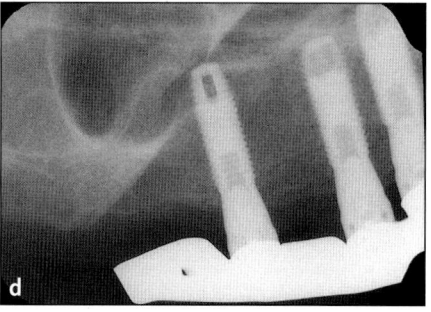

Figs 20-1d and 20-1e No loss of bone graft height is discernible within the sinus.

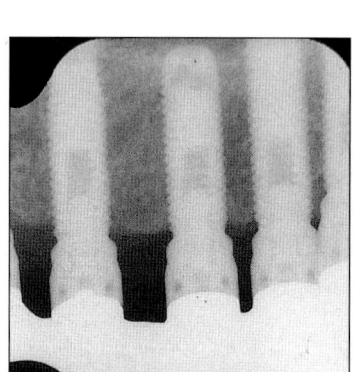
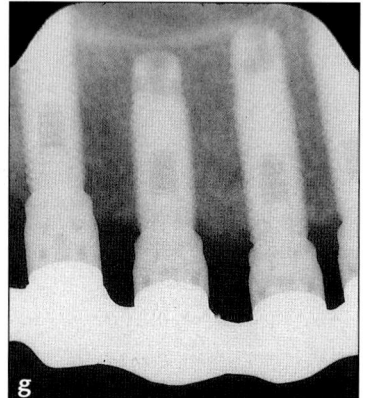

Figs 20-1f and 20-1g Radiographic views demonstrate stable sinus and alveolar bone levels in another patient 7 years after combined iliac grafting.

Fig 20-2a The nasal and sinus cavities are still veiled by the elevated nasal and sinus mucosa with the maxilla in a downfractured Le Fort I position. (Figs 20-2a to 20-2e courtesy of Dr Louisa Gallegos, Denver, Colorado.)

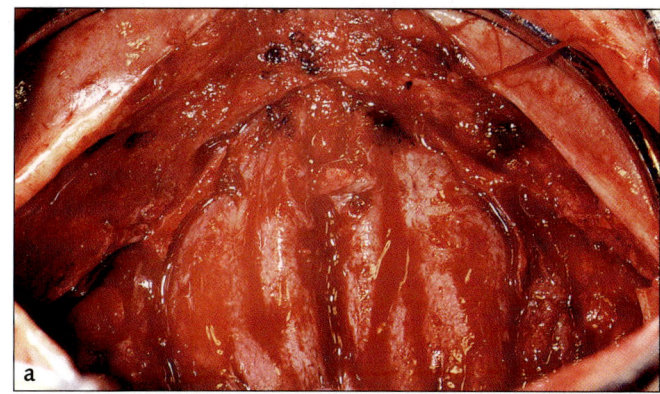

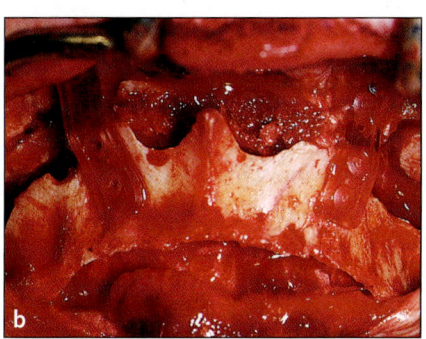
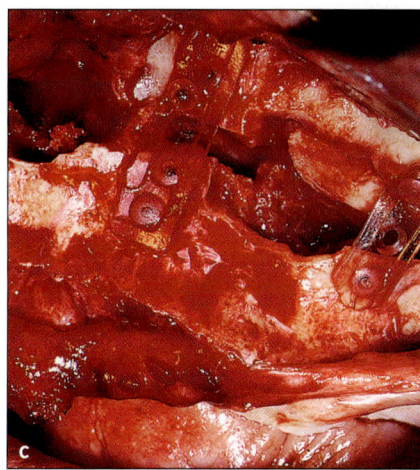
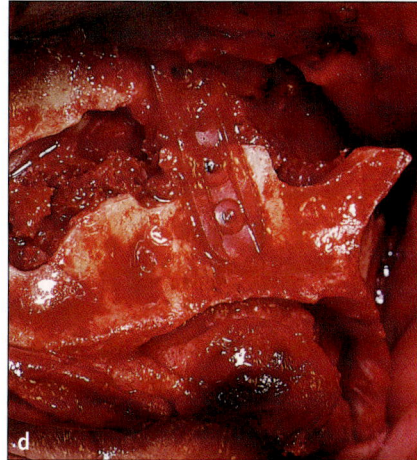

Figs 20-2b to 20-2d Following maxillary advancement and sinus and nasal grafting, resorbable bone plates are used to fix the position of the maxilla forward about 5 mm and downward about 10 mm.

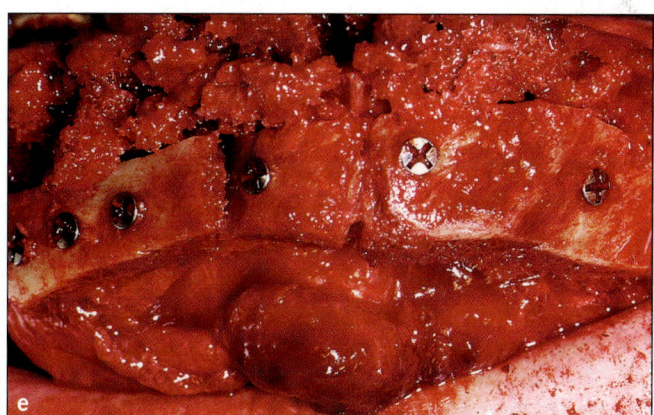

Fig 20-2e The maxilla is then reconstructed by about 5 mm of lateral augmentation and some vertical anterior augmentation of the alveolus.

5. Rigid fixation is applied using resorbable bone plates and screws to establish a down and forward maxillary position (Figs 20-2b to 20-2d).[5] Average movement is 5 mm forward and 5 mm down.
6. Following placement of "internal" fixation of the maxilla, particulate bone is used to augment the sinus floor, and struts of corticocancellous block bone and cancellous marrow are used to augment the maxilla laterally over the resorbable fixation (Fig 20-2e). Unlike the internal fixation, this external grafting is fixated with titanium screws, so that they can be accessed for removal at a later stage.

7. Blocks of corticocancellous bone are interposed into the gap created by maxillary advancement between the pterygoid plate and posterior maxilla to help prevent maxillary relapse.[6]
8. Because the maxilla is tilted inferiorly by several millimeters, care should be taken to interpose particulate bone graft in the nasal fossa and block graft anteriorly. Sometimes block bone can be partially supported by a retained anterior nasal spine (see Fig 20-2b).
9. Barrier membranes should be used selectively since membrane exposure increases the risk of infection.[7]
10. Implant placement should be deferred until after the graft has incorporated, usually about 6 months later, to improve stability and location. Simultaneous implant placement requires that at least a portion of the host basal bone is engaged and therefore should be reserved for less resorbed cases.[8] If bone resorption is uneven, excess bone from one site can be used to supplement areas of excess resorption. Such secondary bone graft "redistribution" shapes and restores alveolar form.
11. Wound closure is accomplished using resorbable sutures in all three layers (periosteal, subcutaneous, and mucosal). Mucosal wound closure should be passive.
12. For implant placement, it is important to make the incision 3 to 4 mm crestal into the fixed palatal tissue. A palatally related guide stent should be used. In most cases, eight implants are placed. The best bone for implant placement is in the sinus grafted areas.
13. Six months after placement (ie, 1 year after iliac bone grafting), implants are exposed through the original palatal-crestal incision, and releasing incisions are made posteriorly.
14. As wound closure progresses around the arch, the entire facial flap advances forward. The wound is closed from anterior to posterior.
15. Final restorative procedures begin 3 weeks after implant exposure, whether for a fixed hybrid or an overdenture prosthesis.

Classification of Edentulous Maxillae and Suggested Treatment Protocols

Multiple physiologic and biomechanical variables obviously make it impossible to follow the same surgical approach in every case. To help the surgeon negotiate these various factors, other authors have devised classification systems that correspond to specific treatment protocols. Previous classifications have been based on the residual bone available for implants or as a descriptive gradation of bone resorption.[9–11] The classification that follows describes suggested treatment approaches based on bone availability.

There are four types of *edentulous* maxillae: the orthognathic maxilla and the moderately, severely, and extremely atrophic maxilla. Treatment for these four types of atrophy is presented in Box 20-1.

The goal of classification is to define sensible and realistic treatment protocols. Establishing a classification system for osseous morphology defines the favored method of using available bone to fixate to, to derive vascular supply from, and to inductively grow new bone around. The goal is to obtain sufficient bone mass for dental implant restoration that is orthoalveolar or reduces cantilever to the restorative scheme.[12–14] To obtain a favorable restorative result in spite of variable bone graft incorporation or bone graft resorption or even relapse of the advancement osteotomy, the treatment protocols are designed to achieve relatively small corrections in each of three planes of space. When advancement of the maxilla is modest, relapse is less likely.[15] When vertical alveolar augmentation is not excessive, dimensional change from late remodeling and implant loading is more likely to be moderate.[16] When the regenerated sinus bone is repositioned anteriorly for a more favorable biomechanical position, implant load-bearing capacity is more stable.[17] When this protocol is followed in the treatment of the resorbed maxilla, bone graft longevity is improved because the basal strut of

BOX 20-1 Classification of edentulous maxillae and suggested treatment protocols

I. Orthognathic (ie, mildly atrophic) maxilla. Does not require vertical grafting; requires only minor grafting laterally; may or may not require sinus grafting. After grafting, four to eight implants can be placed in preparation for a fixed restoration (see chapter 27). In the absence of vertical resorption, overdenture abutments may not be indicated.

Treatment protocol:
Sinus grafting, implant placement with immediate loading (Figs 20-3 and 20-4).

II. Moderately atrophic with moderately retrodisplaced maxilla and severe lateral loss, but minimal vertical resorption (ie, narrow or knife-edged alveolar ridge) (Fig 20-5).

Treatment protocol:
Split alveolar bone grafting or lateral veneer grafts combined with sinus grafting (see chapter 21), OR Le Fort I osteotomy and sinus, nasal floor, and lateral alveolar grafting followed by implant placement (delayed is preferred) (Fig 20-6). A maxilla with 4-mm retrognathia can achieve a stable Class I orthognathic position.

III. Retrodisplaced maxilla with severe horizontal and vertical loss (Figs 20-7a to 20-7g).

Treatment protocol:
Le Fort I osteotomy for maxillary advancement; sinus, nasal floor, and alveolar ridge grafting; interpositional downgrafting followed by delayed implant placement. A fixed hybrid denture is possible, but an overdenture is recommended if the anterior cantilever is too great (Figs 20-7h and 20-7i).

IV. Retrodisplaced maxilla with extreme basal atrophy and sinus and nasal floor dehiscence or reverse architecture. Total absence of alveolar ridge with basal bone resorption. Anterior ablation only (combination syndrome) or anteroposterior ablation (the so-called flat maxilla) (Fig 20-8a).

Treatment protocol:
For total vertical loss anteroposteriorly, the position of the maxilla can be improved only by means of Le Fort I downgraft, primarily to increase bone mass. Implant load-bearing capacity will be almost entirely limited to the sinus-grafted locations (Figs 20-8b to 20-8e).

---

maxillary bone, the foundation of the bone graft, remains *central* in all planes of space.

If an ideal gingival profile restoration is desired, a Le Fort I distraction may need to be combined with sinus bone grafting (see chapter 24) (see Fig 20-6). In the vast majority of maxillary atrophic cases, however, an acceptable biomechanical and esthetic restoration can be accomplished with a modified Le Fort I downgraft alone.

chapter 20 Le Fort I Downgraft with Sinus Elevation

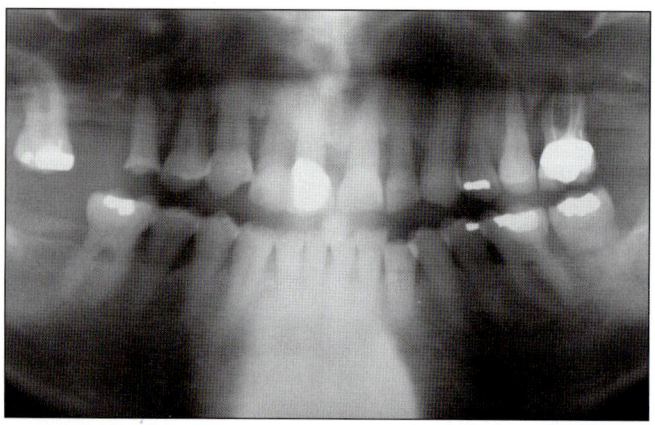

Fig 20-3a A 50-year-old man presents with severe bone loss around the remaining maxillary dentition.

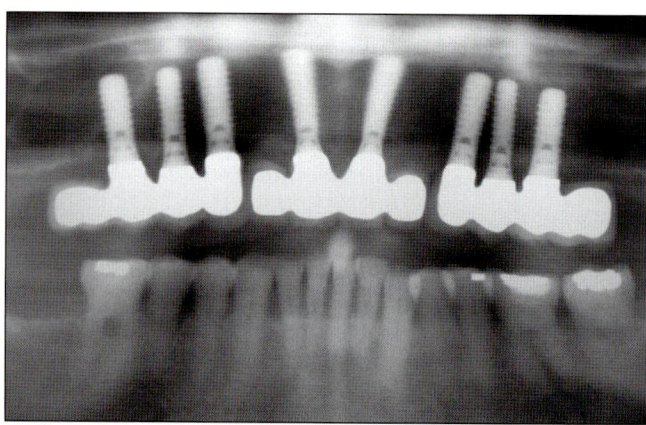

Fig 20-3b The final restoration, following immediate provisionalization and minor sinus intrusion grafting. The maxilla was in Class I arch relation.

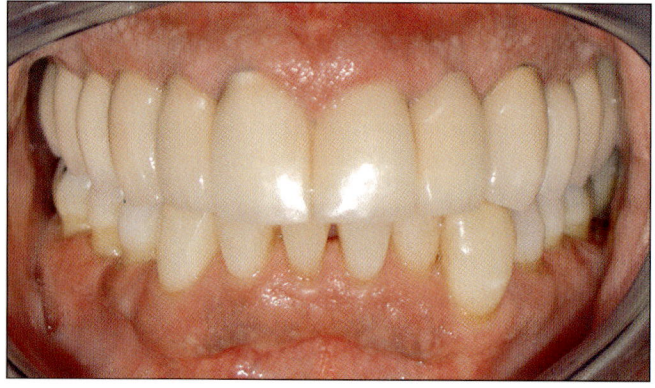

Fig 20-3c Final restoration. (Courtesy of Dr Curtis Becker, DDS, Denver, Colorado.)

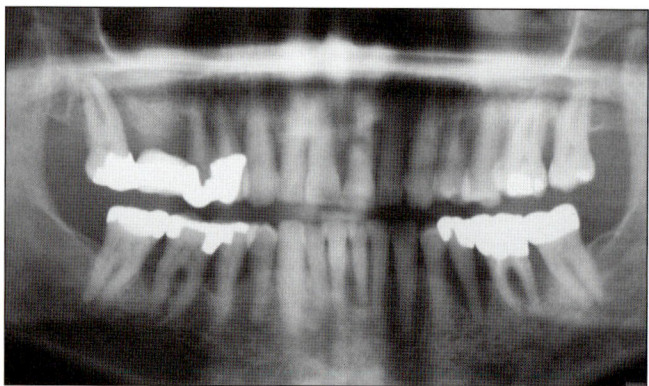

Fig 20-4a A 65-year-old patient with severe periodontal disease treated with implants and sinus elevation on the day of dental extraction with immediate provisionalization.

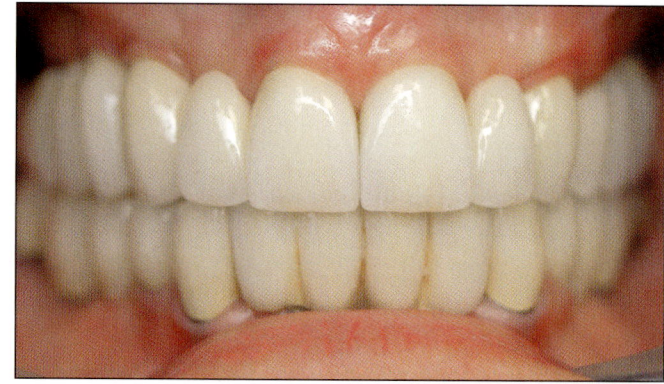

Fig 20-4b Final outcome 3 years post-restoration showing maintenance of arch relation and esthetic alveolar form. (Courtesy of Dr Lee Kuhlke, Englewood, Colorado.)

Classification of Edentulous Maxillae and Suggested Treatment Protocols

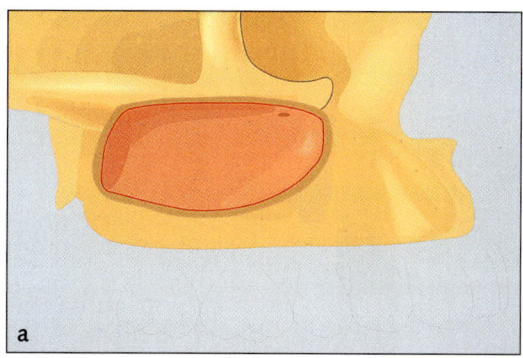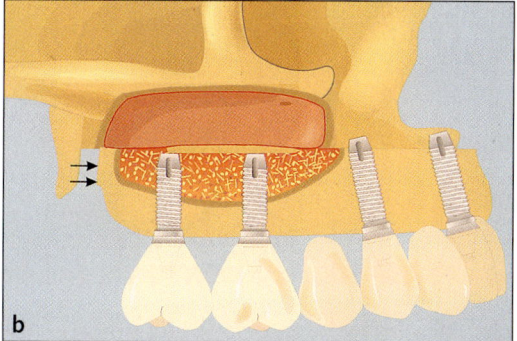

Figs 20-5a and 20-5b Downward and forward movement of the maxilla with sinus grafting. Implants are best placed in a staged approach 6 months after grafting.

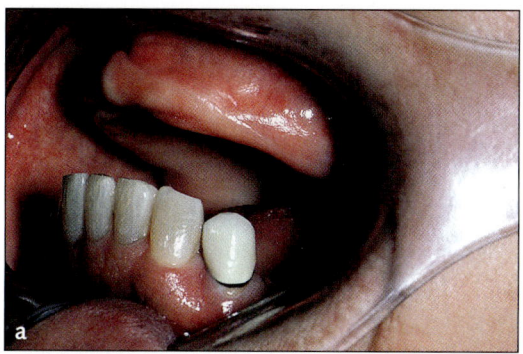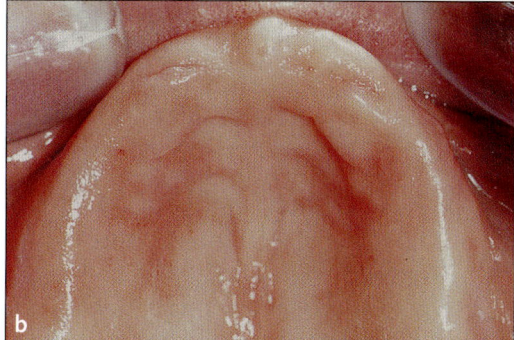

Figs 20-6a and 20-6b Class III edentulous maxilla in a 55-year-old patient who wore a complete maxillary denture opposite natural mandibular dentition for 22 years. (Courtesy of Dr Lee Kuhlke, Englewood, Colorado.)

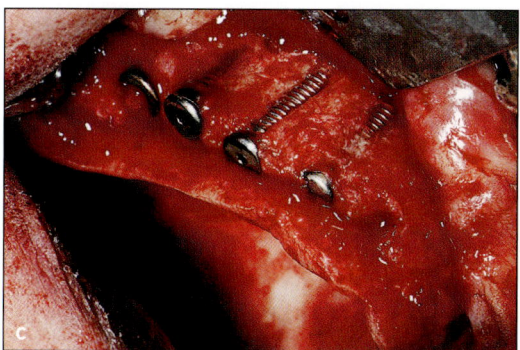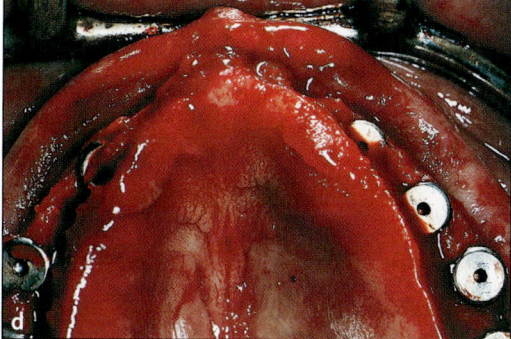

Figs 20-6c and 20-6d Le Fort I advancement and lateral and sinus grafting with simultaneous placement of posterior implants.

Fig 20-6e Stable final restoration 4 years after bone graft reconstruction.

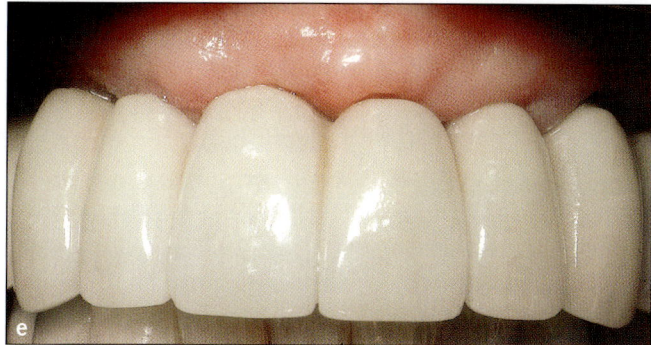

247

Chapter 20: Le Fort I Downgraft with Sinus Elevation

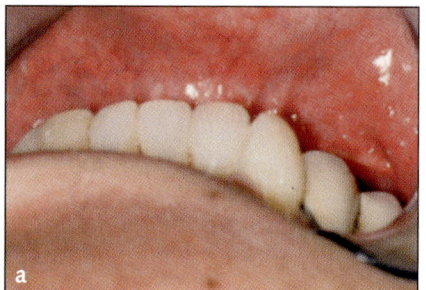
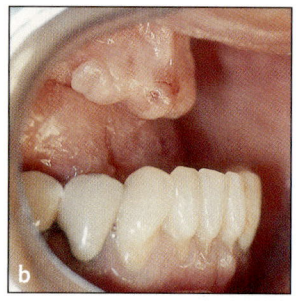

Fig 20-7a Complete absence of maxillary alveolar projection is evident in this preoperative clinical photograph of the patient with the maxillary denture removed.

Fig 20-7b Preoperative lateral view showing severe maxillary retrodisplacement.

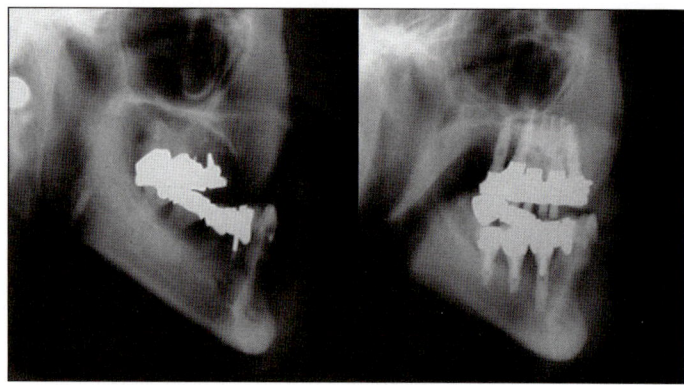

Fig 20-7c Preoperative cephalograph *(left)* showing a 15-mm retrognathic maxillary position. A cephalograph taken 4 years postsurgery *(right)* indicates near Class I implant placement for the modestly cantilevered prosthesis.

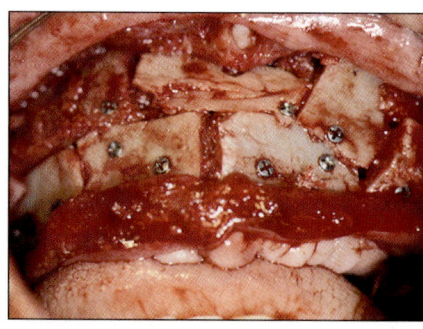

Fig 20-7d The Le Fort I downfracture bone graft technique that was used for the maxilla preserved the sinus and nasal membranes and was followed by sinus and nasal floor grafting with overlay corticocancellous grafting around the arch.

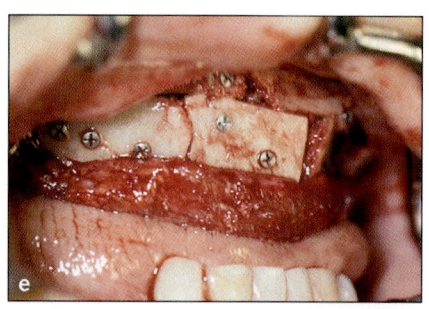
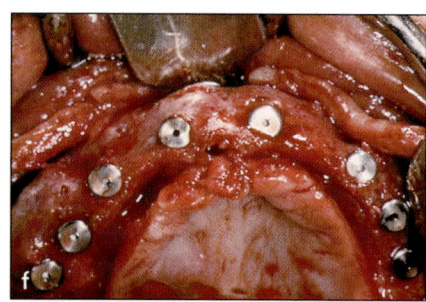

Fig 20-7e About 10 mm of anterior projection was gained via combined maxillary advancement and augmentation, still short of a Class I relation.

Fig 20-7f Implant placement 6 months after bone graft reconstruction.

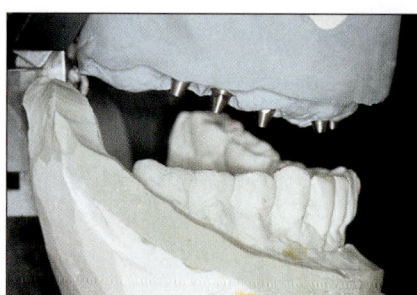
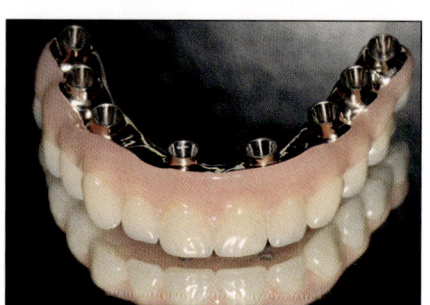
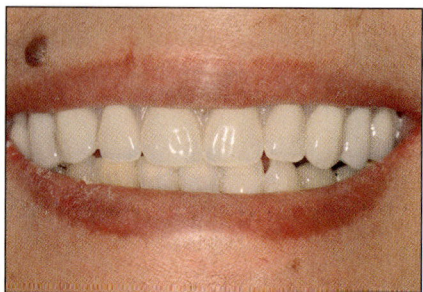

Fig 20-7g Articulated master working conical abutment cast at correct vertical dimension of occlusion demonstrates relative maxillary retrognathia as well as increased interarch space posteriorly.

Fig 20-7h Completed acrylic-fused-to-gold fixed partial denture. Note the horizontal cantilever of 5 to 8 mm around the arch. (Courtesy of Dr Aldo Leopardi, Greenwood Village, Colorado.)

Fig 20-7i The completed implant-borne prosthesis provides lip support for improved esthetics. (Courtesy of Dr Aldo Leopardi, Greenwood Village, Colorado.)

Classification of Edentulous Maxillae and Suggested Treatment Protocols

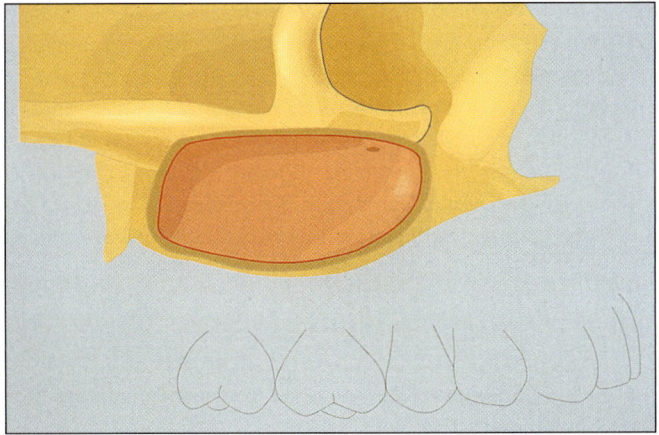

Fig 20-8a In the highly resorbed maxilla, where there is paper-thin bone, the defect involves not only vertical ablation but significant maxillary retrognathia and may involve dehiscence of the nasal floor.

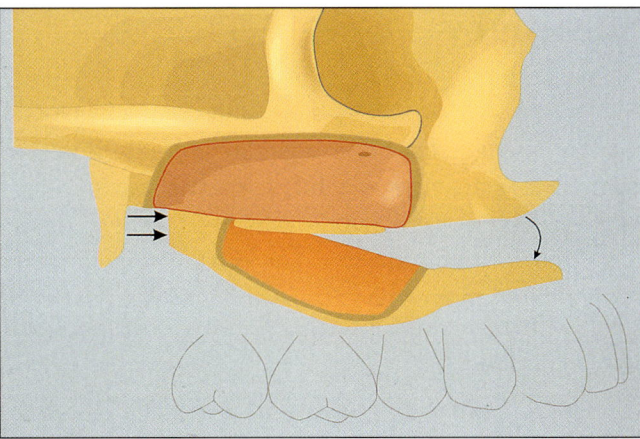

Fig 20-8b The maxilla in this case needs to be downgrafted as well as advanced. Care should be taken to preserve the anterior nasal spine for use as a strut to graft to, if possible.

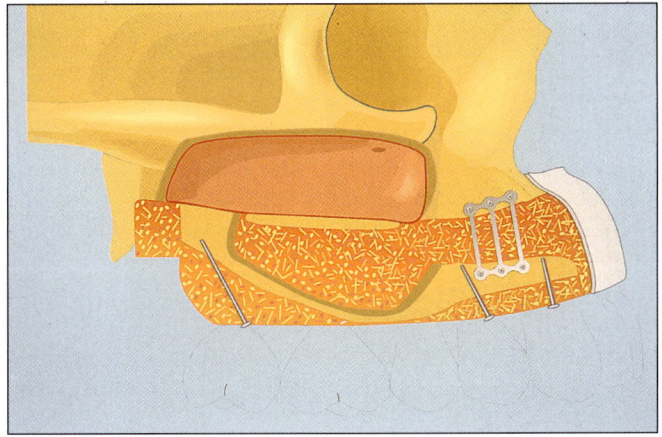

Fig 20-8c Following advancement of the maxilla, lateral fixation is accomplished with resorbable bone plates.

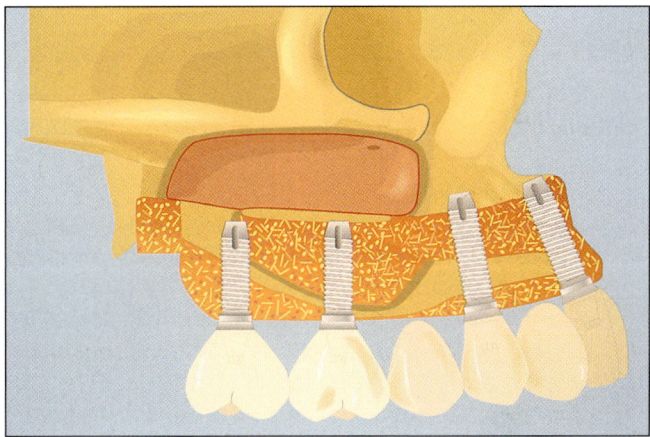

Fig 20-8d Sinus and lateral grafting and barrier membranes can then be used to complete the augmentation. Implant reconstruction follows 6 months later.

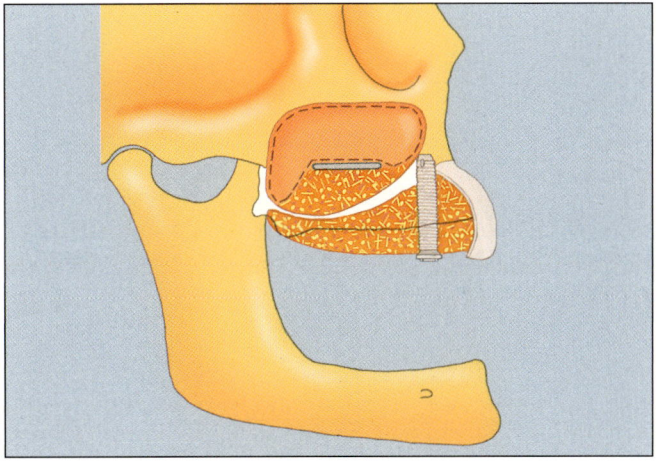

Fig 20-8e Excessive vertical grafting makes complete revascularization of the graft more difficult and wound dehiscence and graft loss more likely.

Summary

The Le Fort I interpositional bone graft derives its biomechanical strength for the support of implants from the sinus bone graft. The edentulous maxilla can often be restored with a fixed hybrid prosthesis depending on the extent of bony atrophy. The modest inferoanterior advancement that can be achieved provides an excellent framework for augmentation. Bone grafting using corticocancellous bone harvested from the ilium is maintained 10, 15, and 20 years with rare late-term implant loss. Prosthetic restoration is established on the most volumetrically dependable maxillofacial bone graft—the sinus floor bone graft.

References

1. Farrel CD, Kent JN, Guerra LR. One stage interpositional bone grafting and vestibuloplasty in the atrophic maxilla. J Oral Surg 1976;34:901–906.
2. Keller EE, Eckert SE, Tolman DE. Maxillary anterior and nasal one-stage inlay composite bone graft: Preliminary report on 30 recipient sites. J Oral Maxillofac Surg 1994;52:438–447.
3. Jensen OT, Shulman LB, Block MS, Iacono VJ. Report of the sinus consensus conference of 1996. Int J Oral Maxillofac Implants 1998;13(special issue):11–45.
4. Jensen OT. Guided bone graft augmentation. In: Buser D, Dahlin C, Schenk R (eds). Guided Bone Regeneration in Implant Dentistry. Chicago: Quintessence, 1994:235–261.
5. Pietrzak WS, Verstynen ML, Sarver DR. Bioabsorbable fixation devices, status for the craniomaxillofacial surgeon. J Craniofac Surg 1997;8:92–96.
6. Bell WH. Ridge augmentation as an aid in jaw surgery. In: Bell WH, Proffit WR, White RP (eds). Surgical Correction of Dentofacial Deformities. Philadelphia: Saunders, 1980:1425–1433.
7. Jensen OT, Greer RO, Johnson L, Kassebaum D. Vertical guided bone-graft augmentation in a new canine mandibular model. Int J Oral Maxillofac Implants 1995;10:335–344.
8. Blomqvist JE, Alberius P, Isaksson S. Sinus inlay bone augmentation: Comparison of implant positioning after one- or two-staged procedures. J Oral Maxillofac Surg 1997;55:804–810.
9. Jensen O. Site classification for the osseointegrated implant. J Prosthet Dent 1989;61:228–234.
10. Cawood JI, Stoelinga PJ, Bonus JJ. Reconstruction of the severely resorbed (Class VI) maxilla: A two-step procedure. Int J Oral Maxillofac Surg 1994;23:219–225.
11. Brånemark P-I, Zarb GA, Albrektsson T (eds). Tissue-Integrated Prostheses: Osseointegration in Clinical Dentistry. Chicago: Quintessence, 1985.
12. Bell WH. Revascularization and bone healing after anterior maxillary osteotomy: A study using adult rhesus monkeys. J Oral Surg 1969;27:249–255.
13. Bell WH, Levy BM. Revascularization and bone healing after posterior maxillary osteotomy. J Oral Surg 1971;29:313–320.
14. Bell WH, Fonseca RJ, Kennedy JW, Levy BM. Bone healing and revascularization after total maxillary osteotomy. J Oral Surg 1975;33:253–260.
15. Bell WH. Le Fort I osteotomy for correction of maxillary deformities. J Oral Surg 1975;33:412–426.
16. Davis WH, Delo RI, Ward WB, Terry B, Patakas B. Long term ridge augmentation with rib graft. J Maxillofac Surg 1975;3:103–106.
17. Boyne PJ, James RA. Grafting of the maxillary sinus floor with autogenous marrow and bone. J Oral Surg 1980;38:613–616.

chapter 21
Trans-Alveolar Sinus Elevation Combined with Ridge Expansion

Daniel R. Cullum, DDS
Ole T. Jensen, DDS, MS

The horizontally deficient alveolar process can be widened simultaneously with sinus floor elevation using a trans-alveolar approach. Though alveolar height can be developed within the sinus using bone grafts placed via a lateral approach, trans-alveolar sinus elevation using osteotomes is a well-founded technique.[1-9] This chapter describes a combined ridge expansion/trans-alveolar sinus floor elevation procedure, both at individual sites and as a complete or contiguous sinus floor elevation.

Ridge Resorption

Alveolar resorption includes loss of both vertical and buccal dimension but is mostly a width deficiency phenomenon. This has been managed with *(a)* block or particulate bone grafting using guided bone regeneration; *(b)* ridge-split grafting[10]; or *(c)* distraction osteogenesis to transport an alveolar segment.[11] All of these methods re-establish alveolar width (and/or height) without taking advantage of the capacity of the sinus graft.

Ridge Expansion

Horizontal bone loss without prominent sinus pneumatization or in regions anterior to the sinus can be reconstructed by sectioning the buccal bone plate and moving it facially to restore normal ridge dimension. Placement of the implant is then restoration-driven for optimal function and esthetics. The ridge expansion technique must use a partial-thickness flap or a flapless approach, which maintains periosteal investment of the lateral cortex and crestal lamella.[2,12] A palatally placed split-thickness incision allows for movement of attached tissue to cover the expansion site, improving both vestibular depth and the width of crestal attached tissue. The *bone flap* is then manipulated laterally to restore buccal arch form and provide for axial alveolar inclination of subsequently placed implants.

The principles of maintaining periosteal blood supply and an adequate buccal plate thickness (minimum 1.5 mm) are critical to avoiding bone resorption. Animal studies have shown complete resorption of the buccal segment when the periosteum is stripped away.[13] The use of tapered implants is recommended because they conform to the shape of the expansion defect, reducing the risk for fracture detachment of the bone plate. After expansion, the result is an intra-alveolar defect like an extraction site, which heals without bone grafting by endosteal proliferation from the surrounding bone walls.[14] Osseous ridge expansion has also been used in combination with subepithelial connective tissue grafts placed crestally to address soft tissue demands in the esthetic zone. The technique can be used in both the mandible and maxilla.

Ridge Expansion and Trans-Alveolar Sinus Elevation

Rationale

In cases where the sinus is prominent and ridge expansion alone will not restore appropriate alveolar dimension, ridge expansion is combined with simultaneous sinus elevation incorporating the principles introduced above. However, combining ridge expansion and trans-alveolar sinus elevation requires a significant change in surgical mindset. The surgeon must imagine the alveolus as a book standing on end that is then opened. Through this open book (trans-alveolar), the binding (sinus floor) is elevated (upfractured) using an osteotome. Combined alveolar and sinus floor therapy is less invasive than a combined sinus graft and ridge augmentation.

Localized management of the sinus floor

The techniques described here develop an expanded intrabony cavity with an intact periosteal blood supply followed by the immediate upfracturing of the antral floor.[15] Apical floor upfracture and elevation using the osteotome that corresponds in diameter to the implant allows elevation of 2 to 3 mm. Bruschi et al[15] modified the technique using a palatal floor infracture for predictable elevation of 4 to 5 mm at each implant site. Greater elevations have been reported[16] with 4 mm or less of remaining bone height but with a noted increase in technical demands and a slightly reduced success rate (91.4%). The technique advocates the use of a no. 64 beaver blade malleted into the palatosinus floor; when freed, it is intruded at planned implant locations. The medial sinus floor and sinus membrane are moved together like a trap door, creating a new sinus floor. Bone gathered from around the periphery is moved apically while the intrabony cavity is left to heal without bone grafting, like an extraction site.

Wound closure is completed at the anterior release by re-approximating the flap to the periosteal margin for a submerged healing protocol. Alternatively, a single-stage (transgingival) protocol calls for anterior and apical repositioning of the flap and modified finger flap development for interproximal primary closure.

Contiguous sinus floor elevation

For extensive maxillary alveolar defects requiring vertical sinus elevation of more than 5 mm, a contiguous sinus floor protocol can be used. This involves upfracturing the sinus floor across the entire defect to produce a new bony roof. When there is only 3 to 4 mm of residual alveolar height available, it is still possible to perform progressive expansion and contiguous sinus floor elevation. It is not necessary to graft the intra-alveolar portion of the bone cavity or, if it is intact, the elevated bony floor. However, the intrasinus portion should be grafted if the membrane has been elevated without a bony roof. This will maintain space during healing, as in a lateral wall approach. While simultaneous implant placement is possible in this setting, primary stability is less predictable and may require delayed implant placement after a 4-month healing period. A staged approach is recommended to reduce the risk of nonintegration. The advantage of this technique over a lateral grafting approach is shorter treatment time, reduced patient discomfort, and restoration of the buccal arch dimension.

Implants are placed in submerged fashion and allowed to integrate for a period of 4 to 6 months. The greater the proportion of implant surface area in native alveolar bone, the shorter the healing interval required. Implants can typically be uncovered after 4 months followed by a period of healing for the soft tissues. Additional healing and progressive loading should be considered for larger elevations that have minimal alveolar support. Single-stage placement is possible when initial implant stability is adequate.

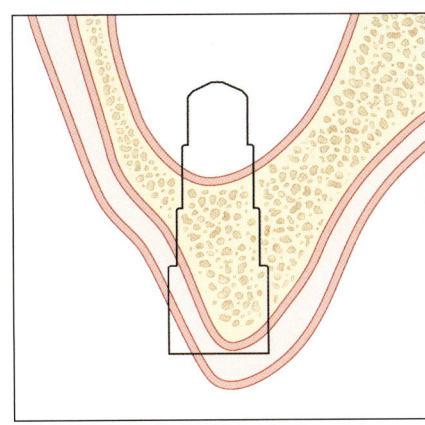

Fig 21-1 Inadequate alveolar width and height.

Sinus elevation simultaneous with tooth removal

This technique can be further modified when it is accomplished at the time of tooth removal. Both the extraction site and the adjacent edentulous areas can be treated with a trans-alveolar approach. First, a rongeur is used to harvest the interradicular bone. Next, a bony trough is developed in continuity with the extraction site using a ridge expansion technique if the alveolus is narrow, and a stepped osteotome technique if it is of adequate width. The sinus floor is then upfractured along the entire length of the combined cavity using blunt osteotomes or a contiguous sinus floor elevator. The harvested bone and collagen can be placed into the intrasinus portion for space maintenance during healing. This technique allows for sinus floor elevation of 3 mm over an extraction site and as much as 10 mm in adjacent edentulous areas. Elevation of a large continuous portion of the sinus floor allows for higher elevation overall and reduces the potential for sinus membrane perforation (see chapter 6).

Indications and Contraindications

Residual alveolar dimensions vary greatly. When traditional endosteal implants are used, 10 mm of alveolar *height* is probably needed for adequate long-term stability. Based on this, the following protocol is proposed for maxillary reconstructive procedures in ridges as narrow as 3 to 4 mm:

- For a bone height of 5 to 7 mm, ridge expansion with localized management of the sinus floor (osteotome apical upfracture or palatal floor infracture) with simultaneous implant placement
- For a bone height of 3 to 5 mm, ridge expansion with contiguous sinus floor elevation and simultaneous implant placement with or without intrasinus bone grafting
- For a bone height of 1 to 3 mm, a lateral approach with onlay and/or particulate bone grafting of the alveolar ridge with delayed implant placement.

This protocol adds subtlety to diagnosis and treatment of the various bone mass deficiencies associated with the sinus. Ridge expansion combined with sinus elevation is strongly indicated for mild to moderate horizontal bone loss (Fig 21-1). For this approach, a residual ridge width of 3.5 to 4 mm and a minimum alveolar height of 3 to 5 mm to the sinus floor are required for adequate intra-medullary bone volume. Bone quality is also an important factor to consider. If the ridge lacks medullary bone, sectioning and expansion become more challenging and the potential for fracture or resorption increases. Osteoporotic bone risks instability or fracture. Vertigo has been reported in patients who have undergone site development treatment with the osteotome technique.[17,18] The condition is generally self limiting but could require further management with an Epley maneuver.

With more severe bone loss in the posterior region, the margin of the zygomatic buttress becomes involved in mobilization of the bone flap. Bone sounding or computerized tomography (CT) scans can aid in preoperative assessment, but operative decision making is paramount. For patients with conditions such as diabetes that compromise bone healing, the vascularized bone flap is preferred

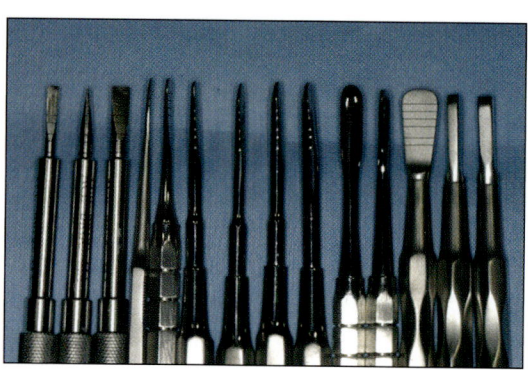

Fig 21-2 Instrumentation for ridge expansion and sinus elevation.

over free block grafts as wound healing is less susceptible to soft tissue dehiscence.

Surgical Considerations

Surgical experience with traditional osteotome techniques is mandatory for a successful treatment outcome. Operating from a sitting position with an armrest and hand support is advisable, because a stable base is needed to control malleting force. Attention to tactile, visual, and auditory cues is necessary for bone manipulation. In addition to gentle, progressive, and repetitive bending, an intrabony incision may be required for a beveled vertical release to avoid sudden fracture of the buccal plate. Sinus floor perforation can be avoided by careful attention to the muting of the sharp note of the mallet ring as the apical bone begins to mobilize and progressive mobilization of the bony floor with osteotomes of increasing diameter until the largest diameter is used for elevation. Surgical templates may be used for site planning and intermittently during site development. However, they must be designed to avoid impingement from the osteotomes and/or the bone flap as it is mobilized.

Surgical Procedure

After an appropriate preoperative assessment and standard preparation with chlorhexidine mouth rinse and antibiotics, intravenous and local anesthesia are administered with the patient in a semi-reclined position. Two assistants are generally required for retraction, support, and instrumentation. A series of graduated dull-edged chisels, "D"- shaped osteotomes, tapered blunt osteotomes, straight flat cutting osteotomes, a site-specific final implant osteotome, rotary instrumentation, and a surgical mallet may be used during site preparation (Fig 21-2).

Flap design

A buccal-based palatal incision is developed just above the level of the periosteum using the no. 64 beaver blade (Figs 21-3a and 21-3b). The split-thickness flap is designed to extend anteriorly, with marginal release at the mucogingival junction; it can be further extended with a vertical release located one tooth anterior to the site. Posteriorly, the flap should extend to about one or two teeth distal to the site. If no posterior teeth are present, the flap should extend to the tuberosity with lateral or vertical release. Care is taken to avoid perforation of the flap, especially at the attached tissue junction. The palatal aspect of the ridge may be exposed with split-thickness dissection, or bone sounding may be used to determine the inclination of the palatal vault. With experience, the procedure can be completed with minimal flap development.

Bone incision

Using the no. 64 beaver blade as a chisel, the residual alveolar ridge is sectioned with a gentle malleting action. The no. 64 blade is malleted in an anteroposterior direction to a point just short of the sinus floor (see Fig 21-3a). The residual ridge should be at least 3.5 to 4 mm thick for bone regeneration. Initial ridge expansion begins in the sectioned ridge below the sinus floor and may require an anterior or posterior intrabony release. The no. 64 blade is angled at 45 degrees toward the facial aspect of the alveolus so as to keep the facial cortical plate intact.

Surgical Procedure

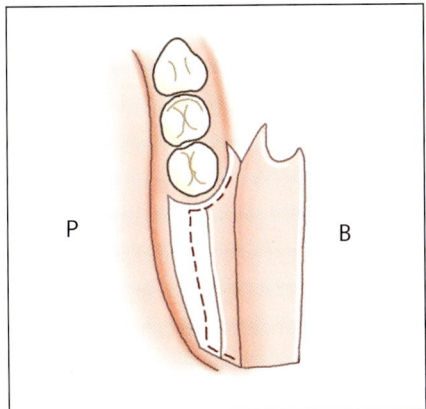

Fig 21-3a Buccal-based flap design and bone incision. (P, palatal B, buccal.)

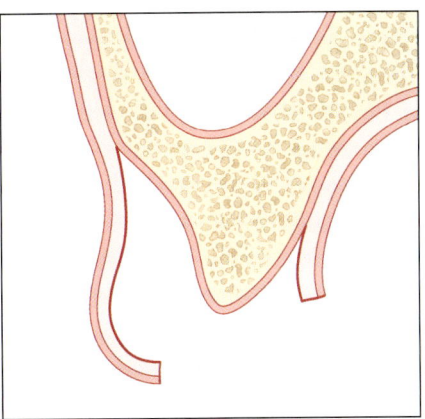

Fig 21-3b Palatal split-thickness incision and buccal dissection.

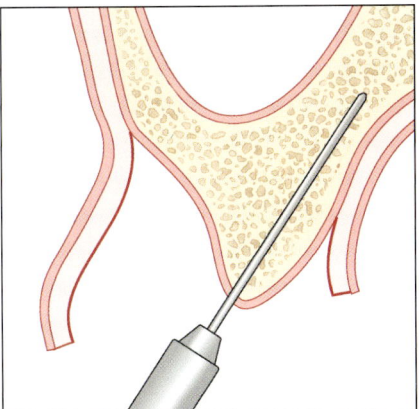

Fig 21-3c Palatal bone incision.

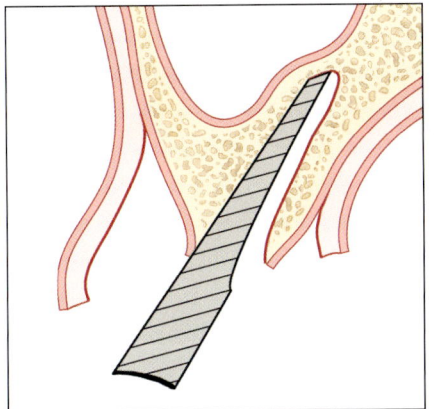

Fig 21-3d Ridge expansion and palatal bone mobilization.

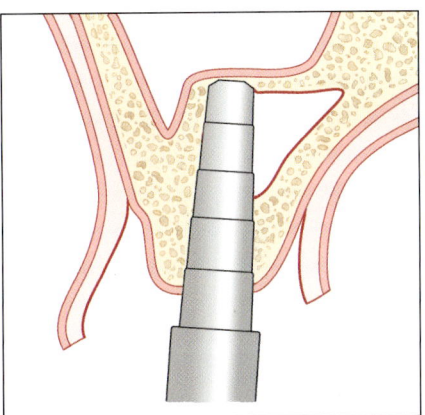

Fig 21-3e Following progressive ridge expansion, sinus floor elevation is accomplished with the largest diameter (final site) osteotome.

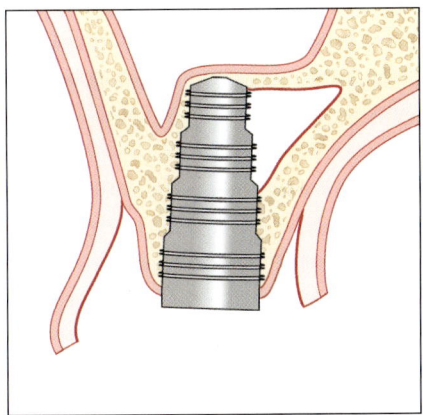

Fig 21-3f Implant in position following vertical and horizontal site development.

Localized management of the sinus floor

Here the technique varies according to the anatomy and approach. For localized management of the sinus floor, elevation up to 3 mm can be accomplished with gentle osteotome upfracture at individual implant sites, increasing osteotome diameter after progressive ridge expansion. If 3 to 5 mm of elevation is required, the beaver blade is used for vertical sectioning of the palatosinus floor at the future implant site, paralleling the exposed palatal vault (Fig 21-3c). An elevator or blunted bone chisel is used to infracture the palatosinus floor (Fig 21-3d). Progressive dilation and expansion of the ridge and elevation of the sinus floor are completed with osteotomes. A small pledget of collagen inserted in the bone defect cushions the force of the osteotome. Elevation to the final height should be avoided until it can be completed with the final osteotome of appropriate diameter. This procedure elevates the sinus floor, creating a new bony roof and an intrabony cavity (Fig 21-3e). The implant is placed (Fig 21-3f), and the expansion cavity is then filled with a collagen sponge and closed at the vertical incision and, if possible, over the expansion site *without bone grafting*. Normal healing in the ridge expansion gap, without primary closure or grafting of the intra-bony cavity, has been demonstrated through histologic evaluation.[12] A 5-year patient follow-up of this technique is demonstrated in Fig 21-4.

chapter 21 Trans-Alveolar Sinus Elevation Combined with Ridge Expansion

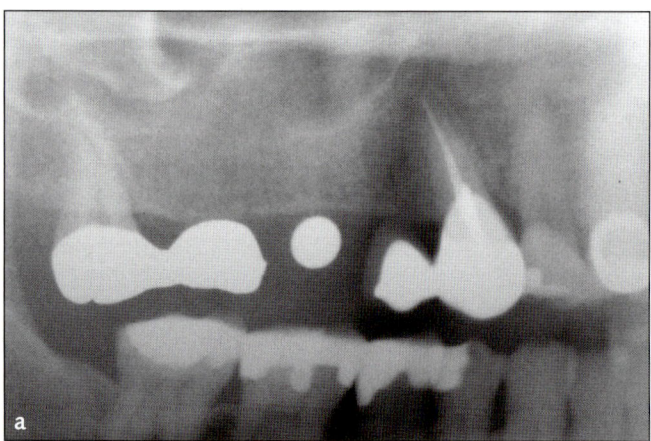
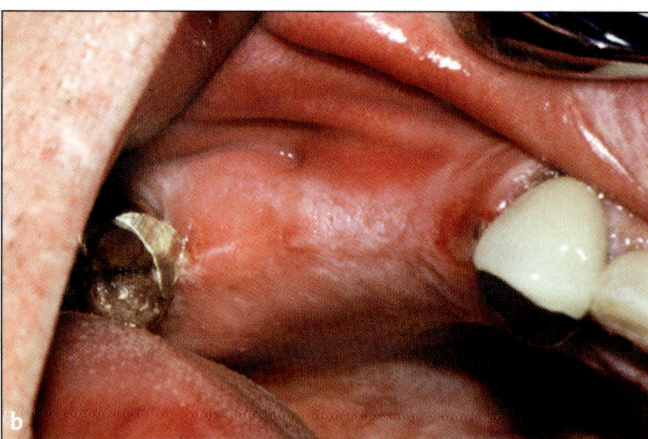

Fig 21-4a and 21-4b Preoperative radiographic and clinical appearance of a patient who has lost the right maxillary premolars and first molar.

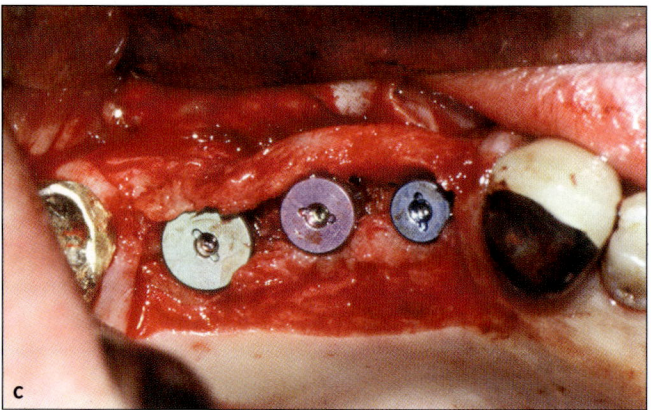
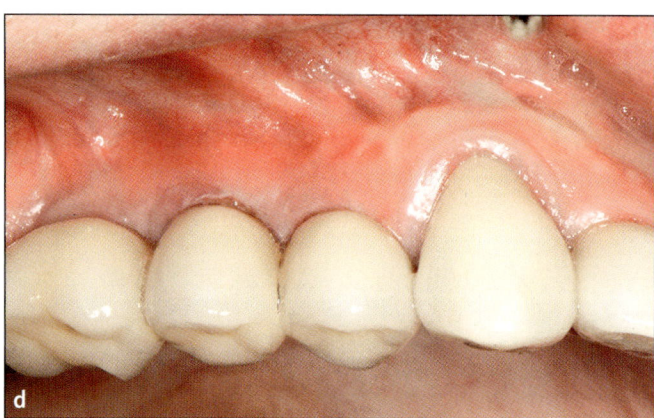

Fig 21-4c Site appearance following split-thickness flap, palatal bone incision, and palatal elevation procedures. Three implants (13 mm long with diameters of 6.5, 5.5, and 4.5 mm) are placed with intact periosteum over the bone flap. The bone expansion gap is filled with collagen.

Fig 21-4d Five-year clinical result.

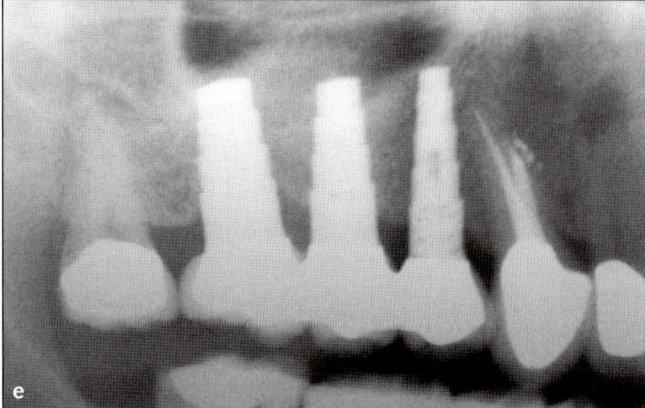
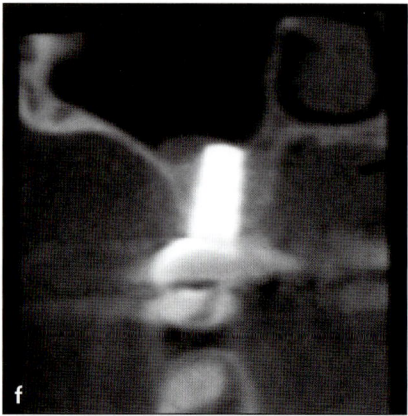

Fig 21-4e Five-year postoperative radiograph.

Fig 21-4f Five-year CT scan demonstrating bone over the first molar implant site.

Surgical Procedure

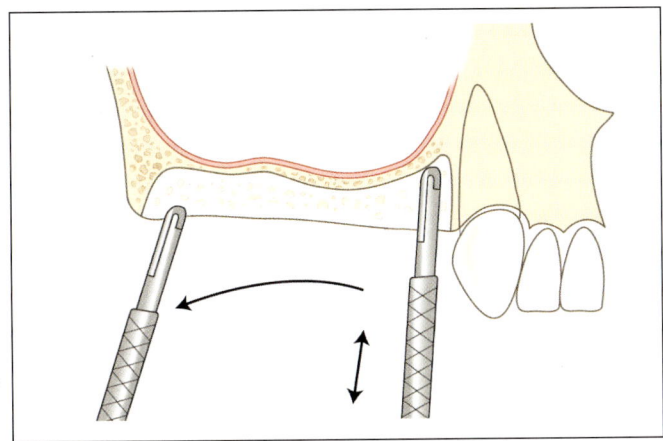

Fig 21-5a Bone incision traverses the site just below the sinus floor.

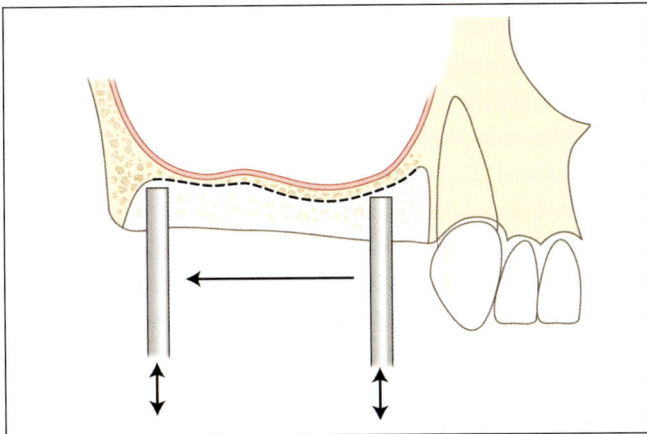

Fig 21-5b The ridge is expanded and the sinus floor is mobilized, though not elevated, with sequential stepping of the osteotome across the roof of the bone cavity.

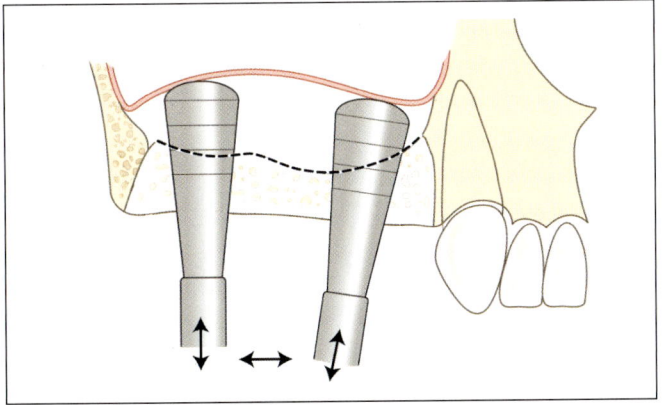

Fig 21-5c The ridge is expanded to the desired width, and the bone floor is mobilized across the floor and elevated.

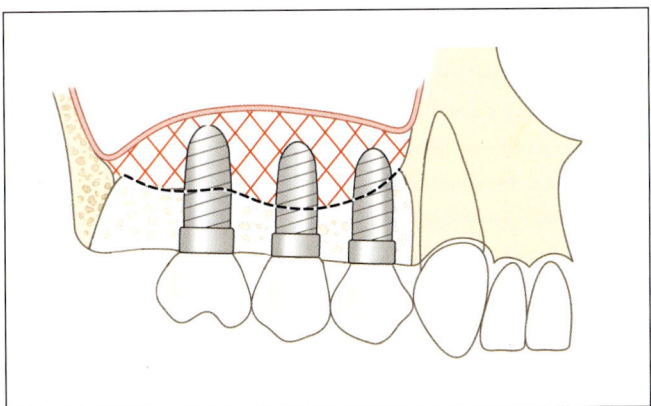

Fig 21-5d Implants are placed in the elevated sinus floor, and grafting is performed as needed.

Contiguous sinus floor elevation

Contiguous sinus floor elevation requires the use of a beaver blade to section the alveolus along the length of the posterior maxilla, just short of the antral floor (Fig 21-5a). Blunted monobevel chisels or "D"-shaped osteotomes are then used to expand the bone flap into a 2-mm anteroposterior trough. The sinus floor is then sequentially fractured (though not elevated) across the entire length of the sinus floor (Fig 21-5b). The contiguous sinus floor is incrementally fractured by malletting with a 2-mm flat osteotome. Meanwhile, the ridge is expanded to 3 mm, and the sinus floor fracture is completed using a 3-mm flat osteotome. The ridge is then expanded to its final width, and the sinus floor is elevated across the entire length of the sinus using a contiguous sinus floor elevator or round-ended osteotome (Fig 21-5c). Crestal implant locations are indexed on the palatal aspect with a cutting osteotome or round bur. A small pledget of collagen is inserted in the bone defect prior to the use of each osteotome to cushion its force. Tactile sensitivity, sound (volume and tone) changes, and visual cues are necessary to avoid sinus perforation. Marrow from the tuberosity and/or local particulate graft material is then placed into the elevated bony cavity. The intra-alveolar portion, which does not require bone grafting, is filled with collagen and heals by endosteal proliferation from the margins of the bone flap. Implants are then seated 1 or 2 mm short of maximum sinus elevation (especially if screw-type implants are used) (Fig 21-5d). A nose-blowing test is used intermittently throughout the procedure to assess the integrity of the sinus membrane. Small tears can be patched with collagen. Larger

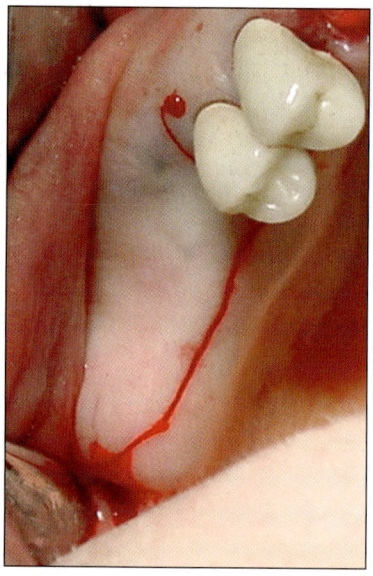

Fig 21-6a Incision design begins at the tuberosity region medially and extends anteriorly on the palatal aspect of the ridge. A lateral papilla-sparing incision continues across the alveolus and then anteriorly, with a marginal release at the mucogingival junction.

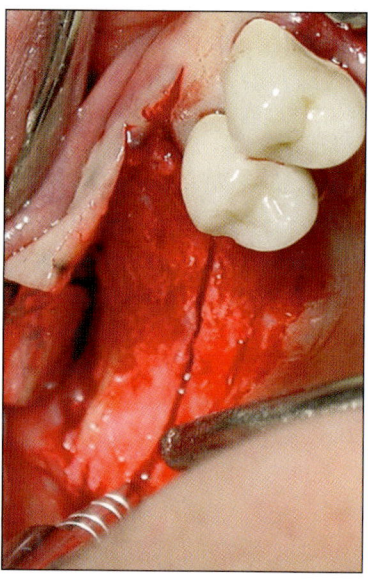

Fig 21-6b Split-thickness dissection and vertical bone incision (1 mm short of the antral floor) are completed.

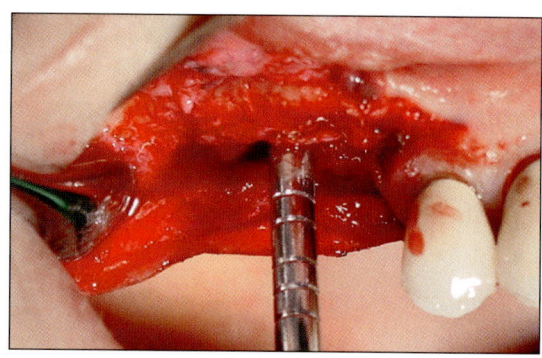

Fig 21-6c After ridge expansion, a flat osteotome is used sequentially to stepfracture the sinus floor, mobilizing it without elevating it.

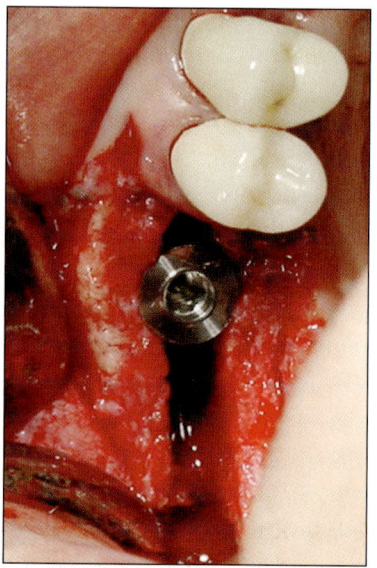

Fig 21-6d After additional ridge expansion, the sinus floor is again mobilized and then elevated at the desired expansion across the anteroposterior extent of the defect. A 6.5 × 13 mm implant is placed, exposing the intrabony gap and bone flap.

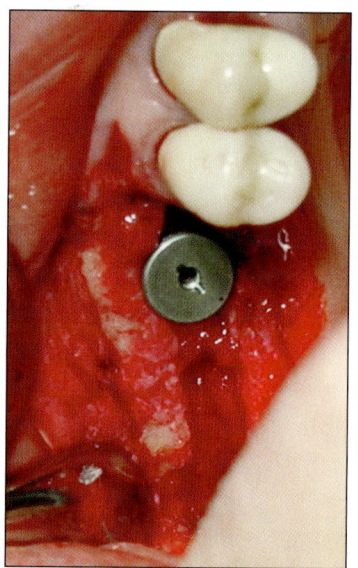

Fig 21-6e The implant cover screw is placed, and the intrasinus portion is loosely grafted with particulate and autogenous bone for space maintenance. Collagen is placed in the intra-alveolar portion. The flap is repositioned for a submerged healing protocol.

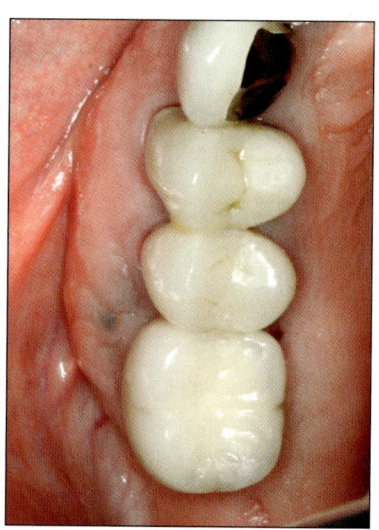

Fig 21-6f Twenty-eight month postoperative clinical result.

Surgical Procedure

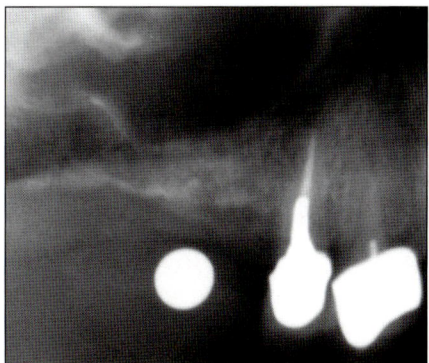

Fig 21-6g Preoperative radiograph with 5-mm marker.

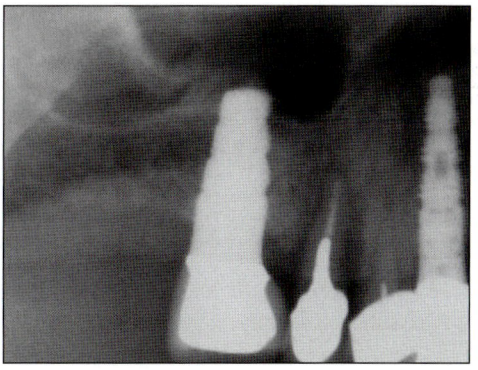

Fig 21-6h Twenty-eight month postoperative radiographic result.

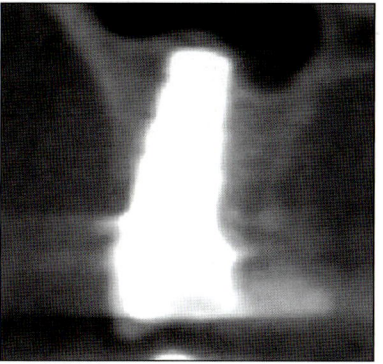

Fig 21-6i Postoperative CT scan demonstrating bone over implant and intact facial bone level.

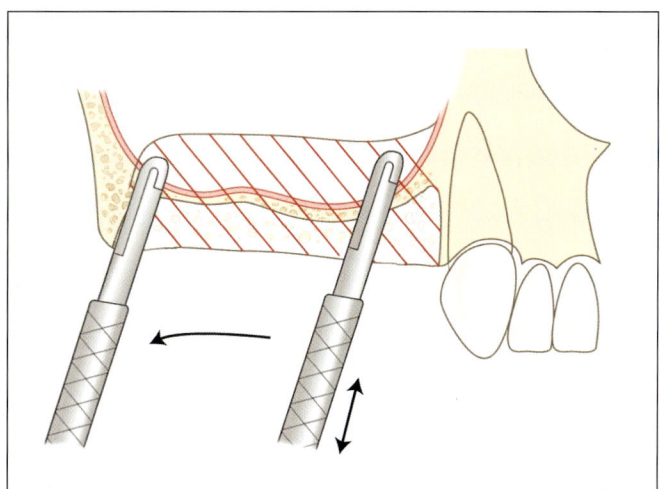

Fig 21-7 Contiguous palatal bone incision.

tears also are patched and, with adequate mobilization, may be grafted short of the passive maximum elevation to avoid displacement of the graft material into the sinus cavity. A case with a 28-month follow-up is shown in Fig 21-6.

When there is less than 5 mm of alveolar height below the sinus floor, this approach can be modified by extending a palatal bone incision over the length of the ridge expansion defect (Fig 21-7). Manipulation of the palatal bone in continuity with the sinus floor is thereby facilitated. The site is then developed with an intact bony roof across the entire defect. This modification offers the potential for greater elevation capacity and at the same time carries less risk of breaching the sinus membrane. At some point, consideration of a lateral wall approach should be done—probably at about 1 to 3 mm. Figure 21-8 shows the use of a single-stage protocol with anterior and apical flap repositioning to increase attached tissue and finger flap development for primary closure.

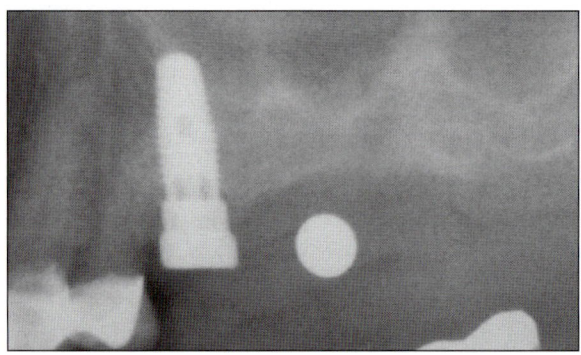

Fig 21-8a Preoperative radiograph with a 5-mm marker.

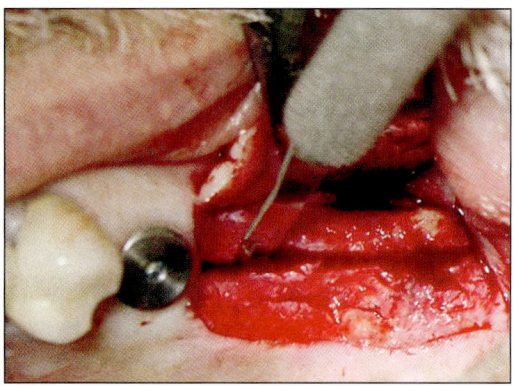

Fig 21-8b Palatal split-thickness incision and initial ridge expansion incision with beaver blade, demonstrating angulation of palatal bone incision.

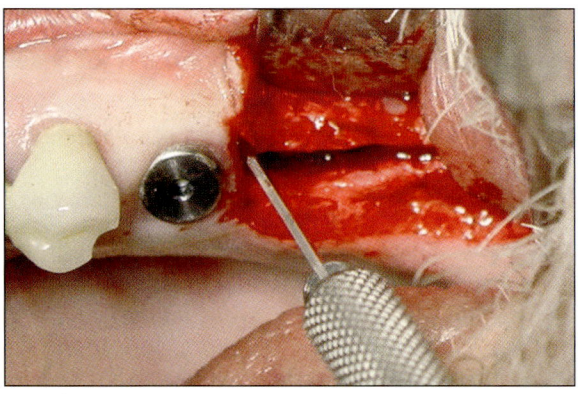

Fig 21-8c Beaver blade demonstrating facial intrabony beveled release incision.

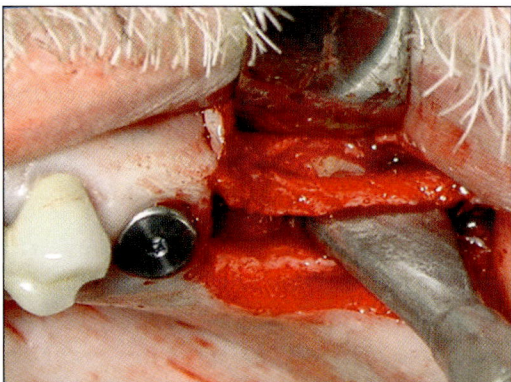

Fig 21-8d After additional ridge expansion and elevation of the palatal floor, a contiguous sinus floor elevation is accomplished.

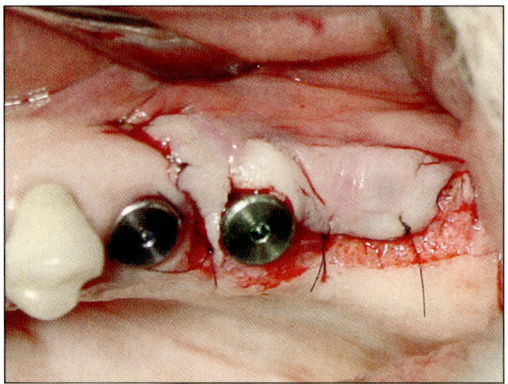

Fig 21-8e Immediate postoperative result with anterior and apical repositioning and anterior-based finger flap. Transgingival healing cap is in place.

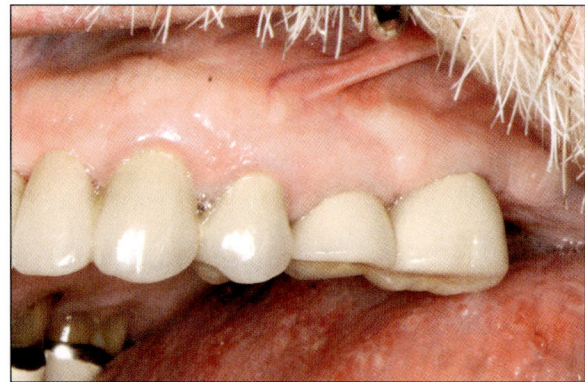

Fig 21-8f Thirty-month postoperative clinical result.

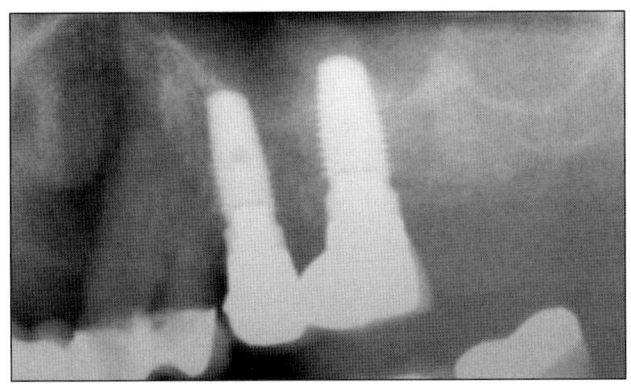

Fig 21-8g Twenty-one month postoperative radiograph.

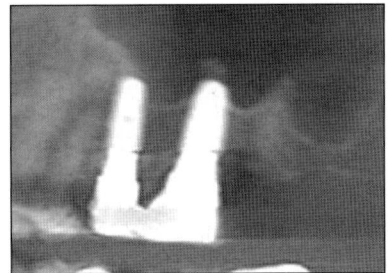

Fig 21-8h Thirty-month postoperative CT scan.

Avoiding Complications

The protocol described in this chapter for alveolar bone volume expansion, if followed, will prevent the complication of buccal wall resorption. Wound healing in alveolar split bone grafts is variable, sometimes resulting in scar incleftation, graft nonincorporation, or graft resorption. This technique avoids the use of graft in favor of local alveolar bone manipulation, making infection, graft extravasation, and volumetric instability much less likely.

Summary

Combined ridge expansion and sinus bony floor elevation constitute an excellent option for implant site development. The use of a palatal incision and a partial-thickness flap augments crestal attached tissues and improves vestibular depth. The use of a vascularized bone flap helps to prevent bone resorption of the expanded buccal plate and enables endosteal proliferation. The need for grafting materials is negligible, leading to a shorter healing interval. Buccal expansion restores lost alveolar dimension and establishes the implant in an axial position at the same time as vertical bone is forming in the sinus. The technique is endosteal, vascularized, and host cell–vital—a rarity when it comes to jawbone-manipulated osseous wounds.

References

1. Boyne PJ, James R. Grafting of the maxillary sinus floor with autogenous marrow and bone. J Oral Surg 1980;38:613–618.
2. Tatum H. Maxillary and sinus implant reconstruction. Dent Clin North Am 1986;30:209–229.
3. Summers RB. A new concept in maxillary implant surgery: The osteotome technique. Compend Contin Educ Dent 1994;15:152–162.
4. Summers RB. The osteotome technique: Part 2—The ridge expansion osteotomy (REO) procedure. Compend Contin Educ Dent 1994;15:422–436.
5. Summers RB. The osteotome technique: Part 3—Less invasive methods of elevating the sinus floor. Compend Contin Educ Dent 1994;15:698–704.
6. Summers RB. A new concept in maxillary implant surgery: The osteotome technique. Compend Contin Educ Dent 1995;16:1090–1099.
7. Fugazzotto PA. Immediate implant placement following a modified trephine/osteotome approach: Success rates of 116 implants to 4 years in function. Int J Oral Maxillofac Implants 2002;17:113–120.
8. Reiser G, Rabinovitz Z, Bruno J, Damoulis PD, Griffin T. Evaluation of maxillary sinus membrane response following elevation with the crestal osteotome technique in human cadavers. Int J Oral Maxillofac Implants 2001;16:833–840.
9. Winter A, Pollack A, Odrich R. Sinus/alveolar crest tenting (SACT). A new technique for implant placement in atrophic maxillary ridges without bone grafts or membranes. Int J Periodontics Restorative Dent 2003;23:557–565.

10. Massimo S, Baldoni M, Zaffe D. Jaw-bone enlargement using immediate implant placement associated with a split crest technique and guided tissue regeneration. Int J Periodontics Restorative Dent 1992;12:463–473.
11. Oda T, Sawaki Y, Ueda M. Alveolar ridge augmentation by distraction osteogenesis using titanium implants: An experimental study. Int J Oral Maxillofac Surg 1999;28:151–156.
12. Scipioni A, Bruschi GB, Calesini G. The edentulous ridge expansion technique: A five year study. Int J Periodontics Restorative Dent 1994;14:451–459.
13. Nosaka Y, Kitano S, Wada K, Komori T. Endosseous implants in horizontal alveolar ridge distraction osteogenesis. Int J Oral Maxillofac Implants 2002;17:846–853.
14. Scipioni A. Bone regeneration in the edentulous ridge expansion technique: Histologic and ultrastructural study of 20 clinical cases. Int J Periodontics Restorative Dent 1999;19:269–277.
15. Bruschi GB, Scipioni A, Calesini G, Bruschi E. Localized management of sinus floor with simultaneous implant placement: A clinical report. Int J Oral Maxillofac Implants 1998;13:219–226.
16. Winter AA, Pollack AS, Odrich RB. Placement of implants in the severely atrophic posterior maxilla using localized management of the sinus floor: A preliminary study. Int J Oral Maxillofac Implants 2002;17:687–695.
17. Pennarocha M, Perez H, Garcia A, Guarinos J. Benign paroxysmal positional vertigo as a complication of osteotome expansion of the maxillary alveolar ridge. J Oral Maxillofac Surg 2001;59:106–107.
18. Saker M, Ogle O. Benign paroxysmal vertigo subsequent to sinus lift via closed technique. J Oral Maxillofac Surg 2005;63:1385–1387.

chapter 22
Osteotome Technique for Site Development and Sinus Floor Augmentation

Robert B. Summers, DMD

The osteotome technique was developed to compress soft maxillary bone. Improved initial fixation obtained from bone compression of the osteotomy walls leads to better primary stabilization, which is key to osseointegration, especially in types 3 and 4 bone.[1] Healing of osteocompressive surgery is rapid and uneventful.

The underlying biologic principle of bone compression osteoplasty is to increase the mineral density *intraalveolarly* by osseous deformation and trabecular microfracture. The net effect of this process is to increase the stiffness of the bone (Fig 22-1). Bone stiffness increases parabolically to a fatigue maximum, which is considered bone "strength." Once a new microarchitecture heals within the alveolus, the increased mineral density becomes not just mechanically but also biologically operative. A third biomechanical variable, that of cross-linked type I collagen, is not affected directly by osteotome expansion and remains the one independent stiffness variable not improved with regard to ultimate alveolar bone strength.

To systematize surgical bone compression, a set of osteotome instruments (Implant Innovations Inc) with concave tips and tapered shape has been designed for this procedure (Fig 22-2). In type 4 bone, these instruments create an osteotomy for implants from 3.3 to 5.0 mm in diameter. The intention is to conserve bone by displacing it laterally to form a dense wall.[1,3–5] In contrast, drilling in areas of inferior bone quality does not improve the site and results in increased failure rates.[6]

The osteotome technique was first presented at the annual meeting of the Academy of Osseointegration in San Diego in 1993. This lecture was followed by publication of a four-part series on the osteotome technique in the journal *Compendium* in 1994–95.[1,3–5] Shortly afterward, a multicenter study was organized to quantify the experiences of clinicians.[7]

Nine surgeons at eight centers participated in this clinical study. Autografts, allografts, and xenografts were used, both separately and in combination, but the types and ratios were determined by the individual clinician. Graft materials did not influence implant survival. Preoperative bone height was recorded. The implants were loaded 5 to 11 months following placement. Implants had various shapes and surfaces, including machined, titanium plasma-sprayed, and hydroxyapatite. Overall, 174 implants were placed in 101 patients.

The most important factor influencing implant survival in the study was the amount of pre-existing bone height from the crest to the sinus floor. Implants placed in 4 mm

chapter 22 Osteotome Technique for Site Development and Sinus Floor Augmentation

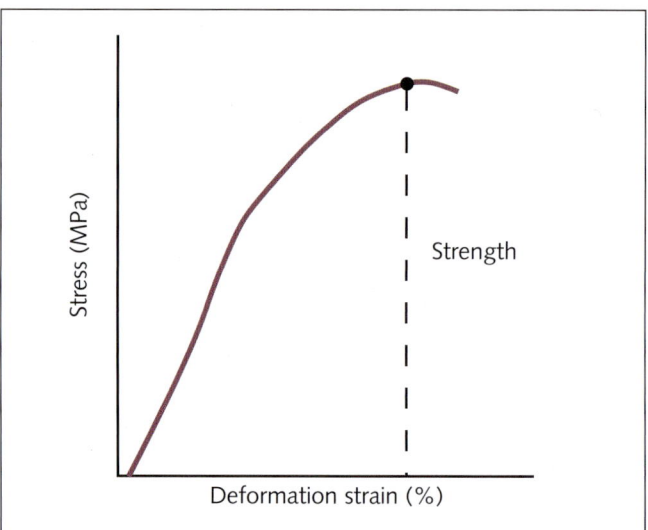

Fig 22-1 Bone compression osteoplasty increases mineral density by osseous deformation and trabecular microfracture. (Redrawn with permission from Banse.[2])

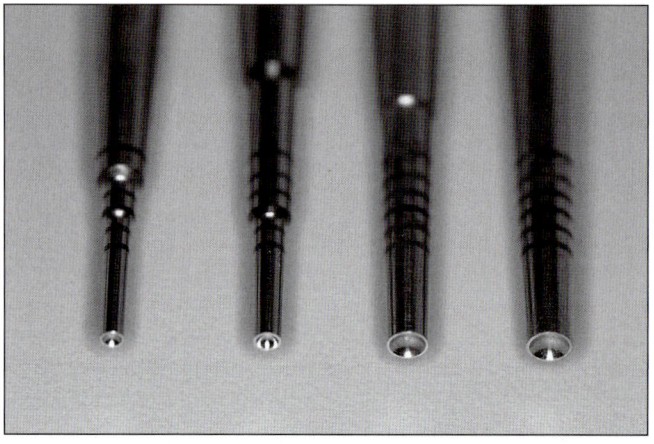

Fig 22-2a Summers osteotomes 1 to 4 *(left to right)*. Bone is carried in a superior direction by the concave tips. The tapered shape repositions osseous material laterally.

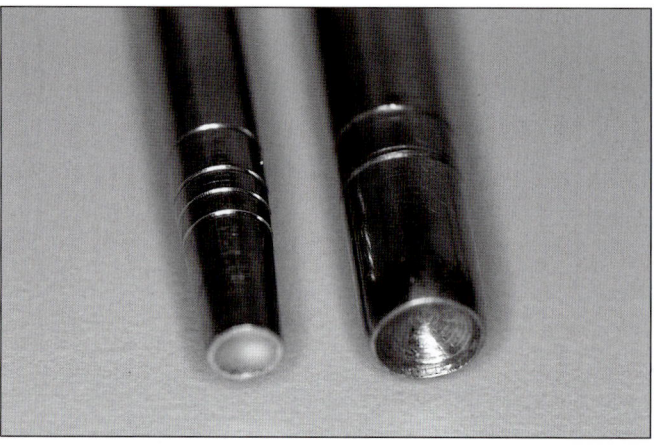

Fig 22-2b Larger-diameter Summers osteotomes: no. 5 *(left)* for 5-mm-diameter implants and FS (future site) *(right)* for staged sinus floor elevation.

or less pretreatment bone showed an 85.7% survival rate. When the ridge height prior to surgery was 5 mm or more, implants had a success rate of 96% or greater (see chapter 5).

Except those 6 mm in diameter, all implant diameters achieved greater than 90% survival rates after an average loading period of 20.2 months. Three of the eight failures occurred prior to loading. Only two late failures (ie, occurring more than 12 months after loading) were reported. The overall success rate was 95.4%. Final restorations included single units, splinted segments, and overdentures. No significant complications were reported.

All clinicians observed increased bone augmentation heights that varied from 1 to 7 mm. No correlation was found between the type or combination of graft materials, the quantity of materials used, and the ultimate increase in visible bone height. It should be noted that this was a retrospective study. While very encouraging, a larger prospective study is still needed.

Osteotome Technique

The osteotome technique requires a two-person team. The protocol is to insert a series of osteotomes of successively larger diameter until full depth is reached, if possible. The surgeon positions and guides the instrument with both hands. One hand creates a rest and maintains stability while the other hand gently rotates and applies pres-

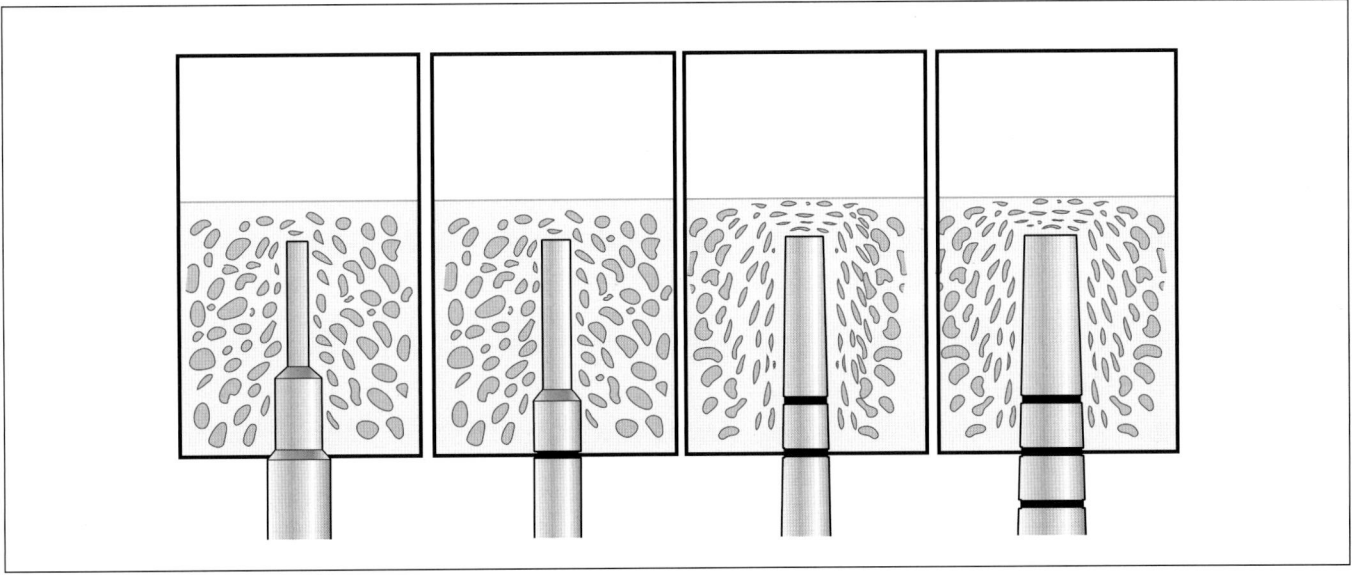

Fig 22-3 Once the osteotome reaches the bone to the 10-mm mark, the tip of the next larger instrument can be introduced without a drill. If necessary, drilling can be used at any point to facilitate the procedure and ease entry of the subsequent instrument.

sure with the osteotome. Meanwhile, the second member of the team uses a gentle malleting technique. The surgeon turns the instrument after each push or stroke of the mallet to prevent the tip from binding in the bone. The osteotome must be maintained in a precise axial position as it is turned. The osteotomes are kept lubricated, but irrigation is not required.

To form a round osteotomy, side-to-side movement of the instrument must be eliminated. The surgeon should maintain constant visual contact with the osteotome and the operative site throughout the procedure. Body or head movement, including reaching for a mallet, decreases tactile sensation and causes inadvertent movement of the osteotome. The surgeon must focus on maintaining the position of the instrument while allowing the assistant to mallet or transfer the next successive osteotome to the surgeon's hand.

The assistant's role is critical. Each strike of the mallet is applied to the osteotome in exactly the same path that it is held, and only after a specific verbal instruction to do so is given by the surgeon. Off-angled malleting causes the osteotome to migrate and creates an elliptical osteotomy, which compromises initial fixation.

When the site is well lubricated and the osteotome is slightly loose, it will advance much more readily. Hard malleting is avoided, and embedding the osteotome too firmly can have a jarring effect on the patient. The surgeon places restraining pressure on the osteotome to prevent it from advancing more than 1 mm with each impact of the mallet. This is particularly important under the sinus, since an instrument that is not held back to some degree can perforate the sinus floor without warning.

If, after several light mallet strikes or pushes, the osteotome does not advance, the surgeon can go back to a smaller-sized instrument or use a drill (Fig 22-3). It is often surprising how easily a smaller osteotome penetrates an area after the larger instrument has been used. In this situation, restraint of the smaller instrument is of paramount importance. The surgeon cannot rely on denser bone quality or a different malleting sound to identify when the sinus floor has been reached. Taking accurate preoperative radiographs and maintaining precise control of the penetration are critical.[8-10]

A drill can be used at any step to increase the diameter of the osteotomy or deepen the preparation as needed.[11] Drilling is always used with caution and at the lowest possible speed. Reproducing a consistent angle of penetration in the posterior maxilla with a drill is extremely challenging because of loss of tactile sensitivity in soft bone, limited access, and blocked sight lines. Compounding these problems are the irrigation stream and handpiece torquing. With osteotomes, vision of the surgical site is better, and no heat is produced as the instrument penetrates the bone.[1]

A practice session in advance of live surgery can represent the difference between successful and mediocre results, especially in small bone volume sites. Over the past decade, presurgical training in the osteotome technique has emphasized the team concept. Hands-on exercises using balsa blocks, hardened foam materials, and animal bone to simulate type 3 and type 4 bone are extremely valuable. Each team member alternately assumes the role of the surgeon and of the assistant handling the mallet.

Ridge Expansion Osteotomy

Edentulous maxillary segments are often narrow in a buccopalatal dimension, thus limiting the number of good sites available for incremental drilling and increasing the complexity of grafting required. Thin ridge areas may force the surgeon to overangulate the implant, which must follow ridge morphology. To address these limitations, the use of tapered osteotomes takes advantage of the inherent flexibility of cancellous maxillary bone, gently displacing it in a lateral direction. As the successive tapered osteotomes are inserted, bone moves laterally, providing wider sites with denser osteotomy walls. Bone is conserved internally in the ridge. This procedure is known as the *ridge expansion osteotomy*.

The ridge is widened with tapered osteotomes that match implant diameter. Implants can be inserted axially with more upright positioning and good fixation. With this procedure, bone is expanded gradually in a controlled fashion. Unlike chisels or wedge-shaped instruments, tapered osteotomes are less likely to cause abrupt ridge fracture.[2] The pace of the procedure is slow to allow each instrument to remain in place for a minute or two before the next-larger instrument is inserted. Limited drilling can be employed to facilitate the procedure. The final instrument is left in place until the moment before the implant is seated since the ridge will flex back to its original position unless it is internally supported by the osteotome or the implant.

Osteotome Sinus Floor Elevation

During osteotome surgery, the surgeon will often find that the osteotomy is deeper than the original preoperative radiographic measurement of the area from the crest to the sinus floor. Probing demonstrates that the sinus floor is not perforated, though it is elevated as much as 2 mm.[1,4] This procedure, termed *osteotome sinus floor elevation*, allows placement of the next-larger implant without the invasiveness of a conventional sinus elevation.[12,13]

Clinical experience with sinus floor elevation has shown no discernible difference in surgical sequelae compared with simple bone compression. Morbidity is equivalent to routine osteotomy, and outcomes are good. With this approach, a minimum of 8 mm of residual ridge height is needed preoperatively for 10-mm implants. One advantage of this procedure is that bone may be added through the sinus floor elevation site.[1,4] The versatility of bone grafting by this method is obvious, including augmentation of smaller residual ridges and providing a greater volume of the available grafted space for implants. Complications are negligible.

Bone-added osteotome sinus floor elevation

The protocol for using the sinus-directed osteotomes is not to enter the sinus cavity itself. In this procedure, repositioned bone particles and trapped fluid create a hydraulic effect, thus moving the sinus floor and the membrane upward. The advantage of this approach to bone grafting is that the osteotome creates a predictable quantity of particulate material, which then forms a hydraulic plug. Although type 4 bone requires no drilling, drilling and osteotomes can be used in combination without sacrificing the outcome of the procedure. This technique ensures accurate and consistent control over the ultimate height of the grafted space with reduced chance of membrane perforation (Fig 22-4).

In the bone-added osteotome procedure, pressure on trapped fluid and particulate graft creates a blunt force over an expanded area that is larger than the osteotome tip. The membrane is less likely to tear under this type of pressure, which has a fluid consistency, than it is under direct application of force from a hard surgical instrument.[14–18] Experience over a 14-year period has shown that the incidence of membrane tears is low when the technique is carefully executed. The few tears that occur are associated with the small-tipped instruments (no. 1 or no. 2) or a narrow-diameter depth probe. Nkenke et al[19] reported 1 tear in 22 osteotome grafting procedures that were viewed with an endoscope from inside the sinus.

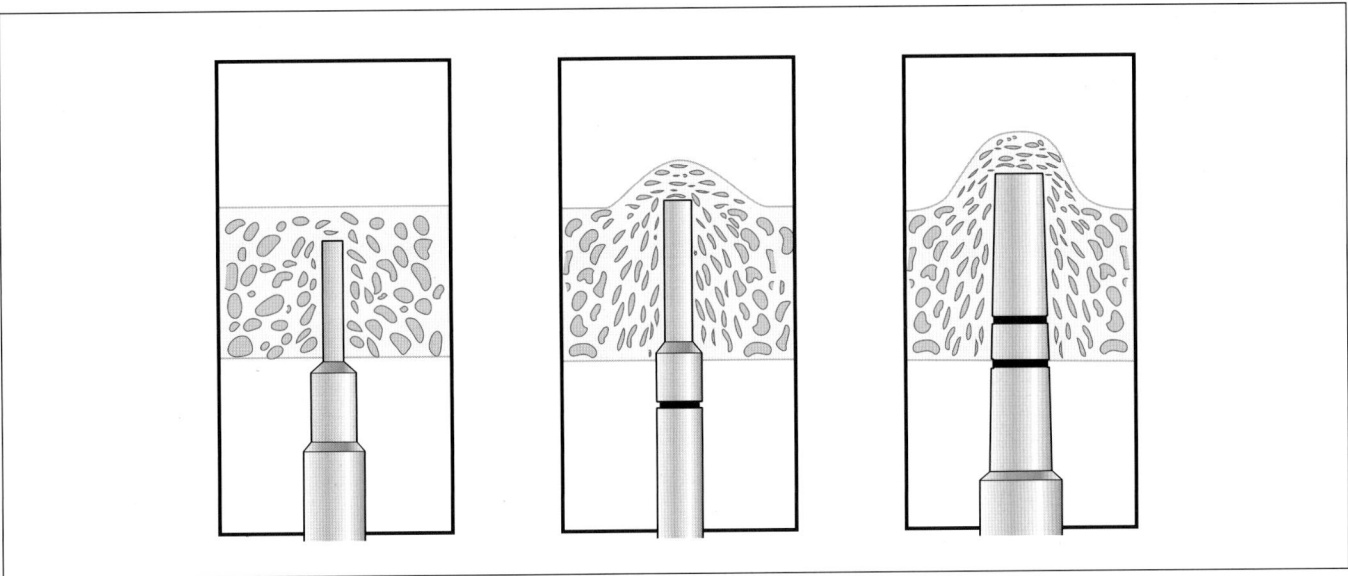

Fig 22-4 Osteotome sinus floor elevation requires precise measurement of the height and width of available bone. Insertion of the instrument is restrained so that the tip does not penetrate beyond the sinus floor. The osteotomes do not directly contact the sinus membrane. In situ bone and trapped fluids form a cushion between the instrument tip and the membrane.

With lateral window procedures, membrane perforation rates as high as 44% have been reported. These tears can be associated with postoperative complication.[18]

During bone graft intrusion, a small tear in the membrane can be patched by carefully introducing soft bone fragments into the osteotomy and then, using a larger osteotome, pushing the fragments upward. This method usually seals off the perforation. Another variation is to use a piece of collagen membrane followed by bone graft. A broad, blunt depth probe is recommended. Probing to check for a perforation is performed with the lightest possible pressure. The Valsalva maneuver, if used, must be performed cautiously as well, since this also can lead to perforation.

During bone grafting, the superior margin of the residual ridge with the dense graft plug above it can be viewed through the osteotomy. Generally, bleeding from the prepared site is minimal, providing that the local anesthetic contains vasoconstrictor. If calcified material is used, the elevation can be evaluated on a radiograph. A successful elevation usually is rounded and of uniform density. The implant functions as the final osteotome, pushing the graft material and the membrane to their final height.[3]

Once osteotome bone grafting is mastered, the sinus floor can be elevated from 3 to 7 mm with simultaneous placement of the implant.[20,21] A variety of graft materials yield equally successful results,[21] and there is no need to open a distant site. Autogenous bone is pushed through the original floor or additional fragments can be harvested from the adjacent area.

Autogenous bone alone has some shortcomings, including resorption,[22,23] so the preference is to supplement autogenous bone with a calcified resorbable material. Nonresorbable hydroxyapatite is not a good choice for simultaneous implant placement because it does not support early implant integration. Decalcified materials are a valid option, but they do not show up well on an immediate radiograph. Of greater importance than the choice of a specific grafting material is the need to maintain sinus membrane integrity. There is long-term evidence that most approved materials will eventually calcify in a tented space above the sinus floor. Boyne has shown that the intact tented space without bone graft is capable of spontaneous calcification.[23]

A minimum pretreatment bone height is needed to ensure adequate fixation of the implant in the residual bone, given that the grafted area provides no immediate support (Fig 22-5). After approximately 3 months, the implant gains stability from osseointegration in the ridge as well as formation of bone in the graft space. Initially, at least 5 mm of ridge height under the sinus was proposed for an implant 10 mm or longer.[3,4] More recently, 8-mm flare-shaped implants have shown the same consistent success in 4-mm preoperative ridges (unpublished data). A

chapter 22 Osteotome Technique for Site Development and Sinus Floor Augmentation

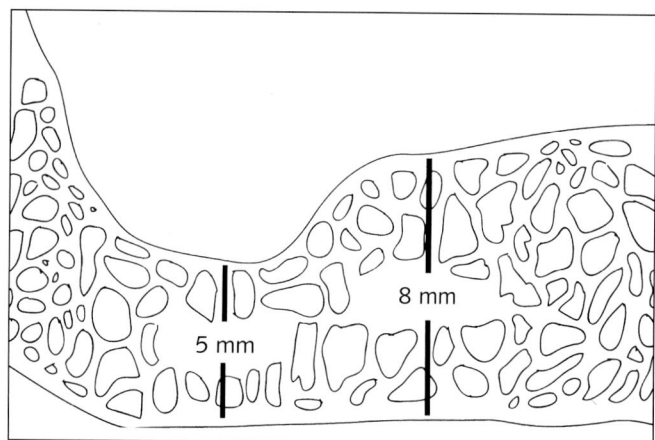

Fig 22-5 Typical bone dimensions for using the bone-added osteotome sinus floor elevation. A 5-mm site can be altered to support a 10-mm implant. An 8-mm presurgical location can be deepened for a 12- or 13-mm implant. (Illustration courtesy of Implant Innovations Inc.)

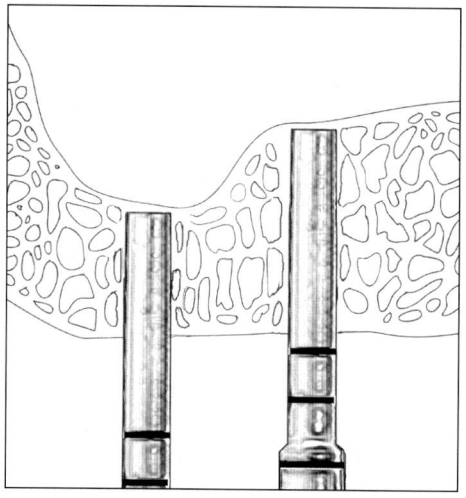

Fig 22-6a Bone-added osteotome sinus floor elevation procedure. Summers osteotome no. 1 inserted to the sinus floor. Hand pressure or light malleting is recommended. If drilling is needed, the drill stops 2 mm from the estimated position of the sinus floor.

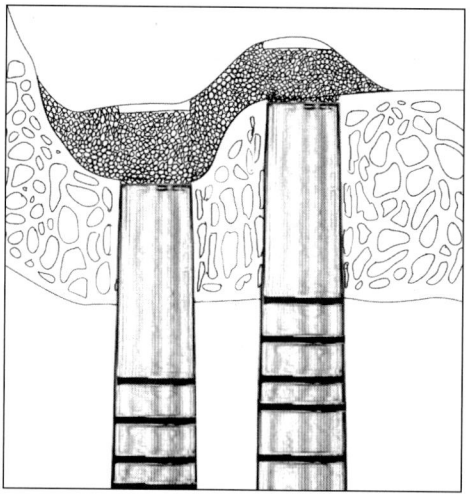

Fig 22-6b The osteotomy is widened, and successive osteotomes are seated to the sinus floor. After the floor is upfractured, a prepared bone mix is added into the osteotomy. The no. 3 or 4 osteotome is used to gently advance the material into the sinus.

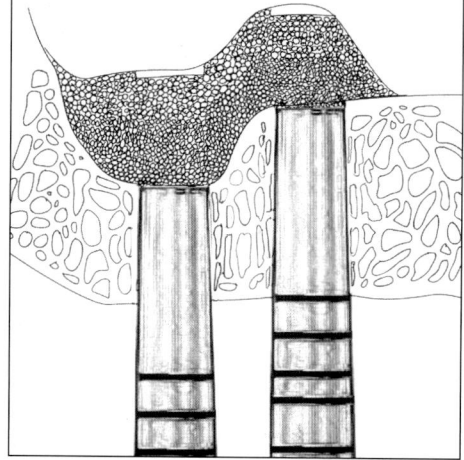

Fig 22-6c With the addition of each measured load of bone, the largest-sized osteotome previously used is reinserted to the sinus floor. Overloading the osteotomy with graft material without reinserting the osteotome is to be avoided.

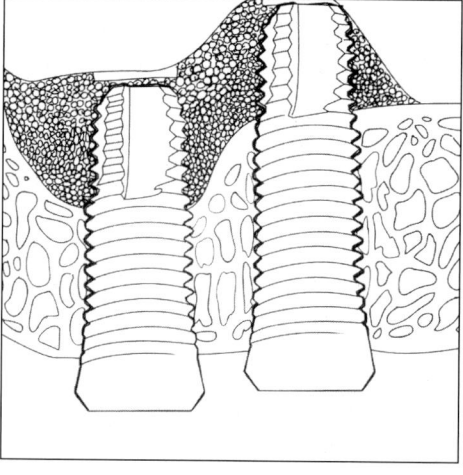

Fig 22-6d When the antral floor is displaced, the graft moves freely, thus elevating the intact membrane. The implant serves as the final osteotome to push up the membrane to its ultimate height. (Illustrations 22-6a to 22-6d courtesy of Implant Innovations Inc.)

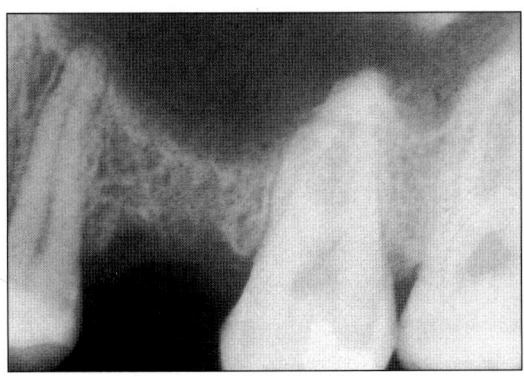

Fig 22-7a Case 1. An accurate long-cone radiograph reveals approximately 5 mm of bone height between a concave crest and the sinus floor.

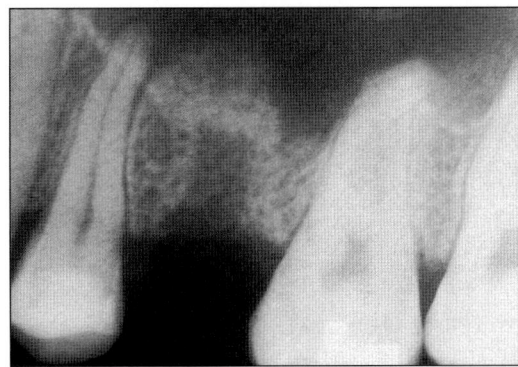

Fig 22-7b A small round bur has dimpled through the crest. Summers osteotomes nos. 1 to 5 have been successively inserted to the sinus floor. Several loads of xenograft mixed with autogenous chips have been pushed through the osteotomy. The tented membrane is visible on an immediate radiograph.

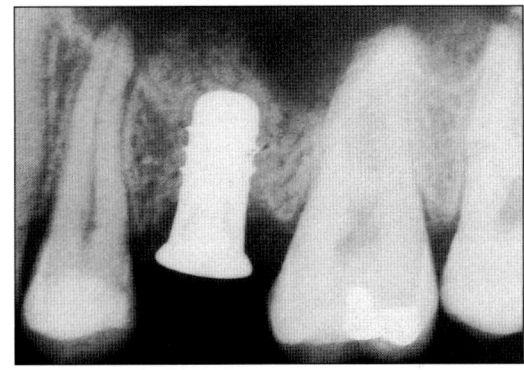

Fig 22-7c A 4.8- by 8-mm textured-surface implant (Straumann) is tightly fixed in the site. The tented area has been elevated further by seating the implant. The implant is the final osteotome.

tapered implant compresses the crestal bone more efficiently to increase initial stability and is therefore preferred to implants of uniform diameter, which have no apical stop.

Variations of this technique have been described, but the fixation requirements remain the critical factor.[24,25] Simplicity of removal of the fixture mount is paramount when choosing an implant that is fixated in only 4 mm of native bone. It may be helpful to loosen and then partially retighten the mount prior to delivering the implant to the site. A variety of implant designs and surfaces can achieve excellent results as long as the basic surgical requirements of instrumentation and graft handling are followed.

Approaching the sinus floor is the key step in bone-added osteotome sinus floor elevation. If drilling is needed, a pilot drill stops 2 mm from the floor, and the no. 1 osteotome is reinserted (Fig 22-6a). If the instrument does not penetrate with hand pressure or light malleting, the drill is advanced into the site an additional millimeter. This step requires only a few revolutions. A radiograph with a depth indicator in place provides valuable information. If the radiograph shows the drill at the depth of the sinus floor, additional drilling is contraindicated (Fig 22-6b).

Each load of bone graft adds about 1 mm to the elevation (Fig 22-6c). The graft material is inserted directly into the osteotomy. The no. 3 osteotome creates a slightly undersized osteotomy for a 3.75-mm-diameter implant. The no. 4 osteotome is designed for a 4.0- or 4.1-mm-diameter implant, and the no. 5 is designed for a 4.8- to 5.0-mm-diameter implant (Figs 22-6d, 22-7, and 22-8).

chapter 22 Osteotome Technique for Site Development and Sinus Floor Augmentation

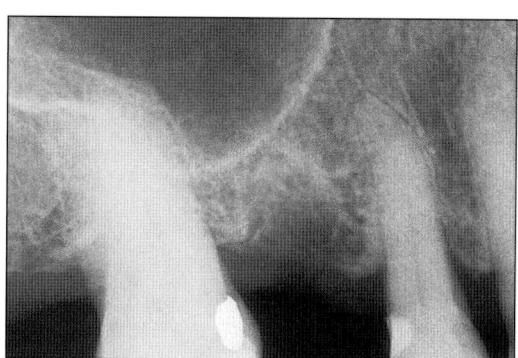

Fig 22-8a Case 2. Preoperative radiograph of the atrophic ridge and poor bone healing of a socket 6 months after extraction.

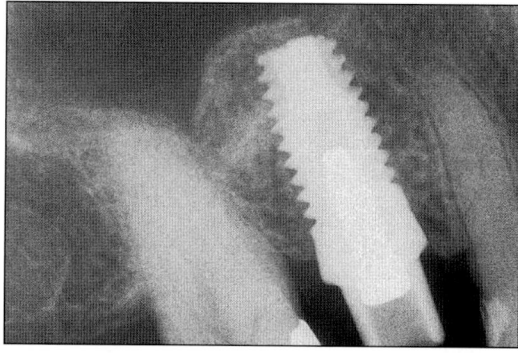

Fig 22-8b A 5.0- by 13-mm implant and abutment (Implant Innovations Inc) 3 months after the bone-added osteotome sinus floor elevation. Note the dense convex grafted space above the original sinus floor.

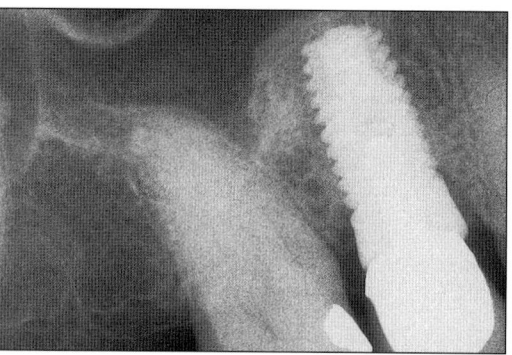

Fig 22-8c Five-year result showing minimal shrinkage of the sinus floor elevation.

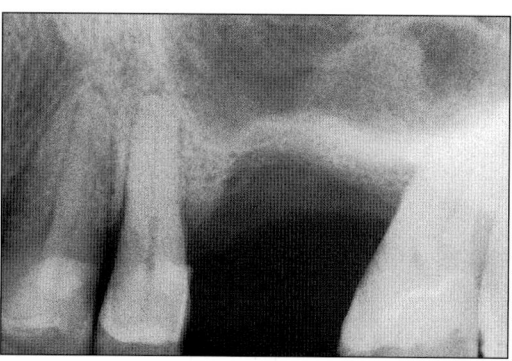

Fig 22-9a Case 3. Residual bone height of 2 mm under the sinus floor.

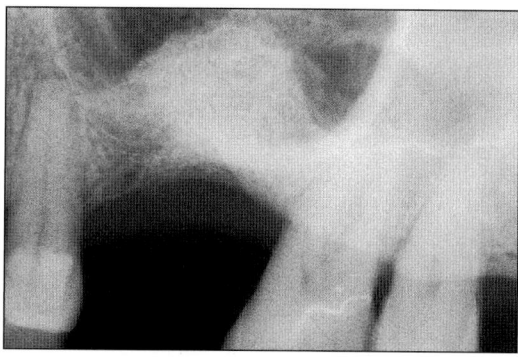

Fig 22-9b The FS and no. 5 Summers osteotomes are used to infracture the crest. Xenograft material is added incrementally. The osteotome displaces graft material, creating broad even pressure on the membrane without actually touching it.

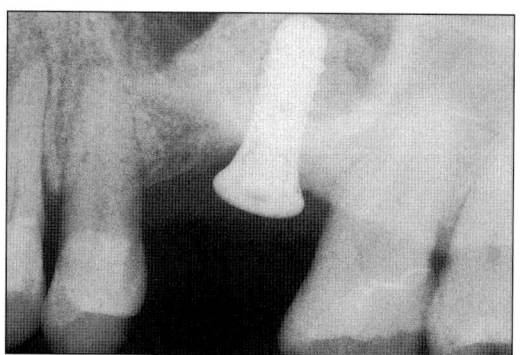

Fig 22-9c Six months later, the implant is placed.

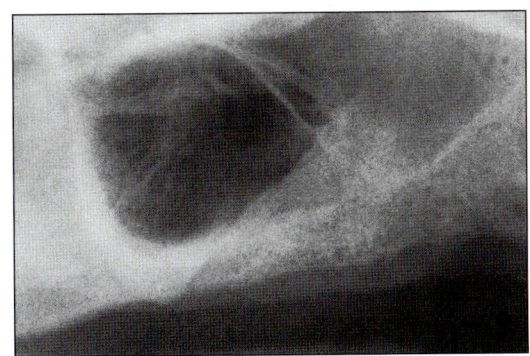

Fig 22-10a Case 4. Preoperative view of the right maxillary sinus. A crestal approach is used with the nos. 4, 5, and FS osteotomes. Xenograft material is inserted, along with a collagen barrier.

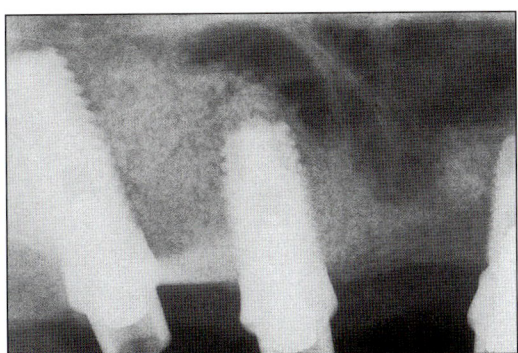

Fig 22-10b External hex implants and abutments (Implant Innovations Inc) in place under a provisional splint.

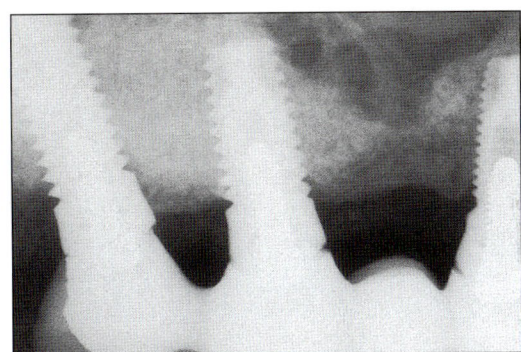

Fig 22-10c Five-year follow-up. Note: Patient is a vegan whose diet consists mostly of uncooked vegetables, nuts, and hard breads.

Staged sinus floor elevation

A technique for sinus floor augmentation with delayed implant placement was introduced by Tatum (Alabama Implant Study Group, 1977). This technique described a crestal approach, but within a few years Tatum, Boyne, and others[27,28] routinely entered the sinus from a lateral approach.

Using a large-sized osteotome designed to infracture the crest after limited use of drills or trephines,[4] the osteotome staged sinus floor elevation technique intrudes the crestal bone and allows grafting to proceed without disturbing the sinus membrane. This protocol is less traumatic than a lateral wall procedure. The crestal entry creates a "socket" that heals rapidly. A round bur is sufficient to score the bone. Also, a collagen membrane rather than a nonresorbable barrier is used over the sinus entry (Figs 22-9 and 22-10).

Conclusion

The osteotome technique is a useful and predictable procedure for simultaneous or delayed implant placement that offers some advantages over other techniques. Using a team approach and following proven guidelines, the sinus floor can be elevated with a method that is less invasive than lateral wall osteotomy. Other advantages of osteotome surgery are compression of poorly organized bone, widening of the ridge, and greater control of instrumentation in the posterior compared to drilling into types 3 and 4 bone. The osteotome technique eliminates the need for a separate donor site. Morbidity is less than that associated with the lateral approach. At present there are no reports in the literature of untoward results associated with osteotome surgery. The osteotome technique is the most widely used approach for minor sinus augmentation and is now taught in graduate training programs. This simple, straightforward approach must be considered an important innovation in implant dentistry.

References

1. Summers RB. A new concept in maxillary implant surgery: The osteotome technique. Compend Contin Educ Dent 1994;15:152–160.
2. Banse X. When density fails to predict bone strength. Acta Orthop Scand Suppl 2002;73:6.
3. Summers RB. The osteotome technique: Part 2. The ridge expansion osteotomy (REO) procedure. Compend Contin Educ Dent 1994;15:422–436.
4. Summers RB. The osteotome technique: Part 3. Less invasive methods of elevating the sinus floor. Compend Contin Educ Dent 1994;15:698–708.
5. Summers RB. The osteotome technique: Part 4. Future site development. Compend Contin Educ Dent 1995;16:1090–1099.
6. Jaffin RA, Berman CL. The excessive loss of Brånemark fixtures in type IV bone: A 5-year analysis. J Periodontol 1991;62:2–4.
7. Rosen PS, Summers R, Mellado JR, et al. The bone added osteotome sinus floor elevation technique: Multicenter retrospective of consecutively treated patients. Int J Oral Maxillofac Implants 1999;14:853–858.
8. Artzi Z, Parson A, Nemcovsky CE. Wide-diameter implant placement and internal sinus membrane elevation in the immediate postextraction phase: Clinical and radiographic observations in 12 consecutive molar sites. Int J Oral Maxillofac Implants 2003;18:242–249.
9. Summers RB. Conservative osteotomy technique with simultaneous implant insertion. Dent Implantol Update 1996;7:4–53.
10. Lazzara R. The sinus elevation procedure in endosseous implant therapy. Current Opinion Periodontol 1996;3:178–183.
11. Davarpanah M, Martinez H, Tecucianu J, Hage G, Lazzara R. The modified osteotome technique. Int J Periodontics Restorative Dent 2001;21:599–607.
12. Boyne PJ, James RA. Grafting of the maxillary sinus floor with autogenous marrow and bone. J Oral Surg 1980;38:613–616.
13. Misch CE. Maxillary sinus augmentation for endosteal implants. Organized alternative treatment plans. Int J Oral Implantol 1987;4:49–58.
14. Ziccardi VB, Betts NJ. Complications of maxillary sinus augmentation. In: Jensen OT (ed). The Sinus Bone Graft. Chicago: Quintessence, 1999:201–208.
15. Wannfors K, Johansson B, Hallman M, Strandkvist T. A prospective randomized study of 1- and 2-stage sinus inlay bone grafts: 1 year follow-up. Int J Oral Maxillofac Implants 2000;15:625–632.
16. Jensen OT, Shulman LB, Block MS, Iacono VJ. Report of the Sinus Consensus Conference of 1996. Int J Oral Maxillofac Implants 1998;13(suppl):5–45.
17. Khoury F. Augmentation of the sinus floor with mandibular bone block and simultaneous implantation: A 6-year clinical investigation. Int J Oral Maxillofac Implants 1999;14:557–564.
18. Schwartz-Arad D, Herzberg R, Dolev E. The prevalence of surgical complications of the sinus graft procedure and their impact on implant survival. J Periodontol 2004;75:511–516.
19. Nkenke E, Schlegel A, Schultze-Mosgau S, et al. The endoscopically controlled osteotome sinus floor elevation: A preliminary prospective study. Int J Oral Maxillofac Implants 2002;17:557–566.
20. Komarnyckyi OG, London RM. Osteotome single-stage dental implant placement with and without sinus elevation: A clinical report. Int J Oral Maxillofac Implants 1998;13:799–804.
21. Moy PK, Lundgren S, Holmes RE. Maxillary sinus augmentation: Histomorphometric analysis of graft materials for sinus floor augmentation. J Oral Maxillofac Surg 1993;51:857–862.
22. Garg AK. Current therapy in augmentation grafting of the maxillary sinus for placement of dental implants. Dent Implantol Update 2001;12:17–22.
23. Boyne PJ. Analysis of performance of root-form endosseous implants placed in the maxillary sinus. J Long Term Effects Med Implants 1993;3:143–159.
24. Fugazzotto PA. Immediate implant placement following a modified trephine/osteotome approach: Success rates of 116 implants to 4 years in function. Int J Oral Maxillofac Implants 2002;17:117–120.
25. Toffler M. Osteotome mediated sinus floor elevation: A clinical report. Int J Oral Maxillofac Implants 2004;19:266–273.
26. Block MS, Kent JN. Maxillary sinus grafting for totally and partially edentulous patients. J Am Dent Assoc 1993;124:139–143.
27. Smiler DG, Johnson PW, Lozada JL. Sinus lift grafts and endosseous implants. Dent Clin North Am 1992;36(1):151–186.
28. Chanavaz M. Maxillary sinus: Anatomy, physiology, surgery, and bone grafting related to implantology—11 years of surgical experience (1979–1990). J Oral Implantol 1990;16:199–209.

chapter 23
Piezoelectric Bone Surgery for Sinus Bone Grafting

Tomaso Vercellotti, MD, DDS
Myron Nevins, DDS
Ole T. Jensen, DDS, MS

Over the last half century, applications of ultrasonic instrumentation in bone surgery have largely failed, particularly in light of reports of their substantial ineffectiveness or even negative influence on the healing process. Studies comparing different types of instruments (ultrasonic instrument, bur, and scalpel) have obtained conflicting results based on a variety of experimental protocols.[1–5] Several authors[6] explored the possibility of using ultrasonics in maxillary sinus surgery, but the effort was curtailed because of insurmountable difficulties. Significant limiting factors include the failure of traditional ultrasonic instruments to cut bone structures that are more than 1 mm thick and a tendency for excessive overheating leading to necrosis. However, recent scientific-technologic research of bone's response to mechanical stimuli, particularly ultrasonic vibration, has led to a new and highly effective technique for osteotomy and osteoplasty called *piezoelectric bone surgery*.[7–12]

The revolutionary properties of piezoelectric surgery have simplified many common osseous surgical procedures, including sinus bone grafting.[13–17]

Piezoelectric Bone Cutting

The piezosurgery device has certain fundamental characteristics that make it safer and more precise than the instruments (manual and motorized) traditionally used in bone surgery. Morphologic and histomorphometric studies have found that tissue responds better to piezosurgery than to the drill.[18,19] The extreme precision and safety of the method are assured by:

- Micrometric cutting action produced by microvibrations, 20 to 60 μm in width at a frequency of 29 KHz, able to effectively cut mineralized structures but remain completely inactive on soft tissues. The total cut selectivity, which has been demonstrated by histologic studies, constitutes the principle advantage of this method.
- Absence of macrovibrations permits better handle control, thus assuring completely safe access to the most difficult anatomic zones and high cut precision.
- Cavitation with the cooling saline solution that is generated from the characteristic ultrasonic vibrations produces tiny spraying particles of water that keep the area cool and free of blood, thus avoiding overheating of the tissues and allowing optimal intraoperative visibility.

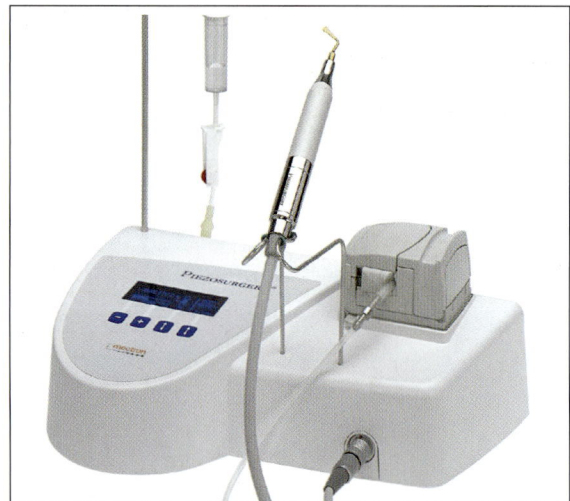

Fig 23-1a Mectron piezosurgery unit.

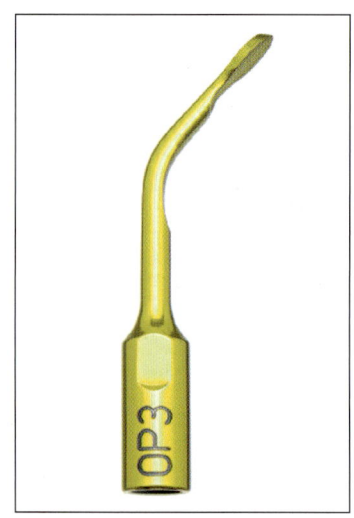

Fig 23-1b Osteoplasty insert.

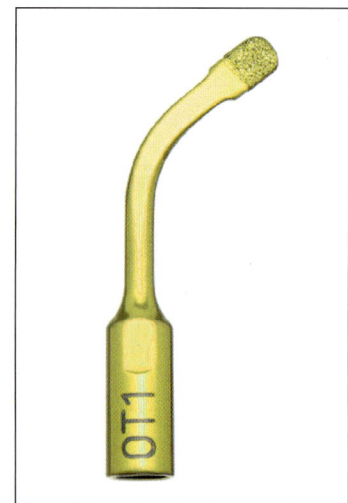

Fig 23-1c Osteotomy insert.

It is important to emphasize that the piezoelectric technique requires a different manual skill from that of the traditional manual and motorized instruments. This skill must be learned. The principal cause of iatrogenic lesions in the soft tissue is incomplete skill development on the part of the operator.

Piezosurgery harnesses electronic control of specific ultrasonic vibrations to remove bone mineral without overheating, in a manner comparable to deep bone "cutting."[20] The ultrasonic cutting action occurs in proportion to the level of mineralization of the bone. The ultrasonic device contains a saline cooling system similar to ultrasonic cavitation, except with modulated cutting power (Fig 23-1a). It also uses a number of different scalpel-like attachments that operate at specific modulated frequencies to selectively remove mineralized tissue, leading to a nearly bloodless osseous field. The microvibration fractures mineral apatite away from collagenous material with remarkable micrometric cutting precision. Since it generates no friction, it requires only light manual pressure.

Three different "scalpels" or inserts are used for a maxillary sinus antrostomy. Each insert is designed to perform a specific function. The *cutting* insert (Fig 23-1b) is designed to reduce wall thickness overlying the sinus. The *smoothing* insert (Fig 23-1c) features a diamond surface for creating the window once the bone thickness approaches 1 mm. Finally, *noncutting* inserts are used for separation and elevation of the membrane. Each of the inserts can be set at two different power modes: *bone mode* is appropriate for cutting hard tissue and *special mode* is appropriate for manipulating nonhard tissue.

Piezoelectric Sinus Antrostomy

A lateral approach to the sinus cavity is generally used,[21–23] although a crestal approach from inside the implant osteotomy site is also an option.[24–27] The lateral approach can be executed via osteoplasty removal of the lateral wall or the osteotomy window technique.

Lateral window technique

The lateral wall osteoplasty involves the gradual thinning of the bony wall to expose the endosteal surface of the sinus membrane. When the wall has been thinned to a point just short of the sinus membrane (ie, 0.2 to 0.3 mm), the osteoplastic insert with rapid traction movement is used to separate the membrane from the bone (Fig 23-2a). This thinning technique allows the surgeon to monitor progress toward the sinus cavity based on the differences in bone color. It also makes it possible to see the abating buttress and septa within the sinus.

Some sinus floors are divided in half by a septum. The safest surgical approach is to make separate mesial and distal windows (Fig 23-2b) and elevate the sinus membrane into two separate graft areas. When necessary, an incomplete septum can be resected to enable complete membrane elevation.

In summary, the piezoelectric osteoplasty technique follows this sequence:

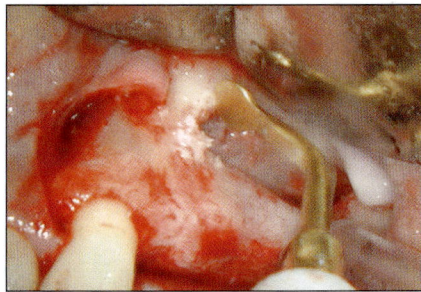

Fig 23-2a Piezoelectric lateral wall osteoplasty technique.

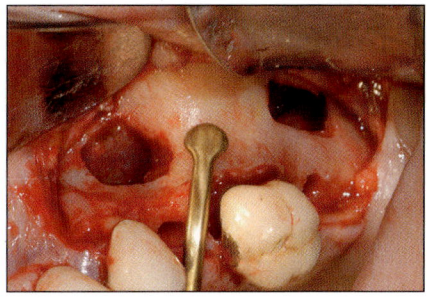

Fig 23-2b Opening of two bony windows in the sinus wall.

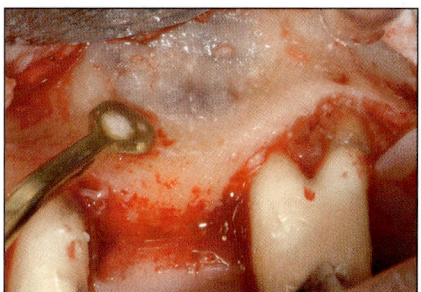

Fig 23-2c Thinning of the lateral sinus wall.

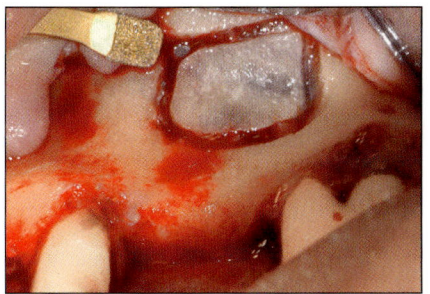

Fig 23-2d Design of the window frame.

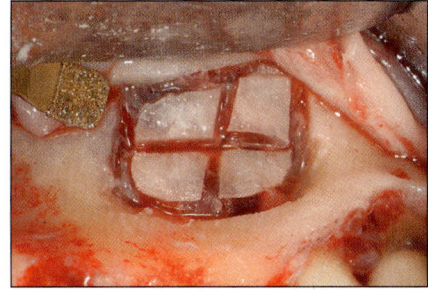

Fig 23-2e Four-part division of the bony window.

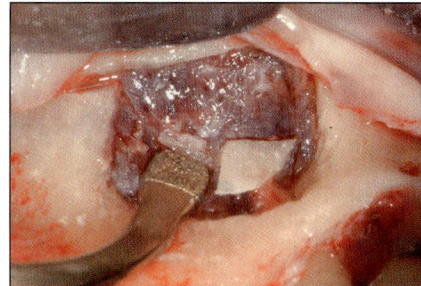

Fig 23-2f Removal of the piece of the bony window.

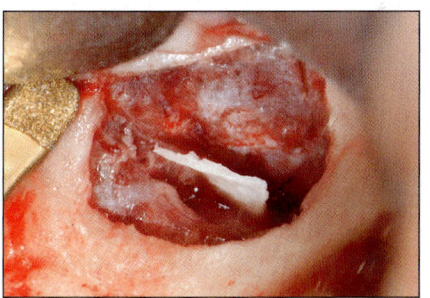

Fig 23-2g Exposure of the sinus septum.

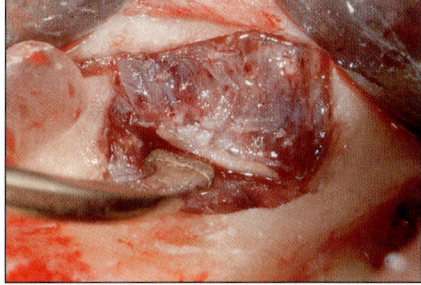

Fig 23-2h Elevation of the sinus membrane.

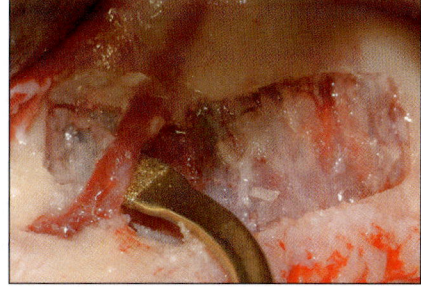

Fig 23-2i Preservation of intact intraosseous artery by use of the piezoelectric instrument.

1. The lateral sinus wall is thinned just to the point where the sinus membrane (including the septa) are visible (Fig 23-2c).
2. The bony window is outlined (Fig 23-2d).
3. The bony window is divided via a four-part osteotomy (Fig 23-2e), and all bone fragments are removed until the septum has been exposed (Fig 23-2f).
4. The sinus membrane is elevated in the lower and upper compartments (Figs 23-2g and 23-2h).
5. Piezoelectric osteotomy is accomplished, the septum is removed, and bone grafting material is placed.

One of the principal advantages of piezosurgery is its facility to cut and remove mineralized tissue without damaging soft tissue. When thinning bone with osteoplasty, intrabony arterioles are routinely preserved, and in some cases the vessel is left intact (Fig 23-2i).

chapter 23 Piezoelectric Bone Surgery for Sinus Bone Grafting

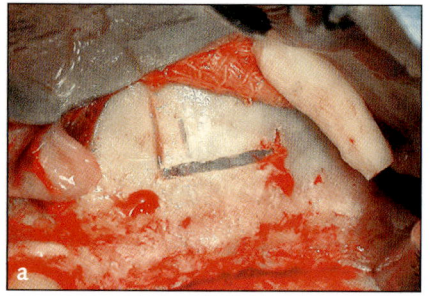

Fig 23-3a Initial outline of the bony window with piezoelectric osteotomy.

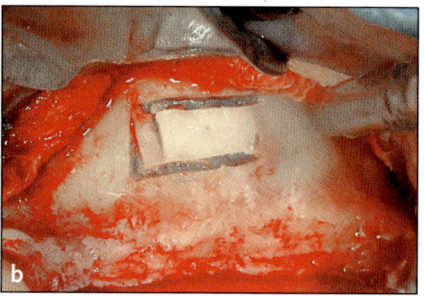

Fig 23-3b Completed osteotomy.

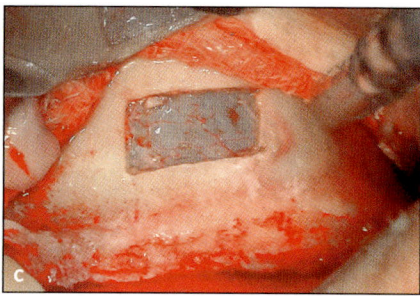

Fig 23-3c Exposure of the sinus membrane after the removal of the bone.

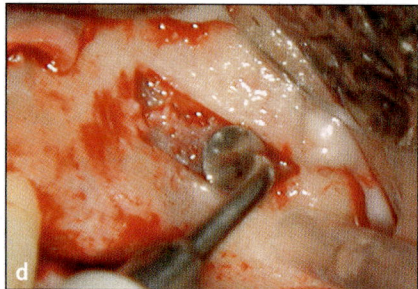

Fig 23-3d Elevation of the membrane with piezoelectric instrument.

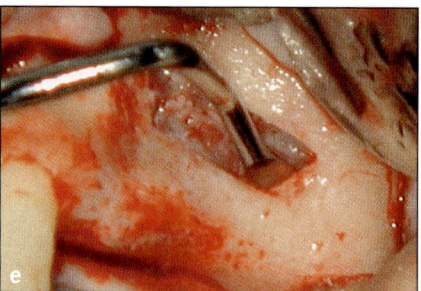

Fig 23-3e Elevation of the membrane using a manual elevator.

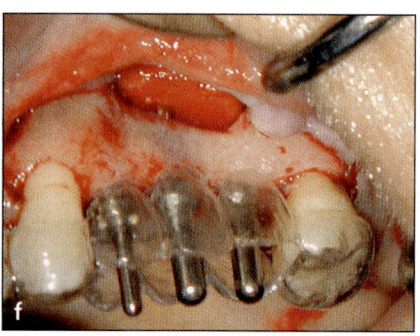

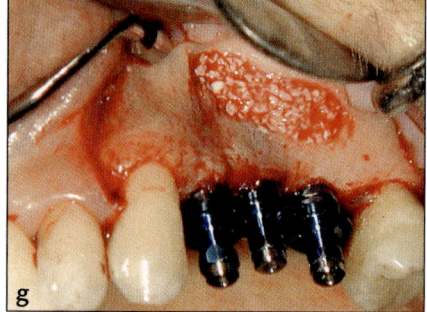

Figs 23-3f and 23-3g Successive phases of implant positioning.

Piezoelectric Antrostomy by Osteotomy

Osteotomy implies complete removal of the lateral sinus wall. This technique uses a diamond insert to cut through the bone, reaching the membrane without any internal pressure. When the surgical procedure is performed properly, no damage will occur to the sinus membrane (Figs 23-3a and 23-3b). The antrostomy is carried out with a pushing movement, making the insert work off-angle vertically. The insert is moved constantly, as it is possible to tear the membrane if care is not used. Any risk of overheating the membrane is minimal and will decrease with experience. Once the outline of the antrostomy is made, care should be taken to remove the spicula of bone or sharp edges at the margins of the osteotomy. Spiculae are easily removed using the same diamond insert. At this point, transparent bony wall adhering to the sinus membrane becomes mobile and is removed (Fig 23-3c).

Fig 23-4a Crestal approach using piezoelectric surgery.

Fig 23-4b Result of single implant positioning by piezoelectric crestal approach.

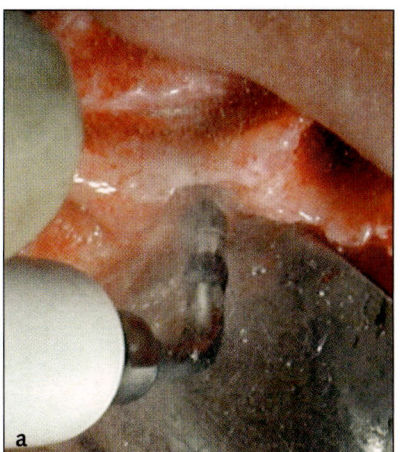
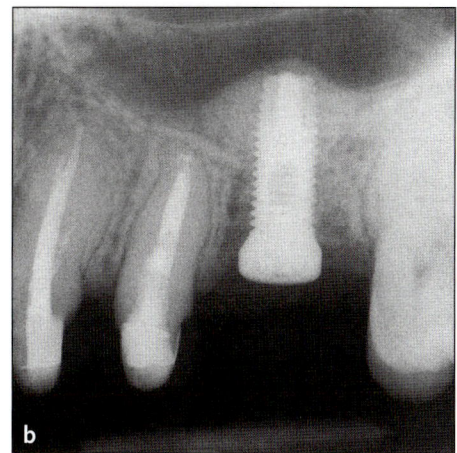

Membrane separation

Once the membrane has become exposed, it can be separated away from the sinus cavity using a special non–bone cutting insert that has an inverted cone shape. This shape allows for easy insertion at the bony margin and gentle separation of bone from the membrane as the rounded edge is advanced at low power. The procedure begins approximately 2 mm from the bony wall resting on the membrane and is performed rapidly without pausing in any one place to avoid overheating (Fig 23-3d).

Membrane elevation

After the initial membrane separation step, the elevation procedure can be accomplished with hand instruments. If, as sometimes happens, the membrane adheres to the sinus floor, it can be released using the piezoknife, either through the crest or at the sinus floor, following the technique used for septa ablation or crestal approach osteotomy technique (Figs 23-3e to 23-3g).

Piezoelectric Membrane Elevation by Crestal Approach

The osteotome technique allows for limited intraoperative control, especially when bone atrophy is significant. The crestal approach for sinus membrane elevation[26–29] requires acute tactile sensitivity to avoid perforation of the membrane. Sinus floor upfracture can also lead to perforation of the membrane. When type 4 bone is present and residual bone volume is insufficient to ensure primary implant stability, a delayed approach is needed (see chapter 22). Conversely, when bone quality is very good, a manual osteotome procedure may be difficult for a conscious patient to tolerate.

In rare cases, piezoelectric surgery can facilitate execution of an osteotomy via a crestal approach. The piezoelectric crestal osteotomy is made using the rounded diamond insert (OT4). Nevertheless, the majority of the single-implant sinus lift elevation procedures are usually performed via a small lateral window (Fig 23-4a). At this point, bioglass is inserted in the osteotomy site, followed by the use of the OT4 insert under bone mode until the bioglass is intruded beneath the sinus membrane. Bone chips are then gathered from an adjacent site using the OP3 insert to harvest bone and grafted in manually using the osteotome. The implants can then be placed in standard fashion.

The piezoknife facilitates the crestal osteotome approach by thinning out the sinus floor prior to use of the osteotome in more dense bone and by improving tactile manipulation in type 4 bone (Fig 23-4b).

Collection of bone chips

The piezoelectric osteoplasty technique allows for collecting bone chips by reducing cooling irrigation and keeping the surgical aspirator adjacent to the surgical site. The chips are placed in a glass Dappen dish and mixed with an

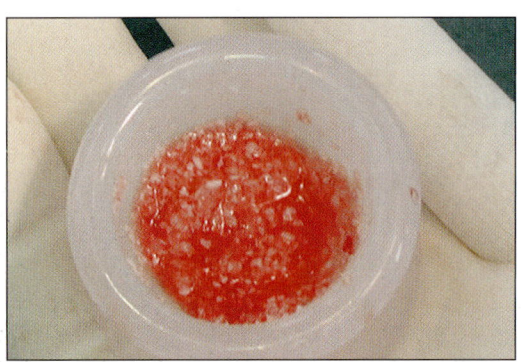

Fig 23-5 Bone chips collected by osteoplasty.

alloplast to serve as a bone graft composite (Fig 23-5). When a sufficient quantity of bone chips cannot be collected using the osteoplastic technique, bone may be harvested from the zygomatic process or the mandible. In the largest sinus cavity, the autogenous bone is combined with a mineral graft material.

Conclusion

Piezoelectric bone surgery is a simple, precise, and safe ultrasonic technology that improves on standard techniques used to perform the sinus bone graft. Piezosurgery is especially helpful for use in the maxillary sinus graft procedure where antrostomy access is made with minimal risk to the sinus membrane. Osteoplastic bone collection results from the antrostomy itself or is easily obtained adjacently, in many cases eliminating second site surgery. Intraoperative visibility is improved with piezosurgery as well because of saline solution cavitation, which reduces traumatic blood flow from bony wound margins. Maxillary sinus graft surgery is a highly predictable procedure[28–32] now significantly improved technically and perhaps biologically by the use of piezoelectric surgery. The cavitation of the saline solution that occurs during the piezoelectric osteotomy reduces the intraoperatory bleeding, increasing surgical visibility compared to the bur osteotomy technique.

References

1. Aro H, Kallioniemi H, Aho AJ, Kellokumpu-Lehtinen P. Ultrasonic device in bone cutting. A histological and scanning electron microscopical study. Acta Orthop Scand 1981;52:5–10.
2. Horton JE, Tarpley TM Jr, Jacoway JR. Clinical applications of ultrasonic instrumentation in the surgical removal of bone. Oral Surg Oral Med Oral Pathol 1981;51:236–242.
3. Horton JE, Tarpley TM Jr, Wood LD. The healing of surgical defects in alveolar bone produced with ultraonic instrumentation, chisel and rotary bur. Oral Surg Oral Med Oral Pathol 1975;39:536–546.
4. Mazarow HB. Bone repair after experimental produced defects. J Oral Surg 1960;18:107–115.
5. McFall TA, Yamane GM, Burnett GW. Comparison of the cutting effect on bone of an ultrasonic cutting device and rotary burs. J Oral Surg Anesth Hosp Dent Serv 1961;19:200–209.
6. Torella F, Pitarch J, Cabanes G, Anitua E. Ultrasonic osteotomy for the surgical approach of the maxillary sinus: A technical note. Int J Oral Maxillofac Implants 1998;13:697–700.
7. Vercellotti T. La chirurgia ossea piezoelettrica. Il Dentista Moderno 2003;5:21–55.
8. Vercellotti T, Obermair G. Introduction to piezosurgery. Dentale Implantologie Parodontologie 2003;7:270–274.
9. Boioli LT, Vercellotti T, Tecucianu JF. La chirurgie piézoélectrique, une alternative aux techniques de chirurgie osseuse. Inf Dent 2004;86:2887–2893.
10. Vercellotti T. Chirurgia Piezoelettrica: Invenzione Italiana. Giornale dell'odontoiatra. 30 September 2004.
11. Siervo S, Ruggli-Milic S, Radici M, Siervo P, Jager K. Piezoelectric surgery. An alternative method of minimally invasive surgery [in German]. Schweiz Monatsschr Zahnmed 2004;114:365–377.
12. Lambrecht JT. Intraoral piezo-surgery [in German]. Schweiz Monatsschr Zahnmed 2004;114:28–36.

13. Vercellotti T. Piezoelectric surgery in implantology: A case report—A new piezoelectric ridge expansion technique. Int J Periodontics Restorative Dent 2000;20:358–365.
14. Vercellotti T, Russo C, Gianotti S. A new piezoelectric ridge expansion technique in the lower arch—A case report (online article). World Dent 2000;1:http://www.worlddent.com/2001/05/articles/vercellotit.xml.
15. Vercellotti T, De Paoli S, Nevins M. The piezoelectric bony window osteotomy and sinus membrane elevation: Introduction of a new technique for simplification of the sinus augmentation procedure. Int J Periodontics Restorative Dent 2001;21:561–567.
16. Robiony M, Polini F, Vercellotti T, Politi M. Piezoelectric bone cutting in multipiece maxillary osteotomies. A technical note. J Oral Maxillofac Surg 2004;62:759–761.
17. Vercellotti T, Pollack AS. Piezosurgery: A new device for bone surgery. Part I—Sinus grafting and periodontal surgery. Compendium (in press.)
18. Vercellotti T, Crovace A, Palermo A, Molfetta A. The piezoelectric osteotomy in orthopedics: Clinical and histological evaluations (pilot study in animals). Mediterranean J Surg Med 2001; 9:89–95.
19. Vercellotti T, Nevins ML, Kim DM, et al. Osseous response following resective therapy with a piezosurgery. Int J Periodontics Restorative Dent 2005;6:543–549.
20. Vercellotti T. Technological characteristics and clinical indications of piezoelectric bone surgery. Minerva Stomatol 2004;53: 207–214.
21. Tatum OH. Maxillary sinus grafting for endosseous implants. Presented at the Annual Meeting of the Alabama Implant Study Group, Birmingham, AL, April 1977.
22. Boyne PJ, James RA. Grafting of the maxillary sinus floor with autogenous marrow and bone. J Oral Surg 1980;38:613–616.
23. Jensen OT, Shulman LB, Block MS, Iacono VJ. Report of the Sinus Consensus Conference of 1996. Int J Oral Maxillofac Implants 1998;13(suppl):11–45.
24. Summers RB. The osteotome technique. Part 3—Less invasive methods of elevating the sinus floor. Compend Contin Educ Dent 1994;15:698, 700, 702–704, 710.
25. Summers RB. A new concept in maxillary implant surgery: The osteotome technique. Compend Contin Educ Dent 1994;15:152, 154–156, 158, 162.
26. Bruschi GB, Scipioni A, Calesini G, Bruschi E. Localized management of sinus floor with simultaneous implant placement: A clinical report. Int J Oral Maxillofac Implants 1998;13:219–226.
27. Fugazzotto PA. Immediate implant placement following a modified trephine/osteotome approach: Success rates of 116 implants to 4 years of function. Int J Oral Maxillofac Implants 2002;17: 113–120.
28. Moy PK, Lundgren S, Holmes RE. Maxillary sinus augmentation: Histomorphometric analysis of graft materials for maxillary sinus floor augmentation. J Oral Maxillofac Surg 1993;51:857–862.
29. Lundgren S, Moy P, Johansson C, Nilsson H. Augmentation of the maxillary sinus floor with particulated mandible: A histologic and histomorphometric study. Int J Oral Maxillofac Implants 1996;11:760–766.
30. Tarnow DP, Wallace SS, Froum SJ, Rohrer MD, Cho SC. Histologic and clinical comparison of bilateral sinus floor elevations with and without barrier membrane placement in 12 patients: Part 3 of an ongoing prospective study. Int J Periodontics Restorative Dent 2000;20:117–125.
31. Hallman M, Sennerby L, Lundgren S. A clinical and histologic evaluation of implant integration in the posterior maxilla after sinus floor augmentation with autogenous bone, bovine hydroxyapatite, or a 20:80 mixture. Int J Oral Maxillofac Implants 2002; 17:635–643.
32. Wallace SS, Froum SJ. Effect of maxillary sinus augmentation on the survival of endosseous dental implants. A systematic review. Ann Periodontol 2003;8:328–343.

chapter 24
Le Fort I and Alveolar Distraction Osteogenesis with Sinus Bone Grafting

Ole T. Jensen, DDS, MS
Zvi Laster, DMD

A moderately atrophic, retrodisplaced edentulous maxilla can be distracted to a Class I jaw relation when combined with sinus bone grafting. This treatment approach is particularly recommended in young edentulous female patients who would otherwise be restored with an anterior cantilevered prosthetic approach.[1]

When a sinus bone–grafted maxilla is anteriorized via distraction osteogenesis, the repositioned sinus floor bone mass allows for axial implant development *throughout* the arch, especially in the canine, premolar, and first molar areas. The repositioned incisal area, previously in anterior crossbite, becomes Class I and is freed of any load-bearing necessity, making it available for pontiform gingival development. Biomechanical support for the restoration is adequately obtained posteriorly.[2]

The net effect of maxillary distraction is that a pseudo–Class III jaw relation becomes Class I. The patient regains lip support as well as an esthetic alveolar profile and becomes a candidate for noncantilevered dental restorations for an esthetic emergence.

This technique advances the goal of establishing *orthoalveolar form*, a larger concept that seeks to establish optimal three-dimensional alveolar morphology, including a Class I interarch relation. A retruded atrophic maxilla advanced by distraction corrects the telescoped interarch relation by advancing it to interarch axial alignment (Fig 24-1). The posterior maxilla generally begins in marked crossbite but becomes less so as the maxilla advances. In most patients, posterior crossbite relation is improved or eliminated.[3]

The surgical technique for distraction osteogenesis with sinus bone grafting proceeds as follows:

1. A 3-cm incision adjacent to the sinus is made bilaterally in the maxillary vestibule, extending from about the first molar region to the canine fossa.
2. Mucoperiosteal flaps are reflected superiorly, and bilateral sinus elevation is accomplished through a narrow antrostomy. The entire sinus membrane should be elevated anteroposteriorly about 10 mm.
3. The lateral osteotomy is extended posteriorly to the pterygomaxillary suture and anteriorly to the nasal fossa using a straight osteotome. The pterygomaxillary suture is freed using a curved osteotome bilaterally.
4. A small vertical incision is made in the maxillary frenum to allow access to the nasal septum, which is separated with an osteotome about 2 cm posteriorly.
5. The maxilla is mobilized slightly at the pyriform rim but not downfractured. The atrophic maxilla generally is easy to mobilize, but if not, a trans-sinusal osteotome can be applied to the lateral nasal walls.

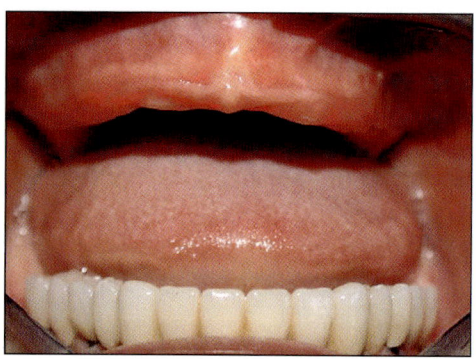

Fig 24-1 Bilateral crossbite comes into axial alignment with maxillary advancement.

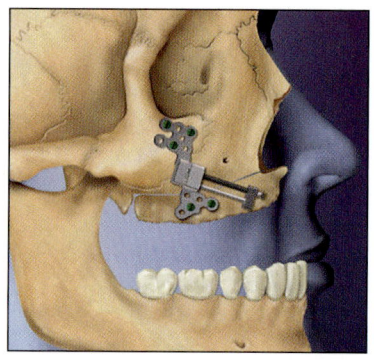

Fig 24-2 Location of distraction plate at the zygomatic buttress.

6. Tibial bone (see chapter 12), possibly expanded with alloplast, is used to augment the sinus floor bilaterally.
7. Distraction appliances (Walter Lorenz) are screwed into place bilaterally (Fig 24-2).[1] The distraction vector should move the maxilla down and forward in approximately a 3:1 ratio. A 15-mm distraction appliance is usually adequate to permit inferior maxillary displacement of about 5 mm.
8. The maxilla is distracted forward about 3 to 4 mm at the time of surgery to establish maxillary *forward* mobility and to ensure proper activation of the distractors. The distractors are then re-adjusted to a nonactivated state, and the wounds are closed with resorbable sutures.
9. The patient's denture is adjusted and relined with a soft liner.
10. After a 1-week period, distraction is initiated at a rate of 1 mm per day, usually in 0.5-mm increments twice per day that are applied by the patient.
11. After 5 to 7 days of activation, the patient returns for denture re-adjustment to accommodate the advancing maxilla. This process is repeated until distraction is complete. The denture is cut back facially so that the buccal flange is completely removed.
12. After a 4-month healing period, the distraction appliance is removed laterally and implants are placed using an anatomic guide stent.
13. An immediate provisional fixed partial denture is placed if implant stability is deemed adequate based on torque and implant stability quotient (ISQ) values.
14. Gingivoplasty is performed anteriorly to develop pontic form for the incisor teeth of the provisional fixed partial denture.
15. After 4 months, the implants are re-checked with resonance frequency analysis (RFA), and the provisional denture is replaced with a definitive porcelain-bonded-to-metal fixed partial denture. (This temporization phase is needed in the event of relapse of the maxillary position.)

Case Reports

Case 1

A 36-year-old woman has worn a maxillary denture since age 18. She presents with a retrognathic maxilla, a pseudo–Class III jaw relationship, a unilateral posterior crossbite, and moderate alveolar atrophy. Maxillary distraction combined with iliac bone grafting using both block and particulate bone is performed according to stereolithographic model planning (Figs 24-3a to 24-3c). The surgery proceeds with placement of bilateral distraction appliances after Le Fort I downfracture, sinus and nasal membrane elevation, and sinus floor bone grafting. The wound is closed with resorbable sutures, and the denture is relined with a soft liner. One week later, distraction is initiated at a rate of 0.5 mm applied twice daily for 9 to 10 days (Figs 24-3d to 24-3k). Four months later, the dis-

Case Reports

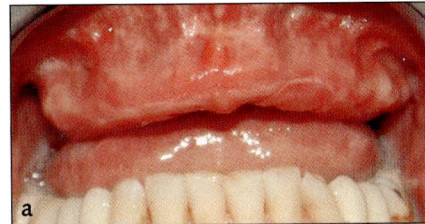

Fig 24-3a Moderate disuse atrophy, posterior crossbite, and modest maxillary retrognathia in a 36-year-old woman who has worn a denture since age 18.

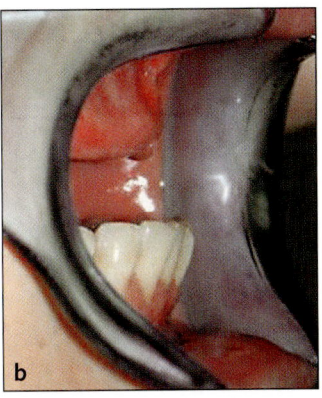

Fig 24-3b The retrognathia, which initially appeared to be mild, is about 7 mm.

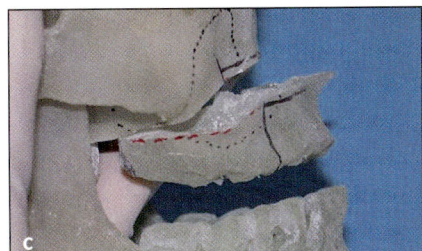

Fig 24-3c Stereolithographic model of sinus (*dotted line*). The maxilla is cut via a low Le Fort I osteotomy and fixed in a 7-mm advanced position.

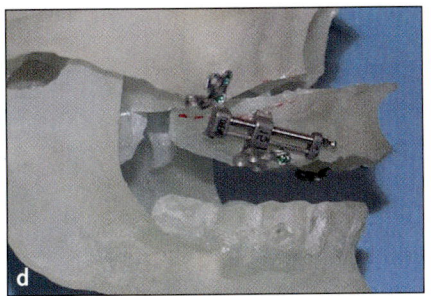
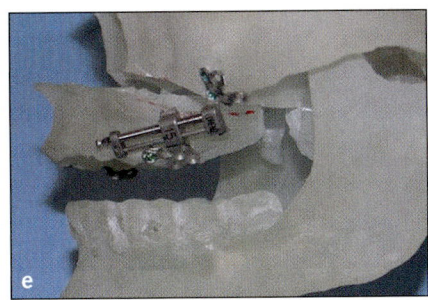

Figs 24-3d and 24-3e The distraction plates are bent and screwed into the model to simulate jaw distraction. The bone plate and placement angle must correspond on each side.

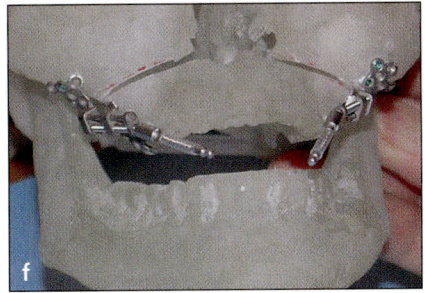

Fig 24-3f The distraction vector is directed downward about 30 degrees from the horizontal osteotomy cut.

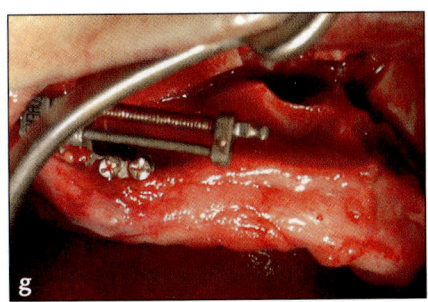

Fig 24-3g Following surgical Le Fort I osteotomy with sinus membrane elevation, the pre-bent distraction bone plate is placed according to the stereolithographic mock surgery.

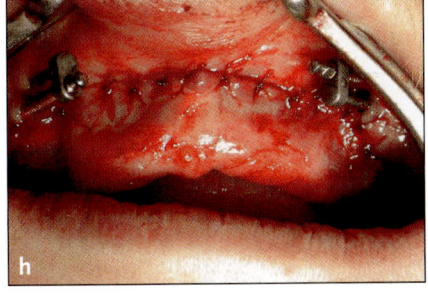

Fig 24-3h Wound closure is designed to allow access to the distraction device activator in each vestibule.

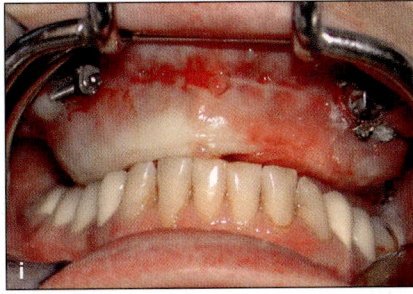

Fig 24-3i Approximately 7 to 8 mm of distraction allow the mandibular teeth to engage the advanced alveolar ridge.

traction appliances are removed, and eight implants are placed. An immediate-load provisional fixed partial denture is placed on six of the eight implants. Pontiform gingivoplasty is performed to develop the anterior gingiva (Figs 24-3l and 24-3m). Four months later, the definitive restoration is placed (Fig 24-3n). Three years later, the axial jaw relationship, the bone height, and implant integration all remain stable (Figs 24-3o and 24-3p).

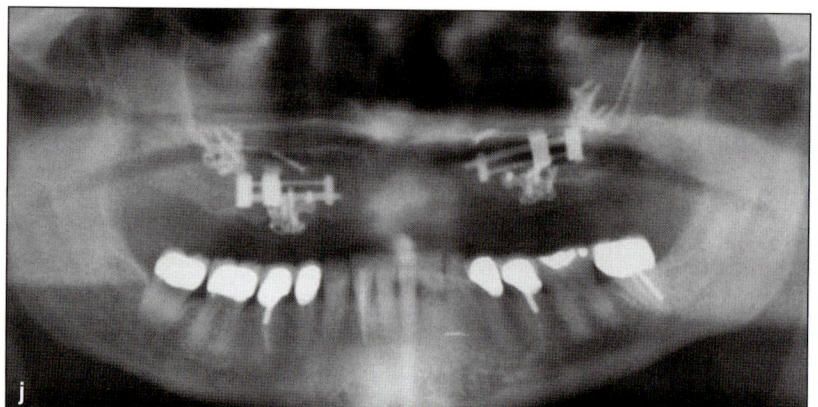

Fig 24-3j Panoramic radiograph of the advanced maxilla with device extension.

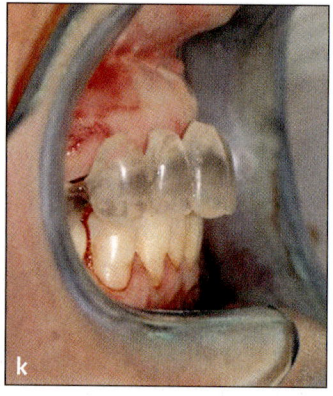

Fig 24-3k Postdistraction guide stent.

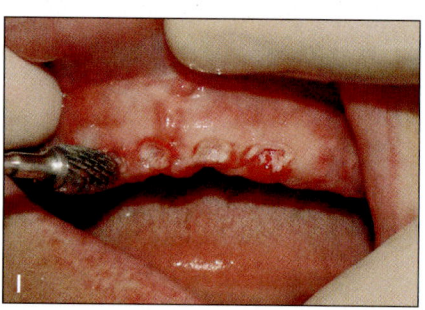

Fig 24-3l Use of the guide stent to determine pontiform gingivoplasty.

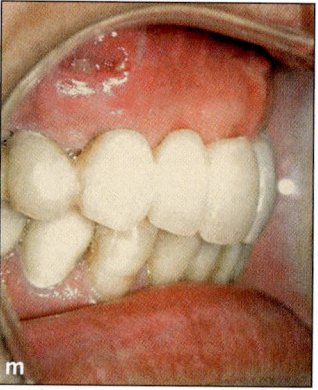

Fig 24-3m Immediate provisional prosthesis placed on six of eight implants.

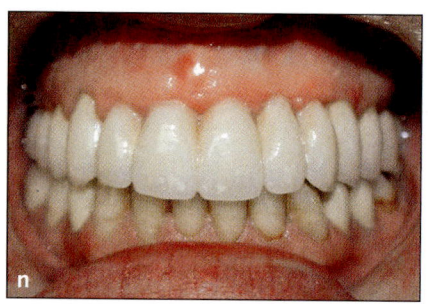

Fig 24-3n Facial view of definitive cross-arch stabilized fixed partial denture in porcelain.

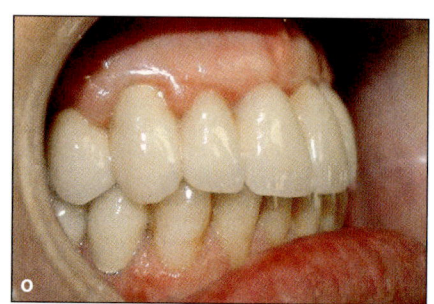

Fig 24-3o Esthetic alveolar projection.

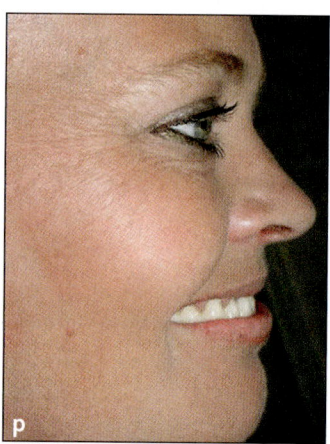

Fig 24-3p Natural alveolar and facial profile. (Courtesy of Dr Louisa Gallegos, Denver, Colorado.)

Case Reports

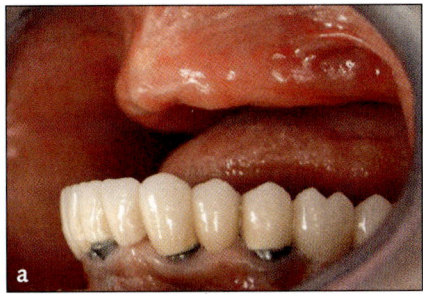

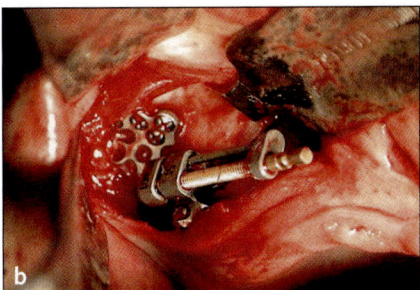

Fig 24-4a Retrodisplaced maxilla with moderate disuse atrophy resulting from 18 years of maxillary edentulism.

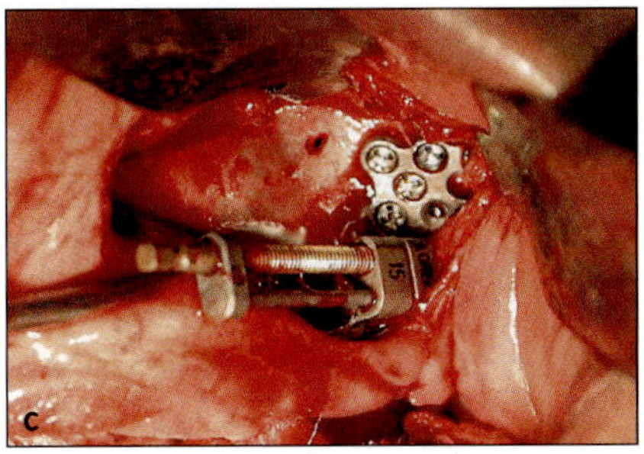

Figs 24-4b and 24-4c Right distractor angles positioned downward and forward. Left distractor angles positioned horizontally.

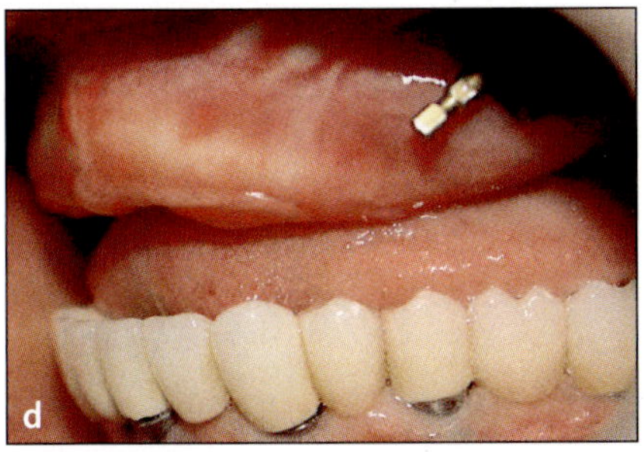

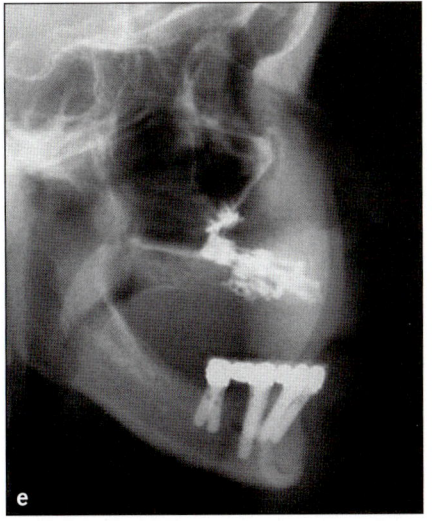

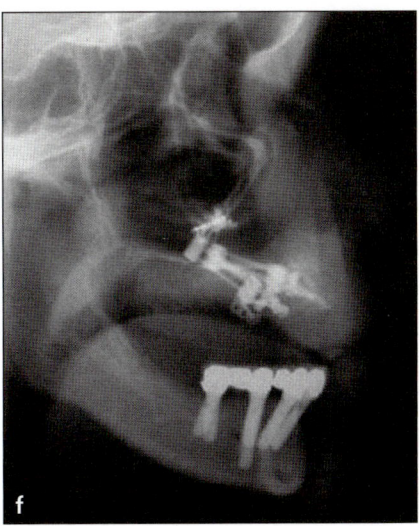

Fig 24-4d Postdistraction maxillary position.

Fig 24-4e Immediate postsurgical cephalogram showing sinus grafts in place and distraction plates activated approximately 2 mm.

Fig 24-4f Completion of 15-mm distraction 2 weeks later. Note maxillary alveolar projection.

Case 2

A 36-year-old woman presents with an edentulous maxilla restored with a complete maxillary denture occluding against an implant-supported fixed prosthesis (Fig 24-4a). During an in-office procedure, a tibial bone graft–xenograft composite is placed onto the sinus floor bilaterally, followed by a Le Fort I osteotomy (without downfracture). Distraction appliances are placed laterally over the sinus-grafted sites (Figs 24-4b and 24-4c). Distraction begins 1 week later and continues for 15 days. The maxilla is moved forward by 15 mm and down by 6 mm (Figs 24-4d to 24-4g). Four months later, eight implants are placed (Fig 24-4h). Because ISQs and insertion torque are low, immediate temporization is not used. Instead, the denture is used for gingival contour development (Figs 24-4i and 24-4j). Four months later, the patient receives a provisional fixed prosthesis (Figs 24-4k and 24-4l).

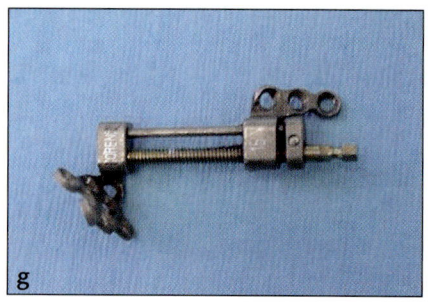

Fig 24-4g After removal 4 months later, the distraction plate shows a distance of 15 mm of distraction.

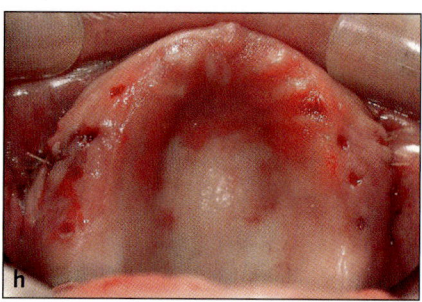

Fig 24-4h Guide stent establishes permucosal implant sites.

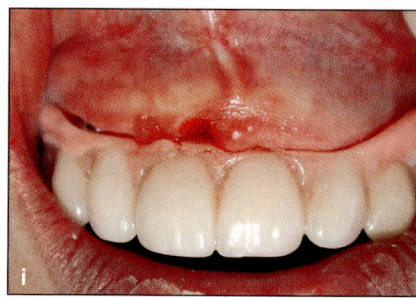

Fig 24-4i The provisional denture conforms to the guide stent and is used to guide the anterior gingivoplasty.

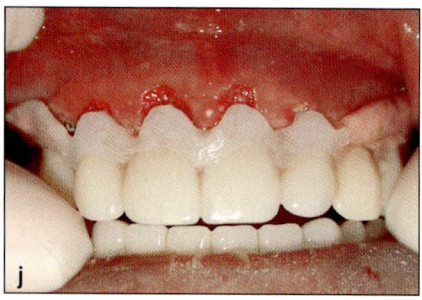

Fig 24-4j Gingival contouring as established by the surgeon.

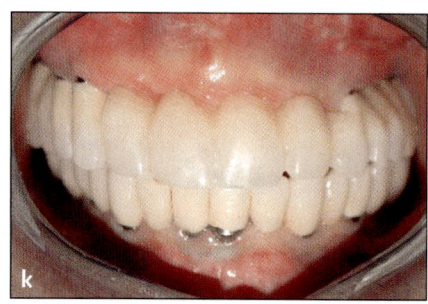

Fig 24-4k The implant-supported provisional prosthesis takes advantage of the anterior gingivoplasty.

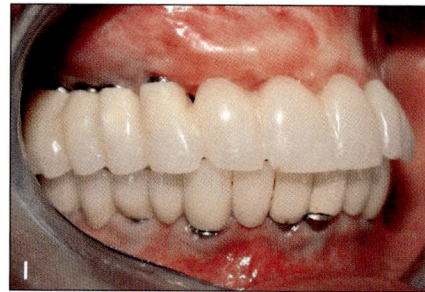

Fig 24-4l Lateral view of provisional prosthesis demonstrating the amount of alveolar projection achieved through distraction.

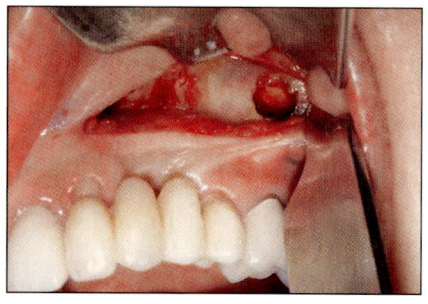

Fig 24-5a An anterior alveolar distraction device encounters the sinus cavity at its posterior margin. Following sinus elevation (above the first molar), the distraction osteotomy is completed without tearing the sinus membrane.

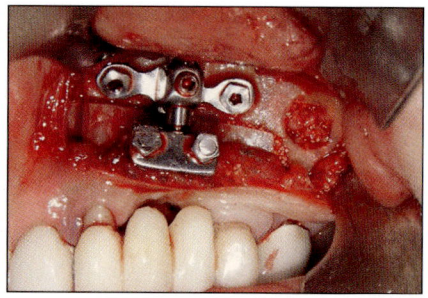

Fig 24-5b After the distraction device (Laster-Mommaerts Crest Distractor, Surgitec) is placed, the sinus is grafted with autogenous bone. The distraction osteotomy site is not grafted.

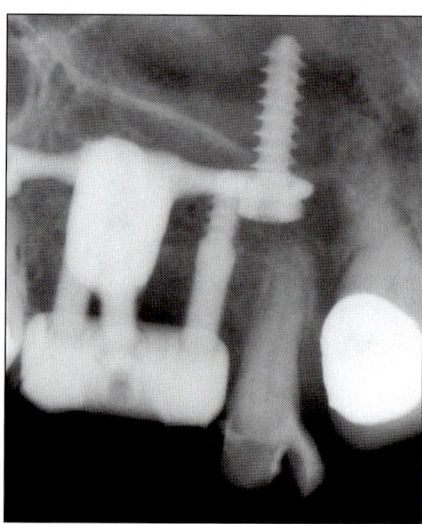

Fig 24-5c Postdistraction radiograph showing bone consolidation both in the distraction gap and in the anterior sinus floor.

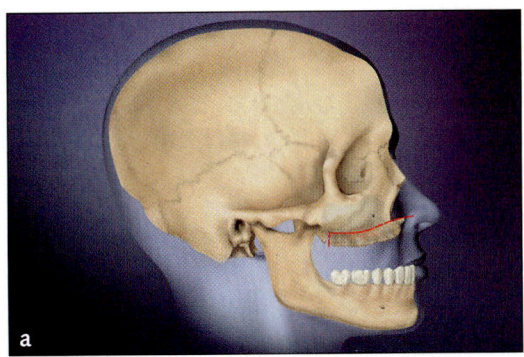
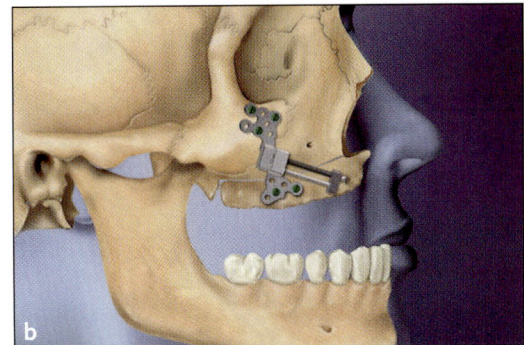
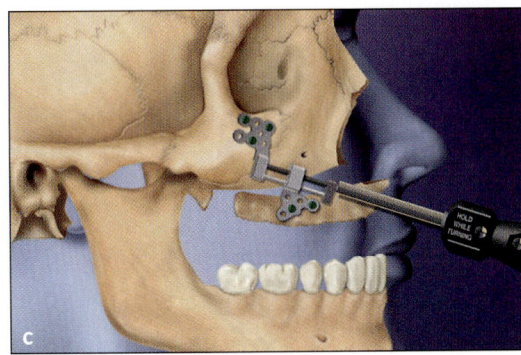
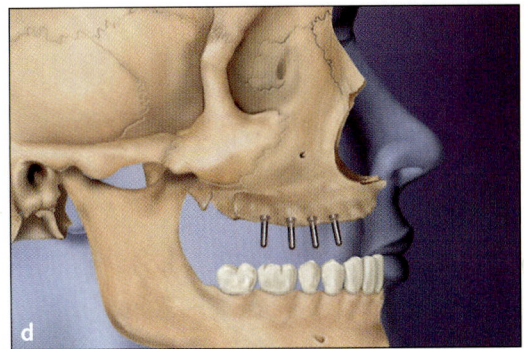
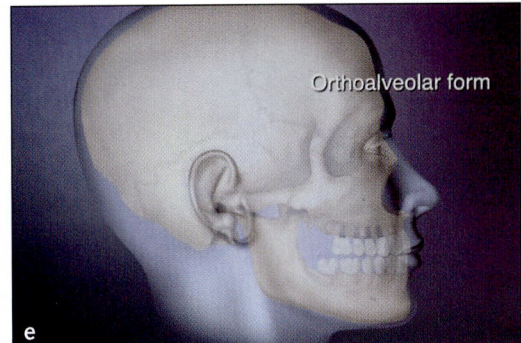

Figs 24-6a to 24-6e Le Fort I distraction technique to recover orthoalveolar form.

Case 3

A 50-year-old woman presents with severe alveolar atrophy for implant therapy with augmentation. Figures 24-5a and 24-5b show a clinical example of alveolar distraction in which the sinus is encountered at the posterior aspect of the segment. When this occurs, sinus elevation with autograft is recommended, but grafting also is needed in the distraction zone, where bone has been regenerated via distraction osteogenesis (Fig 24-5c).

Results

Ten patients consecutively treated with maxillary distraction (Fig 24-6) over a 3-year period are summarized in Table 24-1. Of the 72 implants placed, 2 were lost. The maxilla was stable in all cases with negligible relapse between the provisional and definitive restorations. Six of the patients were treated with orthoalveolar restorations.

TABLE 24-1 Le Fort I distraction osteogenesis with sinus bone grafting in 10 consecutive patients

Patient	Length of advancement (mm)	Type of restoration	No. of implants placed
1	9	Orthoalveolar	8 (1 replaced)
2	15	Orthoalveolar	8
3	17	Orthoalveolar	5
4	18	Fixed hybrid	8
5	15	Orthoalveolar	8
6	25	Fixed hybrid	6 (1 removed)
7	10	Orthoalveolar	7
8	15	Orthoalveolar	8
9	18	Fixed hybrid	8
10	17	Fixed hybrid	6

Summary

A Class III jaw relation resulting from maxillary disuse atrophy can be treated successfully with maxillary distraction osteogenesis in conjunction with sinus grafting. Though the technique must be considered developmental, all restorations and implants in this series remained stable after 1 year without significant maxillary relapse. While 3-year results are favorable, long-term cephalometric comparative data are needed.

References

1. Jensen OT, Leopardi A, Gallegos L. The case for bone graft reconstruction including sinus grafting and distraction osteogenesis for the atrophic edentulous maxilla. J Oral Maxillofac Surg 2004;62:1423–1428.
2. Jensen OT. Combined sinus grafting and Le Fort I procedures. In: Jensen OT (ed). The Sinus Bone Graft. Chicago: Quintessence, 1999:191–200.
3. Jensen OT, Ueda M, Laster A, et al. Distraction osteogenesis. Selected Readings Oral Maxillofac Surg 2002;10(4):1.

chapter 25
PRP and BMP: A Comparison of Their Use and Efficacy in Sinus Grafting

Robert E. Marx, DDS

Platelet-rich plasma (PRP) and bone morphogenetic protein (BMP) represent the only sources of growth factors available to clinicians for sinus augmentation procedures (and other bone regeneration needs) today. Because of its capacity to promote healing in soft tissues as well as in bone, PRP also has indications in nearly all surgical subspecialties of medicine and dentistry.

The three basic biologic elements required for bone regeneration are osteocompetent *cells*, a biologic *signal* for cell proliferation and bone formation, and a *matrix* upon which bone can be formed (Fig 25-1). Both PRP and BMP satisfy these requirements in their own unique ways, which are not exclusive and may even be complementary.

What Are Growth Factors?

PRP

PRP is a concentration of human autologous platelets suspended in a small volume of plasma—hence its name. Platelets initiate all bone and soft tissue healing via expression of seven growth factors: the three isomers of platelet-derived growth factor (PDGFaa, PDGFab, PDGFbb); two isomers of transforming growth factor beta (TGF-β_1 and TGF-β_2); vascular endothelial growth factor (VEGF); epithelial growth factor (EGF); and vitronectin, the cell-adhesion molecule required for cell migration. In the plasma fraction, PRP also contains fibronectin and fibrin, two additional cell-adhesion molecules that also are needed for cell migration.[1]

BMP

Clinically useful BMP is a cloned recombinant human protein that can regenerate bone de novo.[2] There are more than 13 known naturally occurring BMPs, comprising a subgroup in the larger family of growth factors known as *transforming growth factor beta* (TGF-β).[3] In the fetal skeleton, native BMPs are responsible for cell migration and organization and for bone formation. In the adult, BMPs control the process of new bone regeneration associated with osteoclastic resorption and are therefore responsible for maintenance of bone mass and bone remodeling.[4]

How Do Growth Factors Work?

PRP

As noted above, PRP contains seven growth factors (as well as three cell adhesion molecules), whereas BMP is a single growth factor; however, their mechanism of action is fundamentally the same. All such growth factors are

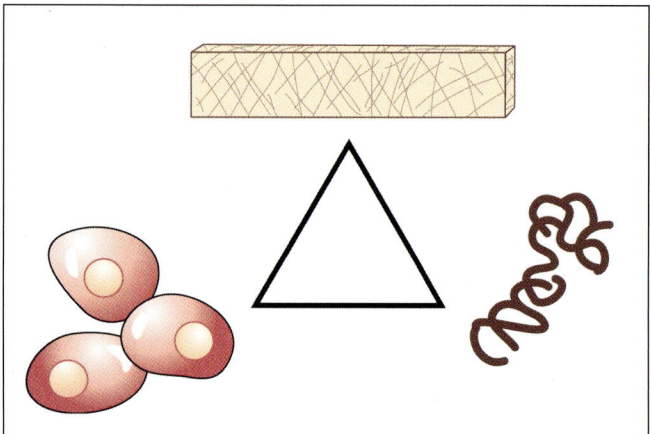

Fig 25-1 The classic triad for tissue bone regeneration: undifferentiated and/or osteocompetent *cells*, signal *proteins*, and a *scaffold* (matrix) upon which bone can form.

either large polypeptides or small proteins of about 25,000 d. They are also dimers, meaning they have two active sites that must be precisely oriented spatially to function as active molecules.[5] These dimers bind to specific cell membrane surface receptors on their target cell. They never enter the nucleus of the cell and, hence, are not mutagenic. Therefore, they cannot create a malignant nor even a benign neoplasia.[6] Rather, they activate two adjacent cell membrane surface receptors via their dimorphic geometry so that their intracytoplasmic portions (these membrane receptors are actually *trans*membrane receptors) are brought into close approximation (Figs 25-2a and 25-2b). The activated transmembrane receptors bind dormant intracytoplasmic transducer proteins together via a high-energy phosphate bond. In turn, the intracytoplasmic transducer proteins detach and float through the cytoplasm to the cell's nucleus, where they activate a specific normal gene or set of genes. The activated gene then codes for the synthesis of specific proteins, resulting in an observed clinical effect (Fig 25-2c). In the case of the three platelet-derived growth factor (PDGF) isomers, the primary biologic effect is mitosis of healing-capable cells. In the case of the TGF-β isomers, the primary effect is cartilage or bone differentiation. In the case of VEGF, it is the specific mitosis of endothelial cells and the formation of type X collagen for vascular basal lamina. In the case of EGF, it is the mitosis of epithelial cells.[7]

BMP

In the case of BMPs, their activity promotes the recruitment, proliferation, and differentiation of marrow stem cells into functioning osteoblasts.[8]

When and How Were They Discovered?

PRP

The technical procedure for concentrating autologous platelets was developed in the 1970s (with the advent of plasmapheresis). In 1990, Knighton et al developed a concentration of homologous human platelets known as *platelet-derived wound healing factor* (PDWHF).[9] In 1998, Marx et al first demonstrated the capacity of true autologous PRP to accelerate bone regeneration.[1] Since then, PRP application has expanded exponentially in specific oral and maxillofacial surgical,[1,10,11] periodontal,[12,13] orthopedic,[14–16] cardiovascular,[17] dermatologic,[18] and cosmetic surgeries.[19,20] Within this short time span, new technology to concentrate platelets efficiently and conveniently has expanded its accessibility to clinicians and thus has broadened its use.

BMP

BMP was discovered in 1965 by Urist,[21] an orthopedic bone researcher, who found that nonviable bone extracts could regenerate viable bone in ectopic sites via a process that he later described as *autoinduction*.[22] Originally, it was thought that large quantities of animal and even human bone could be crushed and serially purified to obtain clinically useful native BMP. However, because bone contains only trace amounts (about 0.25 μg per lb) of BMP, the process required massive amounts of purified animal or cadaver bone, which was not an insurmountable obstacle.

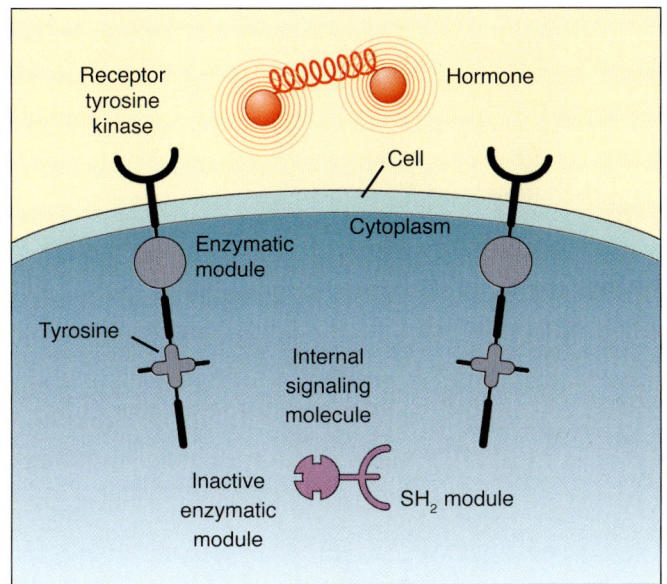

Fig 25-2a The growth factors bind to membrane receptor sites on a target cell. These receptors have both external and intracytoplasmic internal components and are thus termed transmembrane receptors.

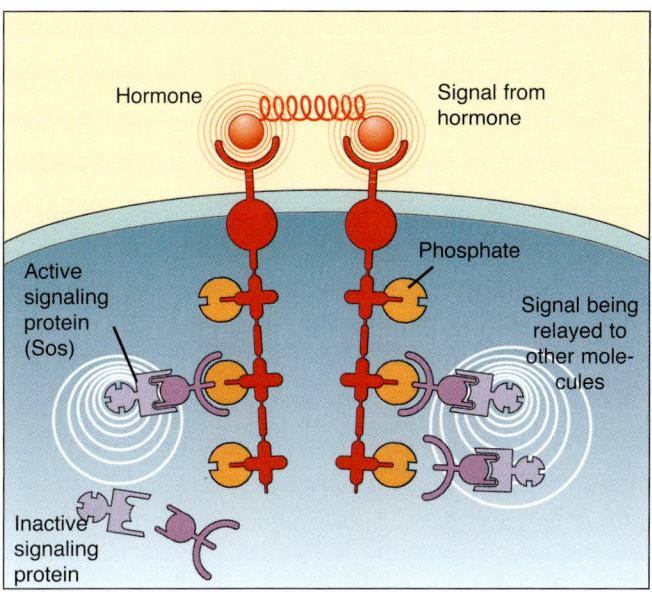

Fig 25-2b Activation of the external receptor site causes a high-energy phosphate bond activation of an intracytoplasmic transducer protein.

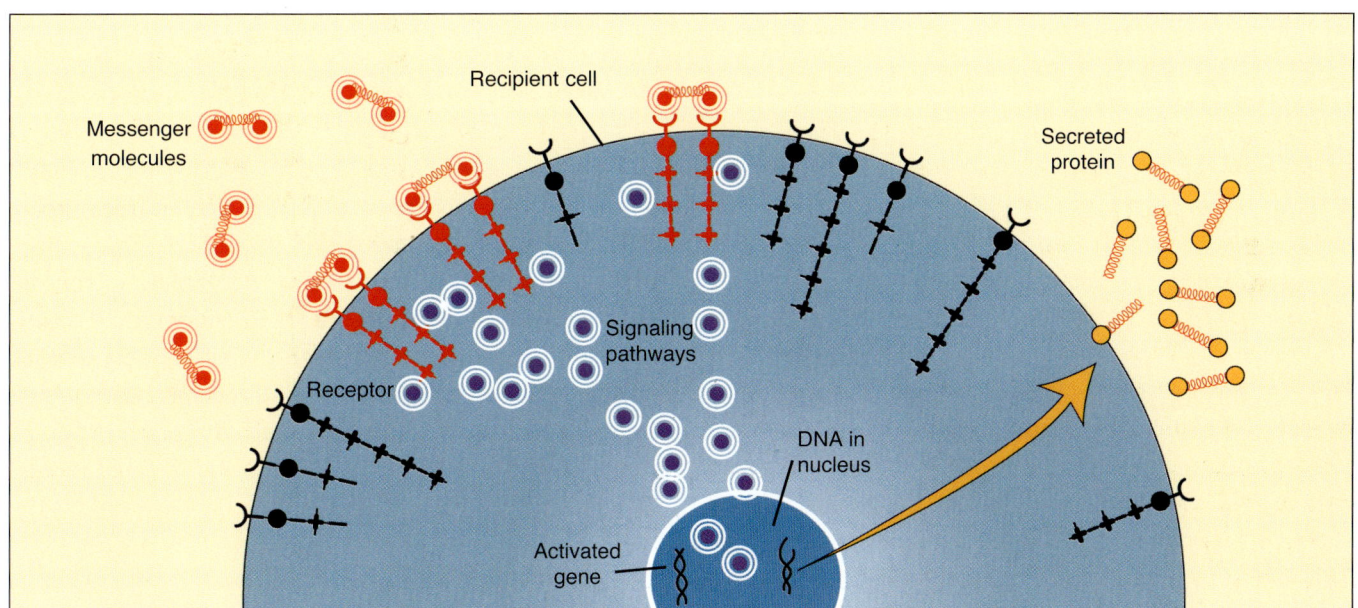

Fig 25-2c The activated signal transducer protein detaches from the transmembrane receptor, floats in the cytoplasm, and enters the nucleus to induce expression of a normal gene.

Nonetheless, the serial purification process could not eliminate all viruses and other animal proteins, and therefore the concept was abandoned. In the 1980s, recombinant technology was used to clone the coding sequence (c-DNA) of two BMPs (BMP-2 and BMP-7), resulting in the clinical availability of 98% pure human BMP in high concentrations (1- to 2-mg/mL).[23] Today, recombinant human BMP-2 (rhBMP-2) in an acellular collagen sponge (Infuse, Medtronic Sofamor Danek) has received Food and Drug Administration (FDA) clearance for two orthopedic indications, and an application is pending for its use in sinus augmentation.

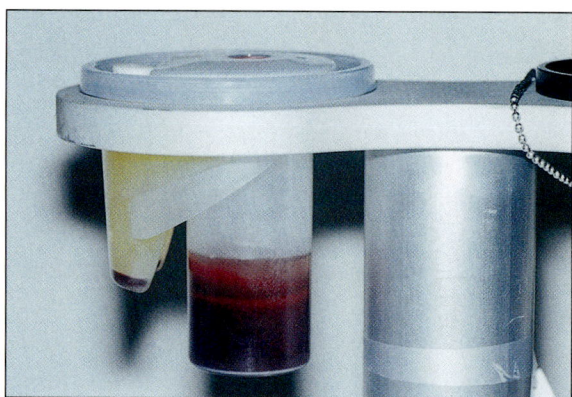

Fig 25-3a After PRP separation, the residual red blood cells are seen here in the chamber to the right, while the chamber to the left shows a red blood cell "button" at the bottom, a thin buffy coat layer just above, and the clear yellow platelet-poor plasma. The concentrated platelets are located in the red blood cell button, the buffy coat, and the bottommost few milliliters of the plasma fraction.

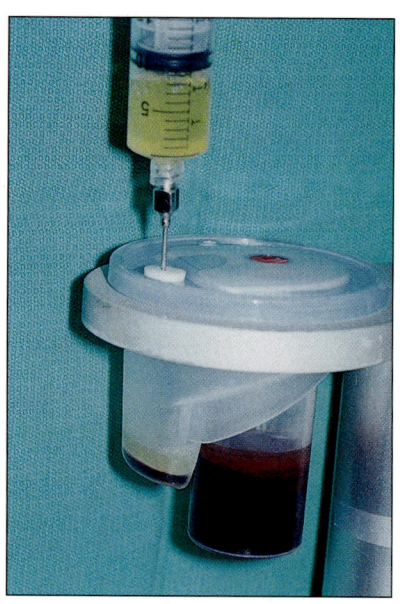

Fig 25-3b The residual volume of plasma is aspirated and will then be squirted back along the side walls and bottom of the canister to suspend the platelet concentrate. This maneuver is performed three times. The subsequent suspension is true PRP.

How Are They Developed?

PRP

PRP is developed by in-office centrifugation devices that concentrate platelets from autologous whole blood. Most devices today use either 20 or 60 mL of whole blood drawn from the patient just prior to the procedure. For example, the sinus graft procedure normally requires about 3 mL of PRP; therefore, the clinician draws 20 mL of whole blood into a syringe containing 2 mL of anticoagulant citrate dextrose-A (ACD-A). The derived 22 mL of anticoagulated blood is then placed into a specific canister containing an additional 1 mL of ACD-A. The canister is placed into a programmed automated centrifuge, where it undergoes a *separation spin* to separate the red blood cells from the white blood cells, platelets, and plasma; this is followed by a *concentration spin,* which concentrates the few residual red blood cells remaining in this fraction, the white blood cells, and the platelets at the bottom of the canister (Fig 25-3a). After centrifugation, which takes approximately 14 minutes, the clinician aspirates the platelet-poor plasma (PPP) (ie, the supernatant) (Fig 25-3b) and then resuspends the platelet concentrate in the remaining 3 mL of plasma (Figs 25-3c and 25-3d). The volume of anticoagulated PRP thus derived has been shown to remain sterile and stable for up to 8 hours. It is stored in a plastic receptacle until it is used at the sinus graft site.[24]

BMP

Recombinant human BMP (rhBMP) is developed in a molecular biology laboratory. To begin, the BMP coding sequence is excised from the parent chromosome via restricted fragment protein enzymes. This c-DNA sequence is then linked to a strong promotor molecule and transfected into a host cell, from which a host cell line is cultured. The host cell line is expanded to create a vat (more than 1,000 L) of rhBMP-producing cells. The host cell line for rhBMP-2 is the Chinese hamster ovary (CHO) cell, a time-tested, contaminant-free host cell that functions as a virtual protein factory. These cells complete the protein to an active state by properly folding the molecule, adding

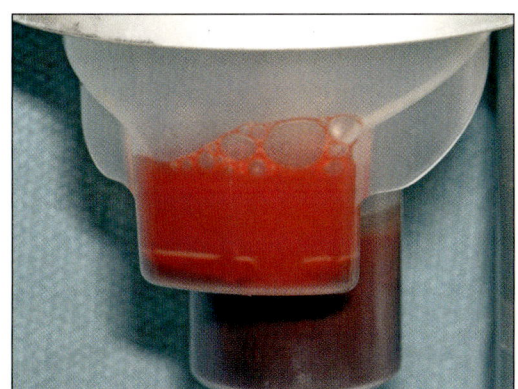

Fig 25-3c Resuspension of the concentrated platelets into PRP is accomplished by ejecting the residual PPP down the walls of the canister three times.

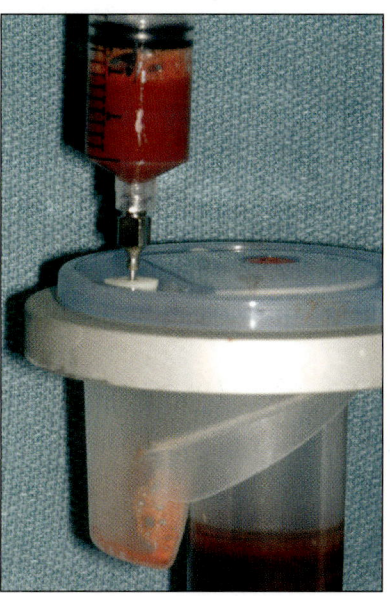

Fig 25-3d The aspirated suspension of PRP is ready for activation and will remain sterile with viable and active platelets for up to 8 hours.

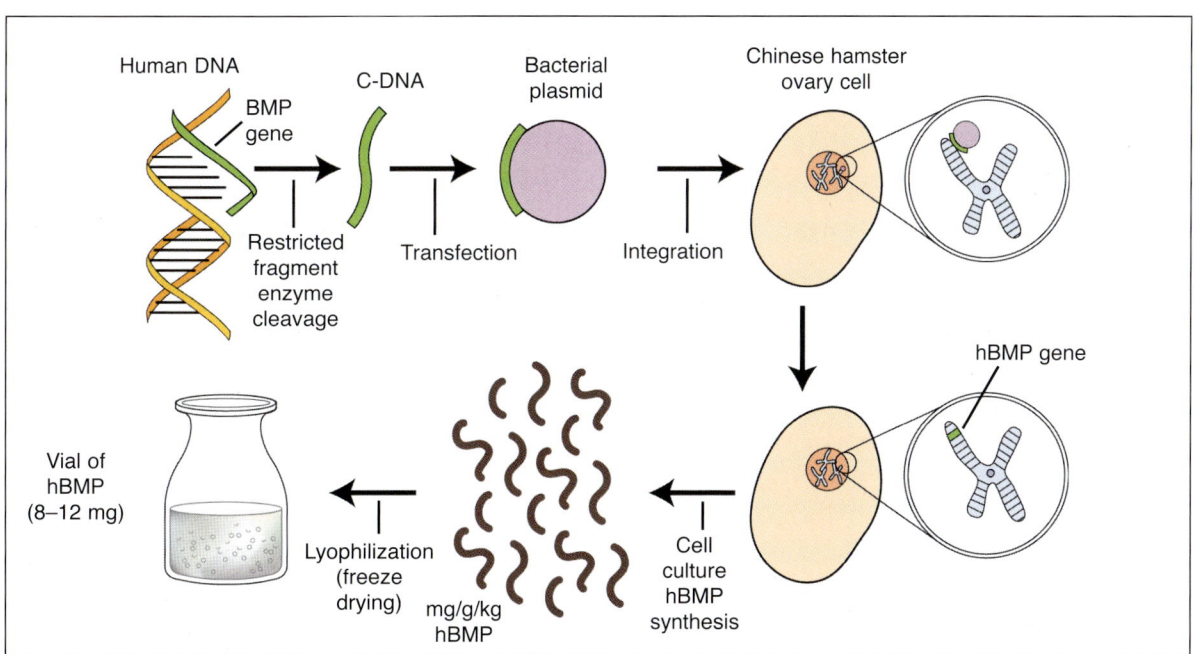

Fig 25-4 Preparation and packaging of rhBMP-2 for clinical use. The sterile vial contains a lyophilized (freeze-dried) powder that is readily soluble in sterile water.

histones and carbohydrate side chains, and dimerizing the amino acid sequence. The resulting rhBMP-2 product is purified from the medium via column chromatography, sterilized via ultrafiltration, and placed in vials for lyophilization (freeze drying) (Fig 25-4). The final product is delivered to the clinician as a white powder that must be reconstituted in sterile water for 5 minutes and then applied to a carrier for a period of 15 minutes to 2 hours for binding to the carrier.[2,23,25]

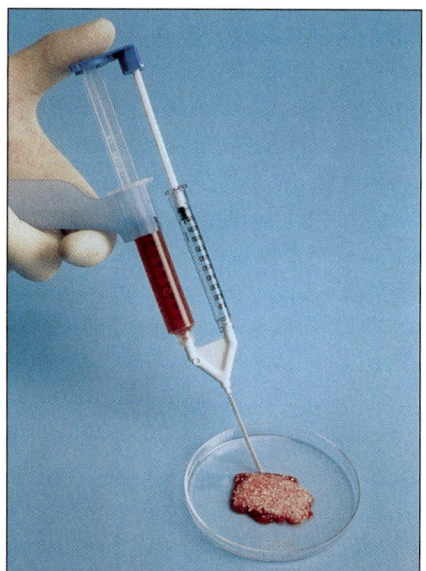

Fig 25-5a The ejection assembly mixes the PRP with the calcium chloride/thrombin solution at a 10:1 ratio so that clotting takes place in 6 seconds or less.

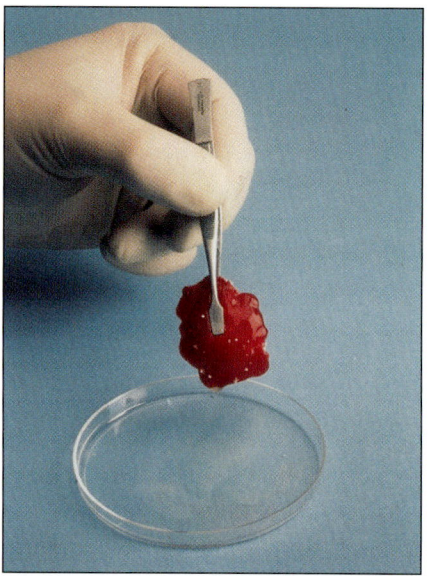

Fig 25-5b Activated PRP congeals bone substitute particles as well as autogenous and allogeneic bone particles for an easy-to-place composite.

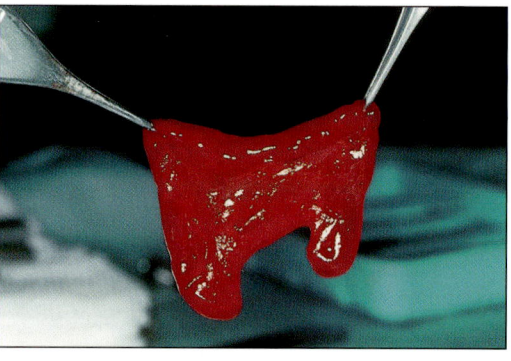

Fig 25-5c A mature PRP membrane can be used in the same manner as any fast-resorbing collagen membrane. However, it is essentially an autologous fibrin membrane that also contains the seven growth factors from the platelets plus the cell adhesion molecules vitronectin, fibronectin, and fibrin itself.

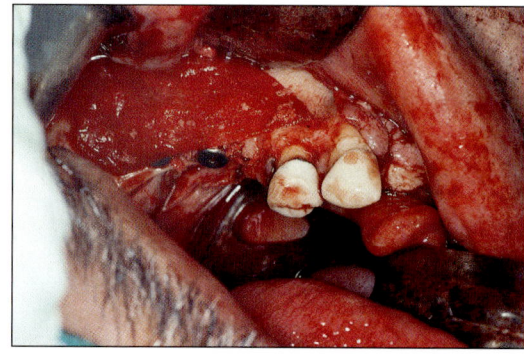

Fig 25-5d Activated PRP placed over a sinus graft window.

How Are They Used in the Sinus Graft Procedure?

PRP

PRP can be combined with any graft material to accelerate bone regeneration. The graft material may consist of autogenous bone, allogeneic bone, bone substitutes, or a composite of these three basic types. However, the anticoagulated PRP must be activated (ie, clotted) beforehand to trigger release of the growth factors from the platelets. Two drops of a solution made of 5 mL of 10% calcium chloride placed into 5,000 units of topical bovine thrombin can be used to activate the PRP. Alternatively, PRP and the activator can be combined in a 10:1 ratio using a so-called double-syringe gun assembly. For this, a 10-mL syringe containing the anticoagulated PRP is attached to a 1-mL

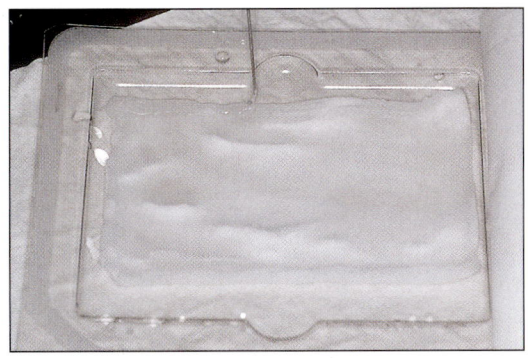

Fig 25-6a Reconstituted rhBMP-2 is used to wet an ACS. Within 15 minutes, 93% of the BMP-2 binds to the sponge.

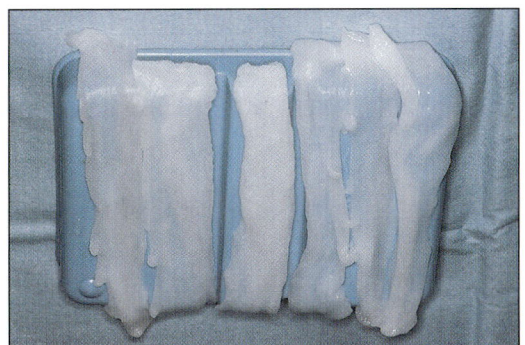

Fig 25-6b The rhBMP-2/ACS composite is usually cut into strips to facilitate placement into the sinus graft site.

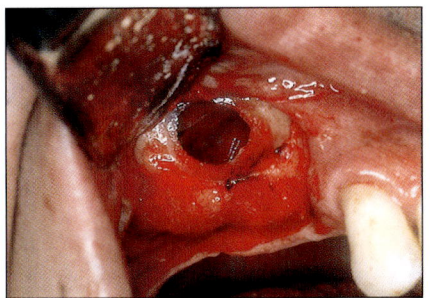

Fig 25-6c Caldwell-Luc standard sinus graft entry and reflected sinus membrane.

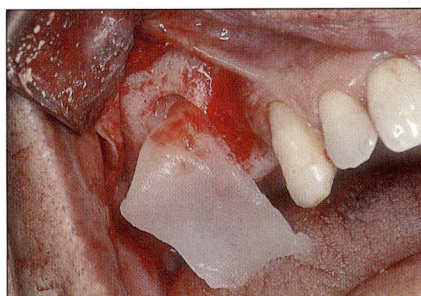

Fig 25-6d The rhBMP-2/ACS composite is layered and compacted into the prepared sinus graft site.

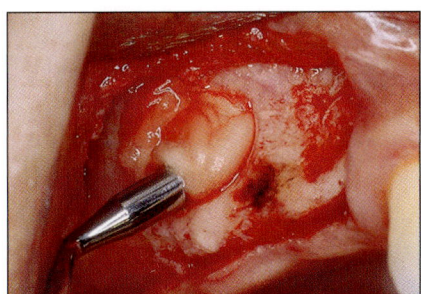

Fig 25-6e As it is compacted, the rhBMP-2/ACS may express some liquid; this will not diminish its bone-inducing capacity.

syringe containing the calcium chloride/thrombin solution, and the two syringes are simultaneously expressed onto the graft (Fig 25-5a). Standard procedure calls for placement of 1 mL of activated PRP into the sinus cavity after the sinus membrane has been elevated; placement of an additional 1 mL into the graft to achieve saturation and adherence of the graft particles and to improve their handling properties (Fig 25-5b); and finally, placement of 1 mL on the graft surface at the sinus wall opening in the same fashion as a membrane would be used (Figs 25-5c and 25-5d). Used in this manner, PRP can be expected to seal small sinus membrane perforations; to accelerate the osteogenesis of any autogenous graft cells; and to accelerate the osteogenesis of cells in the bony walls of the sinus cavity when allogeneic bone, xenogenic bone, or a bone substitute graft is used. PRP also provides a matrix for bone regeneration throughout the sinus graft cavity and promotes the periosteal and soft tissue healing of the mucoperiosteal flap.

BMP

BMP can be expected to form bone on its own, without the addition of any grafting material. As noted earlier, the crystalline white powder of rhBMP-2 must first be reconstituted in sterile water for 5 minutes. For this, 8 mL of sterile water is added to 12 mg of rhBMP-2 to attain a concentration of 1.5 mg/mL.[25] This solution is aspirated into a 10-mL syringe and injected into an acellular collagen sponge (ACS) carrier. A 15-minute waiting period is needed to allow the reconstituted rhBMP-2 to bind to the collagen in the sponge (Fig 25-6a), which is then cut into three strips (Fig 25-6b) and placed individually into the prepared sinus cavity (Figs 25-6c and 25-6d). Some of the liquid in the sponge should be expected to be lost as the sponge is placed; this will not diminish the bone-inducing capacity of the BMP since more than 93% of the protein will be bound to the collagen in the first 15 minutes (Fig 26-6e).[26]

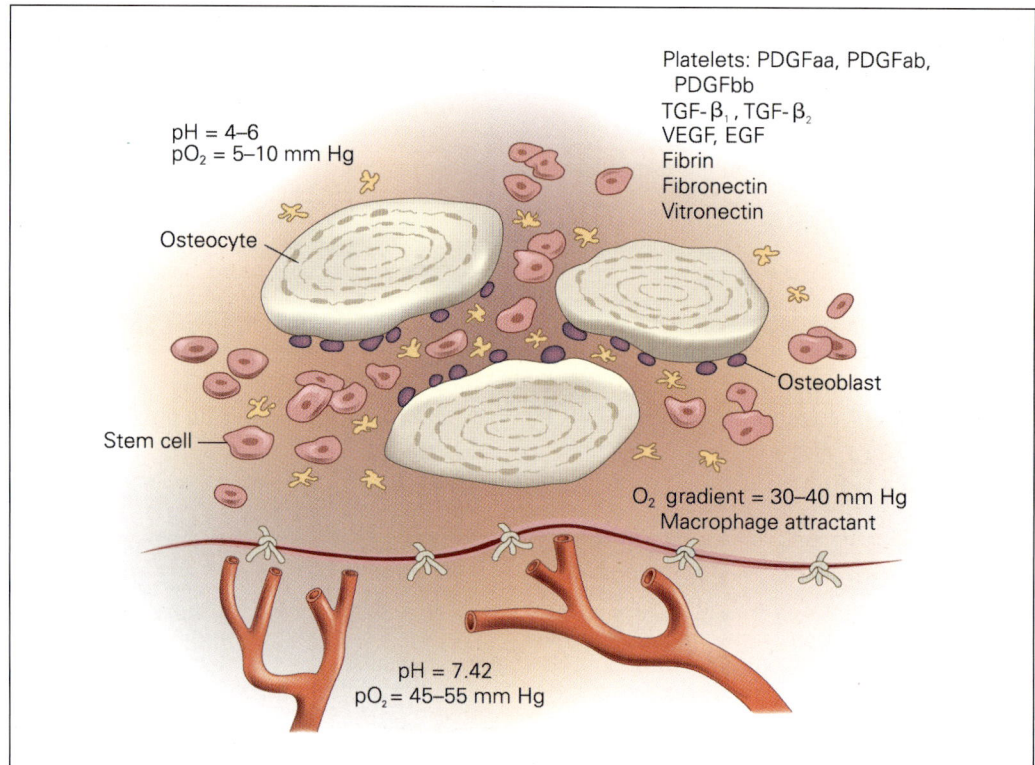

Fig 25-7 The biochemical environment of an autogenous bone graft.

How Do They Regenerate Bone in a Sinus Graft Procedure?

PRP

When autogenous bone is used alone or combined with allogeneic bone or bone substitute, PRP primarily affects the endosteal osteoblast and marrow stem cells of the graft, but it also promotes the osteoprogenitor and vascular endothelial cells of the bony cavity, the sinus membrane, and the mucoperiosteal flap.

Within minutes of activation, the platelets in PRP begin degranulation of their seven growth factors. Within 1 hour, approximately 90% of these presynthesized growth factors are secreted into the graft. After this initial burst of growth factor release, the platelets synthesize and secrete a smaller but steady flow of growth factors throughout their remaining life cycle of about 7 days. The PDGF isomers induce mitosis and hence expansion of the endosteal osteoblasts and marrow stem cell populations. The TGF-β isomers, which are also mitogenic, mainly direct cellular differentiation toward bone formation. (TGF-β is a morphogen as well as a mitogen.) VEGF promotes capillary budding and hence rapid revascularization of the graft. None of the cells in the surgical wound possesses receptors for EGF, which is thus nonfunctional and unnecessary in the sinus graft surgery (Fig 25-7).

The early revascularization of the graft enhances the survival of the osteocompetent cells and promotes their synthesis of osteoid. The PRP-created expansion of the cellular components increases the rate of bone formation and the amount of bone formed. Studies have demonstrated a 19% increase in the amount of bone formed and a 90% increase in the rate of bone formation.[1] In addition, early differentiation of the TGF-β isomers produces a denser and more mature bone, allowing for earlier implant placement and enhanced primary stability. The cell adhesion molecules vitronectin, fibronectin, and fibrin also promote more rapid bone regeneration by providing a matrix (scaffold) upon which cells can migrate and thus a more complete graft that is free of voids (Fig 25-8).

When either 100% allogeneic bone or a bone substitute is used for sinus grafting, the PRP growth factors primarily affect the endosteal osteoblasts and marrow stem cells. The prepared sinus cavity is analogous to a five-wall

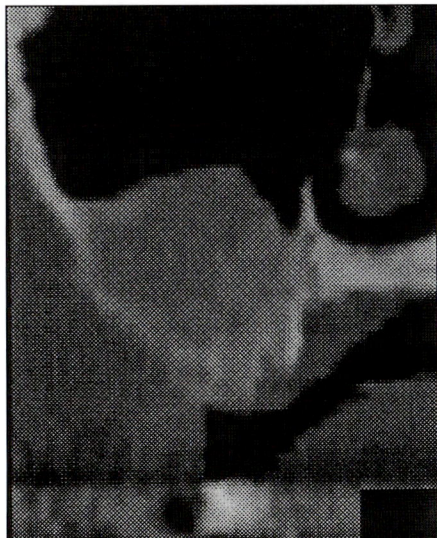

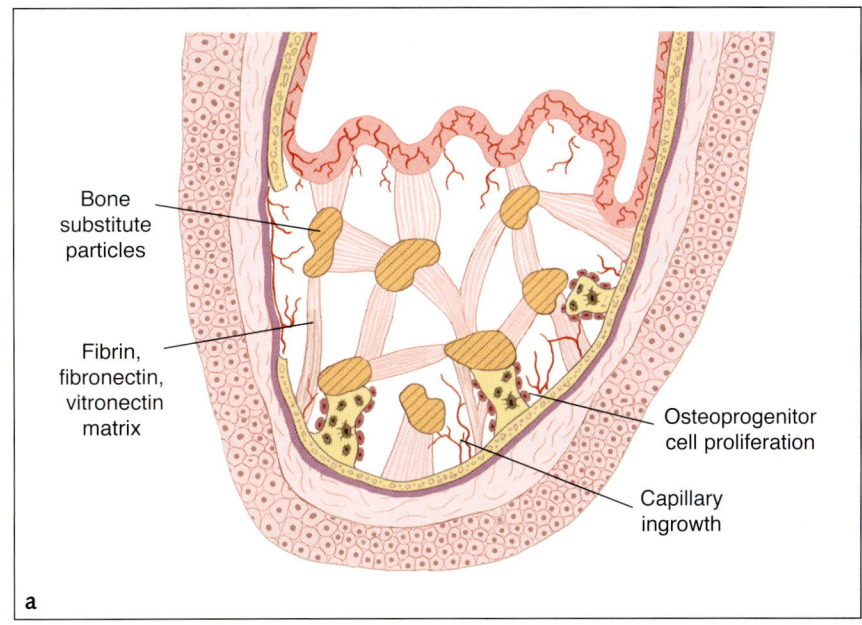

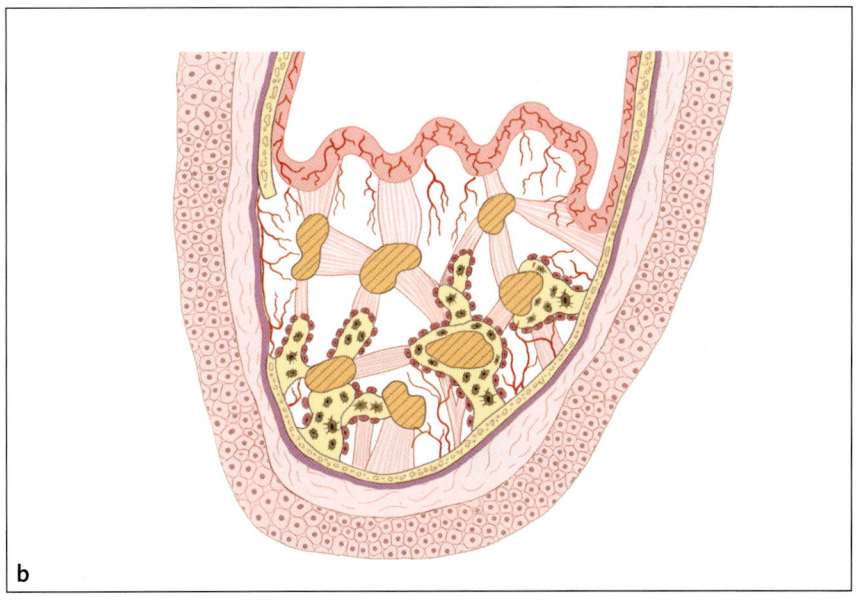

Fig 25-8 *(top, left)* A well-reflected sinus membrane, an autogenous bone graft, and PRP result in rapid bone regeneration and significant volume of bone for placement of the dental implant.

Fig 25-9a *(top, right)* Bone regeneration in a bone substitute graft in the maxillary sinus requires capillary ingrowth into the volume space of the graft, osteoprogenitor cell proliferation, and migration from the surrounding bony walls and then actual bone formation around the bone substitute particles.

Fig 25-9b *(bottom, right)* Since a bone substitute graft requires growth factor–related recruitment of osteoprogenitor cells, their migration, eventual bone formation, and then bone maturation, a longer period of time will be necessary before stable bone develops with a density capable of primary implant stability. Therefore, enhancement with PRP-related growth factors can be of significant value.

bony defect consisting of the sinus floor, the medial sinus wall, the lateral sinus wall, the anterior sinus wall, and the posterior sinus wall at the tuberosity. The only nonbony wall of this cavity is the elevated sinus membrane. The mitogenic effects of the PDGF isomers induce cellular proliferation and migration along the vitronectin-fibronectin-fibrin strands connecting the sinus cavity walls to the nonviable graft material (Fig 25-9a). As they migrate, the TGF-β isomer induces bone differentiation. Osteoid is thus deposited along these cell adhesion strands and on the surface of the graft material, which has adsorbed these cell adhesion molecules (Fig 25-9b).

The mechanism by which bone regeneration occurs in any sinus graft when a nonautogenous graft is used depends on all of these same growth factors and cell adhesion proteins, which it derives from the native blood clot. The difference is that when PRP is used, the rate of bone formation and the amount of bone formed are increased.

TABLE 25-1 Effect of PRP on sinus grafts using autogenous bone, allogeneic bone, and bone substitutes

Graft type (n = 30)	TBA (%) w/o PRP (n = 15)	TBA (%) with PRP (n = 15)	+/– TBA (%)	P value
Autograft	52	78	+26	.005
FDBA	21	36	+15	.01
Bio-Oss	24	39	+15	.01
Pepgen-15	18	23	+5	.01
BioGran	15	21	+6	.05
C-Graft	22	41	+19	.01

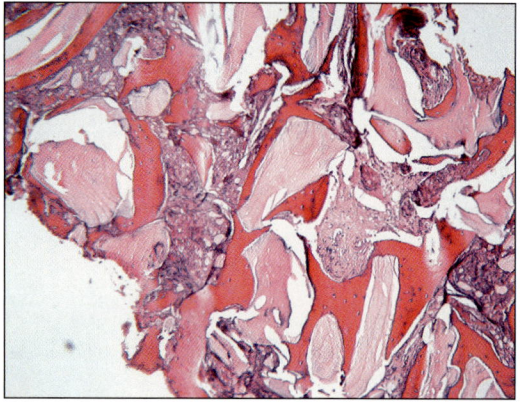

Fig 25-10a Core biopsy specimen from a sinus graft consisting of treated xenogenic bone (Bio-Oss). The area of trabecular bone measured 24% in this specimen. (Hematoxylin and eosin; magnification ×10.)

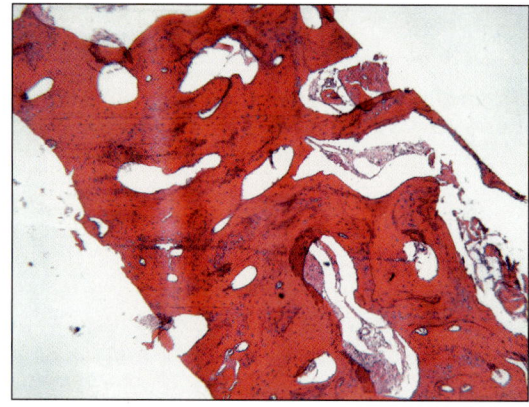

Fig 25-10b Core biopsy specimen from a sinus graft consisting of autogenous tibial cancellous marrow. The area of trabecular bone measured 62% in this specimen. (Hematoxylin and eosin; magnification ×4.)

The same effect has been documented in grafts with allogeneic bone,[27] xenogenic bone,[10,28] and hydroxyapatite preparations.[29] A comprehensive study at the University of Miami Miller School of Medicine's Division of Oral and Maxillofacial Surgery program compared 150 randomized sinus grafts using five different nonautogenous graft materials with and without PRP. The results showed enhancement of a PRP-related viable bone regeneration with all five graft materials. The trabecular bone was observed to be thicker and more mature. The trabecular bone area (TBA) for freeze-dried allogeneic bone (FDBA) improved from 21% to 36%; treated xenogenic bone (Bio-Oss, Osteohealth) improved from 24% to 39%; nonceramic hydroxyapatite (C-Graft, Clinician's Preference) improved from 22% to 41%; treated xenogenic bone with an amino acid sequence added to its surface (Pepgen-15, Dentsply) improved from 18% to 23%; and bioglass (BioGran, Implant Innovations Inc) improved from 15% to 21% (Table 25-1; Figs 25-10a and 25-10b).

BMP

BMP can induce bone without the need for *any* autogenous, allogeneic, xenogenic, or bone substitute product with the exception of a carrier. The ACS is the current state-of-the-art carrier.[2] Once placed into the prepared sinus graft cavity, rhBMP-2/ACS remains active for 3 to 7 days.[23] Like PRP, rhBMP-2 initiates a chain of events leading to bone induction.[30] Initially, the seven growth factors found in the platelets of a natural blood clot incite the proliferation of cells and the migration of blood vessels and stem cells into the ACS (Figs 25-11a and 25-11b).

How Do They Regenerate Bone in a Sinus Graft Procedure?

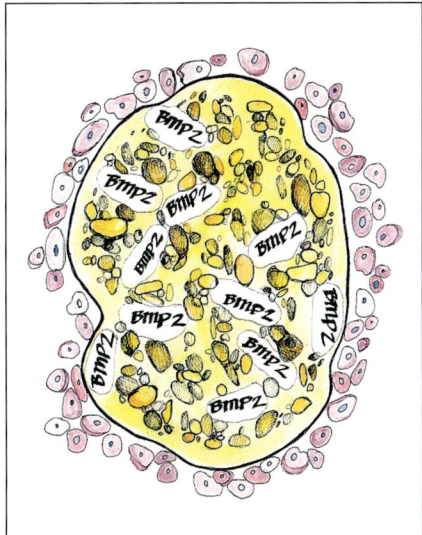

Fig 25-11a Model of rhBMP-2/ACS in a sinus graft surrounded by the cells of the bony maxilla, periosteum, and sinus membrane.

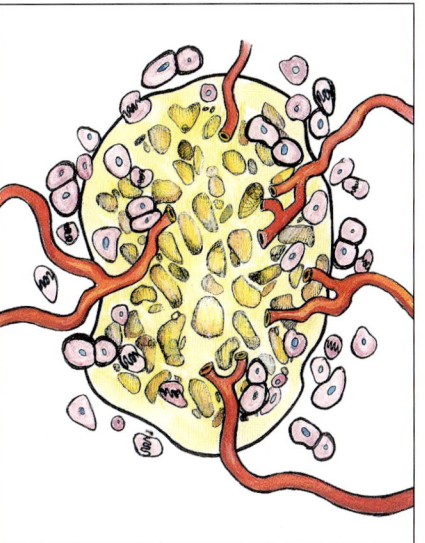

Fig 25-11b The chemotactic, angiogenic, and mitogenic effects of the rhBMP-2 and the inherent blood platelets stimulate a proliferation and differentiation of mesenchymal stem cells, as well as a capillary migration into the ACS.

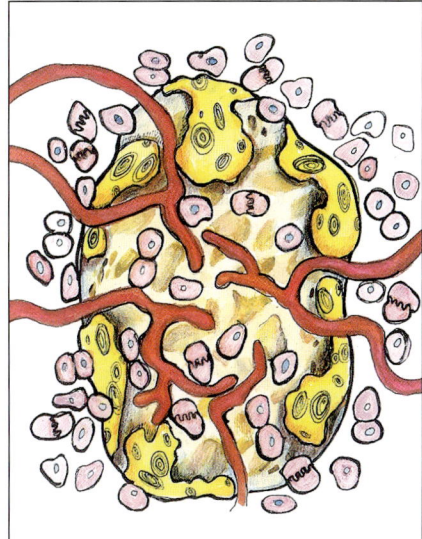

Fig 25-11c Bone formation occurs at the periphery of the sponge, where cells first come into contact with the rhBMP-2.

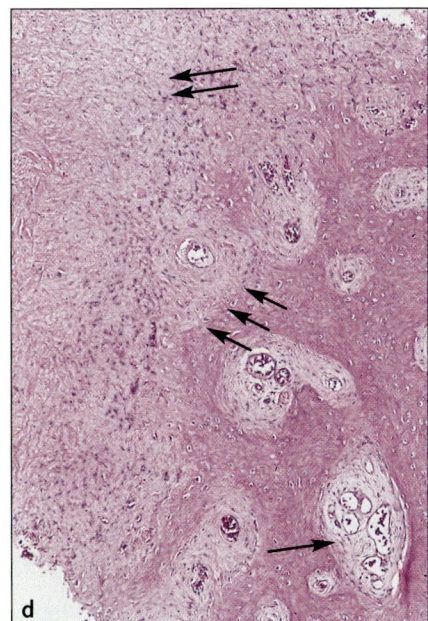

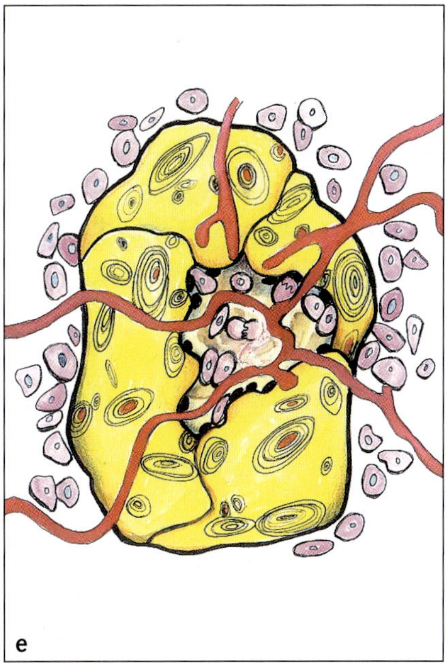

Fig 25-11d Osteoid formation *(arrow)* at the periphery of the ACS *(double arrows)* with a clear line of active cellular proliferation and differentiation *(triple arrows)* progressing centrally.

Fig 25-11e Because initial bone regeneration from an rhBMP-2/ACS graft begins at the periphery, the result is a central void that will dissipate over time and/or function.

This action is triggered by the same biologic mechanism that PRP triggers when it is placed into nonviable graft material, as described earlier. However, when stem cells and endosteal osteoblasts come into contact with the rhBMP-2, they are stimulated to differentiate and actively secrete osteoid. Since cells migrate from the bony walls of the prepared sinus cavity toward the center of the sponge, the initial bone formation occurs at the periphery (Fig 25-11c). The front of active cellular bone progresses centrally (Fig 25-11d). Early immature osteoid formation occurs as early as 1 week postimplantation and proceeds toward the center of the sponge (Fig 25-11e). Bone induced by rhBMP-2 develops slowly and requires 6 months to mature into implantable bone (Figs 25-12a and 25-12b).

chapter 25 PRP and BMP: A Comparison of Their Use and Efficacy in Sinus Grafting

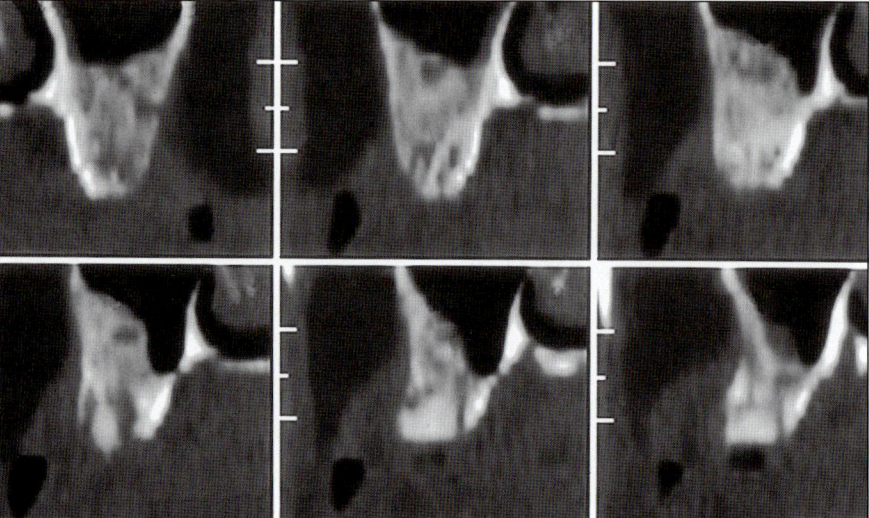

Fig 25-12a Induction of bone regeneration by rhBMP-2/ACS develops somewhat more slowly than an autogenous graft and may, at 4 months, have a low degree of density and/or small voids that will dissipate over time and/or under function.

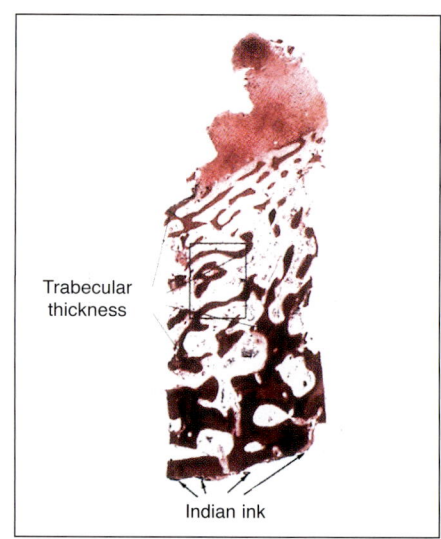

Fig 25-12b Histologic view of a bone core specimen taken from rhBMP-2/ACS–regenerated bone at 6 months.

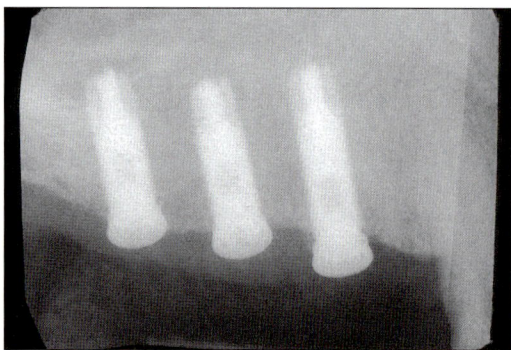

Fig 25-13a Radiographic view of three implants placed into an rhBMP-2/ACS sinus graft accomplished 6 months earlier, demonstrating primary stability but showing incomplete bone mineralization.

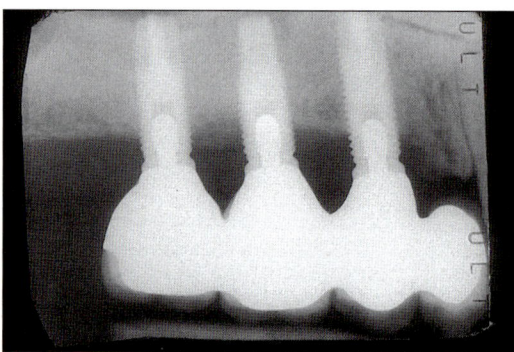

Fig 25-13b Continuing bone mineralization (maturation) following functional loading of the implants placed into an rhBMP-2/ACS sinus graft.

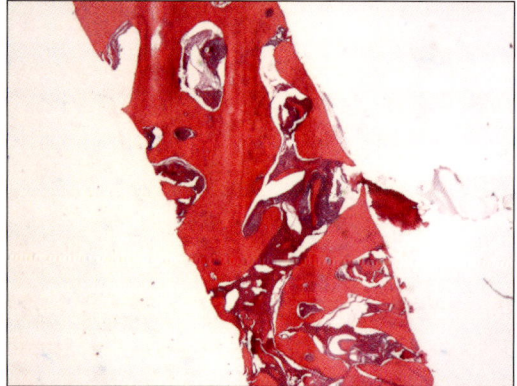

Fig 25-13c Bone core specimen obtained from rhBMP-2/ACS–regenerated bone in a sinus graft.

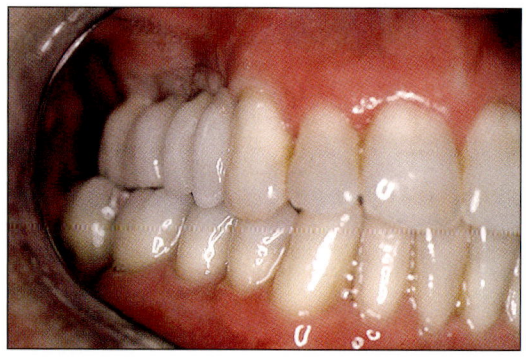

Fig 25-13d Cemented implant restoration in a sinus grafted with rhBMP-2/ACS.

However, once dental implants are placed, bone remodeling and healing proceed normally to achieve osseointegration. As soon as implants are loaded, functional stimulation produces rapid osseous maturation and increased density that is observable radiographically (Figs 25-13a to 25-13d).

Comparison of Advantages and Drawbacks

Proven efficacy in the scientific literature

PRP

As noted earlier, PRP has established documented efficacy in a broad range of oral and maxillofacial reconstructive procedures[1,10,11] (eg, sinus grafting with autogenous,[7] allogeneic,[27] or xenogenic bone[28] or hydroxyapatite[29]; periodontal grafting for root coverage[12]; socket grafting[30]; intrabony pockets[13]; and ridge augmentations,[30] among others),[29,30] in orthopedic medical procedures (eg, orthopedic lumbar fusions,[31] total ankle replacement,[32] and elbow tendinosis,[33] among others), in cosmetic facial surgery,[19,20,34] and in cardiac surgery,[17] all of which attest to the soft tissue and bony healing enhancement properties of PRP. For clinicians who routinely perform sinus grafting procedures of any type, PRP represents an adjunct that will accelerate healing and thus produce more bone sooner while reducing the number of healing-related complications.

BMP

Documentation of the human clinical applications of rhBMP-2 remains much less complete, mostly because of its restricted FDA status. For the sinus graft procedure, three FDA-approved trials have been completed; as of this writing, two have been published[2,35] and a third submitted for publication. In the first trial for which results have been published,[2] four centers accomplished 12 sinus augmentation grafts using 1.77 to 3.4 mg of rhBMP-2/ACS. In each patient, bone regeneration occurred without serious side effects. The results of the second published study[35] documented the concentration (1.5 mg/mL) and dosage (about 24 mg) of rhBMP-2 appropriate for each prepared sinus cavity and demonstrated bone regeneration equal to that of an autogenous graft. The completed multicenter Phase III study has been submitted for publication. In this study, 20 centers accomplished 81 rhBMP-2 sinus grafts and 76 autogenous cancellous marrow sinus grafts. Compared to autogenous bone grafting, rhBMP-2 grafts produced only slightly less bone content (7.83 mm of new bone versus 9.46 mm) but an equal implant survival rate (93%). At present, more documented evidence of the clinical efficacy of rhBMP-2 has been established in orthopedic use, particularly as a replacement for autogenous grafting in lumbar fusions[36] and open fresh tibial fractures,[26] and in cleft palate repair.[37]

FDA approval

PRP

PRP has been cleared by the FDA for use with both autogenous and nonautogenous graft materials and as a wound-healing adjunct. Nearly all commercial PRP devices are now FDA-cleared as well.

BMP

Currently, rhBMP-2/ACS has received FDA clearance only for lumbar fusions and fresh open tibial fractures. Wyeth Pharmaceuticals, the company that produces rhBMP-2, withdrew its FDA application for approval of its use in sinus augmentation surgery in 2002. However, the licensing agent for rhBMP-2, Medtronic Sofamor Danek, obtained Wyeth's consent to resubmit the application to the FDA, where it is under consideration as of this writing. Regardless of its FDA status, rhBMP-2 can be used in the maxillary sinus graft procedure as a so-called off-label indication provided that the patient is fully informed of its current approval status as well as the associated risks, benefits, and cost.

Cost

PRP

The cost of using PRP is calculated based on the initial one-time cost of the commercial device and the per-use cost of the disposable sterile kits. The high-quality PRP devices currently on the market range in price from $2,000 to $5,500. Disposable kits for preparing 3 mL of PRP (the amount required for one sinus augmentation) range in price from $99 to $150, and those for preparing 10 mL of PRP range from $225 to $275.

BMP

The cost of using rhBMP-2 is currently $4,900 for 12 mg (the amount required for one sinus cavity) plus shipping, which ranges from $25 to $50.

Concerns/complications related to use

PRP

The use of PRP warrants very few concerns because it is a preparation of autologous blood that is free of transmissible diseases and is nonimmunogenic. Concerns have been raised, however, about the use of bovine thrombin as an activator, although there has never been a bovine thrombin complication reported in relation to PRP usage.[6] The use of bovine thrombin has led to a concern about Creutzfeldt-Jacob disease (CJD) (commonly referred to as *mad-cow disease*), especially in Europe, where rare cases have been reported of transmission to humans following their consumption of contaminated beef. However, CJD can not be transmitted via blood because the causative agent, a prion, resides only in brain or spinal tissues. Therefore, it can be transmitted only via central nervous system tissues. The few rare cases reported worldwide have been linked to meat contaminated with spinal cord and/or brain tissues. Since blood is not a vector of transmission, bovine thrombin has a safe track record.

The orthopedic, cardiovascular, and neurosurgery literature contains published reports of rare cases linking second-exposure bleeding episodes to bovine thrombin–related coagulopathy.[38] These episodes were actually related to a contaminant found in bovine thrombin preparations prior to 1998 known as bovine factor Va.[39] In each case, the bleeding episode was caused by anti–bovine factor Va antibodies that developed in response to intravascular bovine thrombin and which cross-reacted with human factor Va in these patients.[40] Since then, chromatographic purification has virtually eliminated all traces of bovine factor Va in bovine thrombin.[6] It may reassure clinicians to know that second-exposure bleeding episodes have never been reported in association with PRP activated with bovine thrombin.

BMP

Like PRP, rhBMP-2 has shown little cause for realistic concern. One common observation associated with its use is a greater degree of clinical edema that does not appear to respond to intraoperative steroid treatment, presumably a biologic effect of cell recruitment. This increased edema has been clinically insignificant in the sinus graft procedure since the air space of the sinus readily accomodates it. However, excessive edema threatened the airway in a few cervical vertebral fusions and lengthened the hospital course in a few lumbar fusions.

Some concern has been expressed over the possibility that use of rhBMP-2 will result in the formation of ectopic bone out of the recipient site, particularly in a major organ via the systemic circulation. Such concerns are simply unreasonable since studies indicate that the maximum amount of systemically available rhBMP-2 is 0.1% of the implanted dose and an elimination half-life of 7 minutes.[23] Moreover, this type of reaction has never been seen in any animal model or human case.

Finally, there has been some concern that growth factors in general may cause a neoplasia,[41] since neoplasias produce growth factors to accelerate and sustain their growth and to achieve metastasis. The circular logic behind this fear is that neoplasias produce growth factors, therefore growth factors must produce neoplasias. Following the same logic, we could say that bees produce honey, therefore honey must produce bees. As explained earlier in this chapter, growth factors affect only the cell membrane receptors on the cell surface, not the nucleus, and they express only normal genes, not the abnormal mutant genes found in neoplasias.[42] The tested safety profiles of both PRP and rhBMP-2 show no risk of inducing neoplasias.[7,23,42] Nevertheless, the current product information leaflet concerning rhBMP-2 states that "rhBMP-2 should not be used with extant tumors" (that is, for immediate tumor reconstruction) "and in patients with active malignancies." It may, therefore, be used after tumor treatment in patients who show no signs of persistent disease.

Conclusion

PRP and rhBMP are powerful tools for achieving more predictable outcomes in sinus graft surgeries with less morbidity. Both represent forms of tissue engineering. PRP accelerates soft tissue and bone healing and may be applied to all currently used sinus graft materials to enhance their rate and quantity of bone regeneration. rhBMP is a replacement for bone graft materials that can regenerate viable bone in the sinus graft cavity de novo. Although it has not been fully explored as yet, combining PRP with rhBMP would seem to be the next logical step to overcome the slow and immature bone regeneration associaed with rhBMP.

References

1. Marx RE, Carlson ER, Schimmele SR, Eichstaedt RM, Strauss JE, Georgeff K. Platelet-rich plasma: Growth factor enhancement for bone grafts. Oral Surg Oral Med Oral Pathol Oral Radiol Endod 1998;85:638–646.
2. Boyne P, Marx RE, Nevins M, et al. A feasibility study evaluating rhBMP-2/absorbable collagen sponge for maxillary sinus floor augmentation. Int J Periodontics Restorative Dent 1997;17:11–25.
3. Celeste AJ, Iannazzi JA, Taylor RC, et al. Identification of transforming growth factor β and family members present in bone-inductive protein purified from bovine bone. Proc Natl Acad Sci USA 1990;87:9843–9847.
4. Hogan BL. Bone morphogenetic proteins: Multifunctional regulators of vertebrate development. Genes Dev 1996;10:1580–1594.
5. Israel DI, Nove J, Kerns KM, Moutsatsos IK, Kaufman RJ. Expression and characterization of bone morphogentic protein-2 in Chinese hamster ovary cells. Growth Factors 1992;7:139–150.
6. Marx RE. Platelet-rich plasma: Evidence to support its use. J Oral Maxillofac Surg 2004;62:489–496.
7. Marx RE, Garg AK. The biology of platelets and the mechanism of platelet-rich plasma. Dental and Craniofacial Applications of Platelet-Rich Plasma. Chicago: Quintessence, 2005:3–30.
8. Sampath TK, Maliakal JC, Hauschka PV, et al. Recombinant human osteogenic protein-1 (hOP-1) induces new bone formation in vivo with a specific activity comparable with natural bovine osteogenic protein and stimulates osteoblast proliferation and differentiation in vitro. J Biol Chem 1992;267:20352–20362.
9. Knighton DR, Ciresi K, Fiegel VD, Schumerth S, Butler E, Cerra F. Stimulation of repair in chronic, nonhealing, cutaneous ulcers using platelet-derived wound healing formula. Surg Gynecol Obstet 1990;170:56–60.
10. Rodriguez A, Anastassov GE, Lee H, Buchbinder D, Wettan H. Maxillary sinus augmentation with deproteinated bovine bone and platelet rich plasma with simultaneous insertion of endosseous implants. J Oral Maxillofac Surg 2003;61:157–163.
11. Fennis JP, Stoelinga PJ, Jansen JA. Reconstruction of the mandible with an autogenous irradiated cortical scaffold, autogenous corticocancellous bone graft and autogenous platelet-rich plasma: An animal experiment. Int J Oral Maxillofac Surg 2005;34:158–166.
12. Cheung WS, Griffin TJ. A comparative study of root coverage with connective tissue and platelet concentrate grafts: 8-month results. J Periodontol 2004;75:1678–1687.
13. Hanna R, Trejo PM, Weltman RL. Treatment of intrabony defects with bovine-derived xenograft alone and in combination with platelet-rich plasma: A randomized clinical trial. J Periodontol 2004;75:1668–1677.
14. Slater M. Involvement of platelets in stimulating osteogenic activity. J Orthop Res 1995;13:655–663.
15. Lowery GL, Kuklarni S, Pennisi AE. Use of autologous growth factors in lumbar spinal fusions. Bone 1999;25:47s–50s.
16. Miskra AK, Pavelko T. Treatment of chronic severe elbow tendinosis with platelet-rich plasma. Presented at the American Academy of Orthopedic Surgeons 2005 Annual Meeting, Washington, DC. February 2005.
17. Yamamoto K, Hayashi J, Miyamura H, Eguchi S. A comparative study of the effect of autologous platelet rich plasma and fresh autologous whole blood in hemostasis after cardiac surgery. Cardiovasc Surg 1996;4:9–14.
18. Crovetti G, Martinelli G, Issi M, et al. Platelet gel for healing cutaneous chronic wounds. Transfus Apheresis Sci 2004;30:145–151.
19. Welsh WJ. Autologous platelet gel—Clinical function and usage in plastic surgery. Cosmet Dermatol 2000;11,13:13–19.
20. Powell DM, Chang E, Farrior EH. Recovery from deep-plane rhytidectomy following unilateral wound treatment with autologous platelet gel: A pilot study. Arch Facial Plast Surg 2001;3:245–250.
21. Urist MR. Bone: Formation by autoinduction. Science 1965;150:893–899.
22. Urist MR, Mikulski A, Lietze A. Solubilized and insolubilized bone morphogenetic protein. Proc Natl Acad Sci USA 1979;76:1828–1832.
23. Wozney JM. Biology and clinical applications of rhBMP-2. In: Lynch SE, Genco RJ, Marx RE (eds). Tissue Engineering. Applications in Maxillofacial Surgery and Periodontics. Chicago: Quintessence, 1999:103–123.
24. Marx RE. Platelet rich plasma (PRP): What is PRP and what is not PRP? Implant Dent 2001;10:225–228.
25. Howell TH, Fiorellini J, Jones A, et al. A feasibility study evaluating rhBMP-2/absorbable collagen sponge device for local alveolar ridge preservation or augmentation. Int J Periodontics Restorative Dent 1997;17:124–139.
26. Govender S, Csimma C, Genant HK, et al. Recombinant human bone morphogenetic protein-2 for treatment of open tibial fractures: A prospective, controlled, randomized study of four hundred and fifty patients. J Bone Joint Surg Am 2002;84-A:2123–2134.
27. Kassolis JD, Rosen PS, Reynolds MA. Alveolar ridge and sinus augmentation utilizing platelet-rich plasma in combination with freeze-dried bone allograft: Case series. J Periodontol 2000;71:1654–1661.
28. Camargo PM, Lekovic V, Weinlaender M, Vasilic N, Madzarevic M, Kenney EB. Platelet-rich plasma and bovine porous bone mineral combined with guided tissue regeneration in the treatment of intrabony defects in humans. J Periodontal Res 2002;37:300–306.

29. Mazor Z, Peleg M, Garg AK, Luboshitz J. Platelet-rich plasma for bone graft enhancement in sinus floor augmentation with simultaneous implant placement: Patient series study. Implant Dent 2004;13:65–72.
30. Marx RE, Garg AK. Acceleration of bone regeneration in dental procedures. Dental and Craniofacial Applications of Platelet-Rich Plasma. Chicago: Quintessence, 2005:53–86.
31. Weiner BK, Walker M. Efficacy of autologous growth factors in lumbar intertransverse fusions. Spine 2003;28:1968-1971.
32. Watts JD, Coetzee JC, Pemerey G. The use of autologous concentrated growth factors in fusion rates in total ankle replacements. Presented at the American Academy of Orthopedic Surgeons 2005 Annual Meeting, Washington, DC, February 2005.
33. Sacrponni D. Injected platelet-rich plasma relieves pain and enhances the repair in severe elbow tendinosis. Presented at the American Society of Extracorporeal Cell Technology Annual Meeting, Kansas City, MO, October 2005.
34. Abuzeni PZ, Alexander RE. Enhancement of autologous fat transplantation with platelet rich plasma. Am J Cosmet Surg 2001;18:59–70.
35. Boyne PJ, Lilly LC, Marx RE, et al. De novo bone induction by recombinant human bone morphogenetic protein-2 (rhBMP-2) in maxillary sinus floor augmentation. J Oral Maxillofac Surg 2005;63:1693–1707.
36. Burkus JK, Sandhu HS, Gornet MF, Longley MC. Use of rhBMP-2 in combination with structural cortical allografts: Clinical and radiographic outcomes in anterior lumbar surgery. J Bone Joint Surg Am 2005:87:1205–1212.
37. Chin M, Ng T, Tom WK, Carstens M. Repair of alveolar clefts with rhBMP-2 in patients with clefts. J Craniofac Surg 2005;16:778–789.
38. Christie RJ, Carrington L, Alving B. Postoperative bleeding induced by topical bovine thrombin: Report of two cases. Surgery 1997;121:708–710.
39. Zehnder JL, Leung LL. Development of antibodies to thrombin and factor V with recurrent bleeding in a patient exposed to topical bovine thrombin. Blood 1990;76:2011–2016.
40. Rapaport SI, Zivelin A, Minow RA, Hunter CS, Donnelly K. Clinical significance of antibodies to bovine and human thrombin and factor V after surgical use of bovine thrombin. Am J Clin Pathol 1992;97:84–91.
41. Schmitz JP, Hollinger JO. The biology of platelet-rich plasma [letter, with response by Marx RE]. J Oral Maxillofac Surg 2001;59:1119–1121.
42. Marx RE. The biology of platelet-rich plasma [letter]. J Oral Maxillofac Surg 2001;59:1119–1121.

chapter 26

Zygomatic Implants: A Viable Alternative to the Sinus Bone Graft

Steven M. Sullivan, DDS
Chantal Malevez, MD, DDS
Daniel Henrichson, DMD

Osseointegration of root form implants has revolutionized the treatment of edentulism over the past 40 years. However, treatment with conventional endosseous dental implants is not possible when bone quantity/quality in the posterior maxilla is inadequate. Although sinus grafting is usually undertaken in these patients, the use of the zygomaticus implant is an alternative to the sinus graft that is growing in popularity.

The highly atrophic maxilla presents significant problems for the practitioner undertaking dental rehabilitation. Even more challenging are discontinuity defects such as cleft deformity or maxillectomy defects, which present with gross soft and hard tissue deficiencies.[1] Extensive bone grafting is commonly advocated to create adequate bone mass for placement of dental endosseous implants. Sinus floor inlay and buccal onlay grafting with autogenous bone have been used to treat maxillary atrophy.[2,3] However, bone harvesting is not without morbidity or risk, and grafting requires a lengthy consolidation period of up to 6 months before implants can be placed, with the course of treatment often extending more than 1 year (see chapter 9).[4] Zygomatic implants were introduced by Brånemark in 1989 as an alternative to bone grafting for patients who required shorter treatment time and preferred not to be exposed to the morbidity factors associated with bone harvesting and grafting.

Historical Perspective

Today, edentulous patients have more treatment choices with better outcomes than at any other time in history. Osseointegrated implants and other associated advances in dentistry have made the treatment of the edentulous patient easier for both practitioner and patient. When fully edentulous patients have adequate bone for implant stabilization, they can be predictably restored with titanium endosseous implants and a fixed partial denture. Reported long-term prosthesis stability rates in this situation approach 92%.[5] When patients do not have adequate bone for traditional implant placement, the alternative treatment using the zygomatic implant regimen is prescribed.[6] Recently, a new tricortically fixed implant (Excalibur, MIS Israel) was developed specifically for use within the sinus cavity without the placement of a bone graft. The implant is self-threading and capable of primary stabilization, but a 2-mm-diameter cross screw at the apex provides secondary stabilization.

Various methods of bone grafting in the atrophic maxilla have been evaluated in the literature,[2,6,7] including onlay grafts, inlay grafts, Le Fort I osteotomy with interpositional grafting, and so forth. But each of these treatment modalities requires harvesting from the ilium, cranium, or tibia. The drawback to iliac autogenous bone grafting is donor site morbidity, very often unacceptable to the patient.[8]

A relatively short treatment timeline is one of the greatest advantages of the zygomatic implant technique. Following diagnosis and work-up, two zygomatic implants and four anterior dental implants are placed and allowed to osseointegrate for approximately 6 months. Stage-two surgery (uncovering of the implants) is then performed, and impressions are made. The prosthesis is fabricated and delivered, bringing the total treatment time to approximately 8 months.

The zygomatic implant differs from a traditional dental implant in its extended length of 35 to 50 mm and its unconventional anchorage site, the os zygomaticum.[1,9] However, perhaps the most important difference is that it is not intended to be used as a stand-alone fixture and cannot accommodate a maxillary restoration, but must be accompanied with traditional dental implants in the anterior maxilla. As a general rule, each zygomatic implant must be accompanied by at least two traditional dental implants. This allows for the construction of a semi-circular rigid bar that readily sustains and resists functional loading. Studies have demonstrated a remarkable success rate (97%) associated with the use of the zygomatic implant in the severely resorbed maxilla. Compared with conventional implant modalities, the zygomatic technique demonstrates the highest overall success rate.[8] The zygomatic implant approach satisfies a long-unfulfilled need for a viable grafting alternative to maxillary reconstruction that should be discussed with patients.[10–12]

Patient Selection

A preoperative evaluation is required to assess the amount of bone mass available in the premolar alveolus, the point of zygomatic implant fixation. While patients with relatively severe atrophy of the maxilla are considered prime candidates for zygomatic implant treatment, those with an extremely flat maxilla are not, because inadequate fixation of the implant will lead to initial implant instability and ultimately to implant loss. In addition, adequate bone anterior to the sinuses is needed to accommodate the placement of conventional implants. Thorough radiographic and clinical evaluations are critical in determining whether patients qualify for zygomatic implant placement. Patients with inadequate bone in the anterior maxilla may require supplemental bone grafts harvested locally at the time of zygomatic implant placement. Anterior implants can be placed immediately or in a delayed fashion, depending on the preference of the surgeon and the clinical situation, either in a hospital setting using an intubated general anesthetic or in an office setting under intravenous (IV) sedation and local anesthesia.

Surgical Technique

In the office setting, IV sedation and local anesthesia are quite adequate, but care must be taken to assure that appropriate and profound local anesthesia is obtained. Posterosuperior alveolar blocks with anterior infiltrations and supplemental palatal infiltrations are needed in conjunction with percutaneous zygomaticofacial nerve block.

The aid of appropriately trained assistants is strongly recommended to handle the retraction of the lips and cheeks and the associated armamentaria during the placement of zygomatic implants, which are much longer than conventional implants. Fully edentulous patients are easier to manage than partially edentulous patients because the problem of mandibular teeth interfering with the path of implant placement is avoided.

A crestal incision is made in the anticipated placement site, extending slightly to the palatal and anteriorly to the midline, with a releasing incision made posterior and parallel to the zygomatic buttress. Mucoperiosteal exposure for antrostomy and palatal reflection are accomplished; a short midline releasing incision can be made if additional exposure and retraction are necessary. Adequate reflection along the facial aspect of the zygomatic body facilitates visualization of the instruments as they perforate the lateral cortex on the facial aspect of the zygoma (Fig 26-1a).

The antrostomy should be positioned parallel to the zygomatic buttress, rectangular in shape, and as far lateral as possible to ensure that the implant will be placed parallel to and against the buttress itself. Care should be taken in the reflection of the sinus membrane, and it should be preserved when possible (although some authors do not reflect the sinus membrane). Removal of the bony window is optional (Fig 26-1b).

Reflection of the sinus membrane can be carried out along the entire area of insertion, that is, in the superior and lateral aspects of the sinus, to ensure that soft tissue is

Surgical Technique

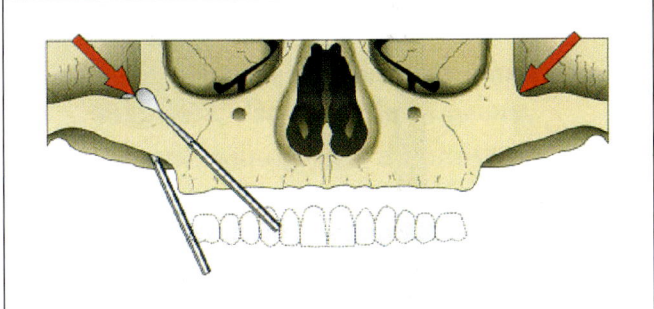

Fig 26-1a Reflection of soft tissues should permit visualization of the zygomatic body and zygomaticofacial nerve. Retraction of these tissues is critical for appropriate visualization during site preparation and implant placement.

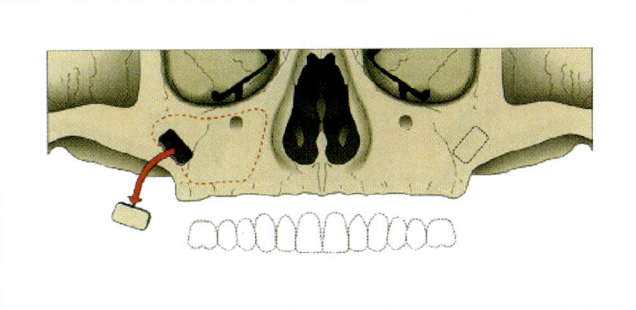

Fig 26-1b The entrance into the sinus should be made as far lateral as possible and parallel to the buttress. The bony window attached to the reflected sinus membrane may be retained or removed.

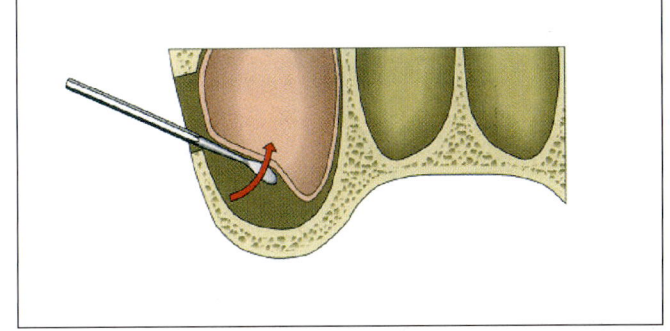

Fig 26-1c The sinus membrane must be thoroughly elevated along the lateral and superior aspects of the sinus to avoid tracking soft tissue into the osteotomy during placement of the implant.

not introduced into the osteotomy site in the body of the zygoma (Fig 26-1c).

A standard osteotomy protocol is followed, although a diameter greater than 3.5 mm is rarely needed since the residual alveolus is often thin and not very dense. The use of a small-diameter osteotomy (ie, less than 4.0 mm) at the alveolar aspect allows for improved stability. The use of drill guides is imperative to prevent laceration of the soft tissue of the lips (Fig 26-1d). Implant length must be properly gauged to prevent palpability of the tip of the implant through the skin (Fig 26-1e). The implant may be placed using a dental implant handpiece or by hand according to the surgeon's preference (Fig 26-1f).

Because it is not visible, the osteotomy site may be difficult to locate in the zygoma. For this reason, it is helpful to use a curved titanium curette to help stabilize and guide the implant into the osteotomy site. If at all possible, the implant should be oriented so that the restorative platform is perpendicular to the alveolus and nearly centered on the residual ridge. This ensures that tongue space will be adequate following prosthetic rehabilitation.

Once the implant has been placed to the proper depth, a 4-mm healing abutment (rather than a healing screw) is placed to facilitate identification of the implant during the uncovering procedure. The healing cap and abutment screwdriver are used to orient the implant into parallel alignment with the cross-arch and anterior implants (Fig 26-1g). Anterior implants should be placed according to standard protocols.

Wounds are closed with a resorbable suture in a continuous fashion. Integration typically takes 3 months but may require as many as 6 months if the anterior implants necessitate bone grafting.

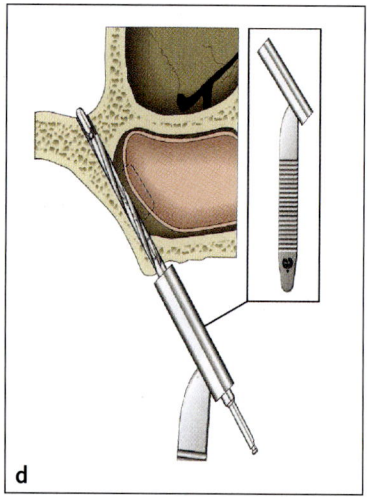
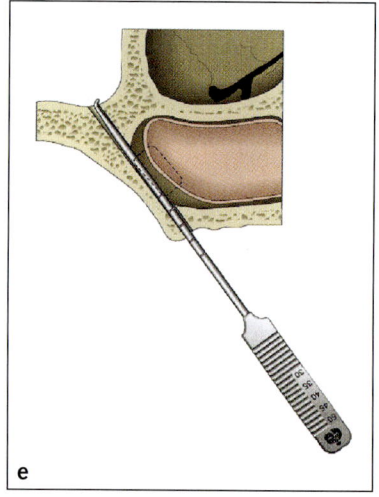
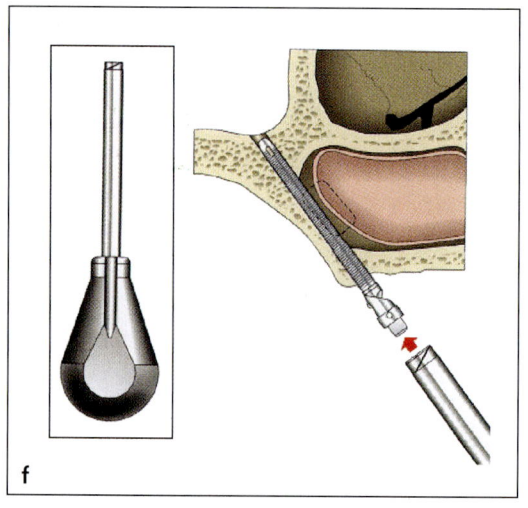
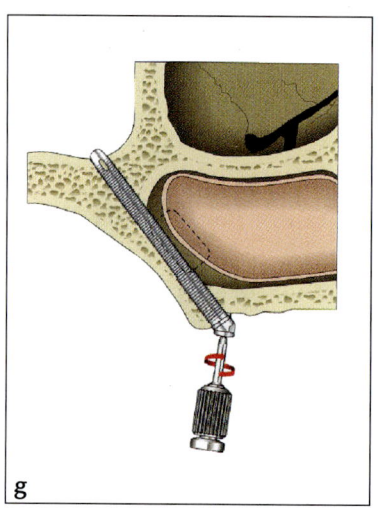

Fig 26-1d Use of drill guides is imperative to prevent inadvertent laceration of the lips.

Fig 26-1e Accurate length measurement will minimize the possibility of placing the implant at a depth that is too shallow, which will make the tip palpable.

Fig 26-1f Placement can be easily accomplished using the hand driver. An implant drill may also be used.

Fig 26-1g The cover screwdriver can also be used to visualize the orientation of the implant in relation to those more anterior and across the arch.

Restorative Considerations

Removable prostheses

Zygomatic implants broaden the number of restorative options. All 20 cases completed by two of the authors (SS, DH) to date have been restored with a removable prosthesis. Locator attachments (Nobel Biocare) and gold bars with retentive O-rings or clips have been used. None of the patients chose to receive a fixed-detachable prosthesis. Medial placement of the zygomatic implant was the most common problem encountered; when this occurs, the palatal aspect of the overdenture prosthesis is bulky and encroaches on tongue space.

Case Studies

Case 1

A 64-year-old man presented with an ameloblastoma of the right posterior maxilla that was confirmed through biopsy (Fig 26-2a). The margin of the lesion could not be seen on the panoramic radiograph (Fig 26-2b), but it was confirmed by a computerized tomography (CT) scan (Fig 26-2c). The right partial maxillectomy extended from the pterygoid plates to the lateral nasal wall (Fig 26-2d).

Immediate implant reconstruction using a left unilateral zygomaticus implant, combined with four root form external hex implants anteriorly, provided adequate support for prosthodontic rehabilitation (Figs 26-2e to 26-2g). The definitive prosthesis was an overdenture with Locator attachments (Fig 26-2h).

Case Studies

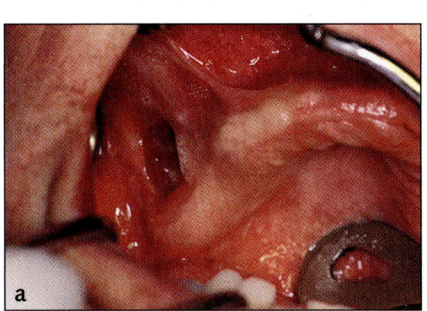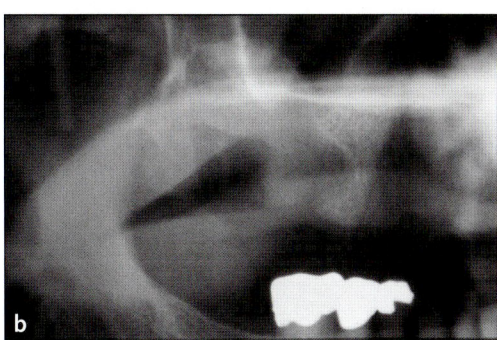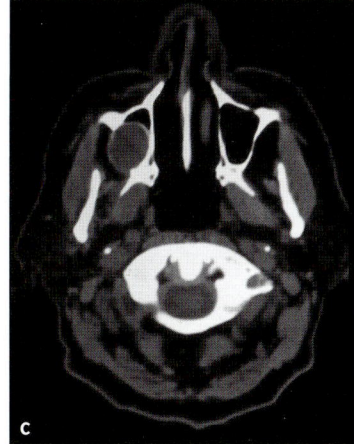

Figs 26-2a to 26-2c An ameloblastoma of the right posterior maxilla required posterior partial maxillectomy. Loss of bony support and vestibular depth compromised denture stability.

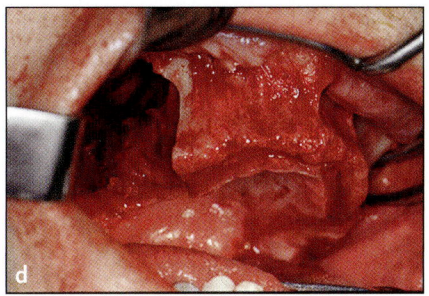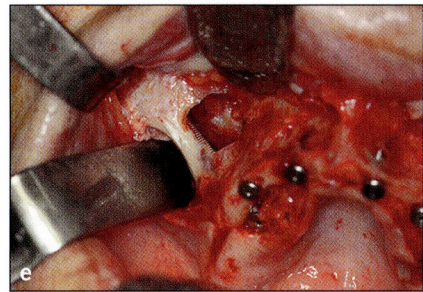

Figs 26-2d and 26-2e Placement of a unilateral zygomatic implant and four root form implants provided prosthetic stability.

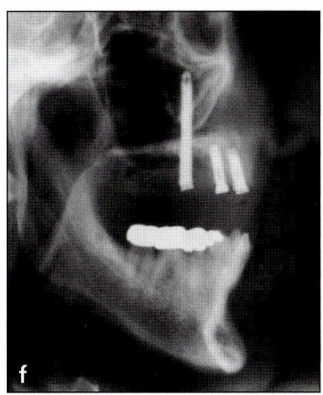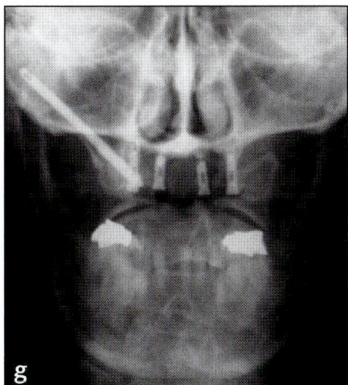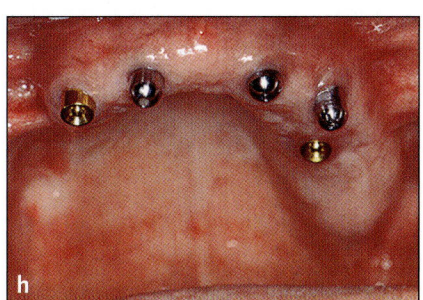

Figs 26-2f and 26-2g Orientation of the zygomatic and anterior implants.

Fig 26-2h Final prosthesis retained by two abutments.

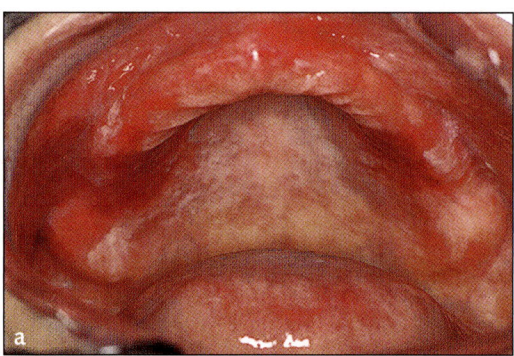
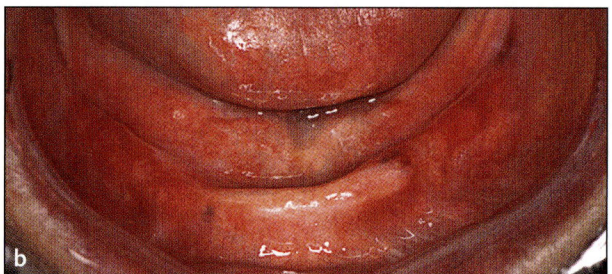

Figs 26-3a and 26-3b Erosive lichen planus compromised denture comfort in this patient.

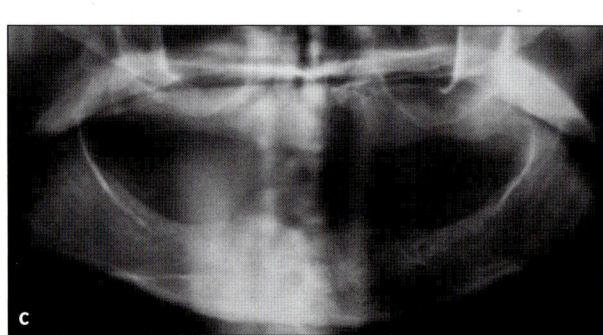
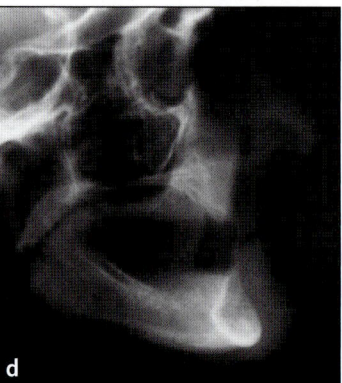

Figs 26-3c and 26-3d Radiographic views of pneumatized sinuses reveal adequate anterior bone volume for implant retention.

Case 2

A 57-year-old woman, seeking denture stability, presented with a long history of erosive lichen planus (Figs 26-3a and 26-3b). Radiographic imaging revealed adequate bone volume in the anterior maxilla for root form implants, but the pneumatized sinuses would require extensive bone grafting (Figs 26-3c and 26-3d). Zygomatic implant therapy was chosen to minimize the amount of surgery and to expedite treatment time.

A standard surgical approach was used to expose the anterior maxilla. Zygomaticus implants were placed bilaterally, and four root form implants were placed in the anterior maxilla. Thread dehiscences were grafted and covered with collected autogenous bone and a barrier membrane (Gore-Tex) (Figs 26-3e to 26-3g).

Five root form implants were placed in the anterior mandible to accommodate a mandibular implant-supported prosthesis. Postoperative imaging revealed a successful surgical result (Fig 26-3h). After 4 months of healing, the prosthetic phase of treatment was completed (Figs 26-3i to 26-3k).

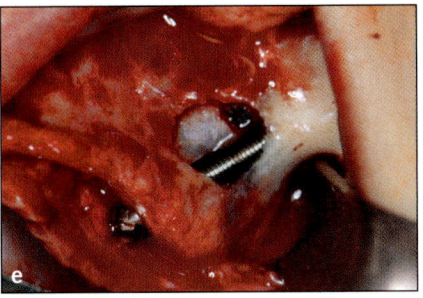 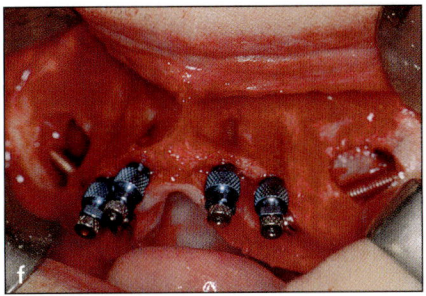 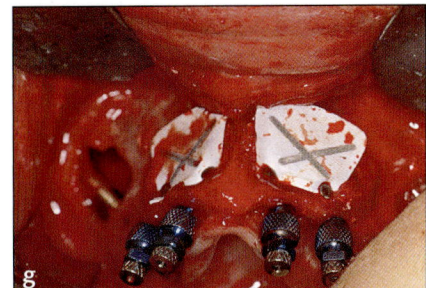

Figs 26-3e to 26-3g Placement of bilateral zygomatic implants with four anterior root form implants were placed. Immediate grafting of thread dehiscences was necessary.

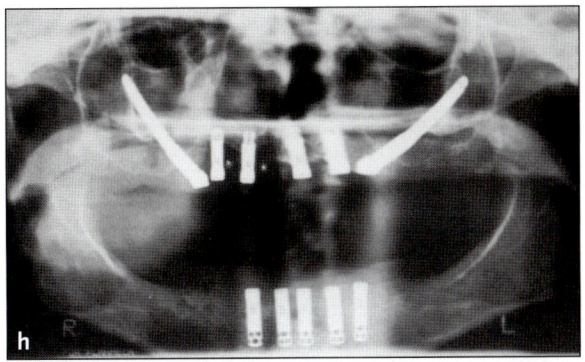

Fig 26-3h Postoperative radiograph showing the maxillary and mandibular implants.

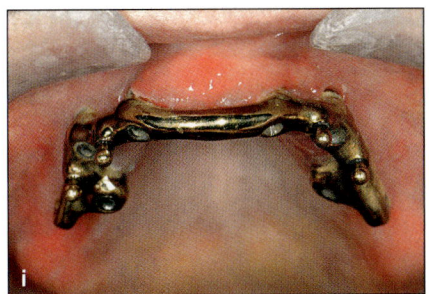 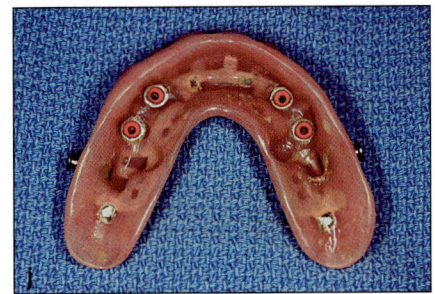 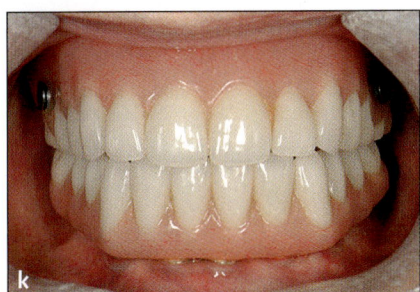

Figs 26-3i to 26-3k Definitive prosthesis is a gold bar with clips and a denture without a palate. The mandibular prosthesis is a fixed-detachable denture.

Fixed prostheses

Zygomatic implants are considered the prime alternative to sinus bone grafting in the atrophic edentulous maxilla when a fixed prosthesis is desired. Fixed prostheses are always challenging in the completely edentulous patient because both esthetic and biomechanical considerations must be addressed. Furthermore, when bone mass is deficient, both of these factors are significantly compromised. Nonetheless, it is usually possible to place two, four, or even six conventional implants anteriorly in most edentulous maxillae despite the presence of significant atrophy.

Some studies suggest that as few as four well-distributed implants are sufficient for maxillary restoration. Long-term osseointegration of only four (usually short) implants in type 3 or 4 bone is generally suspect, however. The addition of zygomatic implants is recommended to provide sufficient biomechanical support for a fixed prosthesis. When the maxilla is extremely atrophic, four zygomatic implants have been used successfully when spaced adequately to form a "quad" foundation to support a fixed prosthesis.

The advantages of a fixed over a removable prosthesis include improved chewing, speaking, and swallowing,

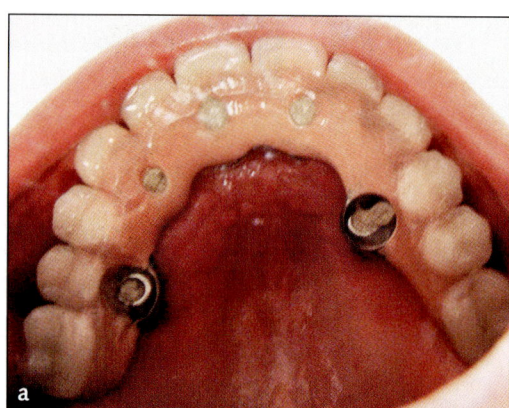
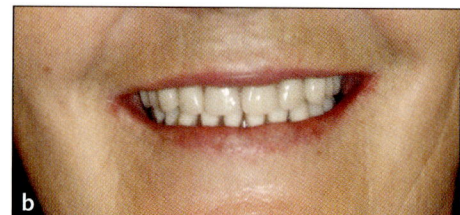
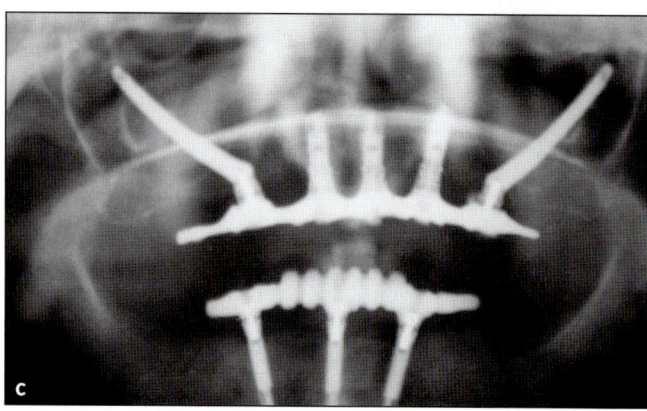

Figs 26-4a to 26-4c Placement of two zygomatic and three conventional implants based on the concepts of "teeth in an hour," guided surgery, and immediate loading.

primarily made possible by the palateless reconstruction. Despite the relatively prominent palatal emergence of the zygomatic implant, patients generally adapt easily, and the bulkiness of the fixed restoration is often diminished as compared to the removable bar clip overdenture attachment.

Treatment planning for a fixed prosthesis with zygomatic implants entails both radiographic (CT scan) and detailed clinical evaluation of patient anatomy. Palpation of the curvature of the sinus wall and the zygoma are essential. Tactile evaluation of the lateral orbital wall, the zygomatic arch, the pterygomaxillary space, and the zygomatic buttress provides visual and sensory cues to correlate with coronal cross-sectional imaging or the preoperative computer software case plan. In the end the surgeon must establish optimal positioning of the zygomatic anchorage to achieve the desired treatment plan or a fixed prosthesis will not be possible.

The surgeon and patient must decide together upon the appropriate treatment plan. The choice of bone graft reconstruction and zygomatic implant reconstruction should be fully discussed. The case for the zygomaticus is a strong one not only because bone graft healing can be avoided, but the morbidity and time course of treatment are more favorable (Figs 26-4 to 26-7). Though the zygomatic approach would appear to be more risky than sinus elevation, a well-trained surgeon will experience much less morbidity with the placement of the zygoma implant than with harvesting of bone from the tibia, hip, or jaw for sinus elevation. The course of healing is much shorter with the zygoma, especially if delayed implant placement is prescribed. Also, recent efforts at early or even immediate fixed provisionalization have been promising. In the future, the use of computer-based planning for the zygoma suggests that the definitive prosthesis can be placed provided there are sufficient anterior implants to maintain primary stability. Zygomatic implants have a very high success rate of 98% (from a multicenter study) to 100%[9] with a follow-up of up to 48 months.

Zygoma implants can also be used in posterior partially edentulous cases, typically with a placement plan of one zygoma implant and two conventional implants. Occasionally, two zygoma implants and only one conventional implant are placed depending on the availability of bone. The fixed prosthesis in this situation can extend from the canine to the second molar without difficulty and can be immediately provisionalized.

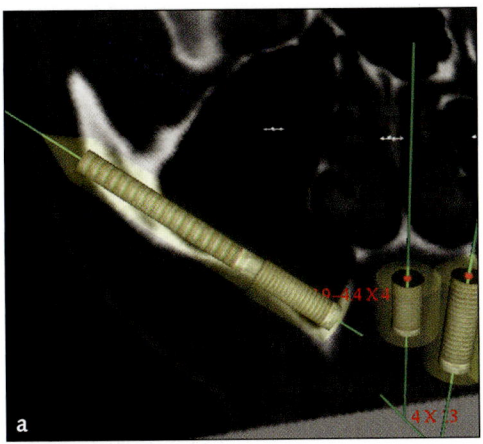
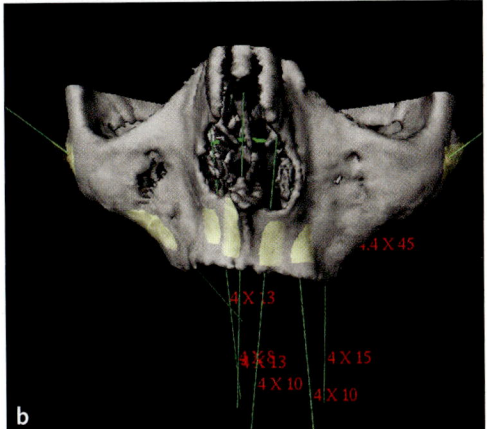

Figs 26-5a and 26-5b Use of software for radiographic treatment planning and positioning of zygomatic implants.

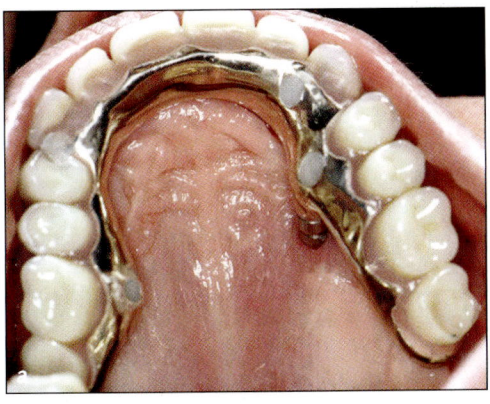
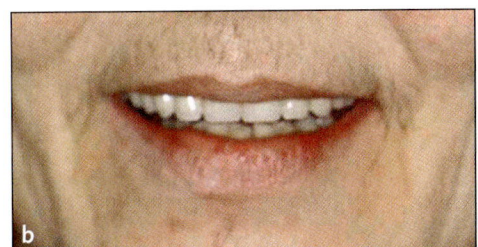

Figs 26-6a and 26-6b Definitive acrylic-gold fixed prosthesis 6 years postrestoration. (a) Occlusal view. (b) Esthetic result.

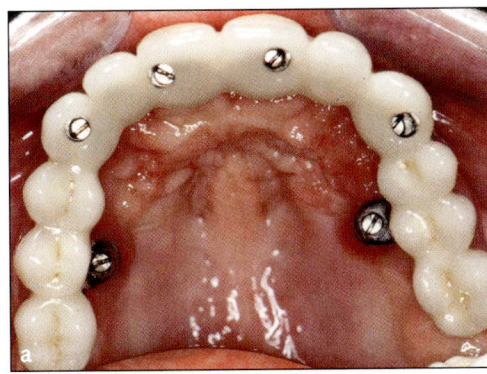
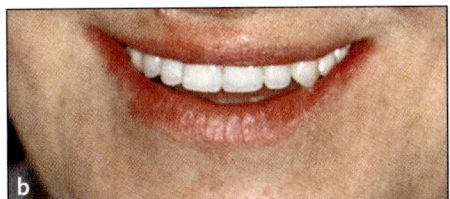

Figs 26-7a and 26-7b Definitive acrylic-porcelain fixed prosthesis. (a) Occlusal view. (b) Esthetic result.

When patients have mandibular dentition or decreased mouth opening, placement of the zygomaticus is more difficult. At some point a limited oral opening may preclude the technical placement of zygomatic implants unless a percutaneous approach is used.

The biomechanical power of the zygomatic anchorage provides the restorative dentist with a strong advantage over conventional implants, making a fixed restoration achievable in what often would otherwise require major bone graft reconstruction.

Potential Complications

A number of complications have been associated with the placement of zygomatic implants, but most can be avoided by following a meticulous surgical technique. Potential complications include pain, infection, excessive bleeding, palpability, zygomaticofacial paresthesia, ocular injury (if the orbit is entered), loss of implants, and sinusitis. Informed consent that includes the possibility of ocular injury is important. Extreme caution should be exercised during implant placement to prevent inadvertent entry into the orbit.

Summary

The introduction of zygomatic implants has expanded the options for restoration of the atrophic maxilla. Treatment time has been shortened, and there is improved patient acceptance. Since 1999, 18 patients have been treated (17 bilaterally and 1 unilaterally) with removable prostheses and followed from 1 to 5 years, resulting in the loss of one implant. All conventional implants (n = 70) placed in the anterior maxilla have been retained as well.

In the fixed restoration setting, two zygomatic implants are supplemented with two to six conventional implants placed anteriorly. For posterior partial edentulism, one zygoma implant and two conventional implants are typically placed. The reported success rate for fixed prosthetic restorations is 100% for 103 implants in 55 patients followed for 0.5 to 4 years.[9]

The learning curve for surgical placement of zygomatic implants is significant, primarily because they involve the use of unfamiliar instrumentation. Because the implants are exceptionally long, the surgeon must have adequate wound exposure and a competent and well-trained surgical assistant. Once appropriate implant angulation through the residual alveolus and along the most lateral aspect of the zygomatic buttress has been mastered, the technique becomes quite routine.

Given that the restorative platform on the zygomaticus is a standard external hex configuration, the prosthetic aspects are straightforward as well. The most significant prosthodontic hurdle to overcome is added prosthetic bulk on the palate when an overdenture prosthesis is used. If a fixed-hybrid prosthesis or a bar O-ring or bar clip prosthesis is used, the palate can be left open.

For patients who require restoration of the atrophic maxilla, zygomatic implant therapy should be considered as an alternative to sinus bone grafting especially when there is a need to minimize the extent of surgery and the treatment time.

Acknowledgment

This chapter includes material contributed by Dr Zvi Laster, Tiberias, Israel.

References

1. Higuchi KW. The Zygomaticus fixture: An alternative approach for implant anchorage in the posterior maxilla. Ann R Australas Coll Dent Surg 2000;15:28–33.
2. Tolman DE. Reconstructive procedures with endosseous implants in grafted bone: A review of the literature. Int J Oral Maxillofac Implants 1995;10:275–294.
3. Li KK, Stephens WL, Gliklich R. Reconstruction of the severely atrophic edentulous maxilla using Le Fort I osteotomy with simultaneous bone graft and implant placement. J Oral Maxillofac Surg 1996;54:542–546.
4. Isaksson S. Evaluation of three bone grafting techniques for severely resorbed maxillae in conjunction with immediate endosseous implants. Int J Oral Maxillofac Implants 1994;9:679–688.
5. Adell R, Eriksson B, Lekholm U, Branemark PI, Jemt T. Long-term follow-up study of osseointegrated implants in the treatment of totally edentulous jaws. Int J Oral Maxillofac Implants 1990;5:347–359.
6. Bedrossian E, Stumpel LJ. Immediate stabilization at stage II of zygomatic implants: Rationale and technique. J Prosthet Dent 2001;86:10–14.
7. Triplett RG, Schow SR, Laskin DM. Oral and maxillofacial surgery advances in implant dentistry. Int J Oral Maxillofac Implants 2000;15:47–55.
8. Boyes-Varley JG, Lownie JF, Howes DG. The zygomaticus implant protocol in the treatment of the severely resorbed maxilla. SADJ 2003;58(3):106–114.
9. Malevez C, Abarca M, Durdu F, Daelemans P. Clinical outcome of 103 consecutive zygomatic implants: A 6-48 months follow-up study. Clin Oral Implants Res 2004;15:18–22.
10. Boyes-Varley JG, Howes DG, Lownie JF, Blackbeard GA. Surgical modifications to the Brånemark zygomaticus protocol in the treatment of severely resorbed maxilla: A clinical report. Int J Oral Maxillofac Implants 2003,18:232–237.
11. Stella JP, Warner MR. Sinus slot technique for simplification and improved orientation of zygomaticus dental implants: A technical note. Int J Oral Maxillofac Implants 2000;15:889–893.
12. Malevez C, Daelemans P, Adriaenssens P, Durdu F. Use of zygomatic implants to deal with resorbed posterior maxillae. Periodontol 2000;33:82–89.

chapter 27
Graftless Rehabilitation of the Atrophied Maxilla Using Tilted and Short Implants and Immediate Function

Bo Rangert, PhD, MechEng
Carlos Aparicio, MD, DDS, DLT, MS
Chantal Malevez, MD, DDS
Edmond Bedrossian, DDS
Franck Renouard, DDS
Paulo Maló, DDS
Roberto Calandriello, DDS

The efficacy of dental implant treatment is well documented, and a number of protocols have been developed to simplify the procedures. Nonetheless, simpler treatment protocols are needed for rehabilitation of the posterior maxilla, where insufficient residual bone volume often makes implant placement difficult. The most obvious solution to this problem—extending distal cantilevers for the positioning of posterior teeth—has been associated with biomechanical problems.[1] Of the various options for implant rehabilitation of the posterior maxilla, sinus grafting is the most popular.

Sinus bone grafting relies on the ossification of autogenous bone grafts or bone substitutes to build new bone for implant anchorage.[2,3] Despite the widespread use of this procedure, however, clinical documentation of its efficacy is inconclusive.[4,5] Moreover, patient acceptance is restricted because of the complexity of the technique, the potential for donor site morbidity, the confusing choices of graft type, and the high cost. The survival rate of implants placed into grafted sites is close to 90%[6–9] (see chapter 8) compared to the 95% to 98% survival rate for implants placed in bone. The new development of oxidized implant surfaces has considerably improved the implant survival rate in grafted bone[10–12] (see chapter 18).

The development of osseoconductive implant biomaterials, such as the oxidized surface,[13,14] offers new possibilities to simplify the treatment protocol for treating patients with maxillary atrophy. As bone forms faster and the amount of bone-implant contact is increased, implants respond more effectively to demanding situations, such as when placed in soft or deficient bone in the maxilla. Furthermore, because of the implant's increased osseoconductivity, stability persists during the healing period. This quality represents a clear improvement over nonactivated surfaces such as a machined-surface titanium implant, which may lose stability during the demineralization phase of bone healing.[15,16] Formation of an early modeling callus that is mechanically resistant is essential for immediate implant function.

The concept of immediate function is scientifically accepted[17] and supported by numerous clinical studies. Providing a stable, fixed provisional prosthesis immediately

Chapter 27: Graftless Rehabilitation of the Atrophied Maxilla Using Tilted and Short Implants and Immediate Function

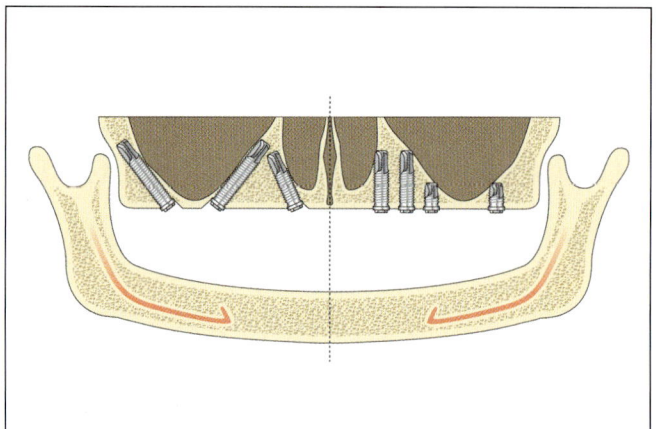

Fig 27-1 By following the anterior sinus wall, tilted implants may be placed in the bone pyramid anterior to the maxillary sinus, where no vital anatomic structures (such as arteries or nerves) are present.

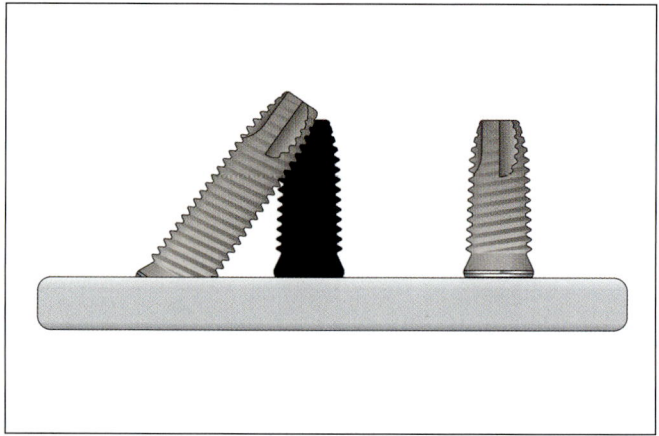

Fig 27-2 The prosthetic load is transferred to the bone via the implant platform (ie, head). Tilting beneath the platform has no influence on the prosthetic support; the position of the platform at the bone crest defines the support point.

after implant placement significantly improves the patient's ability to function and boosts self-esteem. Provided there is high initial implant stability and controlled loading conditions using an osseoconductive implant surface, survival of immediately loaded implants is comparable to that of delayed loading[18–20] and is possible in most clinical situations.

This chapter presents documented clinical protocols for "graftless" rehabilitation of the atrophied maxilla using tilted, zygoma, and short implants and using immediate function. These treatment variations are made possible by recent technologic developments as well as biomechanical analysis.

Avoiding the Sinus with Tilted Implants

The effectiveness of placing implants into the tuberosity area of the pterygoid process is well documented,[21–24] but the technique has been associated with the risk of causing injury to the descending maxillary vasculature.[25] When placed into the retromaxilla, implants are generally tilted anteriorly; however, by tilting them posteriorly, the implants follow the anterior sinus wall and completely avoid the maxillary sinus (Fig 27-1). Cross-arch multi-unit implant placement using this approach extends the prosthetic support posteriorly and anchors the implant in dense bone structures.[20,26–29]

The prosthetic load is transferred to the bone via the implant head or platform. It is the position of the platform at the bone crest, rather than the tilting of the implant beneath the platform, that defines the support point (Fig 27-2). The tilting technique, therefore, provides for prosthetically favorable positioning of the implant heads as well as optimal anchorage in bone. Results of biomechanical analyses[26] and clinical follow-up studies[27,28,30] indicate high survival rates and that the use of tilted implants does not increase bone resorption.

All-on-4

The complete-arch rehabilitation concept known as "All-on-4"[20] uses two posterior tilted implants and two anterior vertical implants to support a complete-arch fixed prosthesis that is placed under immediate function (Fig 27-3). The concept may be applied in either jaw but provides the greatest benefit in the maxilla. Both in vivo implant load analysis and clinical studies demonstrate that four implants are as effective as six for complete-arch rehabilitation of the maxilla.[31,32] Each implant is placed without impinging on adjacent implants. Remarkably, minimal bone volume is needed (Fig 27-4) to establish a 12-tooth fixed prosthesis.[20]

Placement of the posterior implants is facilitated by the use of a surgical guide (Fig 27-5) that is specially designed for precise implant positioning and obtaining the correct

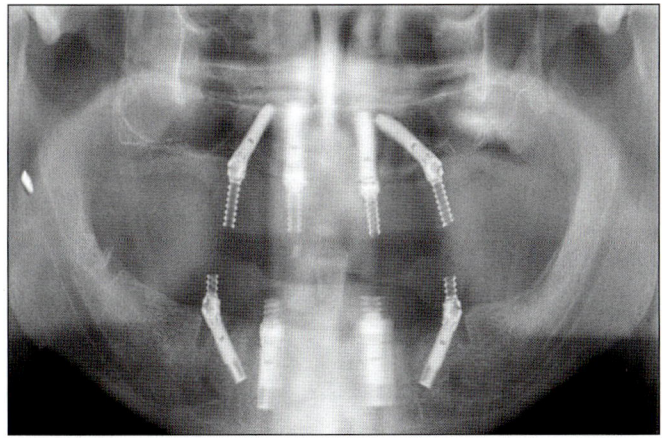

Fig 27-3 The All-on-4 concept uses two posterior tilted implants and two anterior vertical implants to support a complete-arch fixed prosthesis that is placed under immediate function.

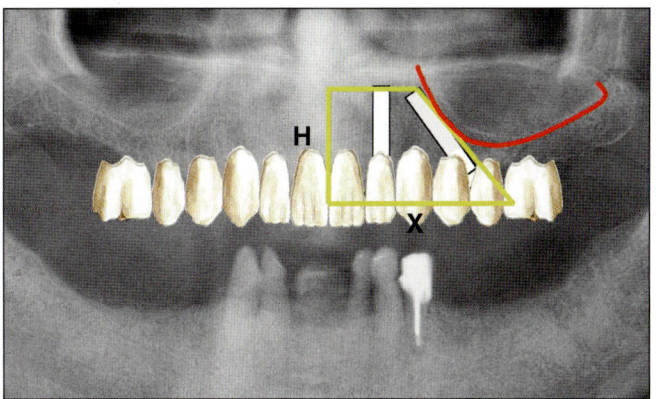

Fig 27-4 The All-on-4 concept can be used to treat varying maxillary atrophy; the determining factor is the position of the posterior implant. The posterior implant head will emerge from different positions at the bone crest, depending on the degree of resorption. The provisional prosthesis should not have more than one cantilever tooth; consequently, the number of teeth under immediate function may be 10 or more, depending on the degree of resorption. (X, crest length > 20 mm; H, height > 10 mm.)

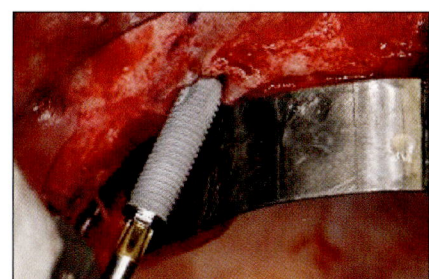

Fig 27-5 A special surgical guide facilitates precise positioning of the implant sites in relation to the opposing jaw and correct tilting of the posterior implant. Tilting the posterior implant makes it possible to position the implant head in the second premolar/first molar region rather than the canine/first premolar region in the case of a vertically placed posterior implant.

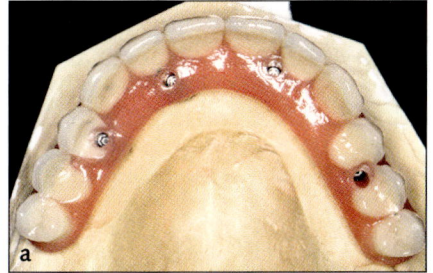

Figs 27-6a and 27-6b The All-on-4 implant arrangement results in a large inter-implant distance and short cantilever lengths. The implant heads and prosthetic screws are placed in prosthetically favorable positions. A high-density, baked all-acrylic prosthesis with titanium cylinders is delivered to the patient within a few hours.

tilt of the posterior implant in relation to the occlusal plane. Tilting makes it possible to place the implant in a canine or first premolar site and yet to position the implant head in the second premolar or even first molar region. Such an arrangement results in a relatively large inter-implant distance and a shortened cantilever length while keeping the implant heads and prosthetic screws placed in prosthetically favorable positions (Figs 27-6a and 27-6b). A high-density, all-acrylic prosthesis with titanium cylinders is delivered to the patient within hours of implant placement (see Fig 27-6b). A more definitive prosthesis may be placed at a later stage. It is estimated that 75% of patients who qualify for maxillary sinus bone grafting could benefit from this procedure.

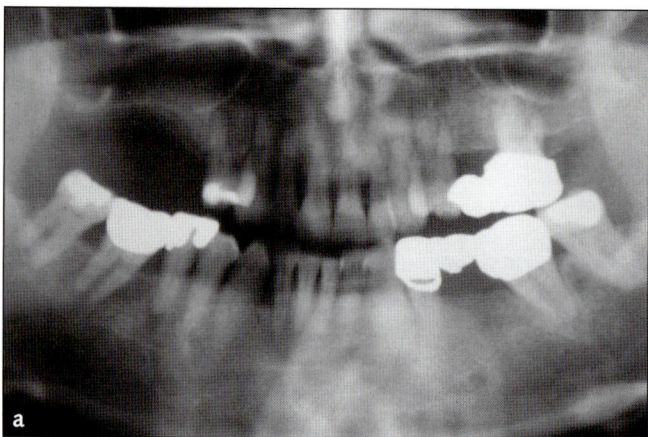
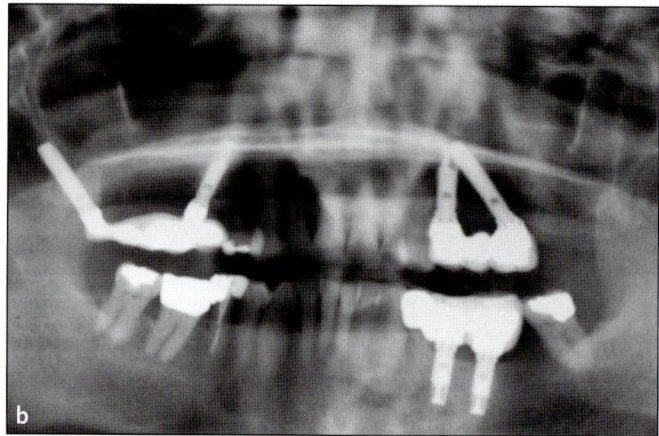

Figs 27-7a and 27-7b Partially edentulous patient treated with tilted implants. The right maxilla has almost no bone posterior to the first premolar. It was successfully treated using one tilted implant at the anterior sinus wall and one in the pterygoid area. The left side benefitted from one straight and one tilted implant following the anterior sinus wall. The mandible was treated with conventional implants.

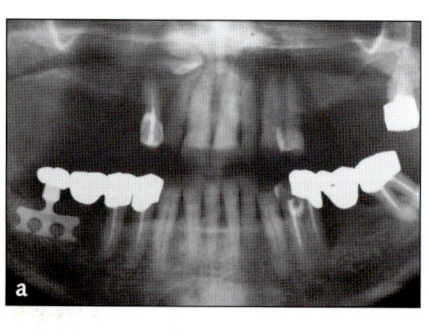
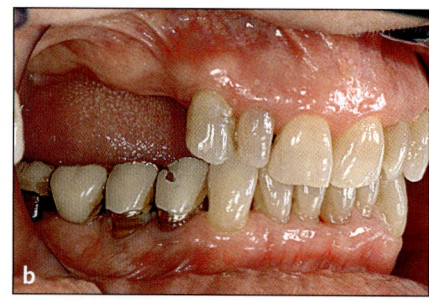
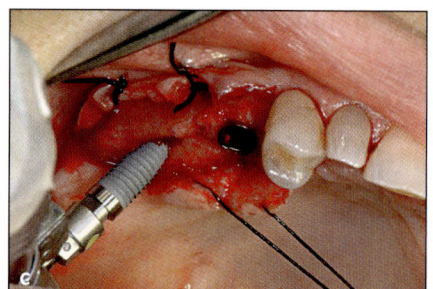
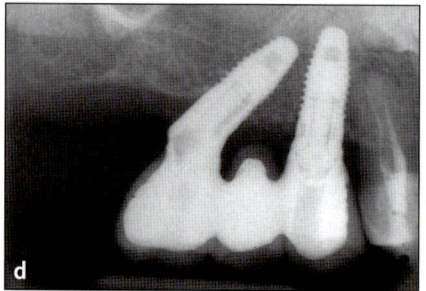
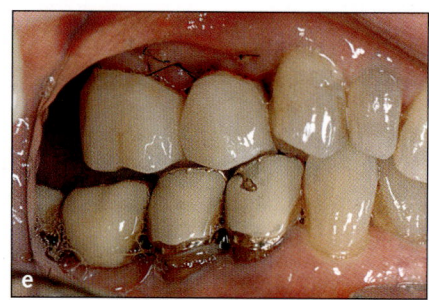
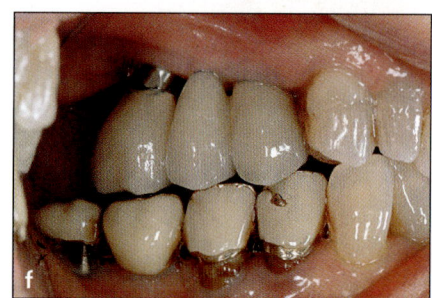

Figs 27-8a to 27-8f Tilting can be combined with immediate function for partial restorations in the atrophied maxilla by using tapered implants with oxidized surfaces. *(a)* Pretreatment panoramic radiograph. *(b)* Severely resorbed maxilla. *(c)* Placement of tilted implant. *(d)* Periapical radiograph after 6 months. *(e)* Provisional prosthesis. *(f)* Definitive prosthesis after 6 months.

Partially edentulous treatment

Restoration of the partially edentulous resorbed maxilla also can be accomplished with the use of tilted implants.[27,30] Partial restorations can be placed under immediate function without cross-arch stabilization,[30] provided that adequate consideration is given to critical load factors.[33] For posterior partial prostheses, tripodization of implants may be an optimum solution for ensuring proper load distribution, although it is not always necessary. For immediate loading in this situation, the reduction of occlusal contacts, particularly the elimination of lateral forces and cantilevers, are means to control the load distribution.

Figures 27-7a and 27-7b document a clinical case in which resorbed maxillary bone is used to anchor tilted implants for optimal prosthetic loading.[27] Figure 27-8 shows how tilting and immediate function are combined for partial restoration of an atrophic maxilla.[30]

Avoiding the Sinus with Tilted Implants

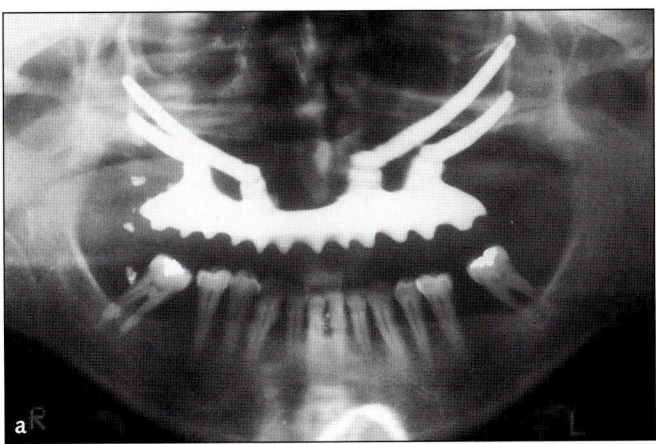 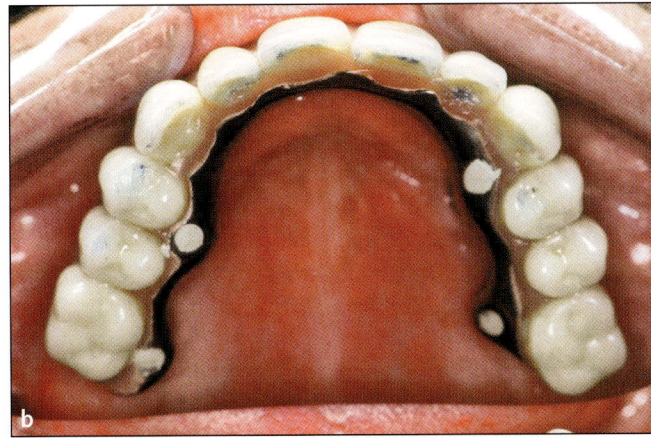

Figs 27-9a and 27-9b Quad zygoma. In patients with severe anterior bone resorption, when the height of bone is less than 10 mm, the two pre-maxillary implants might be zygoma implants emerging at the level of the canine/first premolar.

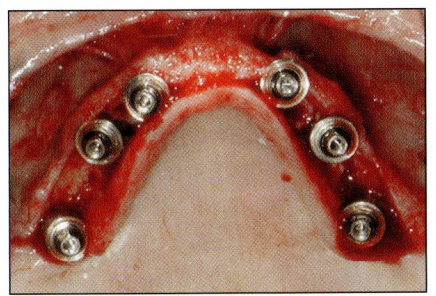 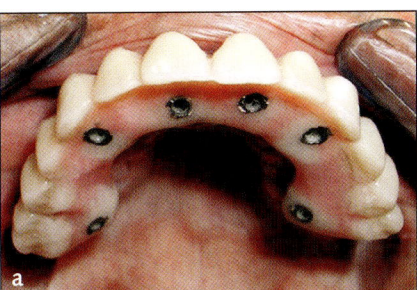 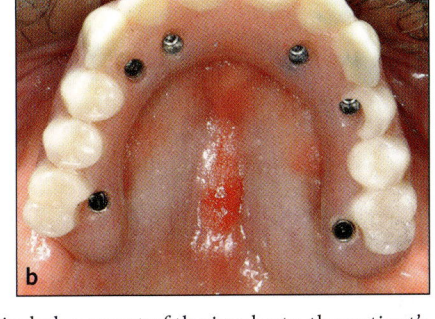

Fig 27-10 Four standard pre-maxillary implants are placed in the canine/central incisor sites as dictated by the surgical stent, and the zygoma implants are placed in the second premolar sites.

Figs 27-11a and 27-11b Following the surgical placement of the implants, the patient's existing denture is converted chairside to an immediate all-acrylic fixed prosthesis (a), which is acceptable until the definitive metal-supported prosthesis (b) is delivered 6 months postoperative.

Zygoma implants

The zygoma implant (see chapter 26) has been used in patients with a moderately to severely resorbed maxilla and has proven successful in supporting fixed prostheses without grafting.[34–37] The off-axis position of the zygoma implant as well as the potential for insignificant crestal anchorage require tripodization or cross-arch stabilization.[38] In situations when the height of anterior bone is less than 10 mm, the two pre-maxillary implants might be zygoma implants emerging at the level of the canine/first premolar (Figs 27-9a and 27-9b). Preliminary results of this "quad zygoma" implant technique are promising.[39] The implant also has been used in immediate function with four standard pre-maxillary implants placed bilaterally in the canine and central incisor sites and zygoma implants placed bilaterally in the second premolar sites (Fig 27-10). The patient's existing denture is converted chairside to an immediate all-acrylic fixed partial denture (Fig 27-11a), which serves until a provisional metal-supported prosthesis is delivered 6 months postoperative (Fig 27-11b). A 100% implant survival rate after 1 year suggests that this immediate function alternative to sinus grafting has considerable potential.[40]

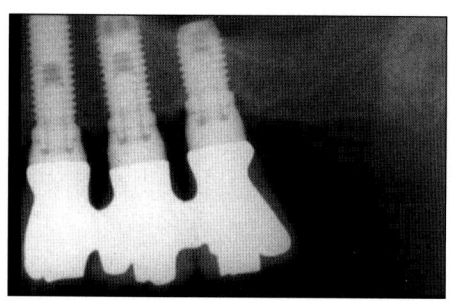

Fig 27-12 Excellent bone stability is demonstrated by these three implants (including one 7-mm-long implant) that were placed 7 years earlier and have remained in function ever since.

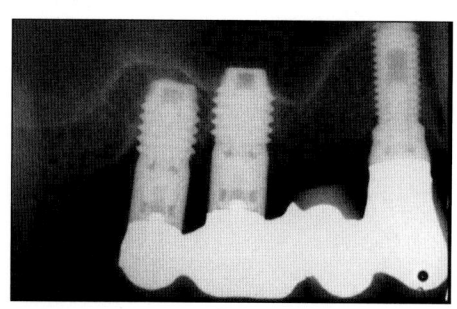

Fig 27-13 Two short (6 mm × 5 mm) implants placed in the sinus 10 years earlier. Note the bone stability around the implant neck.

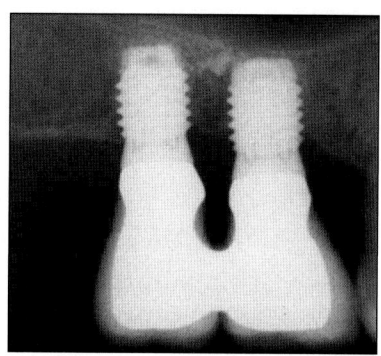

Fig 27-14 Two (6 mm × 5 mm) implants supporting a prosthesis in the posterior maxilla 4 years after loading.

Avoiding Sinus Bone Grafting Using Short Implants

The use of short implants (see Fig 27-1) has long been associated with low success rates.[41–45] However, recent clinical studies indicate that short implants (ie, less than 8.5 mm) that are designed for and achieve high initial stability support most prosthetic restorations quite adequately.[46–50] These clinical findings are supported by theoretical analyses suggesting that long implants often are biomechanically unnecessary, since load transfer between implant and bone often is limited to a few millimeters at the implant's coronalmost point. Bone stress intensity diminishes along the length of the implant body apically, and the effects of loading are often negligible beyond the length of 7 to 8 mm.[51–53]

Most of the implants used in these studies featured modified surfaces for improved osseointegration and resulted in a survival rate of about 95%,[46–50] which compares favorably with the global survival rate (90%)[6–9] of treatment involving bone grafting in preparation for the placement of standard-length implants.

This change of philosophy regarding short implants is a result of improvements in surface morphologies and surgical technique as well as load factor considerations.[33] The oxidized implant surface contributes to the effectiveness of osseointegration.[13,14] Thread anchorage in available cortical bone as well as surgical "underpreparation" improve initial stability.[50] The use of tapered implants may dramatically increase stability, even in low-density bone.[54] There is also speculation that the increased bone flexion of short implants may be an advantage for partial prostheses and lead to reduced lateral forces on the implants.[51]

Figures 27-12 to 27-14 show typical cases in which short implants are used to support a partial prosthesis in a moderately resorbed maxilla.[50] The quantity and position of the implants in these cases are favorable from a loading perspective.[33]

Considerations Related to Graftless Surgery

Graftless rehabilitation of the atrophied maxilla is based on documented biomechanical principles as well as clinical studies. It often offers the possibility of delivering immediate fixed prosthetic function, which is not possible with grafting procedures. Implant survival for these techniques is high (95% to 100%) compared to implants placed in grafted bone (approximately 90%). When comparing different treatment protocols, the overall morbidity (eg, the risk of causing disturbance to the sinus membrane) along with the complication and failure rates for each must be considered. The graftless approach is not only simpler and more appealing to the patient, it is also a safer procedure

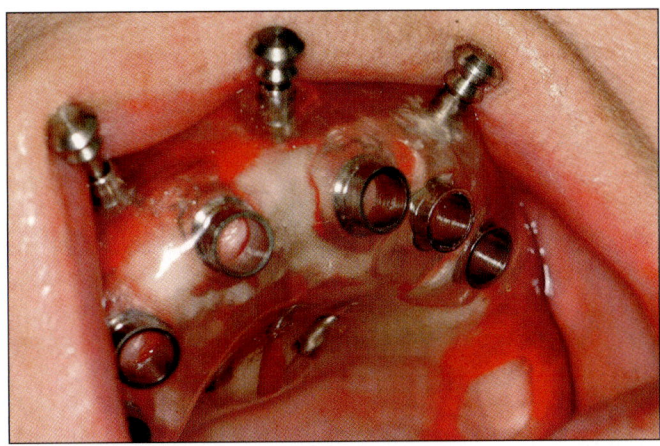

Fig 27-15a Surgical template with the stabilizing pins placed on the maxillary soft tissues for flapless surgery.

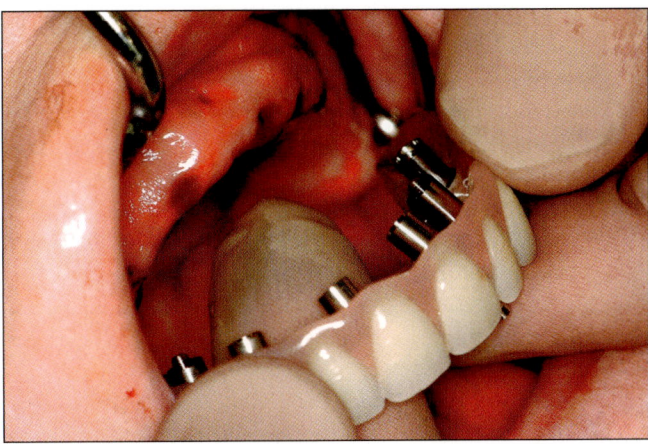

Fig 27-15b The prosthesis is inserted immediately after implant placement.

and a less complex protocol that is nonetheless biomechanically optimal. In contrast, sinus grafting to increase the maxillary bone's load-bearing capacity could be seen as overtreatment.

Recent developments in treatment planning using computerized tomography scanning and virtual planning software increase the potential for graftless procedures. The planning technique makes it possible to place implants even without raising a flap and to manufacture a prefabricated prosthesis for immediate insertion, all with extreme precision (Figs 27-15a and 27-15b).[55–57] This technique increases the potential for immediate function, even in highly resorbed arches.

Conclusion

The use of tilted and short implants is a viable treatment option for graftless rehabilitation of the resorbed maxilla. This new treatment philosophy suggests that sinus grafting may be considered overtreatment in many situations today. Often these graftless protocols may be performed with flapless surgery and immediate function.

References

1. Shackleton JL, Carr L, Slabbert JC, Becker PJ. Survival of fixed implant-supported prostheses related to cantilever lengths. J Prosthet Dent 1994;71:23–26.
2. Jensen OT, Shulman LB, Block MS, Iacono VJ. Report of the Sinus Consensus Conference of 1996. Int J Oral Maxillofac Implants 1998;13(suppl):5–45.
3. Wood RM, Moore DL. Grafting of the maxillary sinus with intraorally harvested autogenous bone prior to implant placement. Int J Oral Maxillofac Implants 1988;3:209–214.
4. Tong DC, Rioux K, Drangsholt M, Bierne OR. A review of survival rates for implants placed in grafted maxillary sinuses using meta-analysis. Int J Oral Maxillofac Implants 1998;13:175–182.
5. Graziani F, Donos N, Needleman N, Gabriele M, Tonetti M. Comparison of implant survival following sinus floor augmentation procedures with implants placed in pristine posterior maxillary bone: A systematic review. Clin Oral Implants Res 2004; 15:677–682.
6. Raghoebar GM, Timmenga NM, Reintsema H, Stegenga B, Vissink A. Maxillary bone grafting for insertion of endosseous implants: Results after 12-124 months. Clin Oral Implants Res 2001;12:279–286.
7. Hallman M, Hedin M, Sennerby L, Lundgren S. A prospective 1-year clinical and radiographic study of implants placed after maxillary sinus floor augmentation with bovine hydroxyapatite and autogenous bone. J Oral Maxillofac Surg 2002;60: 277–284.

8. Wallace SS, Froum SJ. Effect of maxillary sinus augmentation on the survival of endosseous dental implants. A systematic review. Ann Periodontol 2003;8:328–343.
9. Malevez C. Sinus reactions to invasive surgery. In: Jenson OT (ed). The Sinus Bone Graft, ed 2. Chicago: Quintessence, 2006: 115–128.
10. Lundgren S, Brechter M. Preliminary findings of using oxidized titanium implants in reconstructive jaw surgery. Appl Osseointegration Res 2002;3:35–39.
11. Brechter M, Nilson H, Lundgren S. Oxidized titanium implants in reconstructive jaw surgery. Clin Implant Dent Relat Res 2005;7(suppl 1):83–87.
12. Langer L, Langer B. Safety and efficacy of allografts for sinus grafting. In: Jenson OT (ed). The Sinus Bone Graft, ed 2. Chicago: Quintessence, 2006:183–200.
13. Glauser R, Schupbach P, Lundgren AK, Gottlow J, Hämmerle CHF. Machined and oxidized micro-implants retrieved from humans: A comparison using histomorphometry and micro-computed tomography [abstract 64]. Clin Oral Implants Res 2002;13:xxv–xxvi.
14. Ivanoff CJ, Widmark G, Johansson C, Wennerberg A. Histologic evaluation of bone response to oxidized and turned titanium micro-implants in human jawbone. Int J Oral Maxillofac Implants 2003;18:341–348.
15. Rompen E, DaSilva D, Lundgren AK, Gottlow J, Sennerby L. Stability measurements of a double-threaded titanium implant design with turned or oxidized surface. An experimental resonance frequency analysis study in the dog mandible. Appl Osseointegration Res 2000;1:18–20.
16. Glauser R, Portmann M, Ruhstaller P, Lundgren AK, Hämmerle CHF, Gottlow J. Stability measurements of immediately loaded machined and oxidized implants in the posterior maxilla. A comparative clinical study using resonance frequency analysis. Appl Osseointegration Res 2001;2:27–29.
17. Aparicio C, Rangert B, Sennerby L. Immediate/early loading of dental implants: A report from the Sociedad Española de Implantes World Congress consensus meeting in Barcelona, Spain, 2002. Clin Implant Dent Relat Res 2003;5:57–60.
18. Glauser R, Lundgren AK, Gottlow J, et al. Immediate occlusal loading of Brånemark System TiUnite implants placed predominantly in soft bone: 1-year results of a prospective, clinical study. Clin Implant Dent Relat Res 2003;5(suppl 1):47–56.
19. Ganeles J, Wismeijer D. Immediate and early loaded dental implants in single-tooth and partial-arch rehabilitation. Int J Oral Maxillofac Implants 2004;19(suppl):92–102.
20. Maló P, Rangert B, Nobre M. "All-on-4" immediate-function concept with Brånemark System implants for completely edentulous maxillae: A 1-year retrospective clinical study. Clin Implant Dent Relat Res 2005;7(suppl 1):S88–S94.
21. Tulasne JF. Osseointegrated fixtures in the pterygoid region. In: Worthington P, Brånemark PL (eds). Advanced Osseointegration Surgery. Applications in the Maxillofacial Region. Chicago: Quintessence, 1992:182–188.
22. Raspall G, González J, Bescós S, Hueto JA. Pterygomaxillary osseointegrated fixture [abstract]. J Craniomaxillofac Surg 1992; 20:57–58.
23. Graves SL. The pterygoid plate implant: A solution for restoring the posterior maxilla. Int J Periodontics Restorative Dent 1994; 14:513–523.
24. Fernández Valerón J, Fernández Velázquez J. Placement of screw type implants in the pterygomaxillary pyramidal region: Surgical procedure and preliminary results. Int J Oral Maxillofac Implants 1997;6:814–819.
25. Choi J, Park HS. The clinical anatomy of the maxillary artery in the pterygopalatine fossa. J Oral Maxillofac Surg 2003;61:72–78.
26. Krekmanov L, Kahn M, Rangert B, Lindström H. Tilting of posterior mandibular and maxillary implants of improved prosthesis support. Int J Oral Maxillofac Implants 2000;15:405–414.
27. Aparicio C, Perales P, Rangert B. Tilted implants as an alternative to maxillary sinus grafting: A clinical, radiologic, and Periotest study. Clin Implants Dent Rel Res 2001;3:39–49.
28. Aparicio C, Arévalo JX, Ouazzani W, Granados C. Retrospective clinical and radiographic evaluation of tilted implants used in the treatment of the severely resorbed edentulous maxilla. Applied Osseointegration Res 2002;3:17–21.
29. Fortin Y, Sullivan RM, Rangert BR. The Marius implant bridge: Surgical and prosthetic rehabilitation for the completely edentulous upper jaw with moderate to severe resorption: A 5-year retrospective clinical study. Clin Implant Dent Relat Res 2002; 4:69–77.
30. Calandriello R, Tomatis M. Simplified treatment of the atrophic posterior maxilla via immediate/early function and tilted implants: A prospective 1-year clinical study. Clin Implant Dent Relat Res 2005;7(suppl 1):S1–S12.
31. Duyck J, Van Oosterwyck H, Vander Sloten J, De Cooman M, Puers R, Naert I. Magnitude and distribution of occlusal forces on oral implants supporting fixed prostheses: An in vivo study. Clin Oral Implants Res 2000;11:465–475.
32. Brånemark P-I, Svensson B, van Steenberghe D. Ten-year survival rates of fixed prostheses on four or six implants ad modum Brånemark in full edentulism. Clin Oral Implants Res 1995; 6:227–231.
33. Rangert B, Sullivan R, Jemt T. Load factor control for implants in the posterior partially edentulous segment. Int J Oral Maxillofac Implants 1997;12:360–370.
34. Aparicio C, Brånemark P-I, Keller EE, Olive J. Reconstruction of the premaxilla with autogenous iliac bone in combination with osseointegrated implants. Int J Oral Maxillofac Implants 1993; 8:61–67.
35. Stevenson ARL, Austin BW. Zygomatic fixtures. The Sydney experience. Ann Roy Australia Coll Dent Surg 2000;15:337–339.
36. Bedrossian E, Stumpel LJ. The zygomatic implant: Preliminary data on treatment of severely resorbed maxillae. A clinical report. Int J Oral Maxillofac Implants 2002;17:861–865.
37. Malevez C, Abarca M, Durdu F, Dalemans P. Clinical outcome of 103 consecutive zygomatic implants: A 6-48 month follow-up study. Clin Oral Implants Res 2004;15:18–22.
38. Bedrossian E, Stumpel LJ. Immediate stabilization at stage II of zygomatic implants: Rationale and technique. Int J Oral Maxillofac Implants 2000;15:10–14.

39. Malevez C. Clinical outcome of 4 zygomatic implants for the rehabilitation of extremely resorbed edentulous maxillas: A preliminary report. Presented at the 11th International Congress on Reconstructive and Preprosthetic Surgery, Noordwijk, The Netherlands, 21–23 April 2005.
40. Bedrossian E, Rangert B, Stumpel L, Indersano T. Immediate function with the Zygoma implant—A graft-less solution for the patient with mild to advanced atrophy of the maxilla. Int J Oral Maxillofac Implants 2006;(accepted for publication).
41. van Steenberghe D, Lekholm U, Bolender C, et al. Applicability of osseointegrated oral implants in the rehabilitation of partial edentulism. A prospective multicenter study on 558 fixtures. Int J Oral Maxillofac Implants 1990;5:272–281.
42. Jaffin RA, Berman CL. The excessive loss of Brånemark fixtures in type IV bone: A 5-year analysis. J Periodontol 1991;62:2–4.
43. Friberg B, Jemt T, Lekholm U. Early failures in 4,641 consecutively placed Brånemark dental implants: A study from stage 1 surgery to the connection of completed prostheses. Int J Oral Maxillofac Implants 1991;6:142–146.
44. Moy PK, Bain CA. Relation between fixture length and implant failure [abstract 972]. J Dent Res 1992;71(special issue):637.
45. Sennerby L, Roos J. Surgical determinants of clinical success of osseointegrated oral implants. A review of literature. Int J Prosthodont 1998;11:408–420.
46. ten Bruggenkate CM, Asikainen P, Foitzik C, Krekeler G, Sutter F. Short (6-mm) nonsubmerged dental implants. Results of a multicenter clinical trial of 1 to 7 years. Int J Oral Maxillofac Implants 1998;13:791–798.
47. Stellingsmaa C, Meijer HJA, Raghoebar GM. Use of short endosseous implants and an overdenture in the extremely resorbed mandible. A five-year retrospective study. J Oral Maxillofac Surg 2000;58:382–387.
48. Tawil G, Younan R. Clinical evaluation of short, machined-surface implants followed for 12 to 92 months. Int J Oral Maxillofac Implants 2003;18:894–901.
49. Fugazzotto P, Beagle J, Ganeles J, Jaffin R, Vlassis J, Kumar A. Success and failure rates of 9 mm or shorter implants in the replacement of missing maxillary molars when restored with individual crowns: Preliminary results 0 to 84 months in function. A retrospective study. J Periodontol 2004;75:327–332.
50. Renouard F, Nisand D. Short implants in the severely resorbed maxilla: A 2-year retrospective clinical study. Clin Implant Dent Relat Res 2005;7(suppl 1):S104–S110.
51. Pierrisnard L, Renouard F, Renault P, Barquins M. Influence of implant length and bicortical anchorage on implants stress distribution. Clin Implant Dent Relat Res 2003;5:254–262.
52. Meijer HJA, Kuipner JH, Starmans FJM, Bosman F. Stress distribution around dental implants: Influence of superstructure, length of implants and height of mandible. J Prosthet Dent 1992;68:96–102.
53. Akca K, Cehreli MC, Iplikcioglu H. A comparison of three-dimensional finite element stress analysis with in vitro strain gauge measurements on dental implants. Int J Prosthodont 2002;15:115–121.
54. Rompen E, DaSilva D, Hockers T, et al. Influence of implant design on primary fit and stability. A RFA and histological comparison of Mk III and Mk IV Brånemark implants in the dog mandible. Appl Osseointegration Res 2001;2:9–11.
55. van Steenberghe D, Naert I, Andersson M, Brajnovic I, Van Cleynenbreugel J, Suetens P. A custom template and definite prosthesis allowing immediate implant loading in the maxilla: A clinical report. Int J Oral Maxillofac Implants 2002;17:663–670.
56. Wendelhag I, van Steenberghe D, Blombäck U, Glauser R. Immediate function in edentulous maxillae with flapless surgery including a 3-D CT-scan based treatment planning procedure [abstract]. Clin Oral Implants Res 2004;15:lxxiii.
57. van Steenberghe D, Glauser R, Blombäck U, et al. A computed tomographic scan–derived customized surgical template and fixed prosthesis for flapless surgery and immediate loading of implants in fully edentulous maxillae: A prospective multicenter study. Clin Implant Dent Relat Res 2005;7(suppl 1):S111–S120.

Section 4

Looking to the Future

chapter 28
Stromal Stem Cell Preparation from Iliac Bone Marrow Aspirate for Sinus Bone Grafting

Ole T. Jensen, DDS, MS

Historical Perspective

Interest in the osteogenic potential of bone marrow aspirate dates back at least to 1869, when Goujon reported the first use of autologous bone marrow to form bone, and has continued ever since.[1] In the early part of the twentieth century, Chutro demonstrated the use of marrow containing bone graft for long bone fracture repair.[2] McGaw and Harbin later established the role of bone marrow in osteogenic regeneration.[3] Friedenstein and colleagues isolated and cultured what they called "bone marrow fibroblasts" in vitro and later established their osteogenic potential.[4–6] Castro-Maloaspina et al purified these cell populations,[7] and Caplan[8] and Haynesworth et al[9] first identified them as progenitors by their ability to differentiate into osteoblasts, chondroblasts, myoblasts, and diverse other phenotypes. Owen discovered that when transplanted under the capsule of a kidney, these cells produced bone, cartilage, fat, and other tissues.[10,11] Procktop first proposed the term *stromal stem cell* to describe its role as a multipotent precursor cell for nonhematopoietic tissues.[12] (The term it replaced, *mesenchymal stem cell*, is something of a misnomer because it does not allow for the capacity of these cells to become hepatic and neuronal cells.[13,14]) Manjumdar et al then culture expanded these cells and produced a variety of phenotypic progenitors,[15] while Reyes et al determined that the differentiation capacity of osteogenic lineage cells cultured from bone marrow was maintained after as many as 40 doublings.[16,17] According to current estimates, only 2 to 5 stromal stem cells will be found, on average, in every 1 million bone cells,[18] and only 1 in 18,000 nucleated cells is estimated to be a stem cell.[19]

All stromal cells do not perform the same function. In 1999, Pittenger et al reported that only one third of all stromal stem cells are pluripotent (osteoblasts, chondroblasts, and adipoblasts).[20] Muraglia et al confirmed that one third of all bone marrow–derived cell clones are tripotent (osteoblasts, chondroblasts, and adipoblasts) and that the remaining cells are either bipotent (osteoblasts and chondroblasts) or unipotent (osteoblasts).[21] The stromal stem cell population thus is actually comprised of subpopulations of already differentiating cells, and the existence of the stem cell itself remains putative.[22]

Baksh et al introduced a model that suggests that the stem cell "niche" contains heterogeneous stem cell constituents that are quad-, tri-, bi-, or unipotential.[23] The proportion of these phenotypes and the way in which in vitro culturing is carried out determines which cellular constituents elaborate in culture. The stem cell compartment is contrasted with a "committed" cell compartment, both of which are found in bone marrow aspirate. Stem cell compartment cells are multipotent cells that divide either into other stem cells or into precursor (multipotent) cells and then into tri- or bipotent cells. These cell differentiations

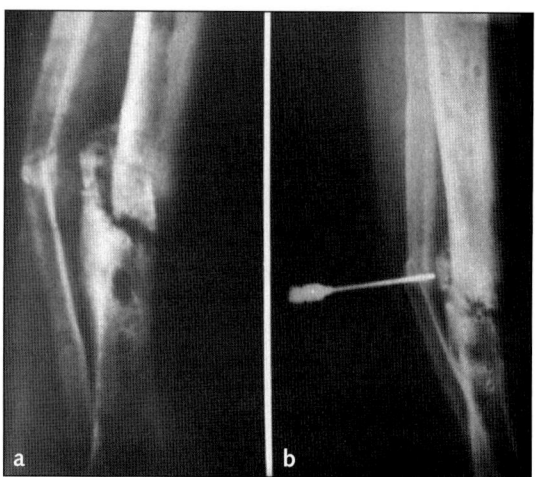
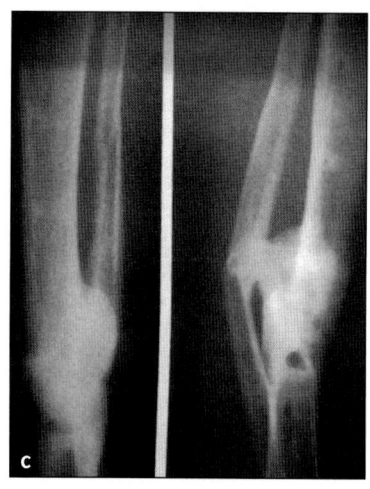

Figs 28-1a and 28-1b *(a)* Lateral radiograph of infected tibia-fibula nonunion fracture 8 months postinjury. *(b)* Posterolateral injection of 85 mL of bone marrow aspirate.

Fig 28-1c Anteroposterior and lateral views of bone healing 8 months after bone marrow injection.

are reversible. But when further differentiation into unipotent progenitor cells occurs, the cells enter the committed cell compartment, where phenotype differentiation is not reversible unless potent inductive cues, such as those delivered by morphogens or growth factors, are present.[23]

Bone-forming stem cells may be characterized as either *adherent* or *nonadherent*. Because they adhere to plastic surfaces and can be easily separated for expansion, adherent stem cells are generally the type obtained for culture. Nonadherent osteoblast lineage cells, the so-called lining cells that appear to be quiescent, recently were reported to be present in peripheral blood in as much as 2% of mononuclear cells. The proportion of circulatory osteoblast-forming cells was found to be greater in growing adolescents than in adults and greater also in individuals with conditions associated with accelerated osseous wound healing, such as a bone fracture repair or bone graft reconstruction.[24]

Osteoblasts are thought to be present in the circulation not only as a source of bone-forming cells, but *primarily* to function through the circulation under certain specific conditions. Osteoblasts gain access to the basic multicellular unit of remodeling via the circulation and not by proximate cell migration from the bone marrow, since the cell-lined compartment is otherwise enclosed.[25,26]

The use of ex vivo cell expansion to produce osteoblasts from bone marrow aspirate is not without functional and practical limitations. Cultured cells may not function entirely like fresh bone marrow aspirate. Hematologic stem cells cultured for hematologic transplantation showed reduced homing efficiency to both bone marrow and spleen. There may be some altered function with expanded stromal stem cells as well. And there is always the practical aspect of laboratory time and cost of cell culturing to be considered (see chapter 25).[27,28]

However, it is clear that, as Yoshikawa et al and others have shown, isolated and cultured mesenchymal stem cells implanted into critical-sized bone defects demonstrate profound osteogenesis.[29-34] Presently, Gao and Caplan,[35] Ueda et al,[36] Schimming and Schmelzeisen,[37] Quarto et al,[34] and others culture marrow cells to differentiate and expand osteoblasts for transplantation (see chapter 25). Early reports, especially in the area of maxillofacial surgery, have been promising. But what of the use of simple autologous bone marrow immediately injected following aspiration into an osseous defect? Might there be a synergistic effect from the multiple cellular constituents of fresh marrow?[34,38,39] Is this simple technique now considered obsolete?

Recent Applications of Bone Marrow Aspirate

The technique of using bone marrow aspirate to treat various maxillofacial defects was developed by Boyne,[40] and although it has never gained widespread acceptance, the technique has been used ever since in oral and maxillofacial reconstruction, alveolar cleft repair, and periodontics.[41]

Fig 28-2 With the patient in a prone or lateral decubitus position, an 11-gauge needle is passed into the bone marrow of the posterior wing of the ilium, just beneath the posterosuperior iliac spine.

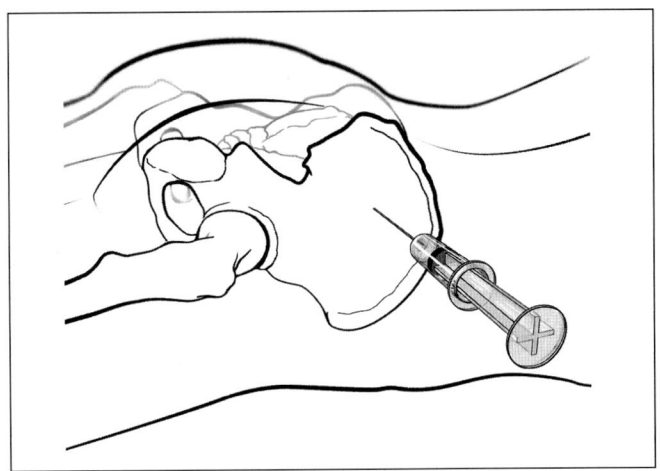

In 1986, Connolly and Shindell reported the results of a study in which they injected 85 mL of autologous bone marrow percutaneously into an 8-month-old infected tibial fracture (Type III B). The fracture was then immobilized with a plaster cast for 6 months, by which time complete repair with exuberant callus formation was observed (Fig 28-1).[18,42] More recently, osseous healing of long bone nonunions using *only* autologous bone marrow aspirate as a graft has been reported in a series of patients, resulting in a 70% to 90% success rate. This finding has been confirmed in animal studies as well.[43–45]

The most productive bone for marrow cell harvest is the posterior ilium, either at the posterosuperior iliac spine or along the superior aspect of the posterior wing (Fig 28-2). Average cell counts of 30,000/dL are obtainable at each of these sites.[18] For maxillofacial surgery, a relatively small volume (about 10 to 20 mL) is needed to ensure adequate cell count. However, centrifuge technology can be used to isolate the cell fraction and thereby reduce transplant volume. Connolly and Shindell reported that cells derived via differential centrifugation increased both the rate and quantity of bone formed, which suggests that osteogenic potential is not disturbed by centrifugation.[18] Concentrating mesenchymal cells into about 2 to 3 mL is a practical requirement for application in areas of limited dimension, such as the sinus floor graft.

Connolly et al found that the use of bone marrow aspirate did not shorten the healing period required for long bone fracture repair, but the procedure was described as safe, less morbid than open wound surgery, and required minimal surgical time.[46] For oral and maxillofacial surgeons, combining marrow cell concentrate with an alloplast recalls the surgical approach used in the 1980s by Salama and Weissman, who mixed Kiel bone (deproteinized calf bone) and marrow aspirate to treat a wide range of orthopedic defects.[47] They found the technique simple, minimally invasive, time saving, less prone to complication, and as effective as standard bone grafting in the vast majority of cases treated.

Bone Marrow Aspiration Technique

With the patient in a lateral decubitus or prone position, the posterior hip is prepped and draped in a sterile manner. The posterosuperior iliac spine is palpated, and a percutaneous needle entry is made 2 cm below the spine and 3 cm lateral to the midline all the way to the bone using an 11-gauge needle (see Fig 28-2). After punching through the cortex, blood is drawn from the marrow space, usually in 2- to 3-mL aliquots. The needle is then redirected without being completely removed, and the process is repeated around the posterior iliac wing. An alternative approach is to insert the needle superior-inferiorly adjacent to the posterosuperior iliac spine, where the cortex is thinner and the marrow space can easily be found with a multiport needle. A 15-gauge needle can be used to aspirate marrow from the anterior iliac crest, which is perhaps the easiest area to access. After 2 mL of blood is withdrawn, the needle is redirected dorsally, caudally, and medially within the marrow space. (Continuous aspiration

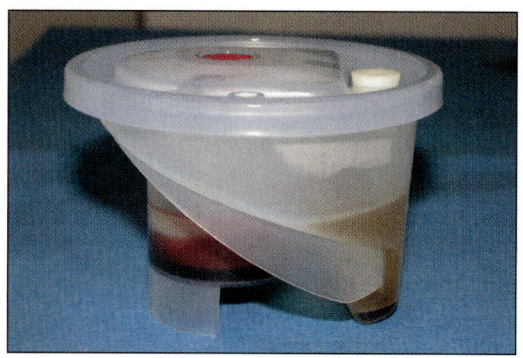

Fig 28-3 Double centrifugation of the aspirate yields a small volume of nucleated cellular fraction.

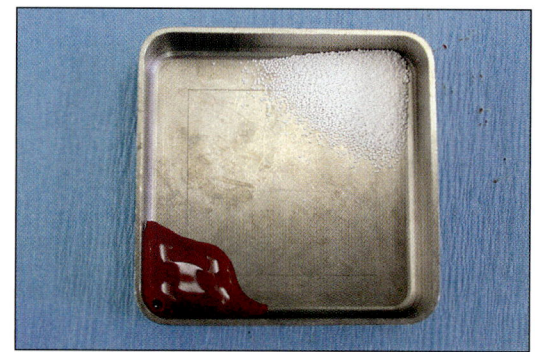

Fig 28-4 The cell concentrate is mixed with β-TCP.

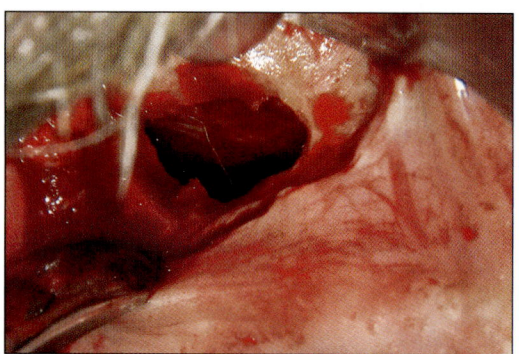

Fig 28-5a Sinus elevation procedure.

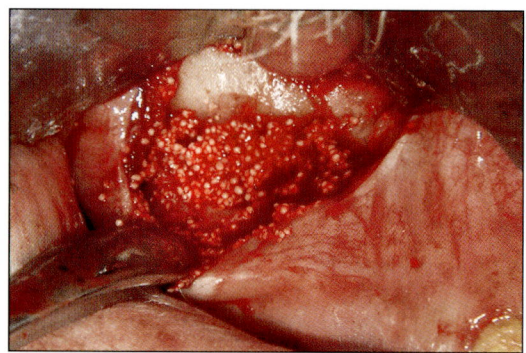

Fig 28-5b Placement of the marrow concentrate–enriched resorbable alloplast into the sinus.

in one site should be avoided because it will yield mostly venous blood.) Most stem cells are derived in the first 2 mL. About 10 mL of aspirate is recommended for most sinus graft situations. The aspirate is then placed into the centrifuge for cell separation.[48,49] Postaspiration discomfort is usually limited to 1 to 3 days.

Stromal cell separation

The centrifuge separates serum and blood and fractionates the cellular residuum, including platelets (Fig 28-3).

Graft preparation

Following cell separation, biphase porous β-tricalcium phosphate (β-TCP) is mixed with the cell concentrate (Fig 28-4). β-TCP has been shown to be a favorable cell attachment vehicle for bone formation.[50–52] The cell preparation is placed beneath the sinus membrane, and the wound is closed with resorbable sutures (Fig 28-5). Dental implants can be placed immediately or 3 to 4 months later, according to standard osseointegration protocols.

This unstudied technique may prove to be as successful as using autograft alone, and it appears to be equally effective in the elderly and younger patient.[53–59]

Summary

Stromal stem cells derived from iliac bone marrow aspirate and concentrated by centrifugation can serve as a promising adjunct to initiate osteogenesis at the sinus floor. Using β-TCP as a space-maintaining carrier, bone harvesting is avoided while autogenous inductivity is preserved.

References

1. Goujon E. Recherches expérimentales sur les propriétés. J Anat 1869;(6):399–412.
2. Chutro P. Greffe osseuse du tibia. Bulletins et mémoires de la Société des chirurgiens de Paris 1918;44:570.
3. McGaw WH, Harbin M. The role of bone marrow and endostium in bone regeneration. An experimental study of bone marrow and endosteal transplants. J Bone Joint Surg 1934;16:816–821.
4. Friedenstein AJ. Osteogenetic activity of transplanted transitional epithelium. Acta Anat 1961;45:31–59.
5. Friedenstein AJ, Chailakhjan RK, Lalykina KS. The development of fibroblast colonies in monolayer cultures of guinea-pig bone marrow and spleen cells. Cell Tissue Kinet 1970;3:393–403.
6. Friedenstein AJ. Osteogenic stem cells in the bone marrow. Bone Miner 1991;7:243–272.
7. Castro-Malaspina H, Gay RE, Resnick G, et al. Characterization of human bone marrow fibroblast colony-forming cells (CFU-F) and their progeny. Blood 1980;56:289–301.
8. Caplan AI. Mesenchymal stem cells. J Orthop Res 1991;9:641–650.
9. Haynesworth SE, Goshima J, Goldberg VM, Caplan AI. Characterization of cells with osteogenic potential from human marrow. Bone 1992;13:82–88.
10. Owen M. The origin of bone cells in the postnatal organism. Arthritis Rheum 1980;23:1073–1080.
11. Owen M. Lineage of osteogenic cells and their relationship to the stromal system. In: Peck WA (ed). Bone and Mineral Research Annual. Vol 3: A Yearly Survey of Developments in the Field of Bone and Mineral Metabolism. Amsterdam: Elsevier, 1985:1–25.
12. Procktop DJ. Marrow stromal cells as stem cells for non-hematopoietic tissues. Science 1997;276:71–74.
13. Schwartz RD, Reyes M, Koodie L, et al. Multipotent adult progenitor cells from bone marrow differentiate into functional hepatocyte-like cells. J Clin Invest 2002;109(10):1291–1302.
14. Simmons PJ, Gronthos S. Isolation, characterization and functional activity of human marrow stromal progenitors in hemopoiesis. Prog Clin Biol Res 1994;389:271–280.
15. Manjumdar M, Thiede M, Mosca J, Moorman M, Gerson S. Phenotypic and functional comparison of cultures of marrow-derived mesenchymal stem cells (MSCs) and stromal cells. J Cell Phys 1998;176:57–66.
16. Reyes M, Dudek A, Jahagirdar B, Kookie L, Marker PH, Verfaillie CM. Origin of endothelial progenitors in human postnatal bone marrow. J Clin Invest 2002;109:337–346.
17. Reyes M, Lund T, Lenvik T, Aguiar D, Koodie L, Verfaillie CM. Purification and ex vivo expansion of postnatal human marrow mesodermal progenitor cells. Blood 2001;98:2615–2625.
18. Connolly JF, Guse R, Tiedeman J, Dehne R. Autologous marrow injection for delayed unions of the tibia—A preliminary report. J Orthop Trauma 1989;3:276.
19. Lucarelli E, Donati D, Cenacchi A, Fornasari PM. Bone reconstruction of large defects using bone marrow derived autologous stem cells. Transfus Apheres Sci 2004;30:169–174.
20. Pittenger MF, Mackay AM, Beck SC, et al. Multilineage potential of adult human mesenchymal stem cells. Science 1999;284:143–147.
21. Muraglia A, Cancedda R, Quarto R. Clonal mesenchymal progenitors from human bone marrow differentiate in vitro according to a hierarchical model. J Cell Sci 2000;113:1161–1166.
22. Kassem M, Kristiansen M, Abdallah M. Mesenchymal stem cells: Cell biology and potential use in therapy. Basic Clin Pharm Toxi 2004;95:209–214.
23. Baksh D, Song L, Tuan RS. Adult mesenchymnal stem cells: Characterization, differentiation, and application in cell and gene therapy. J Cell Mol Med 2004;8(3):301–316.
24. Eghbali-Fatourechi GZ, Lamsam J, Fraser D, Nagel D, Riggs L, Khosla S. Circulating osteoblast-lineage cells in humans. New Engl J Med 2005;352:1959–1966.
25. Canalis E. The fate of circulating osteoblasts. New Engl J Med 2005;352:2014–2016.
26. Hauge EM, Qvesel D, Eriksen EF, Mosekilde L, Melsen F. Cancellous bone remodeling occurs in specialized compartments lined by cells expressing osteoblastic markers. J Bone Miner Res 2001;16:1575–1582.
27. Fibbe WE, Lazarus HM. Mesenchymal stem cells and a hematopoietic stem cell transplantation. In: Atkinson K et al (eds). Clinical Bone Marrow and Blood Stem Cell Transplantation, ed 3. Cambridge: Cambridge University Press, 2004:64–75.
28. Bacigalupo A. Mesenchymal stem cells and haematopoietic stem cell transplantation. Best Pract Res Clin Haematol 2004;15(3):387–389.
29. Yoshikawa T, Ohgushi H, Ichijima K, Takakura Y. Bone regeneration by grafting of cultured human bone. Tissue Eng 2004;10(5/6):688–698.
30. Takagi K, Urist MR. The role of bone marrow in bone morphogenetic protein–induced repair of femoral massive diaphyseal defects. Clin Orthop 1982;171:224–231.
31. Chapman MW. Closed intramedullary bone grafting and nailing of segmental defects of the femur: A report of three cases. J Bone Joint Surg Am 1980;62:1004–1008.
32. Krebsbach PH, Kuznetsov SA, Satomura K, Emmons RV, Rowe DW, Robey PG. Bone formation in vivo: Comparison of osteogenesis by transplanted mouse and human marrow stromal fibroblasts. Transplantation 1997;63:1059–1069.
33. Kuznetsov SA, Krebsbach PH, Satomura K, et al. Single-colony derived strains of human marrow stromal fibroblasts form bone after transplantation in vivo. J Bone Miner Res 1007;12:1335–1347.
34. Quarto R, Mastrogiacomo M, Cancedda R, et al. Repair of large bone defects with the use of autologous bone marrow stromal cells. New Engl J Med 2001;344:385–386.
35. Gao J, Caplan AI. Mesenchymal stem cells and tissue engineering for orthopaedic surgery. Chir Organi Mov 2003;88:305–316.

36. Ueda M, Morimich O, Yoichi Y, Hidehara H. Injectable tissue-engineered bone applied for sinus floor augmentation with simultaneous implant placement. In: Jensen OT (ed). The Sinus Bone Graft, ed 2. Chicago: Quintessence Publishing, 2005.
37. Schimming R, Schmelzeisen R. Tissue Engineering. In: Jensen OT (ed). The Sinus Bone Graft, ed 2. Chicago: Quintessence Publishing, 2005.
38. Burwell RG. Studies in the transplantation of bone. VII. The fresh composite homograft-autograft of cancellous bone: An analysis of factors leading to osteogenesis in marrow transplants and in marrow-containing bone grafts. J Bone Joint Surg 1964; 46:110–140.
39. Burwell RG. The function of bone marrow in the incorporation of a bone graft. Clin Orthop Relat Res 1985;200;125–141.
40. Boyne PJ. Implants and transplants: Review of recent research in this area of oral surgery. J Am Dent Assoc 1973;87:1074–1080.
41. Jackson IT, Scheker LR, Vandervord JG, McLennan JG. Bone marrow grafting in the secondary closure of alveolar-palatal defects in children. Br J Plas Surg 1981,34:422–425.
42. Connolly JF, Shindell R. Percutaneous marrow injection for an ununited tibia. Neb Med J 1986;4:105–107.
43. Connolly JF, Guse R, Tiedeman J, Dehne R. Autologous marrow injection as a substitute for operative grafting of tibial non-unions. Clin Orthop Relat Res 1991;266:259–270.
44. Garg NK, Sanjiv G, Sharma S. Percutaneous autogenous bone marrow grafting in 20 cases of ununited fracture. Acta Orthop Scand 1993;64(6);671–672.
45. Sharma S, Garg NK, Veliath AJ, Subramanian S, Srivastava KK. Percutaneous bone marrow grafting of osteotomies and bony defects in rabbits. Acta Orthop Scand 1992;63(2):166–169.
46. Connolly J, Guse R, Lippiello L, Dehne R. Development of an osteogenic bone-marrow preparation, J Bone Joint Surg AM 1989;71:684–691.
47. Salama R, Weissman SL. The clinical use of combined xenografts of bone and autologous red marrow: A preliminary report. J Bone Joint Surg Br 1978; 60:111–115.
48. Rodgers WB. Bone marrow aspiration. Orthopedics 2003;26 (suppl 5):s560.
49. Muschler GF, Boehm C, Easley K. Aspiration to obtain osteoblast progenitor cells from human bone marrow: The influence of aspiration volume. J Bone Joint Surg Am 1997;79:1699–1709.
50. Matsubara T, Suardita K, Ishii M, et al. Alveolar bone marrow as a cell source for regenerative medicine: Differences between alveolar and iliac bone marrow stromal cells. J Bone Miner Res 2005;20(3):399–409.
51. Kon E, Muraglia A, Corsi A, et al. Autologous bone marrow stromal cells loaded onto porous hydroxyapatite ceramic accelerate bone repair in critical-size defects of sheep long bones. J Biomed Mater Res 2000;49:328–337.
52. Ohgushi H, Goldberg VM, Caplan AI. Repair of bone defects with marrow cells and porous ceramic: Experiments in rats. Acta Orthop Scand 1989;60:334–339.
53. Inoue K, Ohgushi H, Yoshikawa T, et al. The effect of aging on bone formation in porous hydroxyapatite: Biochemical and histological analysis. J Bone Miner Res 1997;12:989–994.
54. Muschler GF, Nitto H, Boehm CA, Easley KA. Age- and gender-related changes in the cellularity of human bone marrow and the prevalence of osteoblastic progenitors. J Orthop Res 2001; 9(1):117–125.
55. D'Ippolita G, Schiller PC, Ricordi C, Roos BA, Howard GA. Age-related osteogenic potential of mesenchymal stromal stem cells from human vertebral bone marrow. J Bone Miner Res 1999;14: 1115–1122.
56. Oreffo RO, Bennett A, Carr AJ, Triffitt JT. Patients with primary osteoarthritis show no change with ageing in the number of osteogenic precursors. Scand J Rheumatol 1998;27:415–424.
57. Shi S, Gronthos S, Chen S, et al. Bone formation by human postnatal bone marrow stromal stem cells is enhanced by telomerase expression. Nat Biotechnol 2002;20:587–591.
58. Simonsen JL, Rosada C, Serakinci N, et al. Telomerase expression extends the proliferative life-span and maintains the osteogenic potential of human bone marrow stromal cells. Nat Biotechnol 2002;20:592–596.
59. Stenderup K, Justesen J, Clausen C, Kassem J. Aging is associated with decreased maximal life span and accelerated senescence of bone marrow stromal cells. Bone 2003;33:919–926.

chapter 29
Tissue Engineering for Maxillary Sinus Augmentation

Ronald Schimming, MD, DMD, PhD
Rainer Schmelzeisen, MD, DMD, PhD

Bone augmentation in preparation for implant placement is usually carried out with autograft, allograft, or alloplast.[1–4] Regardless of the location of the donor site, when autograft is used, the potential for morbidity must be considered. Another consideration is the limited availability of intraoral bone that is suitable for grafting. Alloplastic materials are unsuitable in situations where vascularity is compromised, as is often the case in sinus grafting.

Because it causes little or no donor site morbidity, tissue engineering for bony augmentation of the maxillary sinus floor offers a significant advantage over conventional grafting. Ideally, this procedure is performed under local anesthesia using autologous bone with osteogenic capacity.

Tissue engineering that involves the use of living tissue in vivo represents a new concept in cell culture technology. Compared with conventional cell cultures, the development of engineered tissues depends on the three-dimensional arrangement of cells and the formation or synthesis of an appropriate extracellular matrix, as in a combined alveolar and sinus defect (see chapter 21). Current tissue-engineering methods use resorbable biomaterials, tissue encapsulation, and perfusion cultures and give major consideration to scaffolding of biomaterials to define a three-dimensional shape or to guide matrix formation.[5] Naturally derived and synthetic polymers, composites, ceramics, and bone morphogenetic proteins, as well as cellular systems, are now under study.[5,6] For the sinus graft, a carrier material for maintenance under the sinus membrane is essential.

Periosteum is now known to have cell populations that contain chondroprogenitor and osteoprogenitor cells that can be isolated in tissue culture and used to form cartilage and bone. The use of cultured periosteal cells for tissue engineering to repair bone and cartilage was first described by Rich et al[7] in 1994 and by Breitbart et al[8] in 1998.

Study Design

The clinical procedure described in this chapter was developed using an experimental protocol devised by Sittinger et al[5] in 1996 and by Perka et al[9] in 2000. They reported the technique of segmental bone repair by tissue-engineered periosteal cell transplants with bioresorbable polymer fleece and fibrin scaffolds in rabbits. Eight-millimeter metadiaphyseal ulna defects were created bilaterally and subsequently filled on one side with cell-fibrin beads and on the other with polymers seeded with cells. Identical defects, half of them filled with fibrin beads and polymers alone and the others left untreated, served as controls. Histologic and radiologic scoring for both experimental groups was superior to that of the control groups, which revealed only poor healing indices or, in the case of the untreated defects, did not heal at all. The highest histologic score was obtained in the group with bioabsorbable polymer fleece containing periosteal cells (Fig 29-1).[9]

A prospective clinical study was performed in which tissue-engineered bone transplants were used for maxillary sinus augmentation.[10] Following publication of the results of this clinical study, patients were treated with tissue-engineered bone, both by the authors and by other private practitioners in Germany.

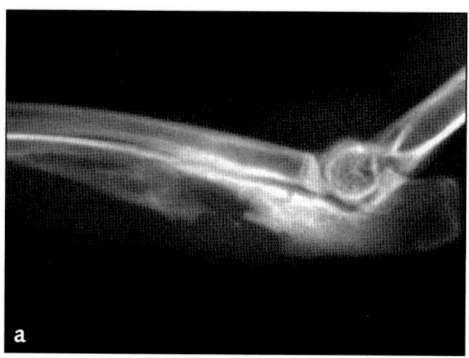 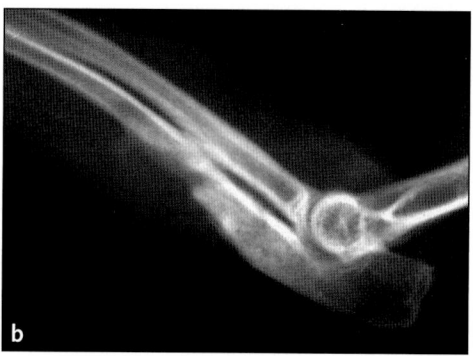

Figs 29-1a and 29-1b Radiologic examination 6 weeks after creation of 8-mm metadiaphyseal ulna defects on New Zealand white rabbits. Defects were left untreated *(a)* or subsequently filled with cell-fibrin beads *(b)*.

Clinical Evaluation

Patients

From June 2001 to June 2002 in the Department of Oral and Maxillofacial Surgery (University of Freiburg, Germany), 27 edentulous patients (17 men, 10 women) with atrophic posterior maxillae underwent surgery for augmentation with tissue-engineered bone in preparation for implant placement. All of the patients exhibited Class IV or V atrophy of the posterior maxilla as defined by Cawood and Howell.[11] In 12 patients, maxillary bone augmentation was performed simultaneous with placement of dental implants in a one-stage procedure. Only patients whose residual maxillary bone showed sufficient vertical ($\geq$ 4 mm) and transverse ($\geq$ 6 mm) dimensions for primary stability of dental implants were selected for the one-stage procedure.

In all remaining patients (n = 15), implant placement was delayed for a period of 3 months after bone augmentation procedures. A bilateral sinus augmentation procedure was carried out in 14 patients, while all other patients (n = 13) underwent unilateral augmentation.

Based on the results of this study, an additional 64 patients were treated by specially qualified private practitioners around Germany, 40 of them in a one-stage and 24 in a two-stage procedure. The follow-up period for these patients was between 8 and 30 months.

Tissue engineering

All procedures, including the harvesting of the periosteum, culturing of the cells, and transplantation of the tissue-engineered graft, were performed according to standards of sterile practice. Under conditions of good manufacturing practice (GMP), periosteal tissue harvested from the lateral cortex of the mandibular angle (1 cm^2) of each patient was used to isolate periosteal cells (Fig 29-2). The periosteum was enzymatically digested with collagenase CLSII (*Clostridium histolyticum*, 333 U/mL) (Biochrom) in DMEM (Dulbecco's modified Eagle's medium)/Ham's F-12 in a 1:1 ratio (InVitrogen). The resulting cell suspension was washed three times with phosphate-buffered saline (PBS) (InVitrogen), and then hemocytometer and trypan blue dye exclusion were used for cell counting and to ensure that cell viability was at least 90% before seeding.[9]

The cells were re-suspended in DMEM/Ham's F-12 (1:1) supplemented with 10% autologous serum, then placed into cell culture flasks and cultured at 37°C with 3.5% carbon dioxide and 95% humidified air. The medium was replaced every 2 days. Upon reaching 70% confluence, the cells were trypsinized (0.02% trypsin, 0.02% ethylenediaminetetraacetic acid [EDTA] in PBS for 5 minutes), and replaced four times at a density of 50 cells/mm^2.

Transplants were prepared as described by Perka et al.[9] Briefly, after four passages, the periosteal cells were once again trypsinized, then suspended in DMEM/Ham's F-12 (1:1) medium and mixed with fibrinogen of human origin (TissueColl, Baxter) in a 3:1 ratio.

The cell suspension was soaked in Ethisorb fleece (Ethicon) and polymerized by the addition of bovine thrombin (TissueColl) that had been diluted with PBS (1:10). The process was completed 6.5 weeks after the harvesting of the periosteal grafts. Subsequently, cell-polymer transplants were cultured for 1 week in DMEM/Ham's F-12 (1:1) medium supplemented with 5% autologous serum, ascorbic acid (50 mg/L), dexamethasone (10^{-7} mol/L) and b-glycerophosphate (10 mmol/L).

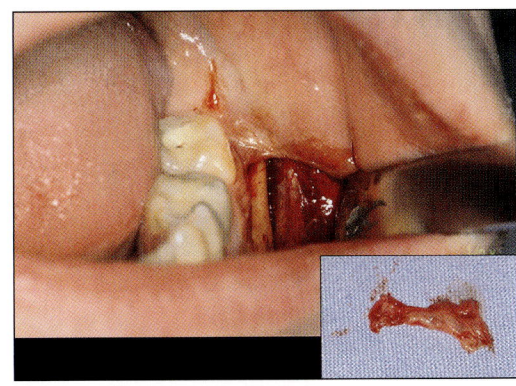

Fig 29-2 Harvesting of the periosteum cells from the mandibular angle under sterile conditions (intraoperative view). The wound is closed primarily.

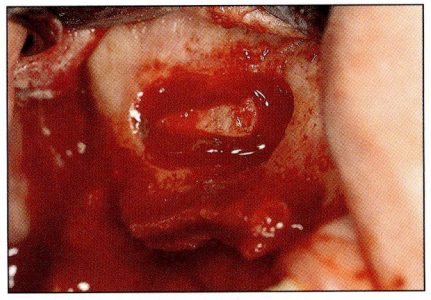

Fig 29-3 Clinical aspect of lateral approach to the posterior maxilla after elevation of the bony window. Because of the knife-edged ridge, a bone-split procedure was performed in addition to the sinus graft.

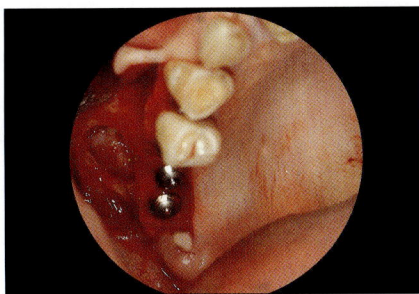

Fig 29-4 One-step procedure with simultaneous application of the grafting material and placement of dental implants.

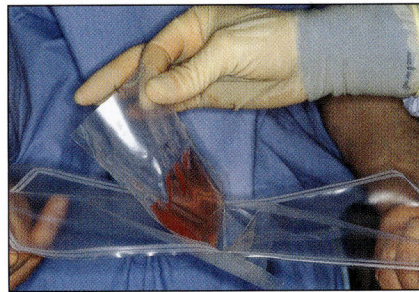

Fig 29-5 The double-coated packs with the grafting material inside allow a sterile bone augmentation procedure.

Surgical procedure

Grafting procedures were carried out in an outpatient protocol under local anesthesia 7.5 weeks after harvesting of the periosteal grafts. Using the lateral approach described by Boyne and James,[12] a supracrestal incision and two vertical incisions extending beyond the mucogingival junction were made, and a full-thickness flap was reflected to gain access to the underlying alveolar bone. An oval-shaped osteotomy was then prepared with rotary instruments under copious sterile saline irrigation. A round, 4-mm-diameter, diamond-coated bur was used to outline the osteotomy window, and then specially designed elevators were used to elevate the sinus membrane (Fig 29-3).[9]

For the one-step procedure, implants were placed according to the ITI surgical protocol (Straumann). The tissue-engineered complex was placed and condensed into the depth of the sinus cavity (Fig 29-4). Using sterile techniques, the scaffolds were prepared in small, double-coated packs, similar to suture material in a nutrient medium, which allows a 48-hour window for transplantation (Fig 29-5). Extreme care must be exercised in handling the scaffolds to avoid destruction of viable cells, and they must remain in the patient's blood until the grafting procedure takes place (Fig 29-6).[9]

For the two-stage procedure, the grafting material was placed into the sinus cavity without the dental implants (Fig 29-7). No membrane was used to cover the augmented area. Primary implant stability was evaluated and confirmed by means of resonance frequency analysis (RFA).[9]

After 3 months, bone biopsies were taken with a trephine and studied via light microscopy (Figs 29-8 and 29-9) prior to implant placement. Panoramic radiography in all cases and computerized tomography (CT) scanning in selected cases were also carried out to evaluate the success of grafting procedures.[9]

Chapter 29: Tissue Engineering for Maxillary Sinus Augmentation

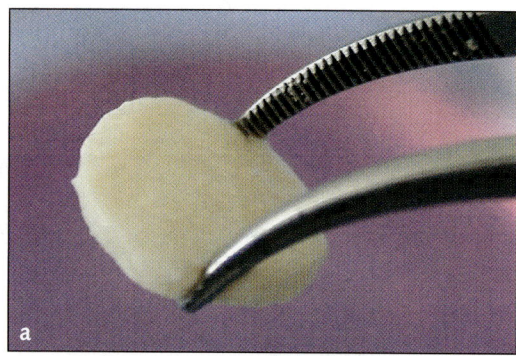
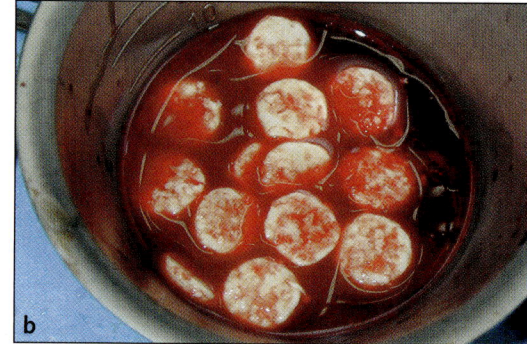

Figs 29-6a and 29-6b An anatomic forceps should be used to handle the scaffolds very carefully *(a)*. The Ethisorb fleece contains approximately 1.5 million viable cells. Until the definitive bone augmentation takes place, the scaffolds are put into a small bowl with patient's blood *(b)*.

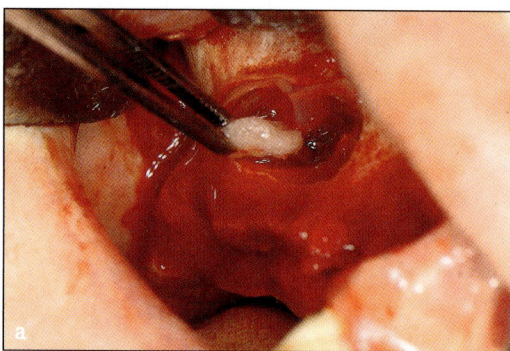
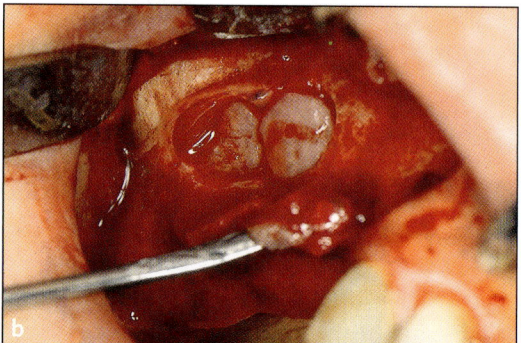

Figs 29-7a and 29-7b Two-step procedure during placement of the grafting material into the sinus.

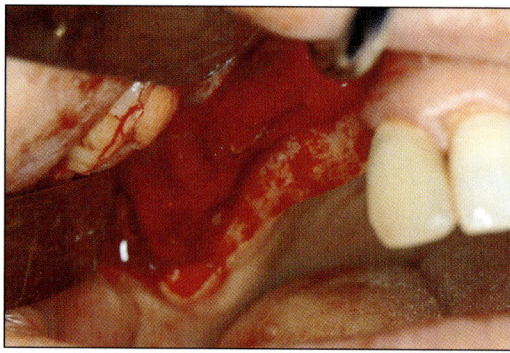
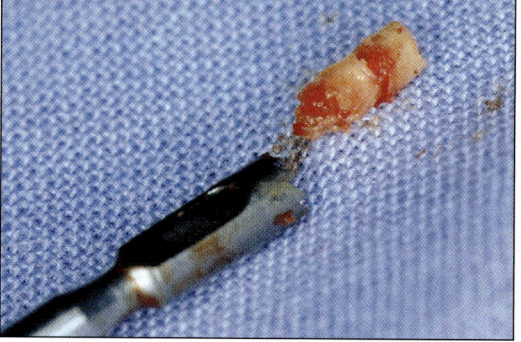

Fig 29-8 Clinical aspect of the alveolar ridge and the lateral wall of the sinus 3 months after augmentation with tissue-engineered bone (same patient as shown in Figs 29-3 and 29-7).

Fig 29-9 In all patients undergoing two-step procedures, bone biopsies using a trephine were taken prior to placement of the dental implants.

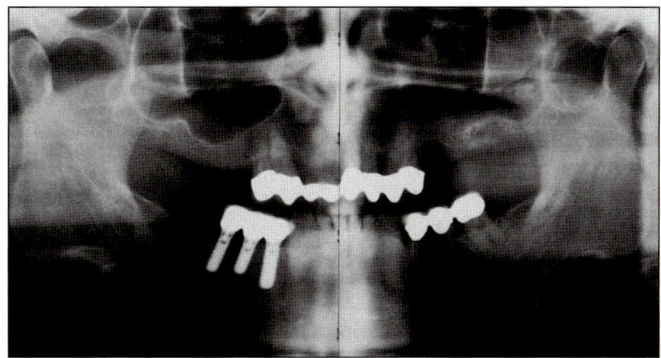

Fig 29-10a Preoperative panoramic radiograph showing the severe atrophy of the edentulous posterior maxilla bilaterally.

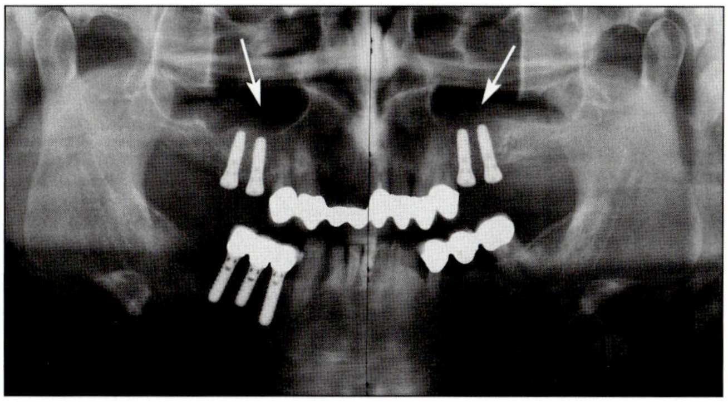

Fig 29-10b Postoperative panoramic radiograph 4 months after augmentation with tissue-engineered bone. Increased density in the augmented material demonstrates further mineralization and bone formation *(arrows)*.

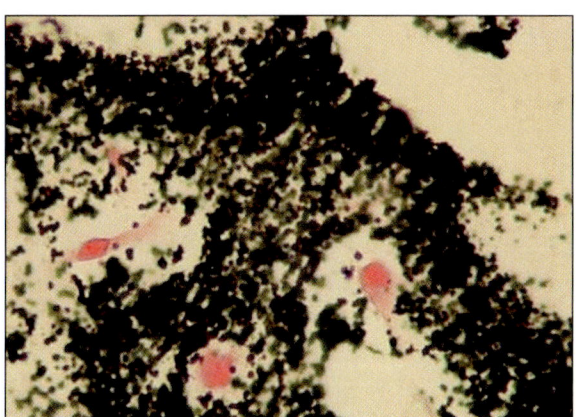

Fig 29-11a Histologic view of tissue-engineered cells on the day of transplantation. The black spots represent the centers of primary calcification and bone formation in the transplant.

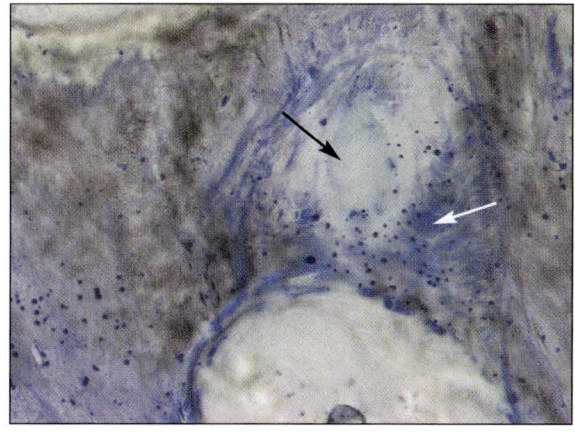

Fig 29-11b Bone biopsy by means of a trephine was processed by resin embedding, diamond sawing, grinding, and staining with toluidine blue. The biopsy specimen shows mineralized trabecular bone *(white arrow)*. Residual biomaterial remains visible between the bone trabeculae *(black arrow)* (magnification ×200).

Results and Complications

Harvesting of the periosteum at the mandibular angle via an intraoral mucosal incision under local anesthesia was well tolerated by all patients. No wound infections or other complications occurred.

In the Freiburg group, the wounds resulting from reimplantation of the engineered tissue and the augmentation of the sinus healed uneventfully in 26 cases. In one patient, graft material and 2 implants had to be removed because of an early infection during the first postoperative days. A total of 70 implants (Straumann) were placed into sinus-grafted areas. All patients subsequently underwent prosthetic rehabilitation with crowns or fixed partial dentures.

In 18 patients, evidence of excellent clinical, radiologic, and histologic results was collected 3 months after augmentation. Compared to the pretreatment situation, the clinical examination showed very good formation of new bone free of any evidence of resorption. These findings were confirmed by radiologic examination (Fig 29-10).[9]

In two-stage cases, the augmented region displayed a bony mass of sufficient size for placement of dental implants with excellent primary stability. Histologically, the bone biopsies from these patients revealed mineralized trabecular bone that contained remnants of biomaterial. Osteocytes in lacunae were observed within the bone substance (Fig 29-11).[9]

In 9 of 18 successfully treated cases, radiologic follow-up of more than 6 months was available, and an excellent outcome under implant-loading conditions was found.

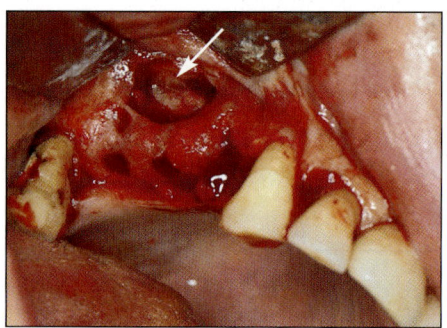 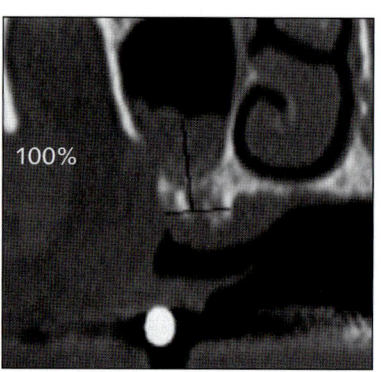 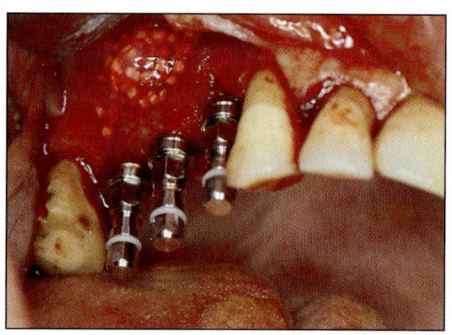

Fig 29-12a Clinical aspect 3 months after augmentation with tissue-engineered bone. No evidence of new bone formation is observed. Replacement/resorption with connective tissue was found, especially at the former base of the maxillary sinus *(white arrow)*.

Fig 29-12b Dental CT scan (coronal slice) with signs of total replacement of the grafting material with connective tissue 3 months after augmentation. Note the defect in the lateral aspect of the maxillary sinus (former bony window).

Fig 29-12c Clinical aspect after placement of three Straumann implants and supplementary augmentation with autologous bone and grafting material.

In the group of private practice patients (n = 53), postoperative healing was uneventful and exhibited no signs of infection or long-term complication. Of the 40 patients in this group who underwent a one-stage procedure, 3 showed insufficient evidence of bone regeneration, and consequently the treatment was deemed unsuccessful. Of the 24 patients treated using a two-stage procedure, 8 revealed insufficient bone formation and an unsuccessful treatment result. (Four patients had a partially successful result.)

In the Freiburg group, an unsuccessful result was found upon clinical examination of eight patients in whom connective tissue had formed in place of new bone 3 months after augmentation procedures (Fig 29-12a). These results were confirmed by dental CT scan (Fig 29-12b). In these patients, no clinical problems or signs of infection had been detected within the 3-month follow-up period.[9]

Augmentation with autologous bone and grafting material was necessary to prepare these patients for dental implant placement (Fig 29-12c).[9]

Conclusion

Ongoing efforts toward the development of tissue-engineered materials are aimed at reducing or eliminating donor site morbidity and gaining materials with mechanical properties equal to or better than those currently in use.[6] Intensive experimentation is taking place to create tissue-engineered hard tissue components such as bone, cartilage, or both.[13–15]

In their search for alternatives to conventional bone augmentation procedures in oral and maxillofacial surgery, Terheyden et al[16] found that applying bone morphogenetic protein to bovine bone material (Bio-Oss, Osteohealth) led to more rapid osseointegration of simultaneously placed implants in animal experiments.

To our knowledge, the studies documented here represent the first demonstration of the feasibility of using a periosteum-derived bony matrix for augmentation in the posterior maxilla in preparation for implant placement. Histology has shown trabecular bone containing viable osteocytes 4 months after augmentation in 30 patients (14 Freiburg group; 16 private practice).

In 19 patients, however, insufficient bone regeneration was found 3 months following augmentation (8/27, Freiburg group; 11/64, private practice group). Sixteen of these patients had received treatment with a two-stage procedure, indicating that residual bone in the posterior maxilla was minimal prior to treatment. In highly atrophic sites, extensive augmentation, and thus a large amount of grafting material, is required. Therefore, a significantly greater amount of tissue-engineered bone was transplanted in these patients than in the patients who qualified for a one-stage procedure. The major questions involved with in vitro tissue engineering of large amounts of tissue such as those used in these 16 cases remain unanswered.

There remains also the critical question of how to supply cells embedded within large cell-polymer constructs while at the same time maintaining sufficient oxygen and nutrients to sustain survival and proliferation, allowing time for the integration of the developing tissue within the surrounding tissue. This may be the main cause for failure, ie, insufficient vascular support of the graft. One possible solution to this problem may be the application of vascular endothelial growth factor (VEGF) to achieve a higher initial angiogenic response and long-term stabilization of capillary-like structures.[17,18]

In these 91 clinical cases, a synthetic biodegradable polymer was used as scaffolding for the three-dimensional tissue-engineered transplant. The scaffold provides a conductive environment for normal cell growth, differentiation, and angiogenesis to allow for rapid integration of the transplanted tissue. Other naturally occurring scaffold materials that could be used for the sinus graft include small intestinal submucosa, acellular dermis, amniotic membrane tissue, cadaveric fascia, and the bladder acellular matrix, all currently in experimental use for soft tissue repair.[19] Upon implantation, these materials have been shown to elicit a host-tissue response that initiates angiogenesis, encourages tissue deposition, and culminates in restoration of structure and function specific to the grafted site. Seeking naturally occurring scaffolds for repair of hard tissue such as maxillary bone may help to overcome the problems encountered in this promising technology.

References

1. Jensen OT, Sennerby L. Histologic analysis of clinically retrieved titanium microimplants placed in conjunction with maxillary sinus floor augmentation. Int J Oral Maxillofac Implants 1998;13:513–521.
2. Lorenzetti M, Mozzati M, Campanino PP, Valente G. Bone augmentation of the inferior floor of the maxillary sinus with autogenous bone or composite bone grafts: A histologic-histomorphometric preliminary report. Int J Oral Maxillofac Implants 1998;13:69–76.
3. Valentini P, Abensur D, Densari D, Graziani JN, Hammerle C. Histological evaluation of Bio-Oss in a 2-stage sinus floor elevation and implantation procedure. A human case report. Clin Oral Implants Res 1998;9:59–64.
4. Yildirim M, Spiekermann H, Biesterfeld S, Edelhoff D. Maxillary sinus augmentation using xenogenic bone substitute material Bio-Oss in combination with venous blood. A histologic and histomorphometric study in humans. Clin Oral Implants Res 2000;11:217–229.
5. Sittinger M, Bujia J, Rotter N, Reitzel D, Minuth WW, Burmester GR. Tissue engineering and autologous transplant formation: Practical approaches with resorbable biomaterials and new cell culture techniques. Biomaterials 1996;17:237–242.
6. Burg KJ, Porter S, Kellam JF. Biomaterial developments for bone tissue engineering. Biomaterials 2000;21:2347–2359.
7. Rich D, Johnson E, Zhou L, Grande D. The use of periosteal cell/polymer tissue constructs for the repair of articular cartilage defects. Trans Orthop Res Soc 1994;19:241–245.
8. Breitbart AS, Grande DA, Kessler R, Ryaby JT, Fitzsimmons RJ, Grant RT. Tissue engineered bone repair of calvarial defects using cultured periosteal cells. Plast Reconstr Surg 1998;101:567–574.
9. Perka C, Schultz O, Spitzer RS, Lindenhayn K, Burmester GR, Sittinger M. Segmental bone repair by tissue-engineered periosteal cell transplants with bioresorbable fleece and fibrin scaffolds in rabbits. Biomaterials 2000;21:1145–1153.
10. Schimming R, Schmelzeisen R. Tissue-engineered bone for maxillary sinus augmentation. J Oral Maxillofac Surg 2004;62:724–729.
11. Cawood JI, Howell RA. A classification of the edentulous jaws. Int J Oral Maxillofac Surg 1988;17:232–236.
12. Boyne PJ, James RA. Grafting of the maxillary sinus floor with autogenous marrow and bone. J Oral Surg 1980;38:613–616.
13. Puelacher WG, Wisser J, Vacanti CA, Ferraro NF, Jaramillo D, Vacanti JP. Temporomandibular joint disc replacement made by tissue-engineered growth of cartilage. J Oral Maxillofac Surg 1994;52:1172–1177.
14. Weng Y, Cao Y, Silva CA, Vacanti MP, Vacanti CA. Tissue-engineered composites of bone and cartilage for mandible condylar reconstruction. J Oral Maxillofac Surg 2001;59:185–190.
15. Abukawa H, Terai H, Hannouche D, Vacanti JP, Kaban LB, Troulis MJ. Formation of a mandibular condyle in vitro by tissue engineering. J Oral Maxillofac Surg 2003;61:94–100.
16. Terheyden H, Jepsen S, Moller B, Tucker MM, Rueger DC. Sinus floor augmentation with simultaneous placement of dental implants using a combination of deproteinized bone xenografts and recombinant human osteogenic protein-1. A histometric study in miniature pigs. Clin Oral Implants Res 1999;10:510–521.
17. Frerich B, Lindemann N, Kurtz-Hoffmann J, Oertel K. In vitro model of a vascular stroma for the engineering of vascularized tissues. Int J Oral Maxillofac Surg 2001;30:414–420.
18. Bouhadir KH, Mooney DJ. Promoting angiogenesis in engineered tissues. J Drug Target 2001;9:397–406.
19. Hodde J. Naturally occurring scaffolds for soft tissue repair and regeneration. Tissue Eng 2002;8:295–308.

chapter 30

Use of Tissue-Engineered Bone Cells for Sinus Augmentation with Simultaneous Implant Placement

Minoru Ueda, DDS, PhD
Yoichi Yamada, DDS, PhD
Morimich Ohya, DDS, PhD
Hideharu Hibi, DDS, PhD

Implant-borne tooth restorations have become a standard of care in modern dentistry. For dental implant placement, the presence of sufficient bone volume is a crucial prerequisite. Predictable bone regeneration of large alveolar defects, such as those resulting from ablative periodontal disease or traumatic injury, pose a significant clinical challenge, particularly when accompanied by significant vertical bone loss. Of the various techniques for reconstructing a deficient alveolar ridge, autogenous bone grafting is predictable, well-documented, and unequivocally accepted as the standard of care. Nonetheless, autografting is sometimes associated with substantial morbidity in the form of infection, malformation, pain, and loss of function.[1] Alternatives to autogenous bone harvesting, such as allograft, xenograft, and alloplast bone substitutes, are associated with other risks and/or potential problems.[2,3] For example, allografts and xenografts carry some risk for disease transmission and have diminished bone-forming capacity. Synthetic materials have a higher incidence of infection, rejection, and extrusion than alloplasts and allografts, and their long-term interaction with host physiology remains uncertain.

Because of these limitations and drawbacks, efforts are underway to find an autogenous alternative to conventional bone grafting that is minimally or non-invasive.[4] A new technology has been developed via tissue engineering to establish a type of "injectable bone" resulting from morphogenesis of osteoinductive cells derived from cell cultures plated onto biocompatible scaffolds and augmented with growth factors.[5] In recent animal studies,[6,7] bone formation was consistently demonstrated in grafted defects using mesenchymal stem cells (MSCs), the growth factors in platelet-rich plasma (PRP), and/or a carrier of beta-tricalcium phosphate (β-TCP). Based on the results of these experimental studies, a human study was conducted using tissue-engineered injectable bone for sinus augmentation simultaneous to the placement of dental implants.

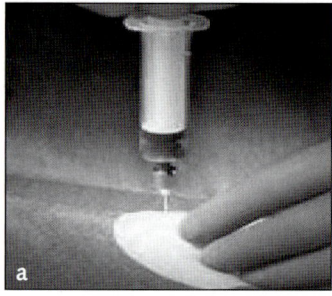
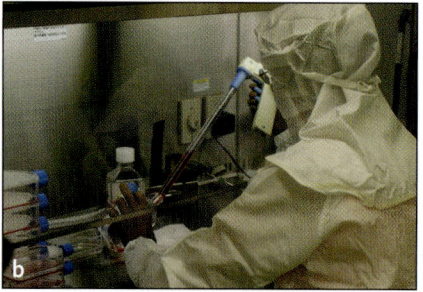
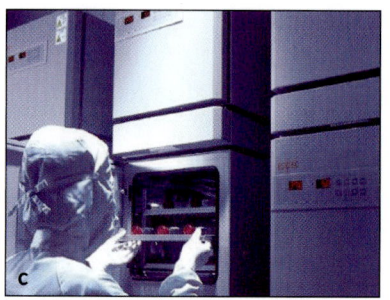
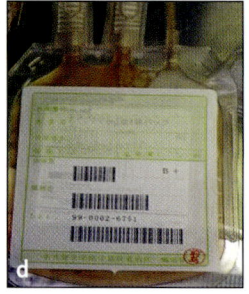
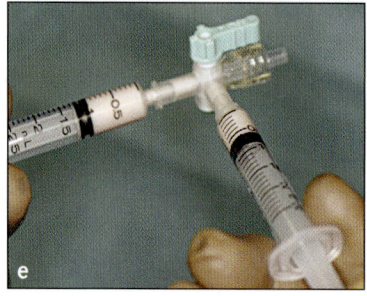
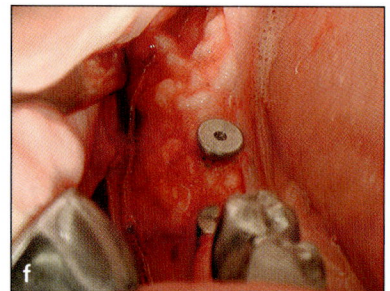

Figs 30-1a to 30-1f Processing of tissue-engineered bone.

Cell-Based Therapy for Sinus Augmentation

Patient selection

Four partially or completely edentulous patients were selected for sinus floor grafting. All patients wore a conventional denture and had retention problems associated with severe maxillary alveolar atrophy. Each had less than 5 mm of residual sinus floor height, necessitating a sinus graft. In three of the patients, a large portion of the residual alveolar arch was deficient in both horizontal and sagittal dimensions. Following routine oral and physical examinations, tissue-engineered bone grafting was accomplished to avoid the need to harvest autogenous bone. In all cases the reconstruction included sinus floor grafting and simultaneous implant placement in the posterior maxilla. All patients were healthy and free of sinus or medical disease. The patients were fully informed about the new bone regeneration method, which had been approved by the Nagoya University Bioethics Committee.

Cell preparation technique

One month prior to surgery, MSCs were isolated from the patient's iliac crest via marrow aspirate (10 mL) (Fig 30-1), according to a reported method.[8] Briefly, the basal medium, low-glucose Dulbecco's modified Eagle's medium (DMEM), and growth supplements (50 mL of serum, 10 mL of 200-mL glutamine, and 0.5 mL of penicillin-streptomycin mixture containing 25 units of penicillin and 25 µg of streptomycin) were obtained from BioWhittaker Molecular Applications. Three supplements were used for inducing osteogenesis: Dexamethasone (Dex), sodium β-glycerophosphate (β-GP), and L-ascorbic acid 2-phosphate (AsAP). These were obtained from Sigma Chemical. The cells were incubated at 37°C in a humidified atmosphere containing 95% air and 5% carbon dioxide. The MSCs were replated at densities of 3.1×10^3 cells/cm^2 in 0.2 mL/cm^2 of control medium. The presence of bone-differentiated cells was confirmed via detection of alkaline phosphatase activity using p-nitrophenylphosphatase as a substrate. The cultured cells were trypsinized and readied for implantation (Fig 30-2).

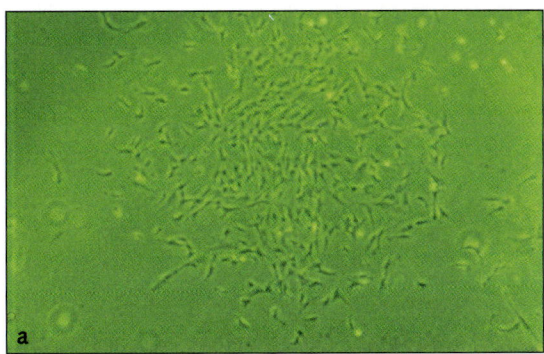 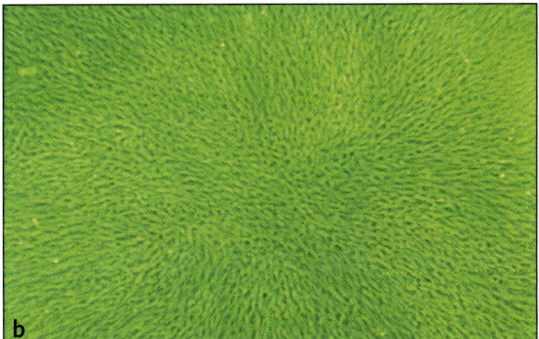

Figs 30-2a and 30-2b Growth process of mesenchymal stem cell (phase contrast microscopy ×200).

Platelet-rich plasma preparation

Preoperative hematologic assessment included a complete blood count (CBC) with platelet levels. PRP was extracted 1 day prior to surgery. The PRP was isolated in a 200-mL collection bag containing anticoagulant citrate under sterilized conditions at the blood transfusion service department. To develop the PRP, the blood was first centrifuged for 10 minutes at 1,100 rpm. Subsequently, the buffy coat (containing the platelets and leukocytes) was taken up. A second centrifugation (2,500 rpm for 5 minutes) was performed to combine the platelets into a single pellet, and the plasma supernatant, which was platelet-poor plasma (PPP), was removed. The resulting pellet of platelets, the buffy coat/plasma fraction (PRP), was re-suspended in the residual 20 mL of plasma to create a platelet gel (see Fig 30-1d). The PRP was stored at 20°C in a conventional shaker until needed.

In a separate sterile cup, human thrombin in powder form (10,000 units) was dissolved in 10 mL of 10% calcium chloride. Next, 3.5 mL of PRP, the MSCs (1.0×10^7 cell/mL), and 0.5 mL of air were aspirated into a 5-mL sterile syringe. In a second 2.5-mL syringe, 500 μL of the thrombin–calcium chloride mixture was aspirated. The cells were re-suspended directly into the PRP. The two syringes were connected with a T-connector, and the plungers of the syringes were pushed and pulled alternately, allowing the air bubble to traverse the two syringes (see Fig 30-1e). Within 5 to 30 seconds, the contents assumed a gel-like consistency as the thrombin affected the fibrin polymerization to produce an insoluble gel.

Surgical technique

Four patients received sinus augmentation surgery under general anesthesia. Sinus grafting followed Tatum's classic description.[9] Briefly, a lateral window was created using a round bur. The window of bone was infractured, and the sinus membrane was elevated from the sinus floor. In the space created, 2.0 to 5.8 g of tissue-engineered bone were inserted in conjunction with simultaneous implant placement. Care was taken to avoid membrane perforation in order to confine the grafting material. No barrier membrane was used over the window. The mucoperiosteal flap was repositioned and sutured in the usual manner. The patients were instructed not to wear a removable prosthesis for 21 days and not to blow their nose for 7 days. Second-stage surgery was performed 5 to 8 months later.

Results

Clinical observations

All of the patients in this study were women ranging in age from 44 to 60 years (mean, 52 years). A total of 21 implants were placed simultaneously with sinus augmentation. None of the patients had postoperative complications aside from normal swelling and inflammation at the surgical sites. Perforation of the sinus mucosa was recorded in one procedure and resulted in minor postoperative nasal bleeding.

At the second-stage surgery, performed after a mean healing period of 5.5 months, a mucosal flap was widely elevated in order to observe the grafted site at the lateral

TABLE 30-1 Patient data and outcome

Patient Age (y)	Sex	Location of implants	Procedure	Vol tissue-engineered bone (g)	No. of implants	Healing period (mos)
51	F	Maxillary right and left 1st and 2nd molars	Maxillary sinus augmentation	5.8	6	6
60	F	Maxillary right 1st and 2nd molars	Maxillary sinus augmentation	2.3	3	5
44	F	Maxillary right 1st and 2nd molars	Maxillary sinus augmentation	2.0	2	6
54	F	Maxillary right and left 1st and 2nd molars	Maxillary sinus augmentation	4.8	10	8

window. All 21 implants were found to be clinically stable and considered successful as defined by complete coverage of the implant up to the cover screw (Table 30-1).

In all cases, sinus-directed implants appeared to be completely covered by newly formed bone. All implants maintained stability 6 months after loading, as tested after removal of the prosthetic reconstruction. Marginal bone resorption did not exceed 1.5 mm.

Radiologic observations

Routine panoramic radiographs clearly revealed the height of the newly formed sinus floor. Radiographic findings suggested integration of the implants within regenerated bone (ie, no bone loss or peri-implant radiolucency).

Computerized tomography (CT) scans carried out 6 months post-insertion showed dense mineralization around the implants; the borderline between the original sinus floor and newly formed tissue was difficult to delineate. Consecutive images clearly revealed anabolic mineralization with the graft sites and subsequent osseous incorporation of the implants. Tissue-engineered cells had formed new bone that resembled the basal bone. No decrease in graft height was observed radiographically.

Case Reports

Case 1

A 51-year-old woman presented with a vertical root fracture of the maxillary right first premolar. The tooth was extracted 8 weeks prior to implant placement (Fig 30-3a). The patient's bone marrow tissue (20 mL) was taken from the iliac crest by syringe 1 month prior to surgery for the cell preparation. On the day of the surgery, the patient was prepared and draped in a conventional manner under sterile conditions. Local anesthesia was used, and a crestal incision was made toward the palatal aspect of the edentulous alveolar ridge. The incision extended beyond the limits of the planned osteotomy because of the amount and position of the attached gingivae. Additional vertical relieving incisions were made in the buccal vestibule to facilitate reflection of a full mucoperiosteal flap. A full-thickness flap was then reflected from the underlying bone. Once the lateral maxillary wall was exposed, a square window was prepared. A round diamond bur was used at slow speed in a high-torque straight handpiece with copious saline irrigation. Meticulous care was taken to avoid perforating the sinus membrane. A 15-mm Ti-Oblast titanium dental implant (Astra Tech) was placed into the prepared implant site (Figs 30-3b and 30-3c). Tissue-engineered bone was then loaded into a syringe and injected into the maxillary sinus. Once the proper position of the implant was confirmed, additional tissue-engineered bone was carefully injected to fill the sinus to the lateral wall as well as any exposed coronal part of the implant (Fig 30-3d). The cell preparation was applied to the surface of the implant as optimally as possible. The periosteum under the buccal flap was relieved until primary mattress sutures could be achieved. Routine postoperative instructions, antibiotics, and analgesics were given. The second-stage surgery was carried out 6 months later. Previously exposed threads were found to be surrounded by newly formed

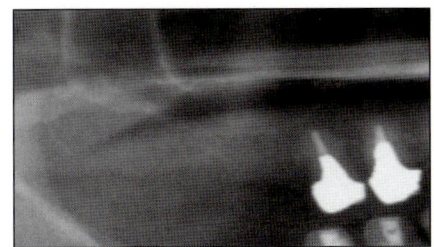
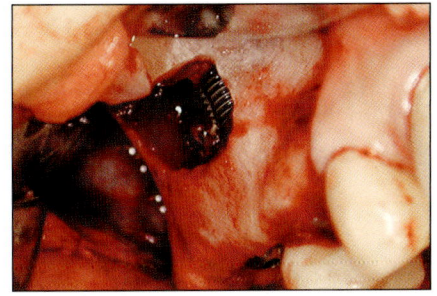
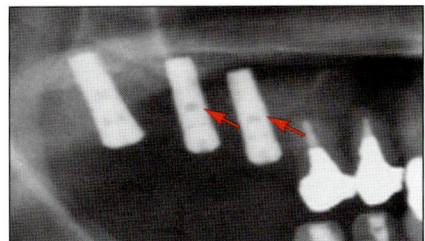

Fig 30-3a Preoperative radiographic view of right maxilla showing very thin residual alveolar bone.

Fig 30-3b Macro view of 15-mm-long TiOblast implant placed into prepared site.

Fig 30-3c Radiographic view of graft area 6 months postsurgery. *Arrows* indicate exposed threads.

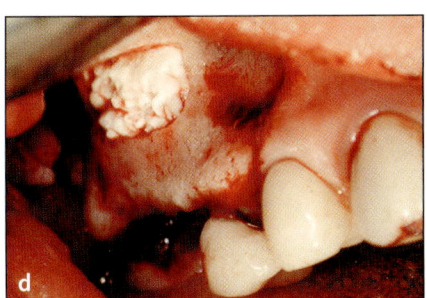
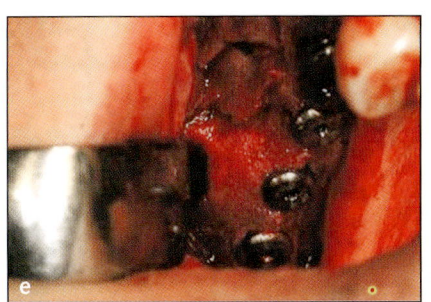

Fig 30-3d Macro view of placement of tissue-engineered bone.

Fig 30-3e Second-stage surgery 6 months after implant placement. Previously exposed screw threads are surrounded by newly formed bone, thus confirming successful osseointegration.

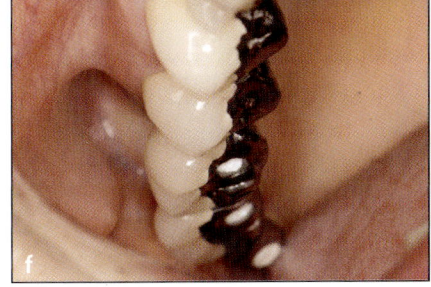
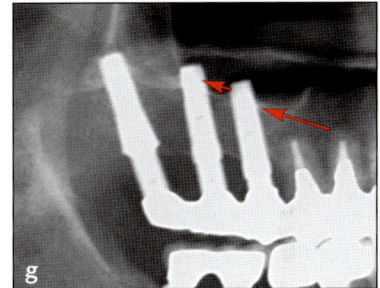

Fig 30-3f Definitive prosthesis with porcelain-fused-to-metal crown.

Fig 30-3g Radiographic view of graft area 30 months postsurgery. Dense alveolar bone *(arrows)* can be observed around the implants.

mature bone, and successful osseointegration was confirmed (Fig 30-3e). A porcelain-fused-to-metal crown was subsequently fitted (Fig 30-3f). The 30-month follow-up examination showed no sign of significant bone loss or any symptoms of implant failure (Fig 30-3g).

Case 2

A 54-year-old woman presented with severe bone resorption of the maxillary alveolar crest. A crestal incision was made in the keratinized tissue to allow for a buccal mucoperiosteal full-thickness reflection of a flap to expose the lateral maxilla. A window was opened laterally, and the sinus membrane was elevated bilaterally. Ten standard 15-mm-length implants were placed around the arch into a thin sinus floor bone that was morphologically deficient in horizontal and vertical dimensions (Fig 30-4a). Sinus-directed implants passed through approximately 5 mm of native bone, leaving at least 8 mm of screw threads exposed (see Fig 30-4a). Tissue-engineered bone was injected around the exposed threads to completely cover them (Figs 30-4b and 30-4c). Horizontal mattress sutures with U stitches were used to create two contact surfaces at least 3-mm thick (first line of closure). No pressure was applied to the surgical area. Healing was uneventful. Sutures were removed after 14 days, and the patient was examined monthly thereafter. Despite the prolonged healing period, the titanium implant remained submerged and the surrounding tissue remained completely healthy without signs of inflammation. At re-entry 8 months later, the grafted

chapter 30 Use of Tissue-Engineered Bone Cells for Sinus Augmentation

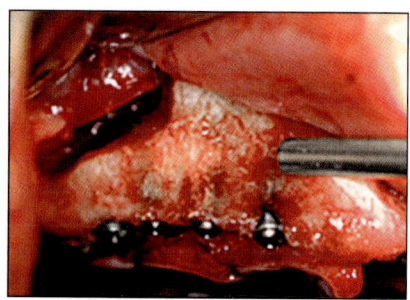

Fig 30-4a Sinus elevation and implant placement.

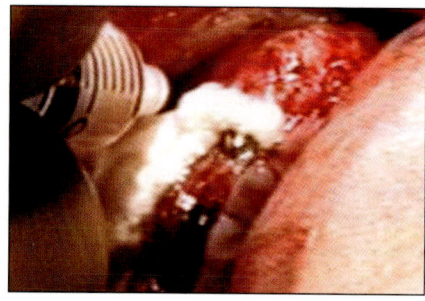

Fig 30-4b Tissue-engineered "bone" applied to the atrophied alveolar ridge.

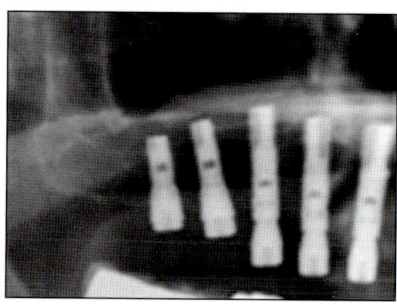

Fig 30-4c Radiographic view of graft area 1 week postsurgery.

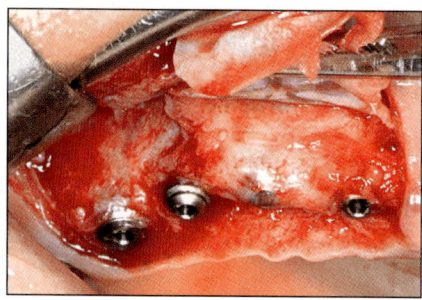

Fig 30-4d Eight months after surgery, the sinus cavity and alveolar ridge show newly formed bone.

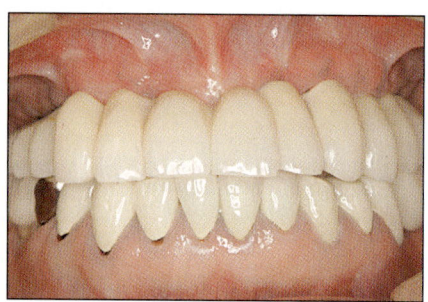

Fig 30-4e Facial view after placement of provisional implant-supported prosthesis.

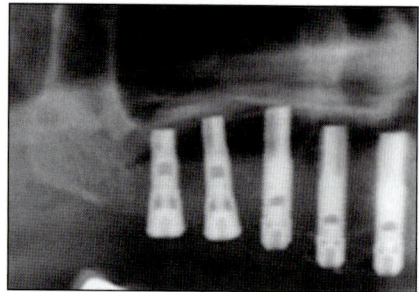

Fig 30-4f Radiographic view of graft area 12 months after surgery, showing dense alveolar bone formed around the implants.

area was observed directly. The maxillary sinus entry site had completely regenerated with hard bone (Fig 30-4d). Newly formed osseous tissue had incorporated the implant and partially covered the cover screws. After placement of the abutment, an implant-supported fixed provisional prosthesis was connected to the abutment, and the flaps were sutured (Fig 30-4e). Nine months later, clinical probing depth measurements did not exceed 2 mm in a firm peri-implant mucosa. After 12 months of loading, periapical radiographs showed bone fill and apparent integration of the previously exposed screw threads (Fig 30-4f).

Discussion

This study evaluated the performance of a one-stage sinus augmentation onlay osteoplasty using MSCs, PRP, and/or β-TCP (tissue-engineered "bone") with simultaneous implant placement. While numerous studies[10–12] have recommended a two-step procedure in patients with less than 5 mm of available alveolar bone height in the posterior maxilla, the results of this investigation suggest that tissue-engineered cells can yield adequate bone volume for simultaneous implant placement. A one-step procedure offers the advantages of reducing the number of surgical procedures and the time needed to complete the implant-supported dental restoration.

Various clinical investigations[13,14] and case reports[15] indicate that, although sinus augmentation can be clinically successful with various grafting materials, autogenous bone nevertheless provides the best osteogenic potential and biomechanical properties to regenerate bone. However, the quantitative limitations of autogenous bone harvested from intraoral sites often force the clinician to combine autograft with other types of grafts in order to obtain adequate amounts of graft material. Alternatives to autogenous bone grafts are inorganic bone mineral and biologically conductive synthetic materials. The osteoconductive properties of synthetic[16,17] materials, within a narrow size range of particles, have been documented in a series of animal studies that demonstrate the formation of bone in protective pouches. Bone was created between the particles and the surrounding tissue fluids through a gelation and corrosion phenomenon arising from the interfacial ion exchange. Autogenous bone, when used as a graft, has an osteogenic potential related to the number of surviving osteoblasts and a potential osteoinductive effect by the release of bone morphogenetic proteins (BMPs) and other growth factors.

Accordingly, recent tissue-engineering approaches attempt to create new bone based on the seeding of expanded osteoblasts onto a porous ceramic scaffold. Due to the slow or nonresorption of hydroxyapatite (HA), these attempts have produced suboptimal results. HA does not have good plasticity, and cellular implants have not been consistent or efficacious with this delivery vehicle. The optimal carrier combines biodegradability with a capacity for receptivity to cultured cells. In this experimental study, a relatively rapid biodegradable calcium phosphate carrier, PRP gel loaded with mesenchymal stem cells, had excellent osteogenic response in vivo. Calcium and phosphorus ions are presumably absorbed into anabolic bone formation. Osteogenic cells function to induce bone tissue, which then organizes in association with the surrounding osseous environment. Use of a combination of PRP, stem cells, and/or β-TCP produces a mature bone tissue in which there is complete resorption, if not absorption of the scaffold. Osseointegration within regenerated bone is observed, both radiographically and clinically, to follow the same pattern as autogenous bone incorporation and is likely to be confirmed with implant retrieval histology. The use of tissue-engineered bone provides a more rapid and effective bone regeneration than bone graft that must be replaced by substitution. The manipulation of tissue-engineered bone is favorable and completely avoids second-site surgery.

These findings conclude that tissue-engineered bone implants elicit true bone regeneration and perform just as well as autogenous bone grafts, with complete disappearance of biomaterial expander and *formation* of new bone in clinically relevant volumes. The ability to inject a tissue-engineered "bone" preparation that solidifies very early within the host and gets replaced very rapidly and seamlessly with bone has powerful implications for the future of oral/maxillofacial and reconstructive surgery. This method represents a breakthrough, albeit only a first step toward customizing tissue-engineered regeneration of bone. In the future, host marrow that is proliferated ex vivo into osteoblasts and then reimplanted into a prescribed biodegradable scaffold will reproduce contoured augmentations, re-establish ablated facial bone structure, reconstruct the periodontal and alveolar process, and osseointegrate dental implants in even the most compromised of settings.

Conclusion

The results of the present investigation indicate that tissue-engineered bone used for maxillary sinus augmentation with simultaneous implant placement in patients provides stable and predictable results and bodes well for the future development of tissue engineering in the coming decade.

References

1. Younger EM, Chapman MW. Morbidity at bone graft donor sites. J Orthop Trauma 1989;3:187–191.
2. Gross JS. Bone grafting materials for dental applications: A practical guide. Compend Contin Educ Dent 1997;18:1013–1036.
3. Misch CE, Dietsh F. Bone-grafting materials in implant dentistry. Implant Dent 1993;2:158–167.
4. Yamada Y, Boo JS, Ozawa R, et al. Bone regeneration following injection of mesenchymal stem cells and fibrin glue with a biodegradable scaffold. J Craniomaxillofac Surg 2003;31:27–33.
5. Langer R, Vacanti JP. Tissue engineering. Science 1993;260:920–926.
6. Yamada Y, Ueda M, Naiki T, Takahashi M, Hata K, Nagasaka T. Autogenous injectable bone for regeneration with mesenchymal stem cells and platelet-rich-plasma. Tissue-engineered bone regeneration. Tissue Eng 2004;10:955–964.
7. Yamada Y, Ueda M, Naiki T, Nagasaka T. Tissue-engineered injectable bone regeneration for osseointegrated dental implants. Clin Oral Implants Res 2004;15:589–597.
8. Pittenger MF, Mackay AM, Beck SC, et al. Multilineage potential of adult human mesenchymal stem cells. Science 1999;284:143–147.
9. Tatum H. Maxillary and sinus implant reconstructions. Clin North Am 1986;30:207–230.
10. Jensen J, Simonsen EK, Sindet-Pedersen S. Reconstruction of the severely resorbed maxilla with bone grafting and osseointegrated implants: A preliminary report. J Oral Maxillofac Surg 1990;48:27–32.
11. Marx RE. Clinical application of bone biology to mandibular and maxillary reconstruction. Clin Plast Surg 1994;21:377–392.
12. Raghoebar GM, Brouwer TJ, Reintsema H, Vanoort RP. Augmentation of the maxillary sinus floor with autogenous bone for placement of endosseous implants: A preliminary report. J Oral Maxillofac Surg 1993;51:1198–1203.

13. Lundgren S, Moy P, Johansson C, Nilsson H. Augmentation of the maxillary sinus floor with particulated mandible: A histologic and histomorphometric study. Int J Oral Maxillofac Implants 1996;11:760–766.
14. Moy PK, Lundgren S, Holmes RE. Maxillary sinus augmentation: Histomorphometric analysis of graft materials for maxillary sinus floor augmentation. Int J Oral Maxillofac Implants 1993;51:857–862.
15. Valentini P, Abensur D, Densari D, Graziani JN, Hammerle CHF. Histological evaluation of Bio-Oss in a 2-stage sinus floor elevation and implantation procedure. A human case report. Clin Oral Implants Res 1998;9:59–64.
16. Furusawa T, Mizunuma K. Osteoconductive properties and efficacy of resorbable bioactive glass as a bone-grafting material. Implant Dent 1997;6:93–101.
17. Schepers EJG, Ducheyne P, Barbier L, Schepers S. Bioactive glass particles of narrow size range: A new material for the repair of bone defects. Implant Dent 1993;2:151–156.

chapter 31
Gene Therapy of Growth Factors for Tissue Engineering and Regenerative Medicine

William V. Giannobile, DDS, DMedSc
Brent Y. Kimball, BS
Li-Xing Man, MD, MSc

Tooth loss, often a consequence of trauma or disease, can lead to the destruction of nearly half of the original tooth-supporting (or alveolar) bone.[1] A variety of techniques have been developed to restore alveolar bone prior to or at the time of dental implant placement, including osseous grafting and guided bone regeneration.[2] However, lack of predictability and an inability to achieve volumetric bone changes beyond the "envelope" of the alveolus limit these reconstructive approaches. Advances in the field of tissue engineering and biomimetics offer significant potential to regenerate craniofacial structures using biologic mediators and matrices that mimic the tissue's original formative processes.[3,4] Tissue engineering of alveolar bone using gene therapeutic approaches may offer potential for optimizing the delivery of growth-promoting molecules at implant osteotomy sites.[5,6] This chapter describes gene delivery methods for regeneration and repair of soft tissue and bone in periodontal, peri-implant, and sinus floor augmentation procedures. The role of bone morphogenetic proteins (BMPs) and platelet-derived growth factors (PDGFs) in dentistry and for reconstructive craniofacial procedures is highlighted.

BMPs belong to the powerful superfamily of transforming growth factor beta (TGF-β) that regulate cartilage and bone formation during embryonic development and regeneration in postnatal life.[7] Recent studies have demonstrated the expression of BMPs during distraction osteogenesis, tooth development,[8,9] and periodontal repair.[10–12] BMP-7, also known as osteogenic protein-1 (OP-1), is a multifunctional member of the BMP family that handles multiple roles in bone formation and regeneration. BMP-7 stimulates bone regeneration around teeth,[13] endosseous dental implants,[14] and in maxillary sinus floor augmentation procedures.[15] Though encouraging, results of recent studies demonstrate only partial or inadequate regeneration, thus highlighting the need for improved methods of growth factor delivery.

Gene Transfer for Clinical Treatment Protocols

Since the half-life of growth factors in vivo is transient (on the order of minutes to hours), complete bone regeneration is not a certain outcome of conventional surgical therapy. Typically, high concentrations of growth factors are required to promote tissue regeneration.[16] Therefore, supplemental local growth factor production via gene transfer may be superior to bolus delivery methods.[17]

In very basic terms, gene therapy refers to the insertion of genes, directly or indirectly, into targeted cells along with a matrix to promote a specific biologic effect in an individual. Typically, the aim is to supplement a defective mutant allele with a functional one, but it can also be used to induce a more favorable host response. Targeting cells for gene therapy requires the use of vectors, or direct delivery methods, to induce transfection.[18] By incorporating DNA in a matrix, gene therapy prolongs the bioavailability of such molecules.[19,20]

Many vector systems are available to deliver DNA sequences of genes of interest, including plasmids, adenovirus, adeno-associated virus, and retrovirus. The choice of vector is based on the duration of delivery and the adverse effects associated with each vector.[21]

Incorporating DNA into scaffolding matrices must allow for transfection of a sufficient number of cells to produce inductive doses of the desired protein.[22] For example, incorporation of PDGF-encoded plasmid DNA into poly(lactic co-glycolic acid) (PLGA) scaffolds showed encouraging results in sustained release of plasmid DNA, which led to transfection of cells and sustained production of the protein of interest for 28 days or longer. In addition, in vivo delivery of the PDGF-encoded plasmid DNA promoted matrix deposition and blood vessel formation in the developing tissue at 4 weeks.[22] In the future, combined DNA and cell therapy may be possible by transducing cells with the DNA of interest to obtain optimal numbers and then seeding the cells in the scaffolds. The cell-gene scaffolds could then be implanted in the wound to provide sustained release for regeneration of tissues and organs.

PDGF-B Gene Therapy for Soft Tissue Wound Healing

Wound healing is a dynamic cellular and biochemical process that is orchestrated by several different growth factors. Cutaneous wound repair follows a sequence of three phases: inflammation, tissue formation, and tissue remodeling. The first two phases require chemotactic signals and cell mitogens such as PDGF, epidermal growth factor (EGF), fibroblast growth factor-2 (FGF-2), and transforming growth factor-2 (TGF-2). One of several critical components of wound repair, PDGF functions variously to induce endogenous growth factors, attract new cells to the wound site, and signal cells to lay down collagen and generate new granulation tissue, all essential to wound repair.

The diabetic wound is particularly difficult to repair, and, because it is deficient in growth factors such as PDGF, standard treatment is often unsuccessful. For this reason, the diabetic wound is optimal for studying the use of gene therapy in wound-healing methods that may have maxillofacial applications. Topically applied PDGF in both animal models and clinical studies has demonstrated only limited success. And while the use of recombinant human PDGF (Regranex, Ortho-McNeil) has achieved variable success in clinical trials of lower extremity and pressure sore wound healing, current clinical experience is often discouraging.[23–25] Recent advances in gene therapy offer alternative ways to apply growth factors. Gene therapy has the potential to create an environment in the diabetic wound where sustained PDGF application can be observed, in contrast to abbreviated temporal exposure that is observed through a topical agent.

A number of methods have been developed for cutaneous gene delivery. One technique to treat wounds involves the use of dermal fibroblasts retrovirally transduced with viral vectors as carriers of the gene for PDGF-B. Lentiviral vectors carrying the PDGF-B gene can also be injected directly into the wound site.

The American Diabetes Association funded a study conducted by the Columbia College of Physicians and Surgeons to explore these methods of PDGF gene application on dermal wounds in diabetic mice.[26] Full-thickness 2- × 2–cm dermal wounds were created on the dorsae of genetically diabetic (db/db) mice. The mice were subsequently treated via application of the PDGF-B gene and observed over 14-, 21-, and 35-day periods. Wound area closure, epithelial gap (the distance separating opposing wound edges), mean vascular density, and mature collagen deposition were quantified. The results demonstrated accelerated healing in the treated wounds compared to controls (Figs 31-1 and 31-2).[26]

Gene therapy as an adjunct to wound healing will be difficult to transfer to clinical application until it has been proven safe, simple, and effective to use.[27,28] Soft tissue wound healing is a complex process that contributes indirectly to graft incorporation in bone graft surgery (see chapter 25). In the future, the best results might be achieved by combining several growth factors timed specifically for

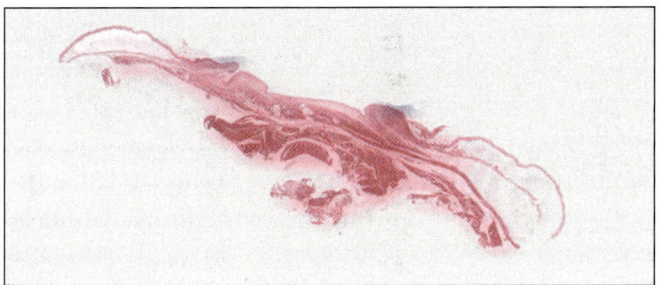

Fig 31-1 Epithelial gap (0.57 cm) from 35-day lentiviral PDGF-B–treated wound demonstrated accelerated closure when compared to control.[26]

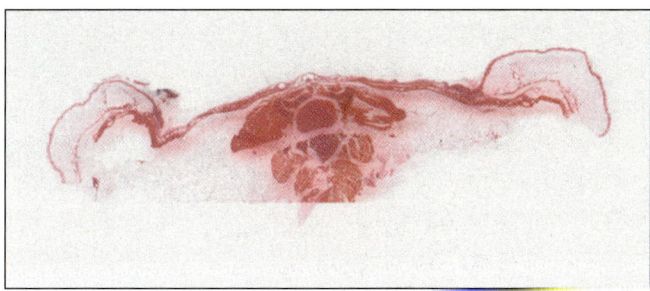

Fig 31-2 Epithelial gap (1.20 cm) from 35-day phosphate-buffered saline (PBS) control wound.[26]

different stages of wound healing.[29] Of the various viral vectors capable of gene delivery, retroviral, adenoviral, and lentiviral vectors hold the most promise for gene therapy in the clinical setting since they yield the most efficient transfections.[26] However, concern over the use of viral vectors remains (see Safety Issues, below).

Gene Therapy for Alveolar Bone–Engineering Applications

The use of topical BMP to promote osteogenesis has been studied in a variety of bony sites over the past 5 years (see chapter 25).[30,31] In the craniofacial complex, an ex vivo approach was used for repair of periodontal alveolar bone; Jin et al[32] used BMP-7 gene transfer to stimulate new alveolar bone, tooth root cementum, and periodontal ligaments. Ad-BMP-7 or its antagonist, Ad-Noggin, transduced syngeneic dermal fibroblasts that were seeded on gelatin carriers and transplanted into large alveolar bone defects (Fig 31-3). Repair of the periodontal defects was observed as a process of rapid chondrogenesis followed by osteogenesis, cementogenesis, and predictable bridging of the bone defect. Conversely, Noggin (competitive BMP antagonist) gene transfer blocked alveolar bone and cementum repair, both in osseous defects and in tissue-engineered cementum.[33] More recently, gene delivery of BMP-7 via an adenoviral vector combined with a collagen matrix was used to repair large alveolar bone defects associated with implants at extraction sockets (Fig 31-4).[34]

PDGF has demonstrated strong potential in regeneration of gingiva,[35] alveolar bone,[36] and cementum[37] in a variety of wound-healing models. Alveolar bone defects treated with adenovirus encoding PDGF-B yielded strong evidence of bone and cementum regeneration beyond that of control vectors, including a nearly four-fold increase in bone bridging and a six-fold increase in tooth-lining cemental repair.[36] In addition, sustained and localized expression of the luciferase reporter gene at the periodontal lesions was confirmed for a period of up to 21 days after gene transfer.

Sonic hedgehog (SHH) also appears to be a key regulator involved in the formation of new bone, both embryologically and in fracture repair. A 45kDa vertebrate homologue of the *Drosophila* segment polarity gene hedgehog, SHH assists in the differentiation of pluripotent mesenchymal stem cells into the osteoblastic lineage by stimulating the expression of a cascade of downstream genes involved in bone development.[38–41] By inducing the expression of multiple BMPs, SHH mimicks the complex mixture of heterodimers normally present in developing bone. In a novel study designed to assess the capacity of SHH to induce new bone formation, Edwards et al[42] combined gingival fibroblasts, fat-derived cells, and mesenchymal stem cells that were transduced with human SHH complementary DNA (cDNA); suspended the cells in an alginate-collagen matrix; and placed the matrix into critical-sized defects in a rabbit model. Gross, radiographic, and histologic assessments of the osseous regenerative capacity of SHH gene–enhanced cells revealed significant bone regeneration at all treatment sites compared to controls.

chapter 31 Gene Therapy of Growth Factors for Tissue Engineering and Regenerative Medicine

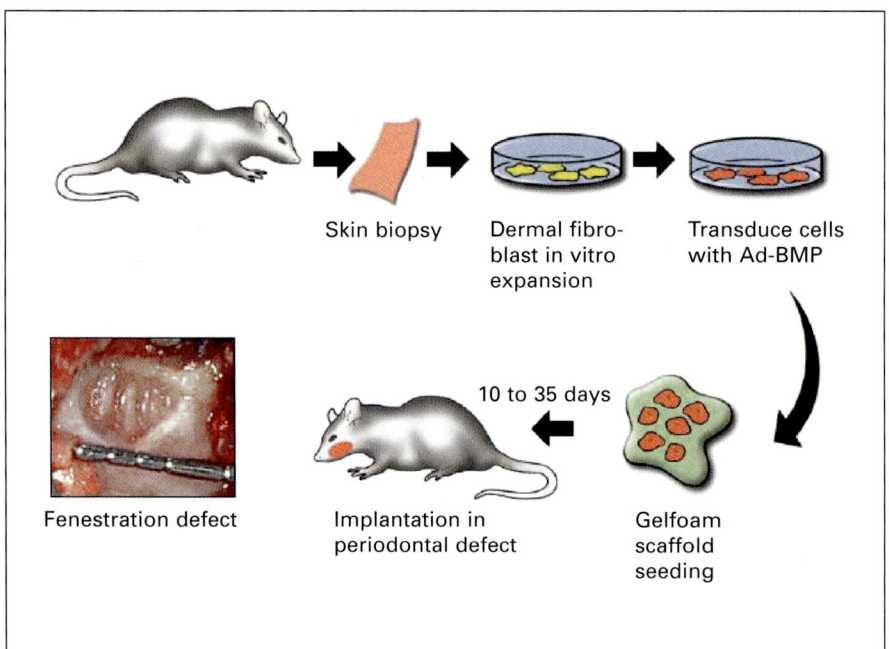

Fig 31-3 Ex vivo gene-targeting model for BMP delivery to alveolar bone defects. Cells are expanded in vitro and then transduced by gene therapy vectors (such as BMP-encoding adenovirus, as shown in the illustration). The transduced cells are then transferred to gelatin scaffolds and transplanted in vivo to periodontal osseous defects to promote tissue engineering of the wounds. (Adapted from Jin et al[32] with permission.)

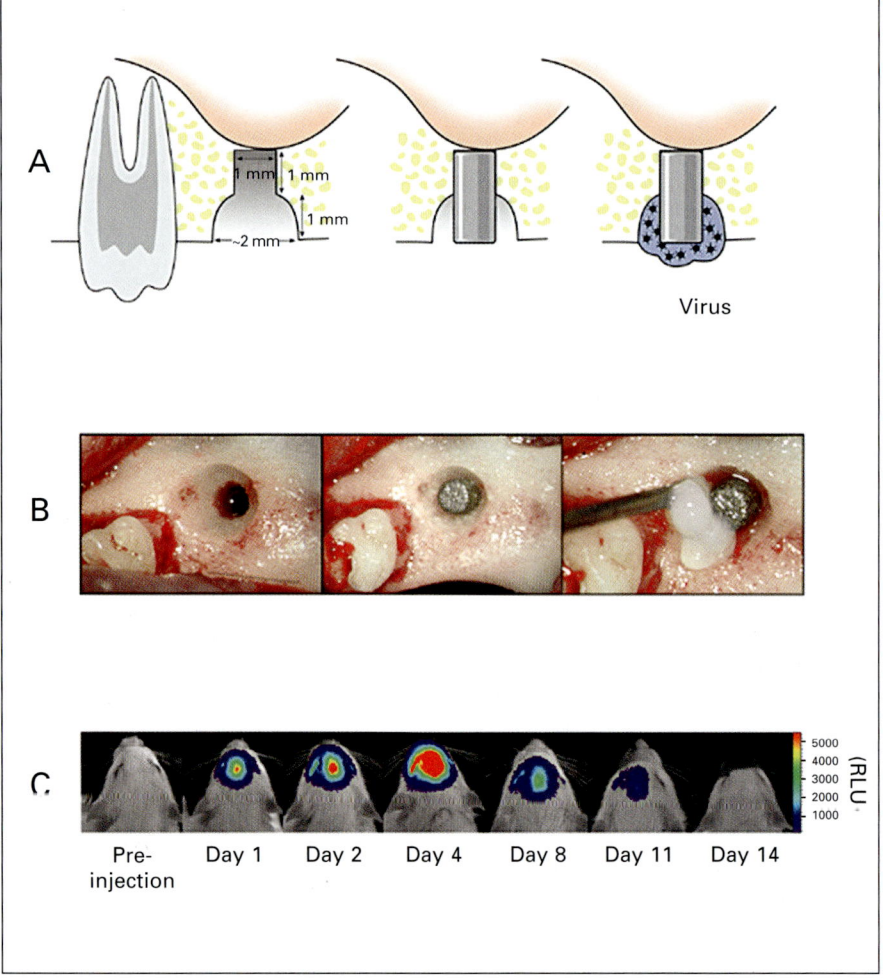

Fig 31-4 In vivo gene-targeting model for dental implant osseointegration. A, Dental implant osteotomy defect model for gene delivery.[35] "Well-type" osteotomy defects are created (A, far left). The titanium dental implant is press fit into position (A, middle), followed by the delivery of a collagen matrix containing either Ad/BMP-7 or Ad/firefly luciferase (A, right). B, High-magnification photographs from the surgical operation corresponding to A, taken at 10× magnification including defect creation (B, far left), dental implant placement (B, middle) and gene delivery (B, right). C, In vivo bioluminescence of gene targeting. In vivo bioluminescence images of a luciferase-treated rat. To localize the signal, color images of the photon emissions were superimposed on grayscale images of the animals, and signals were quantified in relative light units (RLUs). All images were analyzed using the LivingImage software. Distribution of gene delivery is shown beginning at day 1 with the peak expression at day 4. In this case, transgene expression was sustained at measurable levels for 14 days. Photon emissions are measured in RLUs.

Safety Issues

For gene therapy to become a clinical reality for human application in the treatment of disease or injury, safety must be a primary concern. The use of viral vectors for growth factor delivery to bone defects requires evaluation of specific vector biodistribution properties (ie, dissemination of vectors from the osseous site to other extraorthopic tissues and organs). Issues important in biodistribution study in gene transfer medicine development is shown through the determination of target organs for toxicity, germline transmission assessment, and determination of risks of shedding and spreading of vectors in the gene transfer recipient and environment.[32] Various safety assessments have been performed using growth factor transgenes[33] and for bone-sparing agents preclinically[34] demonstrating lack of significant local and systemic toxicity. To address the critical nature of safety for gene therapeutics for the treatment and prevention of disease, the American Society of Gene Therapy developed guidelines that have been reviewed by government regulatory bodies for use in preclinical and human clinical trials.[35] Continued diligence in carefully evaluating both short- and long-term safety of gene therapy vectors will be important if gene therapy will become a viable treatment alternative for bone repair applications.

Future Perspectives

Many advances have been made over the past decade in the reconstruction of complex oral and craniofacial bone defects. In particular, developments in polymeric and ceramic scaffolding systems for cell, protein, and gene delivery have undergone significant growth. A cell-gene scaffolding system has been developed to re-engineer periodontal tissue with successful outcomes.[43] The targeting of signaling molecules or growth factors by gene therapy to the craniofacial complex has led to significant new information regarding bioactive molecules that promote tissue repair in both medicine and dentistry.

A major problem that has been overlooked, however, is modulation of the exuberant host response to microbial contamination plaguing the oral wound environment. To improve the outcomes in regeneration, scientists need to examine dual delivery of host modifiers or use host-modulatory approaches[44] to optimize the results of therapy. Further advancements in the field of gene therapy will continue to rely heavily on multidisciplinary approaches that combine the expertise of engineering, dentistry, medicine, and infectious disease specialists in repairing complex soft and hard tissue wounds.

Acknowledgments

The authors acknowledge the helpful collaboration of Drs Qiming Jin, Mario Taba, Jr, and Christoph Ramseier, and Mr James Sugai. This research was supported by NIH/NIDCR grants DE 13397 and DE 016619 to the University of Michigan, and by a grant to Columbia University from the American Diabetes Association.

The contributions of Drs Arnold S. Breitbart and Salvatore L. Ruggiero are gratefully acknowledged.

References

1. Schropp L, Wenzel A, Kostopoulos L, Karring T. Bone healing and soft tissue contour changes following single-tooth extraction: A clinical and radiographic 12-month prospective study. Int J Periodontics Restorative Dent 2003;23:313–323.
2. Lutolf MP, Hubbell JA. Synthetic biomaterials as instructive extracellular microenvironments for morphogenesis in tissue engineering. Nat Biotechnol 2005;23:47–55.
3. Doll B, Sfeir C, Winn S, Huard J, Hollinger J. Critical aspects of tissue-engineered therapy for bone regeneration. Critical Rev Eukaryot Gene Expr 2001;11:173–198.
4. Alden TD, Beres EJ, Laurent JS, et al. The use of bone morphogenetic protein gene therapy in craniofacial bone repair. J Craniofac Surg 2000;11:24–30.
5. Giannobile WV. Periodontal tissue engineering by growth factors. Bone 1996;19(1 Suppl):23S–37S.
6. Reddi AH. Role of morphogenetic proteins in skeletal tissue engineering and regeneration. Nat Biotechnol 1998;16:247–252.
7. Nakashima M, Reddi AH. The application of bone morphogenetic proteins to dental tissue engineering. Nat Biotechnol 2003;21:1025–1032.
8. Yazawa M, Kishi K, Nakajima H, Nakajima T. Expression of bone morphogenetic proteins during mandibular distraction osteogenesis in rabbits. J Oral Maxillofac Surg 2003;61:587–592.
9. Jensen OT. Exogenous bone morphogenetic protein may improve distraction osteogenesis outcomes. J Oral Maxillofac Surg 2003;61:1505–1506.
10. Aberg T, Wozney J, Thesleff I. Expression patterns of bone morphogenetic proteins (BMPs) in the developing mouse tooth suggest roles in morphogenesis and cell differentiation. Dev Dyn 1997;210:383–396.

11. Amar S, Chung KM, Nam SH, Karataz S, Myokai F, Van Dyke TE. Markers of bone and cementum formation accumulate in tissues regenerated in periodontal defects treated with expanded polytetrafluoroethylene membranes. J Periodontol Res 1997;32:148–158.
12. Thomadakis G, Ramoshebi LN, Crooks J, Rueger DC, Ripamonti U. Immunolocalization of bone morphogenetic protein-2 and -3 and osteogenic protein-1 during murine tooth root morphogenesis and in other craniofacial structures. Eur J Oral Sci 1999;107:368–377.
13. Giannobile WV, Ryan S, Shih MS, Su DL, Kaplan PL, Chan TC. Recombinant human osteogenic protein-1 (OP-1) stimulates periodontal wound healing in class III furcation defects. J Periodontol 1998;69:129–137.
14. Rutherford RB, Sampath TK, Rueger DC, Taylor TD. Use of bovine osteogenic protein to promote rapid osseointegration of endosseous dental implants. Int J Oral Maxillofac Implants 1992;7:297–301.
15. van den Bergh JP, ten Bruggenkate CM, Groeneveld HH, Burger EH, Tuinzing DB. Recombinant human bone morphogenetic protein-7 in maxillary sinus floor elevation surgery in 3 patients compared to autogenous bone grafts: A clinical pilot study. J Clin Periodontol 2000;27:627–636.
16. Bonadio J. Tissue engineering via local gene delivery: Update and future prospects for enhancing the technology. Adv Drug Deliv Rev 2000;44(2–3):185–194.
17. Anusaksathien O, Giannobile WV. Growth factor delivery to re-engineer periodontal tissues. Curr Pharm Biotechnol 2002;3:129–139.
18. Baltzer AW, Lieberman JR. Regional gene therapy to enhance bone repair. Gene Ther 2004;11:344–350.
19. Lieberman JR, Le LQ, Wu L, et al. Regional gene therapy with a BMP-2-producing murine stromal cell line induces heterotopic and orthotopic bone formation in rodents. J Orthop Res 1998;16:330–339.
20. Doukas J, Chandler LA, Gonzalez AM, et al. Matrix immobilization enhances the tissue repair activity of growth factor gene therapy vectors. Hum Gene Ther 2001;12:783–798.
21. Baum BJ, Kok M, Tran SD, Yamano S. The impact of gene therapy on dentistry. J Am Dent Assoc 2002;133:35–44.
22. Shea LD, Smiley E, Bonadio J, Mooney DJ. DNA delivery from polymer matrices for tissue engineering. Nat Biotechnol 1999;17:551–554.
23. Steed DL. Clinical evaluation of recombinant human platelet-derived growth factor for the treatment of lower diabetic extremity ulcers. J Vasc Surg 1995;72:71–81.
24. Robson MG, Phillips LG, Thomason A, et al. Recombinant human platelet-derived growth factor-BB for the treatment of chronic pressure ulcers. Ann Plast Surg 1992;29:193–201.
25. Mustoe TA, Cutler NR, Allman RM, et al. A phase II study to evaluate platelet-derived growth factor-BB in the treatment of stage 3 and 4 pressure ulcers. Arch Surg 1994;129:213–219.
26. Man LX, Park JC, Terry MJ, et al. Lentiviral gene therapy with platelet-derived growth factor B sustains accelerated healing of diabetic wounds over time. Ann Plast Surg 2005;55:81–86.
27. Andree C, Swain WF, Page CP, et al. In vivo transfer and expression of a human epidermal growth factor gene accelerates wound repair. Proc Natl Acad Sci USA 1994;91:12188–12192.
28. Margolis DJ, Crombleholme T, Herlyn M. Clinical protocol: Phase I trial to evaluate the saftey of H5.020CMV.PDGF-β for the treatment of a diabetic insensate foot ulcer. Wound Repair Regen 2000;8:480–493.
29. Fu X, Li X, Cheng B, Chen W, Sheng Z. Engineered growth factors and cutaneous wound healing: Success and possible questions in the past 10 years. Wound Repair Regen 2005;13:122–130.
30. Alden TD, Beres EJ, Laurent JS, et al. The use of bone morphogenetic protein gene therapy in craniofacial bone repair. J Craniofac Surg 2000;11:24–30.
31. Franceschi RT, Yang S, Rutherford RB, Krebsbach PH, Zhao M, Wang D. Gene therapy approaches for bone regeneration. Cells Tissues Organs 2004;176(1–3):95–108.
32. Jin QM, Anusaksathien O, Webb SA, Rutherford RB, Giannobile WV. Gene therapy of bone morphogenetic protein for periodontal tissue engineering. J Periodontol 2003;74:202–213.
33. Jin QM, Zhao M, Economides AN, Somerman MJ, Giannobile WV. Noggin gene delivery inhibits cementoblast-induced mineralization. Connect Tissue Res 2004;45:50–59.
34. Dunn CA, Jin Q, Taba M Jr, Franceschi RT, Bruce Rutherford R, Giannobile WV. BMP gene delivery for alveolar bone engineering at dental implant defects. Mol Ther 2005;11:294–299.
35. Anusaksathien O, Webb SA, Jin QM, Giannobile WV. Platelet-derived growth factor gene delivery stimulates ex vivo gingival repair. Tissue Eng 2003;9:745–756.
36. Jin Q, Anusaksathien O, Webb SA, Printz MA, Giannobile WV. Engineering of tooth-supporting structures by delivery of PDGF gene therapy vectors. Mol Ther 2004;9:519–526.
37. Giannobile WV, Lee CS, Tomala MP, Tejeda KM, Zhu Z. Platelet-derived growth factor (PDGF) gene delivery for application in periodontal tissue engineering. J Periodontol 2001;72:815–823.
38. Spinella-Jaegle S, Rawadi G, Gallea S, et al. Sonic hedgehog increases the commitment of pluripotent mesenchymal cells into the osteoblastic lineage and abolishes adipocytic differentiation. J Cell Sci 2001;114:2085–2094.
39. Hu D, Helms JA. The role of Sonic hedgehog in normal and abnormal craniofacial morphogenesis. Development 1999;126:4873–4884.
40. Kinto N, Iwamoto M, Enomoto-Iwamoto M, et al. Fibroblasts expressing Sonic hedgehog induce osteoblast differentiation and ectopic bone formation. FEBS Lett 1997;404:319–323.
41. Bitgood MJ, McMahon AP. Hedgehog and BMP genes are co-expressed at many diverse sites of cell-cell interaction in the mouse embryo. Dev Biol 1995;172:126–138.
42. Edwards PC, Ruggiero S, Fantasia J, et al. Sonic hedgehog gene-enhanced tissue engineering for bone regeneration. Gene Ther 2005;12:75–86.
43. Jin Q-M, Anusaksathien O, Webb SA, Rutherford RB, Giannobile WV. Gene therapy of bone morphogenetic protein for periodontal tissue engineering. J Periodontol 2003;74:202–213.
44. Taba M Jr, Huffer H, Shelburne CE, et al. Gene delivery of TNFR:Fc by adeno-associated virus vector blocks progression of periodontitits. Mol Ther 2005;10(suppl):1586.

Index

Page numbers followed by "f" denote figures; those followed by "t" denote tables; those followed by "b" denote boxes

A

Abutments, 77
Acellular collagen sponge carrier, 295, 298
Acid-etched implants, 223, 225, 226f, 226t
Acrylic resin, 78
Acrylic resin-porcelain veneers, 82f, 83
Activation→resorption→formation sequence, 35b
Adrenal disorders, 97–98
Age-related bone loss, 19
Alcohol abuse, 97
Alendronate, 95
Algipore, 203
Allergic rhinitis, 104
Allografts
  demineralized freeze-dried bone
    case studies of, 188–193
    description of, 184
  description of, 183
  donors of, 183–184, 184f
  ethylene oxide for, 184
  freeze-dried bone
    bone morphogenetic proteins in, 185
    cortical, 185
    mineralized, 184
    procurement of, 183–185
    safety of, 183–186
    trabecular bone area for, 298
  incorporation of, 27
  infection concerns for
    Creutzfeldt-Jakob disease, 183, 186
    description of, 183, 185–186, 341
    hepatitis, 186
    human immunodeficiency virus, 185–186
    syphilis, 186
  prevalence of, 183
  procurement of, 183–185
  sinus grafting using, 187
  sinus membrane elevation using
    case study of, 189, 189f
    description of, 187, 188f
  sterility of, 184

"All-on-4," 316–317, 317f
Alloplasts
  beta-tricalcium phosphate, 204–206, 205f, 207f
  bioactive glass, 203–204
  hydroxyapatite
    bovine, 137f–138f
    implants coated with, 61
    marginal bone loss using, 202–203
    osteoconductive capacity of, 202, 203f
    sinus membrane caused by, 118
  nonresorbable, 201
  overview of, 201
  resorbable, 201
  summary of, 207
Alveolar bone
  gene therapy applications for, 351, 352f
  height of, implant survival based on, 63t, 263
  tissue engineering of, 349
Alveolar distraction, 131
Alveolar ridge
  advanced vertical bone loss, 76
  atrophic, 174, 175f
  augmentation of
    atrophic ridge, 174, 175f
    calvarial bone grafts for, 174, 175f
    indications for, 5
    onlay grafts for, 176f, 241
    overgraft for, 174, 175f
    sinus grafting and, 131
    vertical, 242f
  expansion of. *See* Ridge expansion.
  height of
    delayed implant placement based on, 47
    description of, 5
    implant survival and, 56–57
    simultaneous grafting and implant placement indications based on, 57, 60b, 61
    sinus augmentation effects on, 64–65
    trans-alveolar sinus elevation and ridge expansion requirements, 253–254
    treatment planning based on, 65
  resorption of, 7, 251
Ameloblastoma, 91f, 309f

Amoxicillin, 153
Ampicillin/sulbactam, 152
Anesthesia
  for tibia bone harvesting, 149, 150f
  for zygomatic implant placement, 306
Angiogenesis
  description of, 14b
  diseases that affect, 19–20
Angiogenic factors, 15
Anterior iliac crest harvesting, 158f–160f, 158–161, 168, 169t
Anticoagulant citrate dextrose-A, 292
Anticoagulants, 93
Antral membrane
  stem cells of, 8
  "tenting up" of, 8
Antrostomy
  lateral
    barrier placement over, 229–231, 230f
    sinus floor elevation by, 64
  piezoelectric
    lateral window technique, 274–275, 275f
    by osteotomy, 276f, 276–277
Antrum
  entrance to, 5
  graft materials in, 5–7
  implant protrusion into, 5–6
Atrophic maxilla
  bone-grafting options in, 305–306
  description of, 305
  graftless rehabilitation of, 320–321
  tilted implants for, 316–318
  zygomatic implants for. *See* Zygomatic implants.
Atrophic nonunion, 27
Autogenous bone
  advantages of, 179, 212
  calvarial. *See* Calvarial bone grafts.
  disadvantages of, 267
  iliac crest. *See* Iliac crest harvesting.
  platelet-rich plasma used with, 296
  resorption of, 267
  sinus grafting using, 212, 346–347
  tibia. *See* Tibia.
Autografts
  advantages of, 212

355

Index

bone mass loss, 20
bone substitute and, 21
incorporation of, 27
osteogenic cells in, 16, 17
osteoinductive properties of, 212
platelet-rich plasma added to, 137, 139
resorption of, 20
Autoinduction, 290
Autologous bone
  advantages of, 129–131, 130t
  biology of, 136–137
  bone morphogenetic proteins in, 129
  bone substitutes used with, 131
  clinical use of, 137–142
  donor sites for, 131–136, 157
  harvesting of, from maxillofacial region sites
    complications of, 133–134
    harvesting procedure, 131–136
    indications for, 131
    mandibular ramus, 134–136
    mandibular symphysis, 133–134
    maxillary tuberosity, 131–132, 132f, 142f
    patient preparation, 131
    risks associated with, 131
    zygoma, 132
    zygomaticomaxillary buttress, 131–132, 132f
  indications for, 131
Autologous bone grafts
  healing of, 130
  healing period for, 141
  from iliac crest, 141
  onlay augmentation with, 130, 136
  particulate, 137
Azithromycin, 153

B

Bacterial sinusitis, 90f
Barrier membranes
  bioabsorbable, 230f, 230–231, 237t
  guided bone regeneration use of, 235, 236f
  history of, 229–230
  nonabsorbable, 235, 237t
  over lateral window, 230f, 230–231
  placement of, 230f
  removal of, 235
  sinus membrane perforation repaired using, 231–232
  stabilization of, 230f, 231
Basic fibroblast growth factor, 14b
Basic multicellular unit remodeling, 27–28, 30, 31f, 35b

Beaver blade, 257
Beta-tricalcium phosphate, 204–206, 205f, 207f, 330, 330f
Bioabsorbable barrier membranes, 230f, 230–231, 237t
Bioactive glass, 203–204
Bio-Oss
  bone formation in sinuses grafted with, 224t
  bone morphogenetic proteins added to, 338
  description of, 138f, 215
Bisphosphonates, 94–95
Bite forces
  in anterior vs posterior region, 42
  description of, 30
Blade implants, 4–5
Block bone grafts
  corticocancellous, 133f
  description of, 56, 59f
  implants used to stabilize, 166
  from mandibular ramus, 134–135
  from mandibular symphysis, 133, 133f
  placement of, 139
  posterior maxillary ridge deficiencies, 139, 140f
Blood vessel formation, 14b, 15f
Bone
  autologous. See Autologous bone.
  lamellar, 28
  microdamage of, 28
  strain windows for, 32
  tetracycline labeling of, 33f
  zygomatic, 121
Bone chips, 277–278
Bone compression osteoplasty, 263, 264f
Bone cores, 135
Bone curettes, 151, 151f
Bone cutting, piezoelectric, 273–274
Bone density
  in osteoporosis patients, 96
  in posterior maxilla, 42
Bone flap, 251
Bone graft(s)
  atrophic nonunion of, 27
  autologous. See Autologous bone grafts.
  block. See Block bone grafts.
  calvarial. See Calvarial bone grafts.
  consolidation of
    description of, 14
    gene therapy for, 19b
    levels of, 22f
    osteogenic cells for, 19b
    osteoporosis effects, 18–20

strategies for, 19b
summary of, 21–22
cortical, 137
corticocancellous block, 133f
cranial, 172–173, 173f
crestal, 76
healing of, 27
iliac. See Iliac bone grafts.
implant-loaded
  description of, 28
  macromodeling effects on, 29
incorporation of, 27
interpositional, 136–137
from mandibular ramus, 134–135
from mandibular symphysis, 133, 133f
membranous, 136
modeling of, 27
nonmechanical factors that affect, 33–34
regional acceleratory phenomenon effects on, 27
remodeling of, 16b
strength of. See Bone strength.
from tibia. See Tibia bone grafts.
trephine, 163, 164f
vital biomechanics for, 28
Bone grafting
  history of, 3
  irradiation before, 93
  osteotome, 267
Bone loss
  advanced, 191f
  age-related, 19
  buccal, 76
  horizontal, 253
  in maxillary sinus, 13
Bone marrow aspirate
  applications of, 328–329
  aspiration technique, 329f, 329–330
  osteoblasts produced from, 328
  from posterior ilium, 329
  stromal cell separation, 330, 330f
  uses of, 327
Bone mass
  definition of, 35b
  description of, 28
  macromodeling effects on, 29
Bone mineral density, 42
Bone modeling
  activation of, 27
  agents that impair, 34
  definition of, 35b
  by drifts, 29f, 29–30
  lag time, 31
  macromodeling, 29

micromodeling, 29–30
remodeling and, 32, 32f
Bone morphogenetic proteins
  adsorption of, to extracellular matrix proteins, 16
  advantages and disadvantages of, 301–302
  applications of, 301
  in autologous bone grafts, 129
  Bio-Oss and, 338
  bone formation and, 19b
  bone regeneration mechanisms, 298–300, 300f
  bone substitutes and, 21
  coding sequence of, 291
  complications of, 302
  costs of, 302
  description of, 12, 289, 349
  development of, 292–293
  discovery of, 290–291
  efficacy of, 301
  FDA approval of, 301
  in freeze-dried bone allografts, 185
  mechanism of action, 290
  osteogenesis promotion by, 351
  recombinant-2, 291, 295
  recombinant-7, 213, 291, 351
    development of, 293–294
    efficacy of, 301
    FDA approval of, 301
  sinus grafting uses of, 295
Bone plate fixation, 243, 243f
Bone regeneration
  bone morphogenetic proteins for, 298–300, 300f
  guided
    barrier membranes in, 235, 236f
    description of, 230–231
    implants placed after, 230
    physiology of, 13
    platelet-rich plasma for, 294, 296–298
    in sinus elevation surgery, 19
Bone remodeling
  after simultaneous implant placement and bone grafting, 60b
  agents that impair, 34
  basic multicellular unit, 27–28, 30, 31f, 35b
  of bone grafts, 16b
  conservation mode, 30
  definition of, 35b
  disuse, 30, 35b
  modeling and, 32, 32f
  osteoclastogenesis for, 16b
  platelet-rich plasma effects on, 19

threshold strain range for, 30
Bone scraper, 132, 135, 136f
Bone strain
  in children vs adults, 31
  decreases in, 43
  definition of, 36b
  implant loading, 31
  levels of, 32
  remodeling and, 28–30
  voluntary amount of, 31
Bone strength
  physical determinants of, 28–29
  vital biomechanical determinants of
    adaptational lag time, 31
    basic multicellular unit remodeling, 30, 31f
    bone modeling by drifts, 29f, 29–30
    combined modeling and remodeling, 32, 32f
    mechanical overload, 30
Bone substitutes
  autografts and, 21
  autologous bone and, 131
  bone morphogenetic proteins added to, 21
  indications for, 129
  platelet-rich plasma growth factors, 296
Bone-added osteotome technique, 266–270
Bone-forming stem cells, 328
Bone-implant contact
  description of, 20
  diabetes mellitus effects on, 97
  surface texture effects, 223
Bovine spongiform encephalopathy, 216–217
Bovine thrombin–related coagulopathy, 302
Bruxism, 76
Buccal bone loss, 76
Buccal flap, 105, 187

C

Caldwell-Luc opening, 4
Calvarial bone grafting, 120, 121f
Calvarial bone grafts, for sinus floor augmentation
  advantages of, 180
  complications of, 178–179
  disadvantages of, 180
  harvesting of, 172–173, 173f
  implant placement after healing of, 178–180
  maxilla reconstruction, 171–178
  osseointegration into, 179–180
  overview of, 171
  rationale for using, 179

  sinus floor grafting, 174, 174f
Cancellous bone
  autologous, 129
  from iliac crest, 161
  sinus augmentation using, 56, 56f
  from tibial plateau, 147, 148f
  volume of, 147
Cantilevers, 75–76
Casts, 75
Cefoxitin, 152
Cell-based therapy, for sinus augmentation
  case reports of, 344–346
  cell preparation technique, 342
  composition of, 341
  overview of, 341
  patient selection, 342
  platelet-rich plasma preparation, 343
  results of, 343–344
  summary of, 346–347
  surgical technique, 343
Chemotherapy, 93–94
Chiapasco classification of posterior maxilla, 47–50
Chorioallantoic membrane assay, 22f
Chronic infection, 112
Chronic sinus disease, 112, 113f
Cluneal nerves, 161, 162f
Concha bullosa, 89, 89f
Conservation mode, of remodeling, 30
Cortical bone, 129
Cortical bone grafts, 137
Corticocancellous block bone graft, 133f
Cranial bone grafts, 172–173, 173f. See also Calvarial bone grafts.
Crestal osseointegration, 43
Creutzfeldt-Jakob disease, 183, 186, 302
Crown height space
  in Chiapasco classification of posterior maxilla, 48f, 48–49
  description of, 43

D

Definitive prosthesis
  acrylic resin occlusal surfaces used in, 78–79
  definition of, 78
  fabrication techniques for
    acrylic resin-porcelain veneers, 82f, 83
    description of, 79–83
    porcelain-fused-to-gold materials for, 83
    removable bar prosthesis, 83, 83f–83f
  try-in, 79
  veneer of, 81–82

Demineralized freeze-dried bone allografts
  case studies of, 188–193
  description of, 184
Deviated septum, 89, 89f
Diabetes mellitus
  bone-implant contact affected by, 97
  complications of, 97
  failed regional acceleratory phenomenon in, 27
  implant survival affected by, 19–20
  periodontitis risks, 97
  sinus grafting contraindications in, 97
Diagnosis, 75–76
Diagnostic casts, 75
Diagnostic waxup, 75
Dimers, 290
Distance osteogenesis, 223
Distraction osteogenesis with sinus bone grafting
  appliances for, 282, 282f
  bone morphogenetic protein expression during, 349
  case reports of, 282–287
  description of, 281
  orthoalveolar form gained by, 281
  results of, 287, 288t
  technique for, 281–282
Disuse bone remodeling, 30, 35b
Donor sites
  autologous bone, 131–136, 157
  sinus grafting, 120
Drifts, 29f

E

Edentulous maxilla
  atrophy of, 49f, 139, 141
  classification of, 244–245, 245b
  description of, 7
  disuse bone remodeling in, 30
  moderately atrophic maxilla, 245b
  orthognathic, 245b
  partially, tilted implants for, 318, 318f
  removable bar prosthesis for, 83, 83f–84f
  retrodisplaced maxilla, 245b
  treatments for, 244, 245b
Endoscopic sinus surgery, 90, 116
Enzyme-linked immunosorbent assay, 185
Epidural catheter, 160f
Epithelial cyst, of maxillary sinus, 111–112, 113f
Ethylene oxide, 184
Expanded polytetrafluoroethylene barrier membrane, 201, 202f
Extraction sockets, 71

F

Fatigue fractures, 28
Fixed prostheses
  removable prosthesis vs, 311–312
  screw-retained, 77–78
  zygomatic implants and, 311–313
Formation drifts, 29f
Fractures
  fatigue, 28
  osteoporotic, 18, 96
Free flap surgery, 50
Freeze-dried bone allografts
  bone morphogenetic proteins in, 185
  cortical, 185
  mineralized, 184
  procurement of, 183–185
  safety of, 183–186
  trabecular bone area for, 298
Freeze-drying, 184–185
Frost, Harold, 37

G

Gene therapy
  alveolar bone engineering uses of, 351, 352f
  definition of, 19b
  ex vivo model, 352f
  future of, 353
  growth factors, 353
  platelet-derived growth factor-B, 350–351
  safety issues, 353
  in vivo model, 352f
  wound healing using, 350–351
Gene transfer, 349–350
Gerdy's tubercle, 147–148, 148f, 150
Gold-palladium cylinders, 79
Graft(s)
  allografts. See Allografts.
  bone. See Bone graft(s).
  interradicular bone intrusion, 67, 68f
  onlay
    alveolar ridge augmentation using, 176f, 241
    autologous, 130, 136
    Le Fort I osteotomy and, 50
  remodeling of, 16b
Graft consolidation
  description of, 14
  gene therapy for, 19b
  levels of, 22f
  osteogenic cells for, 19b
  osteoporosis effects, 18–20
  strategies for, 19b
  summary of, 21–22

Graft consolidation factors, 21, 21t
Graft materials
  block, 56, 59f
  description of, 17–18
  inductor, 12
  in intrusion osteotomy, 8
  particulate, 56
Grafting. See Bone grafting; Sinus grafting.
Graft–woven bone complex, 14, 16, 27
Growth factors
  binding to membrane receptor sites, 291f
  bone formation supported by, 19b
  bone morphogenetic proteins. See Bone morphogenetic proteins.
  definition of, 289
  mechanism of action, 289–290
  neoplasia caused by, 302
  in platelet-rich plasma. See Platelet-rich plasma.
  types of, 14b
  viral vectors for delivery of, 353
Guided bone regeneration
  barrier membranes in, 235, 236f
  description of, 230–231
Guided tissue regeneration, 230

H

Harvesting
  of autologous bone, from maxillofacial region sites
    complications of, 133–134
    harvesting procedure, 131–136
    indications for, 131
    mandibular ramus, 134–136
    mandibular symphysis, 133–134
    maxillary tuberosity, 131–132, 132f, 142f
    patient preparation, 131
    risks associated with, 131
    zygoma, 132
    zygomaticomaxillary buttress, 131–132, 132f
  of cranial bone grafts, 172–173, 173f
  of tibia bone grafts
    anesthesia for, 149, 150f
    cancellous marrow, 147, 150–151
    description of, 120
    ecchymosis secondary to, 152, 152f
    entry site for, 147–148
    Gerdy's tubercle, 147–148, 148f, 150
    graft volume, 154
    incisions for, 150, 150f
    intraoperative medications, 152
    outcome analysis of, 153–155

patient positioning and preparation, 149, 149f
platelet-poor plasma used during, 151, 151f
postoperative recovery and instructions, 152–153
sedation for, 149
sinus augmentation results, 153–154
site morbidity, 154–155
technique for, 150f–151f, 150–151
trephine bone, 163, 164f
Healing
  of bone grafts
    autologous grafts, 130, 141
    description of, 27
    incorporation phase of, 34
    pharmaceuticals' effect on, 34
    strain effects on, 32
    transantral dimension effects on, 46–47
  of xenografts, 217
Hemostatic membrane, for sinus membrane perforation, 106, 107f
Heparan sulfate receptors, 17, 17f
Hepatitis A, 186
Hepatitis B, 186
Hepatitis C, 186
Host bone–graft bone complex
  creation of, 27
  loading between, 28
  stiffness of, 28
  strength of, 28–29
Human immunodeficiency virus screening, 185–186
Hydrocortisone sodium succinate, 98
Hydroxyapatite
  bovine, 137f–138f
  disadvantages of, 347
  implants coated with, 61
  marginal bone loss using, 202–203
  osteoconductive capacity of, 202, 203f
  sinus membrane inflammation caused by, 118
Hydroxycarbonate apatite
  after beta-tricalcium phosphate resorption, 206
  description of, 203–204, 204f
Hyperthyroidism, 97
Hypothyroidism, 97

I

Iliac bone
  characteristics of, 157
  harvesting of. See Iliac crest harvesting.
  osteoconduction of, 157
  trephine bone grafts from, 163, 164f
Iliac bone grafts
  autologous, 141
  disadvantages of, 157
  resorption of, 137
  sinus floor augmentation using
    clinical experience with, 166–167, 168t
    success of, 167
    technique for, 164f–166f, 164–166
Iliac crest harvesting
  anterior, 158f–160f, 158–161, 168, 169t
  antibiotic prophylaxis for, 168
  complications of, 168–170, 169t
  contraindications, 157
  description of, 120, 157
  posterior, 161–163, 162f, 168, 169t
  summary of, 170
  trephine bone grafts from, 163, 164f
Iliohypogastric nerve, 158, 159f
Implant(s)
  abutments for, 77
  acid-etched, 223, 225, 226f, 226t
  antrum protrusion of, 5–6
  below sinus floor, 9
  blade, 4–5
  bone repair of, 9
  bone-implant contact, 20
  configuration of, 6
  criteria for success of, 42
  design of, 43
  efficacy of, 315
  failure of
    bisphosphonates and, 95
    description of, 13–14, 119–120
    osteoporosis and, 96
    periodontal disease and, 120
    smoking and, 95–96, 103
  hydroxyapatite-coated, 61
  loading of
    bone strain associated with, 31
    description of, 20–21
  loss of, 119–120
  machined, 223, 225, 226f, 226t
  migration of, 119f
  occlusal load distribution, 6
  primary stability for, 13–14, 267
  root form, 5
  rough-surfaced, 20, 120, 168t, 196, 197t, 223, 225t
  round cylindrical, 6
  short, 320, 320f
  sinus floor augmentation and
    delayed implant placement, 53–54
    simultaneous implant placement, 54–61, 63–65
    stability considerations, 60b
    surface of implant, 61–62
    survival rates, 61–62, 63t, 178
  sinus floor protrusion of, 6
  stability of, 13–14, 267
  surfaces of
    acid-etched, 223
    bone-implant contact affected by, 223
    clinical experience regarding, 225
    machined, 223, 225, 226f, 226t
    oxidized, 315
    rough, 20, 120, 168t, 196, 197t, 223, 225t
    sandblasted, large grit, acid-etched, 225, 226f, 226t
    smooth, 168t
    success rates based on, 61–62, 196, 197t
    survival of implant based on, 63t, 120, 168t, 223–226, 225t
    titanium oxide–blasted, 225, 226f, 226t
    titanium plasma spray, 212, 225, 226f, 226t
    types of, 20
  survival of
    in augmented sinus, 212
    barrier membrane use and, 236, 237t
    bone height and, 63t, 263
    bone mineral density effects on, 42
    clinical experience regarding, 225
    delay period and, 56
    description of, 13–14
    in diabetes mellitus patients, 19–20
    height of implant and, 42
    osteoporosis effects on, 18–19
    rates, 119, 188, 212
    surface of implant and, 63t, 120, 168t, 223–226, 225t
    when placed simultaneously with bone graft, 55, 63t
  threaded, 43
  tilted. See Tilted implants.
  tissue-engineered, 347. See also Tissue engineering.
  titanium plasma spray-coated, 212, 225, 226f, 226t
  zygoma, 312
  zygomatic. See Zygomatic implants.
Implant placement
  after calvarial bone graft healing, 178
  in bruxism patient, 76

conventional, 44, 45f
crown height space evaluations before, 43
delayed
  with calvarial bone grafts, 180
  in Misch classification of posterior maxilla, 46f, 47
  sinus augmentation and, 53–54, 61, 180, 271
  survival of implants after, 56
illustration of, 139f
immediate
  alveolar bone height requirements for, 57, 60b
  in Misch classification of posterior maxilla, 46
  sinus graft and, 46, 54–60
  survival of implants after, 56, 61
irradiation before, 93
sinus grafting and, 83f
sinus membrane elevation and
  description of, 193–196, 196t
  without bone grafting, 201
submerged, 252
in xenografts, 212
Impression copings, 79
Incisions
  for cranial bone harvesting, 173, 173f
  for iliac crest harvesting
    anterior, 160f, 161
    posterior, 161, 162f
  line opening, after sinus augmentation, 109
  for tibia bone harvesting, 150, 150f
  for zygomatic implants, 306, 307f
Inductor materials, 12
Infections
  after simultaneous sinus graft and implant placement, 46
  after sinus augmentation, 109–111, 110f, 112f
  allograft-related, 183, 185–186
  chronic, 112
  Creutzfeldt-Jakob disease, 183, 186
  description of, 183, 185–186, 341
  hepatitis, 186
  human immunodeficiency virus, 185–186
  oral, 94
  osteotome technique and, 8
  postoperative, 109–111, 110f, 112f
  sinus membrane perforation as cause of, 106
  syphilis, 186
Inferior alveolar nerve, 136
Inguinal ligament, 158, 159f

Integrin, 17, 17f
Interarch axial alignment, 281, 282f
Interpositional bone grafts, 136–137, 250
Interradicular bone intrusion grafts, 67, 68f
Interradicular bone intrusion osteotome technique, 67–70
Interradicular sinus pneumatization, 68f
Intrusion osteotomy
  description of, 8
  graft materials used in, 8

L
Lamellar bone
  drifts of, 34
  micromodeling of, 29–30
  microstrain of, 28
  strength of, 28
Lateral antrostomy
  barrier placement over, 229–231, 230f
  sinus floor elevation by, 64
Lateral cortical plate, 5
Lateral femoral cutaneous nerve, 158, 159f
Lateral fixation, 249f
Lateral sinus window
  barrier placement over, 235–236
  bone formation enhancements secondary to, 236
  description of, 229–231
  evidence to support, 233–236
  implant survival affected by, 236, 237t
Lateral wall osteoplasty, 274, 275f
Le Fort I distraction osteogenesis with sinus bone grafting
  appliances for, 282, 282f
  case reports of, 282–287
  description of, 281
  orthoalveolar form gained by, 281
  results of, 287, 288t
  technique for, 281–282
Le Fort I osteotomy
  description of, 241
  free flap alternative to, 50
  illustration of, 248f
  indications for, 49, 49f
  low-level, 241, 243f
  onlay grafts and, 50
  surgical procedure for, 241–244, 243f
  zygomatic implants vs, 121–122
Levofloxacin, 153
Loading
  of implants
    bone strain associated with, 31
    description of, 20–21
    progressive, 77

of screw-retained fixed-detachable prosthesis, 77
Loma Linda pouch technique, 232

M
Machined implants, 223, 225, 226f, 226t
Macromodeling, 29
Mandibular ramus, 134–136
Mandibular symphysis
  autologous bone harvesting from, 133–134
  complications of, 133–134
Maxilla
  ameloblastoma of, 91f, 309f
  anatomy of, 87
  atrophic
    bone grafting options in, 305–306
    description of, 305
    graftless rehabilitation of, 320–321
    tilted implants for, 316–318
    zygomatic implants for. See Zygomatic implants.
  edentulous. See Edentulous maxilla.
  moderately resorbed
    short implants for, 320, 320f
    zygoma implants for, 319, 319f
  posterior. See Posterior maxilla.
Maxillary first molar
  extraction of, 68f, 73f
  interradicular pneumatization with, 70f
Maxillary pneumatization
  causes of, 33
  description of, 41–42
  imaging of, 88f
Maxillary posterior teeth removal
  buccal bone loss after, 76
  resorption after, 115
  sinus augmentation and, 71
Maxillary sinus
  anatomy of, 87
  antrostomy of, 274
  blood vessels in, 14
  bone loss in, 13
  computerized tomography scan of, 116f
  in edentulous patient, 147
  endoscopic evaluation of, 116–117
  epithelial cyst of, 111–112, 113f
  functioning of, 87
  grafting of. See Sinus grafting.
  intrasinusal osteoma of, 89f
  lining of, 87
  mucocele in, 104, 104f
  mucus retention cyst in, 90f, 103, 104f
  physical evaluation of, 104

pneumatization of. *See* Maxillary pneumatization.
pseudocysts in, 104, 104f
reactions of, to zygomatic implants, 120–122
reconstruction of, 171–176
volume of, 13, 147
Maxillary tuberosity
 autologous bone harvesting from, 131–132, 132f, 142f
 bone removed from, 3, 4f
Maxillofacial region, autologous bone harvesting from
 complications of, 133–134
 harvesting procedure, 131–136
 indications for, 131
 mandibular ramus, 134–136
 mandibular symphysis, 133–134
 maxillary tuberosity, 131–132, 132f, 142f
 patient preparation, 131
 risks associated with, 131
 zygoma, 132
 zygomaticomaxillary buttress, 131–132, 132f
Mechanical overload, 30
Membranous bone grafts, 136
Mental nerve paresthesia, 134
Metallic implants, 4–5
Meteorotropism, 134
Micotic sinusitis, 90f
Microdamage, 28
Microdamage threshold range, 28, 32, 35b
Micromodeling, 29–30
Microstrain, 28
Middle cluneal nerves, 161, 162f
Milled bar, 83
Minimum effective strain range, 35b
Misch classification of posterior maxilla
 conventional implant placement, 44
 delayed implant placement, 46f, 47
 sinus augmentation, 44–45, 45f
 sinus graft and immediate or delayed implant placement, 46f, 46–47
Modeling. *See* Bone modeling.
Modeling threshold range, 29
Molar extractions
 maxillary first, 68f, 73f
 sinus floor intrusion after, 73, 73f–74f
Mucocele, 104, 104f
Mucoperiosteal flaps, 281
Mucoperiosteal reflection, 132
Mucus retention cyst, 90f, 103, 104f
Myocardial infarction, 93

N
Nasomaxillary complex
 benign tumors of, 89, 89f–90f
 malignancies of, 90, 91f
Neoplasia, 302
Nonabsorbable barrier membranes, 235, 237t

O
Occlusal load, 6
Onlay grafts
 alveolar ridge augmentation using, 176f, 241
 autologous, 130, 136
 Le Fort I osteotomy and, 50
Oroantral fistula, 111, 113f
Orthoalveolar form, 281
Orthognathic maxilla, 245b
Orthopantomographic evaluation, 115–116
Osseointegration
 anchorage for, 60b
 into calvarial bone grafts, 179–180
 crestal, 43
 description of, 13
 in extraction sockets, 71
 graft consolidation before, 14
 illustration of, 177f
 osteoclasts for, 16b
 smoking effects on, 96
Osteoblasts
 from bone marrow aspirate, 328
 description of, 328
 formation drifts for creation of, 29f
 recombinant bone morphogenetic protein-2 effects on, 299
Osteoclastogenesis, 15f
Osteoclasts
 Bio-Oss particles and, 215, 216f
 bisphosphonates' effect on, 94
 differentiation of, 16b
Osteoconduction
 description of, 17
 using hydroxyapatite, 202, 203f
Osteogenesis
 bone morphogenetic proteins for promotion of, 351
 definition of, 223
 distance, 223
Osteogenic cells
 from autografts, 17
 description of, 14b
 graft consolidation uses of, 19b
 in osteoporosis, 19

 from periosteum, 16
 sources of, 19b
Osteogenic differentiation, 14b, 15f
Osteogenic protein-1, 349
Osteoid, 299, 299f
Osteomeatal complex
 computerized tomography scan of, 116, 116f
 inflammation of, 106, 108
 narrowing of, 89, 89f
 obstruction of, 109
Osteonecrosis, bisphosphonate-related, 95
Osteopenia, 30, 35b
Osteoplasty
 lateral wall, 274, 275f
 piezoelectric, 274–275, 275f, 277
Osteoporosis
 bone density evaluations, 96
 bone metabolism effects of, 96
 fractures caused by, 18, 96
 graft consolidation affected by, 18–20
 implant failure and, 96
 in postmenopausal women, 18
 sinus grafting in patients with, 96–97
 treatment of, 18–19
Osteoprotegerin, 16
Osteotome bone grafting, 267
Osteotome technique
 bone-added, 266–270
 development of, 263–264
 interradicular bone intrusion, 67–70
 problems with, 8–9
 procedure, 264–266
 sinus elevation using, 266–271
 sinus floor grafting using, 8–9
 sinus perforation during, 8, 45
 summary of, 271–272
Osteotomes, 263, 264f
Osteotomy
 for anterior iliac crest harvesting, 161
 piezoelectric antrostomy by, 276f, 276–277
 ridge expansion, 266
 round, 265
 symphysis graft harvest using, 133, 133f
 trephine bur and sagittal saw for, 134f
 for zygomatic implant placement, 307, 308f
Osterix, 14b
Overlapped flap, 187
Overload, 30

361

P

p24 test, 185
Palatosinus floor, 255, 255f
Pamidronate, 94
Particulate grafts
  autologous, 137
  description of, 56
  from mandibular ramus, 135
Perforation, of sinus membrane
  barrier membranes for, 231–232
  block grafts for, 108
  description of, 8, 45, 105–106, 106f, 231
  graft confinement after, 118
  hemostatic membrane for, 106, 107f
  illustration of, 232f
  infection secondary to, 106
  modified membrane for, 231–232, 233f
  repair of, 131, 231–232
  septa as risk factor for, 108, 108f
  suturing of, 231, 233f
Peri-implant bone, 20
Periodontal disease, 120
Periodontitis, 97
Periosteum
  cell populations from, 333
  harvesting of, 334
  osteogenic cells from, 16
Piezoelectric bone cutting, 273–274
Piezoelectric bone surgery
  advantages of, 275
  antrostomy
    lateral window technique, 274–275, 275f
    by osteotomy, 276f, 276–277
  development of, 273
  membrane elevation by crestal approach, 277–278
Piezoknife, 277
Platelet-derived growth factor
  description of, 14b
  isomers of, 290, 296–297
  platelet-derived growth factor-B, 350–351
  in platelet-rich plasma, 289
  soft tissue wound healing using, 350–351
  treatment uses of, 19b
Platelet-derived wound-healing factor, 290
Platelet-poor plasma, 151, 151f
Platelet-rich plasma
  advantages and disadvantages of, 301–302
  application of, 290
  autografts and, 137, 139
  bone regeneration using, 294, 296–298
  in cell-based therapy for sinus augmentation, 343
  complications of, 302
  costs of, 301
  definition of, 289
  description of, 19b
  development of, 292, 292f–293f
  discovery of, 290
  efficacy of, 301
  FDA approval of, 301
  growth factors expressed by, 289
  mechanism of action, 289–290
  sinus grafting uses of, 294–295
  sinus grafts affected by, 298t
Pneumatic trifurcation, 42
Pneumatization
  interradicular sinus, 68f
  maxillary, 33, 41–42
Poly(lactic co-glycolic acid), 350
Pontiform gingivoplasty, 283, 284f
Posterior ilium
  bone harvesting from, 161–163, 162f, 168, 169t
  bone marrow aspirate from, 328, 328f
Posterior mandible, 134–136
Posterior maxilla
  anatomy of, 41, 42f
  bone in
    composition of, 224
    density of, 42
    residual, 157
    volume of, 42f
  Chiapasco classification of, 47–50
  edentulous areas of, 7
  implants in
    contraindications for, 43–44
    conventional placement of, 44, 45f
    delayed placement of, 53–54
    design of, 43
    immediate placement of, 46f, 46–47, 54–61
    number of, 43
    sinus augmentation before placement of, 44–45, 45f, 53–64
    size of, 43
    treatment planning for, 43, 64f
  Misch classification of
    conventional implant placement, 44
    delayed implant placement, 46f, 47
    sinus augmentation, 44–45, 45f
    sinus graft and immediate or delayed implant placement, 46f, 46–47
  occlusal forces in, 42–43
  resorption of, 41
  sinus grafting in, 315
Posterior teeth
  characteristics of, 43
  maxillary
    removal of, 71, 115
    sinus augmentation and, 71
    maxillary pneumatization caused by loss of, 41
  removable partial denture for, 76
Preoperative assessment, 103–104, 104f
Primary stability, 13–14
Progressive loading, 77
Prostheses. *See* Definitive prosthesis; Provisional prosthesis.
Provisional prosthesis
  abutments, 77
  in bruxism patient, 76
  first-stage, 76–77
  fixed, 77
  removable partial denture, 76
  screw-retained fixed-detachable, 77–78
  second-stage, 77–78
Pseudocysts, 104, 104f

R

Radiotherapy, 93
Receptor activator of NF-kappa B, 16
Receptor activator of NF-kappa B ligand, 16
Recombinant bone morphogenetic protein-2, 291, 295, 302
Recombinant bone morphogenetic protein-7, 213, 291, 351
  advantages and disadvantages of, 301–302
  costs of, 302
  development of, 293–294
  efficacy of, 301
  FDA approval of, 301
Regional acceleratory phenomenon, 27, 34
Remodeling
  basic multicellular unit, 27–28, 30, 31f, 35b
  bone. *See* Bone remodeling.
Remodeling space, 35b
Remodeling threshold, 30
Removable partial denture, 76
Removable prostheses
  bar prosthesis, 83, 83f–83f
  fixed prostheses vs, 311–312
  zygomatic implants and, 308
Resorbable bone plates, 243, 243f
Resorption
  after sinus grafting, 213
  alveolar ridge, 7, 251
  definition of, 35b–36b
  posterior maxilla, 41

of xenografts, 215
Resorption drifts, 29f
Retrodisplaced maxilla, 245b
Ridge expansion
  bone flap for, 251
  osteotomy for, 266
  partial-thickness flap for, 251
  trans-alveolar sinus elevation and
    bone incisions for, 254
    complications of, 261
    contiguous sinus floor elevation, 252, 257–260
    contraindications for, 253–254
    flap design for, 254, 255f–256f
    healing after, 255
    indications for, 253–254
    instrumentation for, 254, 254f
    rationale for, 252
    sinus floor management, 252, 255, 256f
    summary of, 261
    surgical procedure for, 254–260
    tooth removal simultaneously performed, 253
Risedronate, 95
Root replacement technology, 67
Root form implants, 5
Rough-surfaced implants
  bone-implant contact in, 223
  survival rates for, 20, 120, 168t, 196, 197t
Round cylindrical implants, 6
Round osteotomy, 265
RUNX-2, 14b

S

Sandblasted, large grit, acid-etched implants, 225, 226f, 226t
Scarpa's fascia, 159f
Screw-retained fixed-detachable prosthesis, 77–78
Short implants, 320, 320f
Simian immunodeficiency virus, 185
Sinus augmentation
  block grafts for, 56, 59f
  cell-based therapy for
    case reports of, 344–346
    cell preparation technique, 342
    composition of, 341
    overview of, 341
    patient selection, 342
    platelet-rich plasma preparation, 343
    results of, 343–344
    summary of, 346–347
    surgical technique, 343

complications of
  chronic sinus disease, 112, 113f
  description of, 119
  early-postoperative, 105t, 109–111, 110f–111f
  epithelial cyst, 111–112, 113f
  incidence of, 115
  incision line opening, 109
  infection, 109–111, 110f, 112f
  intraoperative, 105–109
  late-postoperative, 111–112, 112f–113f
  membrane perforation, 8, 45, 105–108, 106f
  oroantral fistula, 111, 113f
  potential, 115–118
  sinus membrane perforation, 105–106, 106f, 118
  sinusitis, 108
computerized tomography evaluation before, 104
description of, 333
goals of, 211
implants placed after, 212
  indications for, 44–45, 45f
  lateral approach to, 46
  maxillary posterior tooth removal and, 71
  particulate grafts for, 56
  preoperative assessment, 103–104, 104f
  technique for, 44–45, 45f
  tibial grafts for, 153. See also Tibia, harvesting from.
  xenografts for, 212, 213b
Sinus Consensus Conference, 76
Sinus elevation. See also Sinus floor augmentation.
  allografts for, 187, 188f–189f, 189
  bone regeneration in, 19
  contiguous, 252, 257–260
  description of, 5
  greenstick fracture of sinus floor for, 44–45
  implant placement and
    description of, 193–196, 196t
    without bone grafting, 201
  lateral antrostomy for, 64
  lateral window
    description of, 187, 188f
    implant placement and, 193, 193f
  methods for, 64, 65t
  modified lateral maxillary wall infracture technique for, 61
  osteotomy technique for
    with autogenous bone and xenografts, 63–64
    description of, 8

  piezoelectric, 276f, 277–278
  sinus grafting with, 119–120
  success of, 211
  trans-alveolar, with ridge expansion
    bone incisions for, 254
    complications of, 261
    contiguous sinus floor elevation, 252, 257–260
    contraindications for, 253–254
    flap design for, 254, 255f–256f
    healing after, 255
    indications for, 253–254
    instrumentation for, 254, 254f
    rationale for, 252
    sinus floor management, 252, 255, 256f
    summary of, 261
    surgical procedure for, 254–260
    tooth removal simultaneously performed, 253
  types of, 8
  xenografts and, 217
  for zygomatic implants, 307f
Sinus floor
  atrophic, 10
  dissection of, 172, 172f
  elevation of
    bone-added osteotome, 266–270
    staged, 270f–271f, 271
  grafting of, 174, 174f
  greenstick fracture of, for elevation, 44–45
  implants placed in
    description of, 9
    illustration of, 166f
    protrusion of, 6
  intrusion of
    after molar extraction, 73, 73f–74f
    implant placement and, 71
    osteotome, beta-tricalcium phosphate for, 206, 207f
  localized management of, 252
  pathophysiology of, 9–10, 10f–11f
Sinus floor augmentation
  alveolar bone height gains after, 64–65
  calvarial bone grafts for
    advantages of, 180
    complications of, 178–179
    disadvantages of, 180
    harvesting of, 172–173, 173f
    implant placement after healing of, 178–180
    maxilla reconstruction, 171–178
    osseointegration into, 179–180
    overview of, 171
    rationale for using, 179

sinus floor grafting, 174, 174f
closed, 63–65
crestal approach to, 53
iliac bone grafts for
  clinical experience with, 166–167, 168t
  success of, 167
  technique for, 164f–166f, 164–166
implants with
  delayed placement of, 53–54, 180, 271
  simultaneous placement of, 54–61, 63–65
  stability considerations, 60b
  surface of implant, 61–62
  survival rates for, 61–62, 63t, 178
lateral antrostomy for
  one-step, 65t
  two-step, 65t
methods of, 65t
one-stage technique for
  description of, 53
  indications for, 57
  study of, 335, 335f
osteotomy technique for, 8, 65t
recommendations for, 65
resorption, 137
success rate for, 117
techniques for, 53
treatment-planning chart for, 64f
two-stage technique for
  allografts, 188
  description of, 53, 180–181
  indications for, 57
  study of, 335, 336f
Sinus floor grafting
  implant survival after, 13–14
  osteotome technique for, 8–9
  purpose of, 13
  surgical innovations in, 8–9
Sinus grafting
  autogenous bone for, 212, 346–347
  Bio-Oss for, 224t
  bone morphogenetic protein used in, 12
  contraindications
    adrenal disorders, 97–98
    alcohol abuse, 97
    anticoagulant therapy, 93
    bisphosphonates, 94–95
    cardiac pathologies, 93
    chemotherapy, 93–94
    concha bullosa, 89, 89f
    description of, 87, 115
    deviated septum, 89, 89f
    diabetes mellitus, 97
    intraoral, 92
    irreversible (absolute), 92
    local, 88–92
    medical conditions, 92–98
    mucus cysts, 90f, 103
    myocardial infarction, 93
    nasomaxillary complex tumors, 89, 89f–90f
    nasomaxillary malignancies, 90, 91f
    osteomeatal complex narrowing, 89, 89f
    osteoporosis, 96–97, 103
    potentially reversible (relative), 88–92
    radiotherapy, 93
    rhinosinusitis, 90, 90f
    smoking, 95–96
    thyroid disorders, 97
    tumors, 89, 89f–90f
  description of, 3, 87, 315
  diagnosis before, 75–76
  distraction osteogenesis with
    appliances for, 282, 282f
    case reports of, 282–287
    description of, 281
    orthoalveolar form gained by, 281
    results of, 287, 288t
    technique for, 281–282
  donor site complications, 120
  failure of, 118
  future of, 12
  history of, 129
  illustration of, 88f
  for metallic implants, 4–5
  mucosal inflammation secondary to, 106, 108
  orthopantomographic evaluation before, 115–116
  osseous tissue increases by, 3
  platelet-rich plasma for, 294–295
  in posterior maxilla, 315
  preoperative assessment, 103–104, 104f
  radiographs of, 83f
  sinus endoscopy before, 116
  success rates for, 103, 119
  treatment planning for, 75–76
  in unhealthy sinus, 87–88
Sinus grafts
  bilateral, 141
  block, 56, 59f
  bone height of, 153f
  bone regeneration mechanisms, 296–298
  diagnostic casts before, 75
  failure of, 76–77, 111
  height of, after placement, 120
  implant length for, 43
  indications for, 41–43
  migration of, 106
  particulate, 56
  platelet-rich plasma effects on, 298t
  survival of, 113
  vascularization of, 233–234, 296
Sinus membrane
  elevation of. See Sinus membrane elevation.
  nose-blowing test for integrity testing of, 257
Sinus membrane elevation
  crestal approach, 53, 276f, 277–278
  perforation during
    barrier membranes for, 231–232
    block grafts for, 108
    description of, 8, 45, 105–106, 106f, 231
    graft confinement after, 118
    hemostatic membrane for, 106, 107f
    illustration of, 232f
    infection secondary to, 106
    modified membrane for, 231–232, 233f
    repair of, 131, 231–232
    septa as risk factor for, 108, 108f
    suturing of, 231, 233f
Sinus window
  barrier placement over
    bone formation enhancements secondary to, 236
    clinical efficacy of, 235–236
    description of, 229–231
    evidence to support, 233–236
    implant survival affected by, 236, 237t
  description of, 129, 165f
Sinusitis
  bacterial, 90f
  micotic, 90f
  sinus augmentation–related, 108
Smoking, 95–96, 103, 117
Soldering index cast, 79
Sonic hedgehog, 351
Spark-erosion prosthesis, 59f
Sphingosine-1-phosphate, 14b
Split-thickness flap, 187, 256f
Staphylococcus epidermidis, 186
Stem cell compartment, 327
Strain. See Bone strain.
Stress, 36b
Stromal stem cells
  adherent, 328
  beta-tricalcium phosphate mixed with, 330, 330f
  from bone marrow aspirate, 330, 330f
  discovery of, 327

function of, 327
nonadherent, 328
number of, 327
Sublimation, 184
Superior cluneal nerves, 161, 162f
Surface, of implants
    acid-etched, 223
    bone-implant contact affected by, 223
    clinical experience regarding, 225
    machined, 223, 225, 226f, 226t
    rough, 20, 120, 168t, 196, 197t, 223, 225t
    sandblasted, large grit, acid-etched, 225, 226f, 226t
    smooth, 168t
    success rates based on, 61–62, 196, 197t
    survival of implant based on, 63t, 120, 168t, 223–226, 225t
    titanium oxide–blasted, 225, 226f, 226t
    titanium plasma spray, 212, 225, 226f, 226t
    types of, 20
Syphilis, 186

T
Tetracycline bone labeling, 33f
Threaded implants, 43
Thyroid disorders, 97
Tibia bone grafts
    harvesting of
        anesthesia for, 149, 150f
        cancellous marrow, 147, 150–151
        description of, 120
        ecchymosis secondary to, 152, 152f
        entry site for, 147–148
        Gerdy's tubercle, 147–148, 148f, 150
        graft volume, 154
        incisions for, 150, 150f
        intraoperative medications, 152
        outcome analysis of, 153–155
        patient positioning and preparation, 149, 149f
        platelet-poor plasma used during, 151, 151f
        postoperative recovery and instructions, 152–153
        sedation for, 149
        sinus augmentation results, 153–154
        site morbidity, 154–155
        technique for, 150f–151f, 150–151
        surgical anatomy of, 147–148, 148f
Tilted implants
    "All-on-4" concept, 316–317, 317f
    immediate function and, 318f
    partially edentulous maxilla treated with, 318, 318f
    placement of
        description of, 316, 316f
        surgical guides for, 316–317, 317f
Tissue engineering
    of alveolar bone, 349
    cell-based therapy
        case reports of, 344–346
        cell preparation technique, 342
        composition of, 341
        overview of, 341
        patient selection, 342
        platelet-rich plasma preparation, 343
        results of, 343–344
        summary of, 346–347
        surgical technique, 343
    description of, 333
    methods of, 333
    study of
        clinical evaluations, 334, 335f
        complications, 337–338
        design of, 333, 334f
        results, 337–338
        surgical procedure used in, 335, 335f–336f
        summary of, 338–339
        surgical procedure, 335, 335f–336f
        synthetic biodegradable polymer used as scaffolding for, 339
Titanium oxide–blasted implants, 225, 226f, 226t
Titanium plasma spray-coated implants, 212
Tooth loss, 349
Trans-alveolar sinus elevation and ridge expansion
    bone incisions for, 254
    complications of, 261
    contiguous sinus floor elevation, 252, 257–260
    contraindications for, 253–254
    flap design for, 254, 255f–256f
    healing after, 255
    indications for, 253–254
    instrumentation for, 254, 254f
    rationale for, 252
    sinus floor management, 252, 255, 256f
    summary of, 261
    surgical procedure for, 254–260
    tooth removal simultaneously performed, 253
Transforming growth factor-ß, 16b, 289, 296
Transforming growth factor-2, 350
Treatment planning
    advances in, 321
    alveolar ridge height as basis for, 65
    for posterior maxilla implants, 43, 64f
    sinus grafting, 75–76
Trephine bone grafts, 163, 164f
Trephine sinus intrusion technique, 71, 72f
Tricalcium phosphate, 129, 204–207, 205f, 207f
Tricortically fixed implant, 305
Tschopp approach, 161
Tumor necrosis factor-β, 16b
Type 4 bone, 13–14

U
Ultimate strength, 36b
Unit load, 36b

V
Vascular endothelial growth factor
    bisphosphonates' effect on, 94
    capillary budding promoted by, 296
    description of, 14b, 339
Vasculogenesis, 14b
Vital biomechanics
    bone strength determinants
        adaptational lag time, 31
        basic multicellular unit remodeling, 30, 31f
        bone modeling by drifts, 29f, 29–30
        combined modeling and remodeling, 32, 32f
        mechanical overload, 30
    definition of, 36b
    description of, 28

W
Wnt signaling, 14b
Wound healing, gene therapy for, 350–351
Woven bone
    definition of, 36
    graft–woven bone complex, 14, 16, 27
    micromodeling of, 29–30

X
Xenografts
    bovine spongiform encephalopathy and, 216–217
    conductive efficacy of, 217
    description of, 211
    disease transmission risks, 216–217, 341
    evolution of, 212–216
    healing period for, 217

Index

implants placed in, 212
resorption of, 215
sinus augmentation using, 212, 213b
sinus grafting using, 230f
sinus membrane elevation using, 217
technical considerations for, 213b

Z

Zygoma harvesting, 132
Zygoma implants
  description of, 312
  moderately to severely resorbed maxilla treated with, 319, 319f-320f

Zygomatic implants
  advantages of, 306
  bilateral, 311f
  case studies of, 308–310
  characteristics of, 306
  complications of, 314
  fixed prostheses with, 311–313
  history of, 305–306
  incisions for, 306, 307f
  patient selection for, 306
  preoperative evaluation, 306
  removable prostheses with, 308
  sinus reactions to, 120–122
  summary of, 314
  surgical technique for, 306–307, 307f–308f
  traditional dental implants used with, 306, 311
  training in placement of, 314

Zygomaticomaxillary buttress, autologous bone harvesting from, 131–132, 132f